Principles and Practice of Radiotherapy Techniques in Thoracic Malignancies

Gokhan Ozyigit • Ugur Selek
Erkan Topkan
Editors

Principles and Practice of Radiotherapy Techniques in Thoracic Malignancies

Springer

Editors
Gokhan Ozyigit
Professor and Chairman
Department of Radiation Oncology
Hacettepe University, Faculty of Med.
Ankara
Turkey

Erkan Topkan
Professor and Chairman
Department of Radiation Oncology
Baskent University School of Medicine
Adana
Turkey

Ugur Selek
Professor and Chairman
Department of Radiation Oncology
Koc University School of Medicine
Istanbul
Turkey

Adjunct Associate Professor
Department of Radiation Oncology
MD Anderson Cancer Center
The University of Texas
Houston, TX
USA

ISBN 978-3-319-28759-1 ISBN 978-3-319-28761-4 (eBook)
DOI 10.1007/978-3-319-28761-4

Library of Congress Control Number: 2016935930

Printed on acid-free paper

This Springer imprint is published by Springer Nature
The registered company is Springer International Publishing AG Switzerland

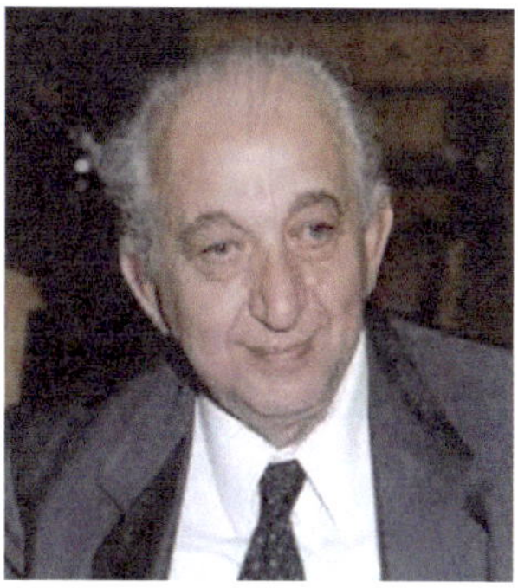

Dedicated to the memory of Professor
Dincer Fırat, MD (1932–2014)

Preface

It is evident that optimal management of thoracic malignancies requires a multidisciplinary team approach through an understanding of functional outcomes with minimal morbidities from the dedicated modalities.

The idea behind the *Principles and Practice of Radiotherapy Techniques in Thoracic Malignancies* is the challenging atmosphere of multidisciplinary care where the radiation oncologists should be closely interacting with the medical oncologists and the surgeons in different degrees based on the type and stage of the malignancies. Therefore, our intent was to provide a summarized, illustrated, and structured method underlying all components of site-specific treatments, from surgical, radiation oncological, and medical oncological perspectives, in order to lead into an evidence-based management pathway equipped with adequate and up-to-date information.

Radiotherapy chapters are arranged with the required illustrated target volume delineations and treatment techniques, including intensity-modulated radiotherapy treatment, stereotactic ablative body radiotherapy, and stereotactic radiosurgery. As detailed surgical techniques are not a part of our oncology residency programs, the specialists who are mainly interested in thoracic malignancies should be equipped with an adequate level of oncological surgery options including the basic knowledge of what goes on under the scar. Therefore, we have included chapters of concise surgical point of views and surgical techniques, as well as clinical chapters with medical oncology perspectives to help in the decision making for the radiation oncology practitioners. Overall, our book covers the general multidisciplinary management including valuable inputs of surgery, radiation, and medical oncology.

We hope "Principles and Practice of Radiotherapy Techniques in Thoracic Malignancies" will meet the need for a practical and up-to-date radiation oncology review of thoracic tumors for residents, fellows, and clinicians of radiation, medical and thoracic oncology, as well as for medical students, physicians, and medical physicists interested in thoracic malignancies.

Ankara, Turkey — Gokhan Ozyigit
Istanbul, Turkey — Ugur Selek
Adana, Turkey — Erkan Topkan

Acknowledgments

The editors are indebted to Corinna Hauser from Springer DE and Bharatwaj M.V. and Sushil Kumar Sharma from SPi Global for their assistance in preparing *Principles and Practice of Radiotherapy Techniques in Thoracic Malignancies*.

We extend our most sincere gratitude to our colleagues and friends at Hacettepe University, Koc University, Baskent University, and University of Texas MD Anderson Cancer Center, as well as our families.

Contents

Contributors

S. Aksoy, MD Department of Medical Oncology, Hacettepe University, Ankara, Turkey

V. Alpan Department of Radiation Oncology, American Hospital, Istanbul, Turkey

S. Bavbek, MD Department of Medical Oncology, American Hospital, Istanbul, Turkey

Y. Bolukbasi, MD Department of Radiation Oncology, U.T. MD Anderson Cancer Center, Houston, TX, USA

Department of Radiation Oncology, Koc University, School of Medicine, Istanbul, Turkey

Department of Radiation Oncology, Baskent University, Adana, Turkey

E. D. Brooks Department of Medicine, Memorial Sloan Kettering Cancer Center, New York, NY, USA

A. P. Cadena Yale University, New Haven, CT, USA

A. K. Cangır, MD Department of Thoracic Surgery, Ankara University, Ankara, Turkey

M. A. Cortez Division of Radiation Oncology, The University of Texas MD Anderson Cancer Center, Houston, TX, USA

E. Dikmen, MD Department of Thoracic Surgery, Hacettepe University, Ankara, Turkey

S. Dilege, MD Department of Thoracic Surgery, Koc University Hospital, Istanbul, Turkey

S. Erus Department of Thoracic Surgery, Koc University Hospital, Istanbul, Turkey

D. R. Gomez Division of Radiation Oncology, The University of Texas MD Anderson Cancer Center, Houston, TX, USA

O. C. Guler Department of Radiation Oncology, Baskent University, Adana, Turkey

M. Gultekin, MD Department of Radiation Oncology, Hacettepe University, Ankara, Turkey

W. Hofstetter Department of Thoracic and Cardiovascular Surgery, The University of Texas MD Anderson Cancer Center, Houston, TX, USA

P. Hurmuz, MD Department of Radiation Oncology, Hacettepe University, Ankara, Turkey

K. Kaban, MD Department of Medical Oncology, American Hospital, Istanbul, Turkey

Y. Kahya Department of Thoracic Surgery, Ankara University, Ankara, Turkey

S. Kirsner, MS Department of Radiation Physics, The University of Texas MD Anderson Cancer Center, Houston, TX, USA

R. Komaki, MD Division of Radiation Oncology, The University of Texas MD Anderson Cancer Center, Houston, TX, USA

X. S. Li Biomedical Informatics at Molecular Match Inc., Houston, TX, USA

Z. Liao, MD Division of Radiation Oncology The University of Texas MD Anderson Cancer Center, Houston, TX, USA

N. Molinas Mandel, MD Department of Medical Oncology, American Hospital, Istanbul, Turkey

Department of Medical Oncology, Koc University Hospital, Istanbul, Turkey

C. Nelson, PhD Department of Radiation Physics, The University of Texas MD Anderson Cancer Center, Houston, TX, USA

S. Niknam Division of Radiation Oncology, The University of Texas MD Anderson Cancer Center, Houston, TX, USA

Y. Ozdemir Department of Radiation Oncology, Baskent University, Adana, Turkey

G. Ozyigit Department of Radiation Oncology, Hacettepe University, Ankara, Turkey

Y. Saglam Department of Radiation Oncology, American Hospital, Istanbul, Turkey

S. Y. Sari, MD Department of Radiation Oncology, Hacettepe University, Ankara, Turkey

J. E. Schoenhals Division of Radiation Oncology, The University of Texas MD Anderson Cancer Center, Houston, TX, USA

U. Selek, MD Department of Radiation Oncology, Koc University, Istanbul, Turkey

Department of Radiation Oncology, The University of Texas MD Anderson Cancer Center, Houston, TX, USA

B. Sepesi, MD Department of Thoracic and Cardiovascular Surgery, The University of Texas MD Anderson Cancer Center, Houston, TX, USA

S. N. Seyedin Department of Radiation Oncology, University of Iowa Hospitals and Clinics, Iowa City, IA, USA

D. Sezen, MD Department of Radiation Oncology, Koc University, School of Medicine, Istanbul, Turkey

S. Tanju, MD Department of Thoracic Surgery, Koc University Hospital, Istanbul, Turkey

E. Topkan, MD Department of Radiation Oncology, Baskent University, Adana, Turkey

X. Wang Institute for Applied Cancer Science, The University of Texas MD Anderson Cancer Center, Houston, TX, USA

J. W. Welsh, MD Division of Radiation Oncology, The University of Texas MD Anderson Cancer Center, Houston, TX, USA

G. Yazici, MD Department of Radiation Oncology, Hacettepe University, Ankara, Turkey

O. Yazici Department of Medical Oncology, Ankara Numune Education and Research Hospital, Ankara, Turkey

B. A. Yildirim Department of Radiation Oncology, Baskent University, Adana, Turkey

Selection Criteria for Definitive Treatment Approach in Thoracic Malignancies: Radiation Oncology Perspective

1

Duygu Sezen, Yasemin Bolukbasi, Erkan Topkan, and Ugur Selek

Introduction

Data depicting regional dose–responses exist from ventilation/perfusions SPECT or tissue density CT series, besides reports of pneumonitis occurring at different constraints and doses/volumes [1–4]. As radiotherapy should have a balance between local control and organ at risk, such as lung and injury risk, the goal in general is ensuring the highest adequate dose possible with acceptable risks to avoid excessive toxicity. So assessment before radiotherapy for radiotherapy-induced injury risk should be a combination of baseline preexisting functional status and evidence-driven knowledge in radiotherapy planning process to design treatment in order to conclude whether the patient could be treated as desired or be treated with modifications in intent with acceptable sacrifice or not be treated at all.

While facing a patient referred for radiotherapy, evaluation to decide the intent of the treatment, such as curative or palliative, is directly related with not only the stage of the thoracic malignancy but also with the general performance status,

D. Sezen, MD
Department of Radiation Oncology, Koc University, School of Medicine, Istanbul, Turkey
e-mail: dsezen@kuh.ku.edu.tr

Y. Bolukbasi, MD
Department of Radiation Oncology, U.T. MD Anderson Cancer Center, Houston, TX, USA

Department of Radiation Oncology, Koc University, School of Medicine, Istanbul, Turkey
e-mail: yaseminb@amerikanhastanesi.org; ybolukbasi@mdanderson.org

E. Topkan, MD
Department of Radiation Oncology, Baskent University, Adana, Turkey
e-mail: docdretopkan@gmail.com

U. Selek, MD (✉)
Department of Radiation Oncology, Faculty of Medicine, Koc University, Istanbul, Turkey

Department of Radiation Oncology, U.T. MD Anderson Cancer Center, Houston, TX, USA
e-mail: ugurselek@yahoo.com, uselek@ku.edu.tr, uselek@mdanderson.org

G. Ozyigit et al. (eds.), *Principles and Practice of Radiotherapy Techniques in Thoracic Malignancies*, DOI 10.1007/978-3-319-28761-4_1

comorbidities, and pulmonary functional reserves. As the preoperative decision process is more clear based on the assessment of estimated perioperative and postoperative lung functions, pre-radiotherapy decision process is more vague at physician disposal, and its borders need to be outlined to become more objective which requires radiotherapy planning process to be included for eligibility [5].

Radiotherapy could be required in many clinical scenarios for lung cancer patients from early to locally advanced and terminal stages of the disease based on the conclusion related with symptoms, pathology, and relevance. Stereotactic body radiation therapy (SBRT) or so-called stereotactic ablative body radiotherapy (SABR) has gained popularity, in mainly medically inoperable early-stage lung cancer cases as well as patients with lung metastases, which delivers very high per day doses to dedicated small areas, besides postoperative, definitive, consolidative, or palliative radiotherapy come into play for more advanced curative intent cases with larger fields necessarily effecting pulmonary volume. Along with lung cancer, other thoracic malignancies like mesothelioma, esophageal cancer, and thymoma management also require pulmonary and cardiac function assessments prior to radiotherapy considering the post-radiotherapy management such as surgery.

Toxicity in normal lung tissue that may occur due to radiotherapy is essentially associated with radiation dose, treatment area, and remaining preserved parenchyma. While high doses are acceptable for small volumes in the lung, low-dose bath to very large parenchyma increases the risk of radiation-induced toxicity. In this context, techniques that are aimed to decrease dose and volume of normal lung tissue that is exposed to radiotherapy are of great importance. Toxicity in lung that may occur due to radiotherapy is described as radiation pneumonitis and it typically arises 2–6 months after radiotherapy. It can be detected as clinically insignificant radiological form without symptoms or as clinically significant with symptoms like persistent nonproductive cough, dyspnea, and fever. In some cases, the risk of radiation pneumonitis can cause difficulty for tumor control by limiting radiotherapy dose that will be prescribed. Patient referred for radiation therapy should be first questioned in terms of underlying pulmonary, cardiac, and autoimmune diseases in order to define whether subclinical damage related to radiation related with the planned treatment might constitute a ground for potential cardiopulmonary problems in the future or might worsen the existing reserves. Similarly, in the presence of interstitial lung disease, acute exacerbation may be observed following the treatment course, and it may lead to a mortal course [6, 7]. In initial assessment severe, active comorbidity could be defined as follows [8]: unstable angina and/or congestive heart failure defined by New York Heart Association class III or IV requiring hospitalization within the last 6 months, transmural myocardial infarction within the last 6 months, acute infection (bacterial or fungal) requiring intravenous antibiotics, exacerbation of chronic obstructive pulmonary disease requiring hospitalization, severe hepatic disease (Child-Pugh Class B/C hepatic disease), HIV positivity with CD4 count <200 cells/μl, and end-stage renal disease on dialysis. On the other hand, justification for considering a patient medically inoperable needs to be based on pulmonary functions for surgical resection of NSCLC including any of the following [9]: baseline hypoxemia and/or hypercapnia; baseline FEV1 <40 %

predicted; baseline exercise oxygen consumption <50 % predicted; severely reduced baseline diffusion capacity; postoperative FEV1 <30 % predicted; severe pulmonary hypertension; diabetes mellitus with severe damage in end organs; severe cardiac, peripheral, or cerebral vascular disease; and severe chronic heart disease.

There is no definitive algorithm regarding functional tests to be implemented before radiotherapy for patients with lung tumors in dedicated intent such as postoperative, definitive radiotherapy alone or chemoradiotherapy, stereotactic radiotherapy, etc. However, literature provides many studies including these patient groups' prescribed different treatments to present their posttreatment functional status in comparison to baseline.

Unfortunately, cancer has an increasing pace and this increase in cancer incidence is driven by cancer diagnosed in mainly older adults, such as a 67 % increase in cancer incidence is anticipated for older adults up to 2030 in comparison to an 11 % increase for younger adults in the United States [10]. This means that more elder cancer patients, who would mostly be medically compromised, will require radiotherapy in coming years. As known, long-term survival in untreated even stage I NSCLC is uncommon with only 6 % overall 5-year survival based on 1,432 patients who did not undergo surgical resection or receive treatment with chemotherapy or radiation in the California Cancer Center registry analysis between 1989 and 2003 [11]. Therefore, radiotherapy should be a role player in even the functionally compromised group of patients to ensure a decline in the proportion of untreated elderly cases with absolute increase in RT use with SBRT introduction (16 % increase) which was converted to an improvement in OS in Amsterdam Cancer Registry cohort [12]. Brunelli et al underlined that most of the patients referred for radiotherapy within this aim, are bearing comorbidities and pulmonary functional problems [5]. In a study, in which Kim et al. examined prognostic effects of pulmonary function reserves before postoperative radiotherapy, the median forced expiratory volume in 1 s (FEV_1) prior to radiotherapy in their cohort of 115 NSCLC patients was 1.68 L and was used to group according to over and below to this value and this value was as a cut off point to stratify patients [13]. Overall survival at 5 years was found to be significantly shorter in cases with low FEV_1 value (35.4 % versus 56.9 %, $p=0.002$). Five-year OS of the low FEV1 group was significantly lower than that of the high FEV1 group (35.4 % versus 56.9 %, $p=0.002$), which continued to be significant in multivariate analysis (HR=2.04, CI, 1.18–3.55, $p=0.011$), without any significant differences in locoregional relapse-free and distant metastasis-free survival and in lung toxicity [13].

Evaluation of Dosimetric Values in Planning

In determining probable radiation-induced lung toxicity, apart from lung function tests, dose–volume values detected during radiotherapy planning are important to consider. The median lung dose (MLD), volume of lung receiving at least 20 Gy (V20), volume of lung receiving at least 10 Gy (V10), and volume of lung receiving at least 5 Gy (V5) are the most significant values, and their lung toxicity-safe limits are known [14]. It is important to use the definitions correctly to calculate dosimetric parameters for risk of radiation pneumonitis such as the volume of normal lung receiving 20 Gy (V20) and the mean lung dose (MLD). Kabolizadeh et al. in the University of Pittsburgh Cancer Institute investigated the dosimetric differences of analysis based on excluding planning target volume [PTV] versus gross tumor volume [GTV] from the total bilateral lung volume [15]. The MLD, V5, V10, V20, and V30 were all slightly but significantly higher with total bilateral lung minus GTV in comparison to minus PTV ($P<0.001$); average MLD was 16.7 Gy and 14.8 Gy; mean V5, V10, V20, and V30 were 51.3 %, 40 %, 28 %, and 21.5 % versus 49.8 %, 38 %, 25 %, and 18.8 %, respectively, while the V20 of four patients with clinical pneumonitis were >27 % versus >23 % when excluding the GTV versus PTV from total bilateral lung volume [15]. This significant difference delineates the necessity to use common definitions of dosimetric information properly to be able to compare or optimize treatment plans to avoid pneumonitis.

Baseline Pulmonary Function

In 2000, Robnett et al. commented on predictors of severe radiation pneumonitis and noted that none of their patients with a good baseline pulmonary function of pretreatment FEV1 ≥2.0 L suffered severe radiation pneumonitis following treatment with conventional radiation fields and doses [16]. Wang et al. studied whether poor baseline pulmonary function might increase the risk of symptomatic radiation-induced lung toxicity (SRILT, grade 2 and higher radiation pneumonitis and fibrosis) or not in their 260 stage 1–3 NSCLC patients treated with conformal radiation therapy based on lung function tests such as $FEV_{1,}$ forced vital capacity (FVC), carbon monoxide diffusion capacity (DLCO), mean lung dose (MLD), presence of chronic obstructive pulmonary disease (COPD), age, performance status, concurrent chemotherapy, etc. in analysis [17]. SRILT occurred in overall 58 (22.3 %) patients and was mainly significantly correlated with advanced age (>65 years old) and MLD, but not with poor pretreatment pulmonary function values which therefore do not constitute a contraindication. Enache et al. demonstrated small reduction of lung function within 7.5 months after 3DCRT which was correlated weakly with dose–volume histogram (DVH) parameters in a similar study in which 11 NSCLC patients (17 %) developed grade 2–3 SRILT [18]; besides, no significant difference was observed before and after radiotherapy spirometer and DLCO values in cases with impaired lung function at setup. Although ongoing randomized RTOG trials such as phase 2 1106/ACRIN 6697 study requested a baseline FEV1 ≥1.2 l or ≥50 % predicted without bronchodilator to be suitable for definitive radiotherapy, there is not a defined consensus everyone accepts (Table 1.1).

As basal pulmonary functions were also evaluated by Takeda et al. in 128 patients treated with 50 Gy (10 Gy/fraction) stereotactic body radiotherapy (SBRT) for their solitary pulmonary metastases or primary lung tumors [19], multivariate analysis revealed high FEV1, female gender, and high V15 as significant independent factors to differentiate between grade –1 and grade 2 RP. Also all grades of radiation

Table 1.1 Lung function guided radiotherapy selection is given below

Class 0	Class I	Class II	Class III	Class IV
FEV1 ≥80 % predicted	FEV1 ≥65–79 % predicted	FEV1 ≥55–64 % predicted	FEV1 ≥45–54 % predicted	FEV1 <45 % predicted
DLCO ≥75 % predicted	DLCO ≥65–74 % predicted	DLCO ≥55–64 % predicted	DLCO 45–54 % predicted	DLCO <45 % predicted
VO_2 max >25 mL/kg/min	VO_2 max 22–25 mL/kg/min	VO_2 max 18–21 mL/kg/min	VO_2 max 15–17 mL/kg/min	VO_2 max <15 mL/kg/min
Able to tolerate even pneumonectomy		Average risk for any surgical intervention	Average risk for any surgical intervention	Very high risk / medically inoperable
			If LVEF ≤50 %, more vulnerable	
Definitive RT or SABR based on clinical requirement	Assessment of regional lung parenchymal function			
	Predicted post-RT FEV1 >30 % and DLCO >35 %		Predicted post-RT FEV1 <30 % and DLCO <35 %	
			Palliative RT or SABR	
	Definitive RT or SABR		Strongly consider mean lung dose <8 Gy and and V20 <10 %	

SABR Stereotactic ablative body radiotherapy, *RT* radiotherapy

penumonitis was found to be dose -volume dependent, while grade 2 pneumonitis rate increased for the group with FEV1 >1.81 and females. Even in the presence of chronic obstructive pulmonary disease (COPD), SBRT might not negatively affect the FEV 1 and DLCO values and can be considered for treatment [20, 21]. Palma et al. studied outcomes after SBRT with severe COPD based on Global Initiative for Chronic Obstructive Lung Disease (GOLD) criteria in their single-institution cohort of 176 stage I NSCLC patients with COPD GOLD III-IV or a predicted postoperative FEV1 of </=40 % [20]. Although COPD severity correlated with overall survival ($p = 0.01$), and despite the poorer pulmonary functioning patients selected for SBRT, mean 30-day mortality was 0 % in SBRT and 10 % in surgery patients with comparable OS [20]. The only clear criteria for patient assessment before radiotherapy to decide whether the treatment would be tolerable or not are dose–volume limitations in the radiotherapy plan which need to be individualized according to clinical features. Therefore, a model to combine known clinical risk factors and dose parameters is expected to give more predictive estimation for SRILT [14, 22, 23]. In QUANTEC study, the MLD to keep the risk of radiation pneumonitis below 20 % was identified as 19.8 Gy without any personal factors taken into account; the generated model identified the presence of comorbidities, middle or lower lobe tumors, and advanced age as negative factors, while surprisingly tobacco usage at the time of diagnosis reduced the risk of radiation pneumonitis [22, 24]. Thus, for the young patient with tumor in upper lobe, without pulmonary disease, who had not taken chemotherapy, and is smoking, the MLD value to keep the radiation

pneumonitis risk under 20 % increases to 27.8 Gy. But in the presence of negative criteria, same risk is identified as 7 Gy. This study is important for contributing pretreatment clinical evaluation and personalizing critical dose limits for radiotherapy. On the other hand, MLD doesn't take into account high-dose areas although it is the most common criteria for determining the risk of radiation pneumonitis. Lyman-Kutcher-Burman (LKB) normal tissue complication probability (NTCP) modeling has emerged as a dosimetric alternative to the MLD. In this model, high dose in small volume seems worse than low dose in large volume. LKB modeling ($n=0.41$) is important especially for comparing different treatment techniques [25].

Not now, but eventually in the near future, a personal genetic profile detailing the most relevant genes would guide to individualize their radiotherapy based on predictive factors [26].

Three-Dimensional Conformal Radiotherapy (3DCRT) and Intensity-Modulated Radiotherapy (IMRT)

IMRT should be strictly quality assured and all required dose parameters should be implemented in planning. Yom et al. documented the retrospective evaluation of treatment-related pneumonitis in MD Anderson Cancer Center cohort of 151 advanced NSCLC patients treated with concurrent chemotherapy and IMRT between 2002 and 2005 and compared rates of pneumonitis for 68 eligible IMRT (median 63 Gy, median GTV 194 mL) patients (after excluding early-stage, major lung resection, prior chest radiotherapy, low dose of <50 Gy, combined IMRT with 3DCRT, without concurrent chemotherapy) with 222 similar 3DCRT (median 63 Gy, median GTV 142 mL) patients [27]. They have revealed the significantly lower rate of ≥grade 3 pneumonitis at 12 months with IMRT despite larger median GTV (8 % versus 32 %, $p=0.002$) which both delineates the ability of IMRT to decrease symptomatic pneumonitis and the importance of strictly quality assured and standardized systems to gain the IMRT benefit. A recent study of Khalil et al. at Aarhus University Hospital pointed out the importance of knowledge-based dose constraints in IMRT planning and investigated three different planning constraints in three phases in their IMRT plans delivered using four to eight beam arrangements [28]; only one dose constraint of V20 <40 % in phase I, a second additional dose constraint of MLD ≤20 Gy in phase II, and a third constraint of V5 ≤60 % in phase III were used. IMRT was associated with a 41 % increase of RP in phases I and II with grade 5 RP in 6 of 37 (16 %), while introducing V5 led to a significant reduction in the lethal pneumonitis to 4 % (2 of 50 patients, $p=0.05$) but did not decrease the incidence of severe (grade ≥3) RP [28]. Chen et al. has recently documented their investigation of the association between absolute volumes of lung spared from low radiotherapy dose and radiation-induced lung injury in 83 patients with lung cancer treated with IMRT at Fujian Medical University [29]. They have studied the bilateral and ipsilateral lung findings for grade ≥2 lung injury including normal lung relative volumes receiving greater than 5, 10, 20, and 30 Gy (V5-30), mean lung dose (MLD), and absolute volumes not receiving more than 5, 10, 20, and 30 Gy

(AVS5-30). With the median follow-up of 12.3 months, lung injury was observed as grade 2 in 18 (21.7 %), grade 3 in 7 (8.4 %), and grade 4 in 2 (2.4 %) cases, where multivariate analysis documented ipsilateral lung AVS5 as prognostic for grade ≥2 lung injury ($P=0.010$, OR=0.272, 95 % CI: 0.102–0.729), and the incidence of grade ≥2 lung injury was shown to be significantly lower with AVS5 of the ipsilateral lung ≥564.9 cm^3 than with AVS5 <564.9 cm^3 ($P=0.008$) (e.g., a functional spared volume with minimum diameter of 10 cm if accepted as a sphere) [29]. Therefore, IMRT can be considered a powerful tool to spare functional parenchymal volume, helping to ensure eligibility for definitive treatments for more patients. Potential effects of advanced radiotherapy techniques on pulmonary function will continue to be a subject of research. Lopez et al. examined the change in pulmonary functions in 250 NSCLC patients who were prescribed 3DCRT, or IMRT or proton therapy [30]. In each one of the three groups, DLCO decreased after the radiotherapy. Although more pronounced decrease in the DLCO was documented when initial DLCO was ≤50 % and gross tumor volume was ≥100 cm^3, no significant difference was found between the three radiotherapy techniques. The effect of thoracic radiotherapy on FEV_1 and FVC was not clarified, but its relationship with DLCO has been apparent. Although DLCO prior to RT was not predictive, DLCO change difference between before and after the treatment was found to be related with the risk and severity of radiation pneumonitis [31]. Recently, along with DLCO, change of nitrogen monoxide (NO) diffusion capacity during radiotherapy is being investigated. The results of these studies might contribute to the evaluation of the patient prior to radiotherapy [32]

Chemotherapy

Chemotherapy agents sequential or concurrent with radiotherapy are known to trigger lung damage. As the concurrent chemoradiotherapy in locoregionally advanced NSCLC is more effective in comparison to sequential chemotherapy and radiotherapy [33, 34], the concurrent combination also increases the toxicity. Assessing patients prior to chemoradiotherapy, especially patients over the age of 65, it is important to consider concurrent chemotherapy with radiation as a potential risk factor for radiation pneumonitis due to an individual patient data meta-analysis identifying carboplatin and paclitaxel (CP) as a major risk factor (odds ratio of 5.52) in comparison to cisplatin and etoposide (EP) [35].

Cardiopulmonary Relationship

A study in patients with inoperable NSCLC and chemoradiotherapy candidates by Semrau et al. supports the pre-radiotherapy individualized assessment to be a whole considering all comorbidities; impairments in cardiopulmonary functions, mainly decreased left ventricular ejection fraction (LVEF ≤50 %), were shown to diminish the overall survival significantly [36], in addition to pulmonary factors as decreased inspiratory VC <60 %, decreased FEV1 <80 % or ≤1,5 l and impairment in DLCO <60 %, although no relationship between basal cardiopulmonary values and toxicity was identified.

Functional Imaging, Assessment, and Prediction

Along with functional assessments, additional parameters that may predict radiation pneumonitis prior to radiotherapy are also investigated. Some studies claim that pretreatment high pulmonary [18F]-2-fluoro-2-deoxyglucose (FDG) uptake (standard uptake value 95-SUV95) can indicate the cases with high risk of radiation pneumonitis. For individuals with average age and the same V30Gy value, in condition of SUV95 = 1.5 when compared to ones with SUV95 = 0.5 risk of grade 2 radiation pneumonitis is increasing 6.9 times [37].

In recent years, for thoracic radiotherapy, studies that aim defining and maintaining the functional lung space have been accelerated. In routine, when planning radiation therapy, keeping total lung dose at minimal levels is aimed. This approach doesn't take into account that lung tissue may be heterogeneous in terms of functionality. However, patients, especially those who smoke, may have different pulmonary ventilation characteristics. In the past, many research showed that determining functional lung areas with the methods such as single-photon emission computed tomography (SPECT), high-resolution computed tomography (CT), and hyperpolarized helium magnetic resonance imaging (^{3}He MRI) can be used in radiotherapy planning [38–41]. In the mentioned studies, healthy lung tissue dose was reduced by adding related techniques that have been reported. But there is no clear data about clinical reflection of these developments. FLAIR study which is planned in cases with stage 3 NSCLC diagnosis who will receive chemoradiotherapy is remarkable in this respect. In this trial, addition to routine radiotherapy plan, by preserving functional lung sections using hyperpolarized ^{3}He MRI cases divided into two arms. The study will be prepared as double-blind randomized, and toxicity evaluation will be done in both groups. This study which will be supported with pretreatment and posttreatment pulmonary function tests and life quality assessment is significant for the functional imaging examinations to become routine [42].

Recent findings encouraged functional parameters to be implemented more into planning and optimization process to reduce the risk of radiation-induced toxicity. Farr et al. in Aarhus University Hospital analyzed their patients whether perfusion single-photon emission computed tomography (SPECT) could predict the risk of RP compared to standard CT-based dose-volume parameters and revealed functional parameters in multivariate analysis to produce superior risk estimates, being all standard CT parameters, except V30, not related to the risk of radiation pneumonitis [4].

Yamamoto et al. tried to avoid highly functional lung regions based on quantifying the pulmonary ventilation in four-dimensional computed tomography (4D-CT) and performing functional treatment planning in their cohort of 15 patients [43]. They gained an average reduction of 1.8 Gy for IMRT ($p<0.001$) and 2.0 Gy for VMAT ($p<0.001$) in the mean dose of high-functional lung and pointed out the potential of functional planning in functional avoidance, especially for critical PTV adjacent to high-functional lung volume.

Immune Parameters

Pretreatment immune parameters have recently been shown in the setting of SBRT to predict for overall survival and toxicity in early-stage NSCLC patients [44], i.e., an elevated pretreatment neutrophil-to-lymphocyte ratio (NLR), platelet-to-lymphocyte ratio (PLR), and neutrophil count and the presence of lymphocytopenia independently predicted for poor OS, while baseline higher NLRs and lower serum albumin levels were shown leading to less treatment-related symptomatic (grade $\geq$2) radiation pneumonitis.

Conclusion

Severity of clinical symptoms caused by untreated tumor progression would probably be complicating the pulmonary functions worse than a carefully assessed, planned, and individually delivered radiotherapy despite poor basal lung functions; therefore the general effort should not only be making the decision to treat or not but also generating a radiotherapy environment to gain the highest effect with the least toxicity [45]. An algorithm for radiotherapy sounds to work leading the way for how to and by which technique to treat but not defining the ones not to be treated. In this context, proposals to basal evaluation and risk assessment were discussed among different groups [46]. Besides, it sounds reasonable to evaluate the expected loss and remaining functional volume to decide the extent we can treat, such as in mesothelioma patients treated following an extrapleural pneumonectomy or pleurectomy/decortication surgery [47]. Eligibility for definitive radiotherapy could be robust based on the predicted post-radiotherapy FEV1 >30 % and DLCO >35 %, to be on the safe side, generated on estimation following patients undergoing a pneumonectomy and can be calculated with following equation "predicted post-resection/radiotherapy FEV1 = current FEV1 × % perfused in uninvolved (≈unirradiated) lung determined by quantitative ventilation/perfusion scan." If the patient is not eligible for a definitive radiotherapy based on lung functions, palliative approach with very limited fields such as stereotactic ablative radiotherapy can be a life a saver.

References

1. Woel RT, Munley MT, Hollis D, Fan M, Bentel G, Anscher MS, et al. The time course of radiation therapy-induced reductions in regional perfusion: a prospective study with >5 years of follow-up. Int J Radiat Oncol Biol Phys. 2002;52(1):58–67. PubMed Epub 2002/01/05. eng.
2. Seppenwoolde Y, Muller SH, Theuws JC, Baas P, Belderbos JS, Boersma LJ, et al. Radiation dose-effect relations and local recovery in perfusion for patients with non-small-cell lung cancer. Int J Radiat Oncol Biol Phys. 2000;47(3):681–90. PubMed Epub 2000/06/06. eng.

3. Zhang J, Ma J, Zhou S, Hubbs JL, Wong TZ, Folz RJ, et al. Radiation-induced reductions in regional lung perfusion: 0.1–12 year data from a prospective clinical study. Int J Radiat Oncol Biol Phys. 2010;76(2):425–32. PubMed Epub 2009/07/28. eng.
4. Farr KP, Kallehauge JF, Møller DS, Khalil AA, Kramer S, Bluhme H, et al. Inclusion of functional information from perfusion SPECT improves predictive value of dose-volume parameters in lung toxicity outcome after radiotherapy for non-small cell lung cancer: A prospective study. Radiother Oncol. 2015;117(1):9–16. Epub 2015/08/21.eng
5. Brunelli A, Charloux A, Bolliger CT, Rocco G, Sculier JP, Varela G, et al. ERS/ESTS clinical guidelines on fitness for radical therapy in lung cancer patients (surgery and chemoradiotherapy). Eur Respir J. 2009;34(1):17–41. PubMed Epub 2009/07/02. eng.
6. Ueki N, Matsuo Y, Togashi Y, Kubo T, Shibuya K, Iizuka Y, et al. Impact of pretreatment interstitial lung disease on radiation pneumonitis and survival after stereotactic body radiation therapy for lung cancer. J Thorac Oncol Off Publ Int Assoc Study Lung Cancer. 2015;10(1):116–25. PubMed Epub 2014/11/08. eng.
7. Nagano T, Kotani Y, Fujii O, Demizu Y, Niwa Y, Ohno Y, et al. A case of acute exacerbation of idiopathic pulmonary fibrosis after proton beam therapy for non-small cell lung cancer. Jpn J Clin Oncol. 2012;42(10):965–9. PubMed Epub 2012/07/25. eng.
8. Protocol N-B. A Phase 1 study of stereotactic body radiotherapy (SBRT) for the treatment of multiple metastases. Available from: https://www.rtog.org/ClinicalTrials/ProtocolTable/StudyDetails.aspx?study=1311.
9. Protocol R. A Randomized phase II study comparing 2 stereotactic body radiation therapy (SBRT) schedules for medically inoperable patients with stage I peripheral non-small cell lung cancer. 2015. Available from: https://www.rtog.org/ClinicalTrials/ProtocolTable/StudyDetails.aspx?study=0915.
10. Smith BD, Smith GL, Hurria A, Hortobagyi GN, Buchholz TA. Future of cancer incidence in the United States: burdens upon an aging, changing nation. J Clin Oncol Off J Am Soc Clin Oncol. 2009;27(17):2758–65. PubMed Epub 2009/05/01. eng.
11. Raz DJ, Zell JA, Ou SH, Gandara DR, Anton-Culver H, Jablons DM. Natural history of stage I non-small cell lung cancer: implications for early detection. Chest. 2007;132(1):193–9. PubMed Epub 2007/05/17. eng.
12. Palma D, Visser O, Lagerwaard FJ, Belderbos J, Slotman BJ, Senan S. Impact of introducing stereotactic lung radiotherapy for elderly patients with stage I non-small-cell lung cancer: a population-based time-trend analysis. J Clin Oncol Off J Am Soc Clin Oncol. 2010;28(35):5153–9. PubMed Epub 2010/11/03. eng.
13. Kim H, Lussier YA, Noh OK, Li H, Oh YT, Heo J. Prognostic implication of pulmonary function at the beginning of postoperative radiotherapy in non-small cell lung cancer. Radiother Oncol J Eur Soc Ther Radiol Oncol. 2014;113(3):374–8. PubMed Epub 2014/12/03. eng.
14. Marks LB, Bentzen SM, Deasy JO, Kong FM, Bradley JD, Vogelius IS, et al. Radiation dose-volume effects in the lung. Int J Radiat Oncol Biol Phys. 2010;76(3 Suppl):S70–6. PubMed Pubmed Central PMCID: 3576042, Epub 2010/03/05. eng.
15. Kabolizadeh P, Kalash R, Huq MS, Greenberger JS, Heron DE, Beriwal S. Dosimetric definitions of total lung volumes in calculating parameters predictive for radiation-induced pneumonitis. Am J Clin Oncol. 2015;38(4):401–4. PubMed Epub 2013/09/26. eng.
16. Robnett TJ, Machtay M, Vines EF, McKenna MG, Algazy KM, McKenna WG. Factors predicting severe radiation pneumonitis in patients receiving definitive chemoradiation for lung cancer. Int J Radiat Oncol Biol Phys. 2000;48(1):89–94. PubMed Epub 2000/08/05. eng.
17. Wang J, Cao J, Yuan S, Ji W, Arenberg D, Dai J, et al. Poor baseline pulmonary function may not increase the risk of radiation-induced lung toxicity. Int J Radiat Oncol Biol Phys. 2013;85(3):798–804. PubMed Pubmed Central PMCID: 3646086, Epub 2012/07/28. eng.
18. Enache I, Noel G, Jeung MY, Meyer N, Oswald-Mammosser M, Pistea C, et al. Impact of 3D conformal radiotherapy on lung function of patients with lung cancer: a prospective study. Respiration. 2013;86(2):100–8. PubMed Epub 2012/11/17. eng.

19. Takeda A, Ohashi T, Kunieda E, Sanuki N, Enomoto T, Takeda T, et al. Comparison of clinical, tumour-related and dosimetric factors in grade 0–1, grade 2 and grade 3 radiation pneumonitis after stereotactic body radiotherapy for lung tumours. Br J Radiol. 2012;85(1013):636–42. PubMed Pubmed Central PMCID: 3479872, Epub 2012/01/19. eng.
20. Palma D, Lagerwaard F, Rodrigues G, Haasbeek C, Senan S. Curative treatment of Stage I non-small-cell lung cancer in patients with severe COPD: stereotactic radiotherapy outcomes and systematic review. Int J Radiat Oncol Biol Phys. 2012;82(3):1149–56. PubMed Epub 2011/06/07. eng.
21. Stephans KL, Djemil T, Reddy CA, Gajdos SM, Kolar M, Machuzak M, et al. Comprehensive analysis of pulmonary function Test (PFT) changes after stereotactic body radiotherapy (SBRT) for stage I lung cancer in medically inoperable patients. J Thorac Oncol Off Publ Int Assoc Study Lung Cancer. 2009;4(7):838–44. PubMed Epub 2009/06/03. eng.
22. Appelt AL, Vogelius IR, Farr KP, Khalil AA, Bentzen SM. Towards individualized dose constraints: adjusting the QUANTEC radiation pneumonitis model for clinical risk factors. Acta Oncol. 2014;53(5):605–12. PubMed Epub 2013/08/21. eng.
23. Vogelius IR, Bentzen SM. A literature-based meta-analysis of clinical risk factors for development of radiation induced pneumonitis. Acta Oncol. 2012;51(8):975–83. PubMed Pubmed Central PMCID: 3557496, Epub 2012/09/07. eng.
24. Jin H, Tucker SL, Liu HH, Wei X, Yom SS, Wang S, et al. Dose-volume thresholds and smoking status for the risk of treatment-related pneumonitis in inoperable non-small cell lung cancer treated with definitive radiotherapy. Radiother Oncol J Eur Soc Ther Radiol Oncol. 2009;91(3):427–32. PubMed Epub 2008/10/22. eng.
25. Tucker SL, Mohan R, Liengsawangwong R, Martel MK, Liao Z. Predicting pneumonitis risk: a dosimetric alternative to mean lung dose. Int J Radiat Oncol Biol Phys. 2013;85(2):522–7. PubMed Epub 2012/05/15. eng.
26. Huang Q, Xie F, Ouyang X. Predictive SNPs for radiation-induced damage in lung cancer patients with radiotherapy: a potential strategy to individualize treatment. Int J Biol Markers. 2015;30(1):e1–11. PubMed Epub 2014/09/30. eng.
27. Yom SS, Liao Z, Liu HH, Tucker SL, Hu CS, Wei X, et al. Initial evaluation of treatment-related pneumonitis in advanced-stage non-small-cell lung cancer patients treated with concurrent chemotherapy and intensity-modulated radiotherapy. Int J Radiat Oncol Biol Phys. 2007;68(1):94–102. PubMed Epub 2007/02/27. eng.
28. Khalil AA, Hoffmann L, Moeller DS, Farr KP, Knap MM. New dose constraint reduces radiation-induced fatal pneumonitis in locally advanced non-small cell lung cancer patients treated with intensity-modulated radiotherapy. Acta Oncol. 2015;54(9):1343–9. PubMed Epub 2015/07/23. eng.
29. Chen J, Hong J, Zou X, Lv W, Guo F, Hong H, et al. Association between absolute volumes of lung spared from low-dose irradiation and radiation-induced lung injury after intensity-modulated radiotherapy in lung cancer: a retrospective analysis. J Radiat Res. 2015;56(6):883–8. Epub 2015/10/09.eng.
30. Lopez Guerra JL, Gomez DR, Zhuang Y, Levy LB, Eapen G, Liu H, et al. Changes in pulmonary function after three-dimensional conformal radiotherapy, intensity-modulated radiotherapy, or proton beam therapy for non-small-cell lung cancer. Int J Radiat Oncol Biol Phys. 2012;83(4):e537–43. PubMed Pubmed Central PMCID: 3923580, Epub 2012/03/17. eng.
31. Lopez Guerra JL, Gomez D, Zhuang Y, Levy LB, Eapen G, Liu H, et al. Change in diffusing capacity after radiation as an objective measure for grading radiation pneumonitis in patients treated for non-small-cell lung cancer. Int J Radiat Oncol Biol Phys. 2012;83(5):1573–9. PubMed Pubmed Central PMCID: 3931002, Epub 2012/07/10. eng.
32. Zarza V, Couraud S, Hassouni A, Prevost C, Souquet PJ, Letanche G, et al. Pulmonary diffusion test to NO and CO time course during thoracic radiotherapy for lung cancer: the CONORT prospective study protocol. Cancer Radiother. 2014;18(5–6):420–4. PubMed Epub 2014/09/11. Evolution de la double diffusion au CO et au NO au cours de la radiotherapie pulmonaire pour cancer bronchique : presentation du protocole de l'etude prospective Conort. fre.

33. Auperin A, Le Pechoux C, Rolland E, Curran WJ, Furuse K, Fournel P, et al. Meta-analysis of concomitant versus sequential radiochemotherapy in locally advanced non-small-cell lung cancer. J Clin Oncol Off J Am Soc Clin Oncol. 2010;28(13):2181–90. PubMed Epub 2010/03/31. eng.
34. Curran Jr WJ, Paulus R, Langer CJ, Komaki R, Lee JS, Hauser S, et al. Sequential vs. concurrent chemoradiation for stage III non-small cell lung cancer: randomized phase III trial RTOG 9410. J Natl Cancer Inst. 2011;103(19):1452–60. PubMed Pubmed Central PMCID: 3186782, Epub 2011/09/10. eng.
35. Palma DA, Senan S, Tsujino K, Barriger RB, Rengan R, Moreno M, et al. Predicting radiation pneumonitis after chemoradiation therapy for lung cancer: an international individual patient data meta-analysis. Int J Radiat Oncol Biol Phys. 2013;85(2):444–50. PubMed Pubmed Central PMCID: 3448004, Epub 2012/06/12. eng.
36. Semrau S, Klautke G, Fietkau R. Baseline cardiopulmonary function as an independent prognostic factor for survival of inoperable non-small-cell lung cancer after concurrent chemoradiotherapy: a single-center analysis of 161 cases. Int J Radiat Oncol Biol Phys. 2011;79(1):96–104. PubMed Epub 2010/03/31. eng.
37. Castillo R, Pham N, Ansari S, Meshkov D, Castillo S, Li M, et al. Pre-radiotherapy FDG PET predicts radiation pneumonitis in lung cancer. Radiat Oncol. 2014;9:74. PubMed Pubmed Central PMCID: 3995607, Epub 2014/03/15. eng.
38. Hodge CW, Tome WA, Fain SB, Bentzen SM, Mehta MP. On the use of hyperpolarized helium MRI for conformal avoidance lung radiotherapy. Med Dosim. 2010;35(4):297–303. PubMed Pubmed Central PMCID: 2975877, Epub 2009/12/01. eng.
39. Ireland RH, Din OS, Swinscoe JA, Woodhouse N, van Beek EJ, Wild JM, et al. Detection of radiation-induced lung injury in non-small cell lung cancer patients using hyperpolarized helium-3 magnetic resonance imaging. Radiother Oncol J Eur Soc Ther Radiol Oncol. 2010;97(2):244–8. PubMed Epub 2010/08/21. eng.
40. Shioyama Y, Jang SY, Liu HH, Guerrero T, Wang X, Gayed IW, et al. Preserving functional lung using perfusion imaging and intensity-modulated radiation therapy for advanced-stage non-small cell lung cancer. Int J Radiat Oncol Biol Phys. 2007;68(5):1349–58. PubMed Epub 2007/04/21. eng.
41. Vinogradskiy YY, Castillo R, Castillo E, Chandler A, Martel MK, Guerrero T. Use of weekly 4DCT-based ventilation maps to quantify changes in lung function for patients undergoing radiation therapy. Med Phys. 2012;39(1):289–98. PubMed Epub 2012/01/10. eng.
42. Hoover DA, Capaldi DP, Sheikh K, Palma DA, Rodrigues GB, Dar AR, et al. Functional lung avoidance for individualized radiotherapy (FLAIR): study protocol for a randomized, double-blind clinical trial. BMC Cancer. 2014;14:934. PubMed Pubmed Central PMCID: 4364501, Epub 2014/12/17. eng.
43. Yamamoto T, Kabus S, von Berg J, Lorenz C, Keall PJ. Impact of four-dimensional computed tomography pulmonary ventilation imaging-based functional avoidance for lung cancer radiotherapy. Int J Radiat Oncol Biol Phys. 2011;79(1):279–88. PubMed Epub 2010/07/22. eng.
44. Shaverdian N, Veruttipong D, Wang J, Schaue D, Kupelian P, Lee P. Pretreatment immune parameters predict for overall survival and toxicity in early-stage non-small-cell lung cancer patients treated with stereotactic body radiation therapy. Clin Lung Cancer. 2015. pii: [Epub ahead of print]:S1525-7304(15)00187-4.
45. Selek U, Bolukbasi Y, Welsh JW, Topkan E. Intensity-modulated radiotherapy versus 3-dimensional conformal radiotherapy strategies for locally advanced Non-small-cell lung cancer. Balkan Med J. 2014;31(4):286–94. PubMed Pubmed Central PMCID: 4318398, Epub 2015/02/11. eng.
46. Miller KL, Shafman TD, Marks LB. A practical approach to pulmonary risk assessment in the radiotherapy of lung cancer. Semin Radiat Oncol. 2004;14(4):298–307. PubMed Epub 2004/11/24. eng.
47. Chance WW, Rice DC, Allen PK, Tsao AS, Fontanilla HP, Liao Z, et al. Hemithoracic intensity modulated radiation therapy after pleurectomy/decortication for malignant pleural mesothelioma: toxicity, patterns of failure, and a matched survival analysis. Int J Radiat Oncol Biol Phys. 2015;91(1):149–56. PubMed Epub 2014/12/03. eng.

Modern Radiotherapy Techniques in Lung Cancer

2

Yasemin Bolukbasi, Duygu Sezen, Erkan Topkan, and Ugur Selek

Introduction

Radiotherapy is a well-established local treatment for locally advanced or medically inoperable early-stage lung cancer. In the last decade, we have an evidence-based understanding of the value of local control and its influence on survival in patients with non-small cell lung cancer (NSCLC), supported by a meta-analysis demonstrating the translation of locoregional control into an absolute 5-year survival benefit of 4.5 % with concurrent chemoradiotherapy [1]. Modern radiotherapy techniques integrating four-dimensional computerized tomography (4D-CT), intensity-modulated radiotherapy (IMRT), and image-guided radiotherapy (IGRT) have allowed incorporation of tumor respiratory motion besides more accurate target definition and improved target conformality with more precise application of high-dose radiation

Y. Bolukbasi, MD
Department of Radiation Oncology, Koc University, School of Medicine, Istanbul, Turkey

Department of Radiation Oncology, U.T. MD Anderson Cancer Center, Houston, TX, USA
e-mail: yaseminb@amerikanhastanesi.org; ybolukbasi@mdanderson.org

D. Sezen, MD
Department of Radiation Oncology, Koc University, School of Medicine, Istanbul, Turkey
e-mail: dsezen@kuh.ku.edu.tr

E. Topkan, MD
Department of Radiation Oncology, Faculty of Medicine, Baskent University, Adana, Turkey
e-mail: docdretopkan@gmail.com

U. Selek, MD (✉)
Department of Radiation Oncology, Faculty of Medicine, Koc University, Istanbul, Turkey

Department of Radiation Oncology, The University of Texas, MD Anderson Cancer Center, Houston, TX, USA
e-mail: ugurselek@yahoo.com, uselek@ku.edu.tr, uselek@mdanderson.org

G. Ozyigit et al. (eds.), *Principles and Practice of Radiotherapy Techniques in Thoracic Malignancies*, DOI 10.1007/978-3-319-28761-4_2

along with enhanced knowledge of organs at risk to avoid as much potential side effects as possible [2, 3]. Proton beam therapy has been under investigation and gaining ground in both locally advanced and early-stage NSCLC [4–6].

In clinical routine, there is no 100 % standardization and consensus to answer the best way to immobilize patients, manage respiratory motion, and integrate IGRT into routine practice, aside from many common departmental justifications and applications. This chapter will focus on the extent of modern radiotherapy techniques for early and local advanced lung cancer treatments where organ motion is dominant and technical options are scarce.

Radiation Treatment Planning

Historically, treatment field design has been based on the correlation of soft tissue and bony landmarks in the two-dimensional (2D) planning era where only clues were anatomic structures visible fluoroscopically. Despite 2D radiotherapy, three-dimensional conformal radiation therapy (3D CRT) providing a 3D model of the patient's anatomy allows accurate tumor and organs at risk delineation. More sophisticated planning, delivery, and on-board imaging systems in the last two decades such as intensity-modulated radiotherapy (IMRT) and image-guided radiotherapy (IGRT) have allowed more targeted delivery of radiotherapy [7].

In order to have an improved dose distribution, the first step is to describe the moving target appropriately with all microscopic extension encompassed in addition to overcome the large interobserver variability [8]. Transition from 2D to 3D and beyond has been studied in dosimetric and clinical studies covering 4D-CT or PET-CT integrated simulation, adequate immobilization, advanced planning, on-board imaging, and precise delivery including stereotactic radiosurgery (SRS), IMRT, or volumetric arc therapy (VMAT).

Positron Emission Tomography (PET-CT) Simulation

PET/CT is an effective imaging modality for the diagnosis, staging, and restaging of cancer patients which combines the complementary information of functional PET images and anatomical CT images in one modality. FDG-PET imaging is achieved through the detection of a pair of γ rays (511 keV each) produced in positron annihilation, which are emitted in 180° to each other [9, 10]. FDG-PET has superior sensitivity and specificity almost 83–91 % for tumor detection compared to computer tomography alone [11]. In terms of radiation treatment planning, the accuracy of tumor targeting can be improved by integrating information from the PET scan into the planning process and this may lead to significant modifications of the treatment strategy and the radiotherapy planning in lung cancer patients [12, 13]. The radiation therapy has evolved toward omitting nonmetastatic lymph node treatment and escalation of curative treatment doses to improve local control as the importance of accurate delineation of tumor volume and decreasing the percentages of interobserver variability has become more important and raised the possibility of incorporation of PET/CT information into target delineation.

Initial attempt in PET-CT trials intended investigating to better define the tumor borders by using a subjective threshold uptake value within the FDG-avid area, such as 40 %, 42 %, or 50 % [12–14]. The heterogeneity of the methods described in the literature makes difficult to establish a universal consensus threshold to optimally use the PET metabolic uptake information in contouring the gross tumor volume (GTV). Caldwell et al. implied the poor representation of the moving tumor based on time-averaged position and shape in a fast CT, asked the possibility of PET imaging to provide a more accurate representation of the 3D volume encompassing patient-specific motion for an individualized integrated tumor volume (ITV), and noted a threshold as low as 15 % of the maximum value, instead of using a set point as 40 % intensity level, could help to estimate true extension of lung cancer [15]. However, Duan et al. recently pointed out that none of the PET-based contours had both close spatial and volumetric approximation to the generated gross target volume (iGTV) of the primary tumor contoured on the ten phases images of 4D-CT and concluded as 3D-PET/CT should not be used for iGTV generation [12].

Aside from inability to generate individualized ITV, PET/CT guidance provided a significant impact on the radiotherapy plans with a range of 30–60 % [10, 16], especially in delineation of GTV in cases with atelectasis and of CT-insignificant nodal areas. Vanuytsel et al. documented in their dosimetric study that PET provided a reduction in GTV with a corresponding reduction on planning target volume (PTV) by 29 ± 18 %, leading to a reduction in the volume of lung receiving at least 20 Gy by 27 ± 18 % [17].

Hanna et al. have assessed the effect of using an additional planning PET-CT scan for GTV definition in their cohort of 28 PET-CT staged NSCLC patients [18] and expressed the improvement of the confidence intervals between observers in defining the GTV using the PET-CT images while the median of the mean percentage of volume change from CT-guided GTV to fusion-guided GTV was found to be −5.21 % for the induction chemotherapy group and 18.88 % for the RT-alone group [18]. Superiority of software registration of PET and simulation CT images in comparison to visual fusion has been pronounced in promoting interobserver consistency in tumor volume delineation [19, 20]; Ashamalla et al. found an increased concordance between the GTVs of two independent observers when co-registered PET data were provided (84 % vs. 37 % had a ≤10 % difference in volume from mean of GTVs with the use of PET/CT) [20]. Therefore, target volume delineation with registered PET/CT could be encouraged to reduce interobserver variability [19–21].

The reduction in volume delineated by PET-CT has also found place in investigating dose escalation [22]; De Ruysscher et al. studied on 21 locally advanced non-small cell lung cancer patient's data of CT and PET-CT-guided delineated volumes and concluded that combined dedicated PET-CT-simulator guidance in delineation could reduce radiation doses of the esophagus and lung in order to allow the possibility for radiation dose escalation while keeping all organs at risk constraints; 55.2 ± 2.0 Gy with CT planning to 68.9 ± 3.3 Gy with the use of PET-CT was feasible [22].

Motion Management

Radiotherapy precision requires reproducibility and reduction of uncertainties in planning and delivery [3, 7]. The optimal definition of the size, shape, and location of gross tumor volume is one of the most important steps in the planning of radiation therapy. Respiratory motion management which is directly related with reproducibility is the major consideration for thoracic tumors [23]. The International Commission on Radiation Units and Measurements (ICRU) report 62 introduced the concept of an internal target volume (ITV) which includes geometric uncertainties due to internal variations in tumor position, size, and shape [24]; the ITV plus setup margin is used to generate the PTV. The AAPM Task Group 76 guidelines [25] listed the methods to take into account and compensate motion by different approaches as encompassing motion with slow CT scanning or combining inhale and exhale breath-hold CT or 4D-CT/respiration-correlated CT, gating respiratory movement with internal or external markers, stabilizing at a phase with breath-hold by self or device control, fixing the diaphragm with abdominal compression for decreasing movement as shallow breathing, and finally real-time tracking. AAPM task group 76 recommended to consider motion management for tumors with more than 5 mm motion, whereas Korreman and Guckenberger advised that gating should be spared for tumors moving more than 13 and 15 mm, respectively [25–27]. Motion quantification, immobilization techniques, and strategies to overcome can vary from institute to institute. Patient selection is important to gain benefit for reducing normal tissue in field and more conformal gross tumor volume coverage. The American Association of Physicist in Medicine Task Group reports and the UK SABR consortium could be used to generate institutional guidelines in regard to motion management preferences [25, 28].

Four-Dimensional CT Simulation (4D-CT)

Currently, four-dimensional CT (4D-CT) is widely used for the simulation of lung cancer as a reliable and effective tool for assessing tumor and organ motion through the entire breathing cycle [10]. Enhanced accuracy in tumor localization could improve tumor control probability as "geometric miss" of the tumor target has been diminished. Several 4D imaging techniques can be used to create an ITV and to determine an approach for motion management. During 4D-CT scanning, respiration wave form is synchronously recorded. One of the common approaches involves recording respiratory signals using infrared-reflecting markers placed on the upper abdomen of the patient during quite free breathing. The markers are illuminated by infrared-emitting diodes surrounding the camera which captures the motion of these markers. The commercial version of this system is produced by Varian Medical Systems under the name real-time position monitoring (RPM) device (Palo Alto, CA). Additional methods to measure abdominal displacement in respiration employ either a strain gauge 41 or a pneumatic bellows system. There are two other methods that use the air inhaled and exhaled by the patient during respiration to produce a respiratory surrogate. Spirometer measures the rate of airflow into and out of the patient's mouth during respiration to obtain a breathing surrogate [29]. Alternatively, a thermocouple has been used to measure the temperature of the air in the patient's mouth to obtain a respiratory surrogate curve [23]. The principle behind the thermocouple method is that air exhaled will be increasingly warmer while the air inhaled is increasingly cooler. These last two methods assume that the 3D motion of the lung is directly correlated to the flow of air in and out of the lung [23]. It has been shown that spirometer does correlate to the internal air content of the CT images, which can be used as a surrogate for internal motion, better than the amplitude of an external marker [25].

Ten respiration phases correlated 3D datasets are commonly derived from a single 4D dataset, and each represents the patient's anatomy during single respiratory phase. Delineation options to generate ITVs from 4DCT scans include: (a) contouring GTV in all phases of 4DCT, (b) contouring GTV in only the extreme phases of respiration, and (c) using maximum intensity projection (MIP) of all phases of the 4D-CT. Maximum MIP is the fastest form of delineation. This set is commonly used to generate ITV for planning purposes [23]; however it is noted to be less accurate than the ten-phase overlap approach for CT [30, 31].

A large analysis of respiration-induced tumor motion in mainly stage III NSCLC patient's reports that principal component of motion was in the superior inferior (SI) direction with 10.8 % of tumors moving greater than 1 cm [32], and motion greater than 5 mm during normal breathing was 39.2 % for SI, 1.8 % laterally and 5.4 % anteroposteriorly [32]. Despite general trends, three-dimensional motions detected in individual patients and groups of patients could be in a range of spectrum [33–35]. In the study of Seppenwoolde et al., gold markers implanted in or near the tumor were tracked with fluoroscopy over multiple 10 breathing cycles in their cohort of 21 patients. and the average amplitude of motion was found to be greatest in the cranio-caudal direction (12 ± 2 mm) in the lower lobes and much smaller in lateral and anteroposterior directions (2 ± 1 mm for both upper and lower lobes) [36]. The most interesting finding of this study was a hysteresis effect between the inhalation and exhalation motion trajectories of the gold markers in 10 of the 21 patients, ranging from 1 to 5 mm [36]. Besides, Seppenwoolde et al. also noted that cardiac beat caused a measurable motion in the range 1–4 mm for 7 of 21 tumors, greatest in the lateral direction, mostly in tumors located near the heart or attached to the aortic arch [36]. Overall, the motion of lung tumor was shown to be extremely complex, patient dependent, and mainly cranio-caudal. Yu et al. studied tumor motion tracking after defining volumes and gross tumor volume delineated by physicians in the end of expiration phase in their cohort of 191 (94 early stage, 97 locally advanced) non-small cell lung tumors using 4D-CT [37]; and the displacement was found to be not volume correlated but was significantly related to the stage and the location of the tumor, such as early-stage lower lobe tumors displaying the largest motion (median 9.2 mm) and upper/mid-lobe tumors exhibiting fairly small motion (median 3.3 mm). Interestingly, motion was mainly in right–left in early stage and cranio-caudally in advanced stage [37]. Underberg et al. studied 31 consecutive patients with stage I lung cancer undergoing 4D-CT scan. They have generated 3 PTV volumes as PTV10bins (a combination of 10 phases), PTV gating (consists 3 consecutive phases that movement was observed plus 3mm) and PTV10 mm (includes 3 consecutive phases that movement was observed plus 10 mm) [38]. PTV 10 mm has the largest PTV volume and PTV gating was even smaller than the others which are 70.5 % of the latter two volumes. This turned into the reduction of the volume encompassing 80 % isodose lines [38]. Lin et al. confirmed in their dosimetric evaluation that PTV free-breathing is larger than PTV gating (387.23 cm^3 vs. 314.41 cm^3) for stage I–III NSCLC patients plan based on respiratory gating [39]. Although gating has proven to reduce margins and facilitate sparing of organs at risk, treatment times can be comparatively longer [30].

Schmidt et al. investigated prospectively how the intrafractional respiratory motion, the interfractional baseline shifts, and the anatomical changes impacted the dose distribution for a group of lung cancer patients and pointed out that anatomical changes were found to have a more important impact on the target dose distribution in comparison to internal target motion (Respiratory tumor motion mainly craniocaudally, 0-13.1 mm; whiletumour baseline shifts, 24 mm in left-right and anterior posterior direction, 18 mm in craniocaudal direction) [40]. Spoelstra et al. have investigated a motion management strategy which uses internal anatomical surrogates such as carina and diaphragm to predict the 3D position of lung tumors [41] and concluded on significant prediction errors with both using carina and diaphragm, depending on tumor position, baseline tumor motion, and respiratory phase that were observed. No appropriate surrogate has been shown to date in literature which is more convenient than using 4D-CT data [41].

Liao et al. documented MD Anderson experience on outcome of the clinical use of conventional CT simulated and 3D conformally treated patients in years compared with 4D-CT-simulated and intensity-modulated treated cases, revealing a significant decrease in treatment-related toxicity and improvement in survival with the latter [42]. As more accurate targeting and margin reduction sound to result in significant dose reduction to lung and heart leading to improved quality of life, 4D-CT seemed to be the key component of dose escalation in lung cancer radiotherapy [42].

In clinical practice, 4D-CT is superior to 3D-CT, with passive FB approach for PTV delineation and treatment planning. 4D-CT recommendations for lung cancer patient's delineation can be summarized as using a combination of MIP with visual validation, ensuring coverage in early-stage I NSCLC but checking the target volume MIP-based ITV on each of the ten phases in advanced stage II and III due to possibility of irregular breathing patterns causing deviations [30].

Breathing Control: Breath-Hold Technique

Patient-performed "deep inspiration breath hold" can be voluntary or assisted by using a spirometer which can be connected to either a screen or video glasses for patient cooperation, which should be reproducible in both simulation and treatment. Its significance in NSCLC has not been established yet aside from case reports [23,

43], while it is a very well-known practice in left breast cancer patients for avoiding doses to heart and coronary arteries [44–46]. Josipovic et al. has presented in their three patients that not all cases could benefit from breath-hold techniques [43]. Berson et al. expressed the advantages of breath hold over free-breathing as decreased requirement for fluoroscopy, decreased motion of internal organs, less time for CT acquisition, and improved patient compliance [47].

Active Breathing Control

Active breathing control has been largely investigated for lung cancer. In University of Florida experience, SBRT on 20 patients were performed with ABC device [48]. The volumes acquired with the ABC device were significantly smaller than the free-breathing volumes (23 % reduction of planning tumor volume), and ABC allowed a reduction of all dosimetric parameters [2.28 % reduction of percentage volume of lung treated to a dose of ≥20 Gy (V20); 10 % reduction of mean lung dose] [48]. Significant differences were found both in SRT and in 3D-CRT, in peripheral and apical lesions [48]. In published dosimetric studies, ABC has the potential to reduce lung toxicity which can result in dose intensification while maintaining the same risk of lung toxicity [49–51].

Gating

Respiratory gating is also a form of breathing control which radiation has been delivered within a predefined phase of respiratory cycle based on 4D-CT scanning [52]. Same external respiratory signal coordinators or internal markers could be used to guide for gating during simulation and treatment. Gating has the similar gains of decreasing target to be treated like the other systems described above [23]. Lin et al. compared 4D-CT-based respiratory-gated (50–75 % and 100 % ex phases) IMRT plan and 3D-CT-based IMRT plans in 17 patients with non-small cell lung cancer [39] and mentioned that the GTV volumes were smaller using 4D-CT gating with lower V10, V20, V30, and V40 lung and mean heart doses without compromising homogeneity and coverage of PTV compared to IMRT plans based on 3D-CT [39].

Summary of Motion Management

The most important disadvantage of breathing control systems was the extension of treatment time when IMRT over 3D-conformal techniques is preferred treatment approach [25, 53]. Breath hold needs a vital patient cooperation and is usually combined with the delivery of 3D-CRT or step-and-shoot IMRT due to the short duration of breath holding less than 30 s. In case, the patients having respiratory problems related with the primary disease could complicate the required compliance of these patients. Individualization and patient selection for a dedicated technique sound to be a rationale approach.

Abdominal Compression

Abdominal compression was the most common immobilization system in stereotactic body radiosurgery before 4DCT era. The aim of the system is to minimize respiratory motion with forced shallow breathing by applying abdominal pressure – pushing down the upper abdomen with a manual or sensorized pressure device during pretreatment imaging and treatment delivery [54–56]. Different immobilization devices are available in the market for clinical use.

Bouilhol et al. analyzed their 4D-CT data of 27 patients with and without abdominal compression to measure three-dimensional tumor motion amplitude [57]. The mean reduction of tumor motion amplitude was 3.5 mm for lower lobe tumors and 0.8 mm for upper/middle lobe locations, which led to a 3.6 cm3 mean reduction of ITV volumes for lower lobe and 0.2 cm3 for upper/middle lobe tumors [57]. Negoro et al. documented significant reduction of the tumor movement with abdominal press from a range of 8–20 mm to a range of 2–11 mm ($p=0.0002$) [58], while acceptable daily setup errors within 5 mm in 90 %, 100 %, and 93 % of all verifications in left–right, anteroposterior, and cranio-caudal directions.

Even the benefit of using AC has been widespread reported previously; recent literature provided conflicting results claiming that AC could cause increased variation in tumor motion [54, 58, 59]. Mampuya et al. has detected larger interfractional variations in tumor motion amplitude in AC group which triggered the risk of under dosing target or overdosing organ at risk [60] and reported lower local control rates with AC in their SBRT series using a bony-structure-based setup (22 patients, 82.5 % without vs. 25 patients, 65.4 % with AC). In current advanced technological environment of image guidance, clinic guidelines include usually a combination of imaging and immobilization system in terms of delivering high dose with high precision rates in contrast to previous series using only a bony-structure-based setup without volumetric imaging [25].

Types of abdominal compression:
(a) Manual
(b) Pressure
(c) Thermoplastic mask system
(d) Elekta BodyFIX™

Image Guidance Technology

External radiotherapy implanted various image guidance strategies in clinic such as kV images, CT on rails, CBCT, etc. [61]. On-board imaging simultaneously acquiring more than one slice became available and these volumetric imaging techniques such as Kv or MV CBCT at treatment setup have provided important anatomic information related to the position and relation of tumor and adjacent organs at risk. kV cone beam has the superiority to provide soft tissue information compared to MV cone beam CT [62]. First aim to use CBCT is to reduce geometric uncertainties with more reliable tumor localization and smaller setup errors [63]. Imaging of regions having high-density materials such as implants could produce artifacts, where MV CBCT could be the preferred CBCT method [62]. The survey evaluating the quality of curative intent radiotherapy for NSCLC in UK revealed 50 % use of CBCT in 2011 which increased to 67 % in 2015 showing required technology to become increasingly accessible nowadays [64].

Schmith et al. measured the daily CBCT scans and documented that the interfraction baseline shifts averaged 5.8–7.8 mm in three directions and some patients showed shifts up to 24 mm [40]. Other series showed varying tumor positions up to 5–10 mm in any directions [65, 66]. Daily image guidance helps to reduce margins to 0.3 cm and was shown to decrease more than 5 mm setup errors from 20–43 % to 6 % when compared to less than daily guidance [67, 68]. Royal Marsden and Odense Universities compared the effect of using different immobilization techniques in thoracic cancer patients with same pattern of image guidance [69], s CBCT at initial three fractions, at 10th, 20th and 30th, fractions. Royal Marsden used standard wing board while Odense University preferred custom vacuum cushions, VacFix™ and a full thermoplastic mask, and the setup uncertainties were found to be similar by using the same CBCT imaging protocol despite the different setup systems [69].

CT on rails is anon on board diagnostic CT located in treatment room and has already been used clinically for quite a few years by mobilizing the table top with patient setup on it from CT on rails to linear accelerator (Linac) [70]. The advantages of CT on rails are obtaining anatomic and volumetric imaging in treatment room, providing CT for dose calculation (planning or treatment evaluation), and good image quality. The in-room CT image can then be fused with the reference CT acquired for planning purposes before the start of the treatment based on soft tissue and bony contrast. Also, in-room CT images can be used to reconstruct dose distributions and may allow image-guided adaptive radiotherapy by adjusting treatment parameters according to variations in the patient's anatomy during external radiotherapy.

Real-Time Tracking

Real-time tracking is also a form of image guidance with the main goal of minimizing the effect of target motion not only between treatments but also during a treatment fraction [25]. Real-time tracking usually needs the shortest time delay between the detection of change of the target and the implementation of the correction [25]. Surrogate markers such as fiducial markers or a subset of target positional information related to anatomic structures are warranted. The Novalis Body System™ (BrainLAB AG, Heimstetten, Germany) and TrueBeam STx are linear accelerators that the IGRT system for target localization implemented, in order to perform setup correction, to monitor the movement of infrared-reflecting markers placed on the patient's skin, and to align internal target based on either bony landmarks or implanted fiducial markers. Treatment interventions can be performed in either adaptive gating of the treatment beam or real-time correction of target offset by using a robotic couch. The CyberKnife system™ (Accuracy Inc., Sunnyvale, CA,) has an X-ray stereoscopic guidance system mounted in the treatment room and it is designed primarily for radiosurgery applications. The CyberKnife system is principally a robotic application of a small X-band linear accelerator. Stereoscopic X-ray imaging system serves for patient setup before treatment and for tracking of target movement during radiation delivery [71]. The robotic arm can move several centimeters per second, so it can easily keep track with tumor motion [71].

Treatment Delivery

Intensity-Modulated Radiotherapy (IMRT)

Chemotherapy and radiotherapy are accepted as standard of care for many locally advanced non-small cell lung cancer (NSCLC) patients. Standard radiation prescription doses have remained 60–66 Gy for more than 30 years except at a couple of comprehensive cancer institutions [2, 10, 72]. Despite the benefits of radiotherapy, local control rates remained poor with standard doses, leading to dose escalation to decrease local failure of disease and to eliminate the primary source for distant metastases [73, 74]. Analysis of seven different Radiation Therapy Oncology Group (RTOG) trials of chemoradiotherapy for locally advanced NSCLC revealed improved survival and locoregional control with dose escalation [74]. The innovations in the radiation therapy of NSCLC such as IMRT and VMAT, compared with previous 3DCRT methods, can deliver higher doses more conformally and precisely to the tumor while minimizing doses to organs at risk. These factors could possibly lead to decreased morbidity and increased local control. However, the preliminary findings of RTOG-0617 comparing standard-dose (60 Gy) versus high-dose (74 Gy) conformal radiotherapy with concurrent chemotherapy for stage IIIA/IIIB non-small cell lung cancer showed no survival benefit of dose escalation with 3D-CRT or IMRT based on enrolling departments awaiting the technical analysis [75]. Although poor prognostic patients were mainly treated with IMRT in RTOG 0617, IMRT exhibited significantly lower pneumonitis which was directly related with lung V_{20} and lower heart V_{40} which was correlated with survival and less toxicity to ensure IMRT patients are more likely to receive full doses of consolidative chemotherapy [76].

In daily clinical practice, 3D-CRT and IMRT could be used in the treatment of early and locally advanced lung cancer. 3D-CRT techniques consist of unmodulated fields directly covering the target, whereas computer-chosen optimized modulated fields were used to generate IMRT [7]. IMRT plans have physical and biological conformality with the help of dose escalation for lung cancer, and studies have shown improvements over 3D-CRT planning with respect to tumor dose escalation and doses to organs at risk (OARs) [73]. Grills et al. performed a planning study for 18 patients with stage I–IIIB. Their aim is to prescribe 70 Gy in IMRT, 3D-CRT, limited 3D-CRT (two to three beams only), and a traditional radiotherapy field consisting elective nodal irradiation [77]. IMRT has a 15 % gain in lung V_{20} and 40 %

in esophageal V_{50}, especially in node-positive patients with the benefit of dose escalation apart from the results in node-negative patients [77].

Although no randomized trial compared conformal therapy and IMRT, a few retrospective studies reported the late outcomes of IMRT. Another retrospective dose-escalating clinical study coming from the Memorial Sloan Kettering underlined favorable local control and survival rates (2-year survival: 58 %) without increasing toxicity (radiation pneumonitis rate: 11 %) in a series of 55 lung cancer patients [78]. A recent clinical analysis from the Netherlands Cancer Institute revealed a 2-year survival of 52 % along with grade 3 or higher toxicity of 35 % [79]. Apart from the studies above, MD Anderson analyzed their stage III patients treated with IMRT and compared them with the historical group; the results revealed significant decrement in pneumonitis and esophagitis but no overall survival benefit [80, 81]. When recurrence patterns were analyzed per field, importantly, no marginal missed were noted [81]. IMRT is the most promising treatment method for dose escalation where local control in lung tumors was shown to be dose dependent [73]. In RTOG-0617, even radiation treatment modality was not randomized; almost half of the patients received IMRT depending on the physician's disposal. The patient quality of life results from randomized dose escalation study, RTOG 0617, showed that patient-reported quality of life is better after IMRT compared to 3D-CRT. This is the first prospective data that indicates that IMRT can lessen the toxicity and improve the quality of life of the patients [82]. The only ongoing randomized trial compares 66 Gy 3D-CRT vs. IMRT for unresected locoregionally advanced non-small cell lung cancer without evidence of hematogenous metastases in recruited 168 patients. The final data collection date for primary outcome measure will be on August 2016 (NCT00520702).

At present, IMRT should be regarded as a promising technique in locally advanced NSCLC. Major concerns regarding IMRT are internal tumor motions consisting of interfraction shifts of the tumor position and interfraction motion due to respiration and cardiac motion. All these changes introduce the difference between the tumor position and the MLC position which is also called the "interplay effect" in the IMRT delivery and may compromise the optimal target coverage. This triggers the question of safe delivery of radiotherapy with developing technology in the era of intensity-modulated radiotherapy (IMRT) and volumetric arc radiotherapy (VMAT). Solutions for motion management were described above in this chapter. To establish a well-working IMRT program for lung cancer patients, 4D-CT or motion management systems have to be used, quality assurance for the clinical workflow is essential, and image guidance is the primary checkpoint for the quality during the delivery. Quality assurance is the other key point for the success of latest techniques of radiation delivery which is a title of another chapter.

Volumetric Arc Therapy

VMAT is a relatively new treatment option which is an arc-based IMRT technique with a full 360° of beam directions available for optimization which helps to reduce monitor units (MUs) and beam-on treatment time. However, increased volumes of low-dose compared to step-and-shoot IMRT (ssIMRT) are a limitation (REF). Preliminary results for treatment plans generated with VMAT optimization have displayed equivalent or superior dose distributions to static gantry IMRT plans [83]. Zhang et al. compared the efficacy of IMRT and volumetric-modulated arc therapy (VMAT) in the treatment of 125 NSCLC patients. The mean total lung, V5 and V10 in the VMAT group were markedly higher than those in the IMRT group; nevertheless the high dose levels V_{20}, V_{30}, and V_{40} in the VMAT group were significantly lower. The lower heart dose volume of VMAT was the only benefit compared to IMRT in contrast to spine and esophagus at-risk volume [61]. Clinical studies suggested that both IMRT and VMAT had significant advantages in the treatment of NSCLC [61, 84]. Dosimetric planning studies suggested that both IMRT and VMAT presented similar results in V20 and V30, representing that they could equally minimize the dose volume to decrease risk of pneumonitis [61, 84]. Holt et al. analyzed coplanar VMAT for stereotactic body radiotherapy (SBRT) with IMRT and provide comparable or better plan quality and dose levels to the skin than IMRT in early-stage lung cancer treatment [85]. Jiang et al. retrospectively analyzed, based on the dose-volume histograms (DVH) of the IMRT, single arc/partial arc VMAT plans respectively [83]. Independent from the arc technique, VMAT plans had higher V5/10 and lower V20/30 and MLD in the total and contralateral lungs compared to IMRT plans [83]. In another dosimetric study, Dickey et al. found that VMAT has the better plan compared to multiple static fields and conformal arcs [86]. Similar results were documented previously by William Beaumont Hospital dosimetric study defining single arc VMAT planning to be highly conformal with significant reduction in lung dose-volume parameters in addition to satisfactory organ at risk doses [87]. Despite the encouraging results, VMAT still has the uncertainties in lung treatment without accounting for breathing (4D cone beam computed tomography, tumor tracking) or preventing excessive tumor motion (abdominal compression, active breathing control, and gating). A combination of traditional conformal radiotherapy and double-arc VMAT called the hybrid RapidArc technique 6 was evaluated by Chan et al. to overcome the lung low-dose bath [84]. Superior dosimetric results were demonstrated when compared with conformal radiotherapy and VMAT alone, while a hybrid IMRT (static plus IMRT beams treated concurrently) technique was noted to demonstrate advantages for reduction of low dose to the lung [88]. Helical tomotherapy, another arc-based IMRT approach, in small series, has also been reported to show equal dosimetric parameters with IMRT-based approach [89]; however low-dose bath and V_5 for normal lung has to be cautiously evaluated as treatment-related deaths due to pneumonitis and acute esophagitis were reported in helical tomotherapy experience [89]. In their series of 37 patients with 56 % overall survival at 2 years, they pointed out the volume of contralateral lung receiving 5 Gy or more to be very prognostic in pneumonitis as rates of pneumonitis were almost 35 % if V5 >60 % and none if less than 60 % [89]. Another data to be taken into consideration for correlation of lower lung doses with pneumonia was by Shi et al. documenting their IMRT experience which revealed rates of pneumonitis to be 29 % if V10 <50 % versus 6 % if below this level [90]. New clinical results have to be waited to evolve with longer follow-up period.

New concept for personalized therapy, which is also named "isotoxic" treatment, is linear dose escalation until the maximum dose constraints for normal tissue such as the esophagus, heart, and normal lung are reached. This approach provides personalized radiotherapy dose [24]. In a prospective study including 166 patients with medically inoperable stage I–III NSCLC treated with a median prescribed TTD 64.8 Gy, Radiotherapy doses were individualized based on normal tissue dose constraints (mean lung dose, 19 Gy; maximal spinal cord dose, 54 Gy) up to a maximal TTD of 79.2 Gy in 1.8 Gy fractions twice daily. Considering that all included stage III patients who received sequential chemoradiotherapy or radiotherapy alone, OS was 21.0 months and also associated with acute and late radiation toxicity [91]. The potential of their approach has been tested in three different randomized trials in the UK (ClinicalTrials.gov Identifier: NCT01836692-Clinical Trial Identifier: ISRCTN12155469- isotoxic, hypofractionated radiotherapy) (ClinicalTrials.gov Identifier: NCT0153799: dose escalation of CHART) (Clinical Trial Identifier: ISRCTN45918260).

Image-Guided Adaptive Radiation Therapy

During external radiotherapy, tumor size, shape, and normal tissue relationships can change due to atelectasis, pleural effusion, and pneumonitis or tumor shrinkage. Those changes suggest that lung cancer treatment could have been improved by renewed contouring and replanning on resimulation or IGRT images such as cone beam CT.

Online plan re-optimization is performing new IMRT plans using daily cone beam images. This process is a compound of segment aperture morphing and segment weight optimization to correct target deformation and monitor unit recalculation respectively [8]. Tvilum et al. compared 52 patients treated with adaptive radiotherapy approach (ART) with non-ART IMRT external treatment [92]; in ART group, patients were tracked by a cone beam, and if the patient will benefit from replanning, they will undergo 4D-CT and new CTV was created with 5 mm margin. At 12 months follow-up, the recurrence rates were 53 % and 35 % in the no ART and ART group respectively [92]. An ongoing prospective, randomized multi-institutional clinical trial, RTOG 1106/ACRIN 6697, is questioning the value and additional benefit of PET/CT adapted boost for patients with large lung tumors with dose escalation aim [93]. This area has just opened a new horizon to be investigated in more clinical studies.

Proton Therapy

Proton is a positively charged hydrogen ion produced by stripping a hydrogen atom off its electron. Electrons were accelerated to a typical energy of 70–250 mega electron volts (MeV) by a synchrotron or cyclotron.

Proton therapy has been investigated in lung cancer treatment in latest years as low entrance dose and depositing maximum energy at Bragg peak with little exit dose. The maximum energy of the protons determines the distal range of Bragg peak. In clinical practice, the combination of various energies of the protons can be superpositioned to cover a specific tumor volume.

Therapy was administered by either "passively scattering" or "beam-scanning technique." Passive scattering proton therapy irradiates the tumor volume as a whole, using collimators and compensators for dose conformality [94]. Beam-scanning technique irradiates the target volume by scanning spot-by-spot with a proton beam, permitting intensity-modulated proton therapy (IMPT) [95]. Until gaining a more robust IMPT and planning upgrade, most institutions treating NSCLC with protons continue to use the passive technique because it is the most widely accessible and less sensitive to breathing motion than beam-scanning technique [94].

In proton therapy, the beams are molded laterally using either apertures or by magnetically scanning a proton beam across the patient in the case of pencil beam scanning [96]. Different from external beam photon radiation, the dose deposition is not uniform in all directions [95]. Protons are sensitive to the electron density of the material through which they pass and cause an uncertainty. In lung cancer, where the difference in electron density between the soft tissue of the chest and mediastinum and the lung is significant, uncertainties in the electron density are a key consideration [96]. Several dosimetric studies have compared proton and photon dose distributions for lung cancer treatment especially for reducing lung oesophagus, brachial plexus, chest wall and heart doses [97–100]. This has been taken as a promising potential to dose intensification and escalation. Despite the most important dosimetric advantage of proton therapy, respiratory tumor motion and size variability during radiotherapy are the main concern for geographical miss. Techniques to overcome tumor motion and interpretation of it for the planning are similar to what is used in proton treatment such as using 4D-CT, respiratory gating systems, body immobilization systems, and internal fiducials. The "smearing technique" can correct planning uncertainties [101]. To perform this technique, compensators are modified to maintain the coverage of target at the expense of some conformity. Beam configurations and margin expansions have to be designed in each beam directions. Also protons have less conformal dose distribution in treating irregular tumor shape compared to photons [102]. The interchange between the intrafractional tumor motion and the scanned proton beam has negative effects on the dose distribution as "interplay effect," which can cause severe under or overdose spot [103–105]. Therefore this effect cannot be compensated by simply adding a surrounding margin in IMPT. This is essential especially for IMPT, in contrast to the single field uniform dose (SFUD) technique, and could lead to completely inhomogeneous dose distributions per field if not planned properly [104, 106, 107]. As PSPT is considered a relatively robust technique [108], robust optimization in IMPT by using the worst-case scenario method sounds to be necessary to take setup and range uncertainties as well as anatomical changes into account during plan optimization [6]. Although repeated imaging and adaptive planning as required are obviously recommended for IMPT, robust optimization in IMPT can reduce the dose variations during treatment compared with PTV-based planning [6].

For SBRT, Loma Linda University has the largest series where respiratory gating and kV imaging was used with 3–5 mm PTV margins [109]; survival rates at 5 years were 18 %, 32 %, and 51 % for 51 Gy, 60 Gy, and 70 Gy in ten fractions, respectively, as well as no pneumonitis reported [109]. In a retrospective clinical study by Nakayama et al., PBT for local advanced lung cancer treatment with median dose of 78.3 Gy provided local progression-free survival of 93.3 % at 1 year and 65.9 % at 2 years with no grade 3 or more toxicity in stage II–III patients [101]. Dose-escalating phase II studies of 74 Gy reported 79.5 % local control and no grade 4–5 toxicity [110]. These promising results were supported by Oshiro et al. [111]. Using concomitant platinum-based chemotherapy with curative intent, Sejpal et al. found that higher doses of proton radiation than 3D-CRT or IMRT could be delivered with a lower risk of esophagitis and pneumonitis [112].

In a randomized phase III trial (RTOG 1308), photon versus proton chemoradiotherapy will be compared for their impact to improve overall survival. A total of 560 inoperable stage II–IIIB NSCLC patients are being planned to be enrolled with 70 Gy using either modality, besides the option to decrease to as low as 60 Gy if the dose constraints to the organs at risk cannot be met [113].

Stereotactic Body Radiotherapy

The principles and practice of stereotactic body radiotherapy (SBRT) or stereotactic ablative body radiotherapy (SABR) have been generated from the knowledge and experience from cranial stereotactic radiosurgery. The definitions of SBRT provided by the American Association of Physicists in Medicine (AAPM) task group 101, the American Society for Radiation Oncology and the American College of Radiology (ASTRO and ACR), Canadian Association of Radiation Oncology-Stereotactic Body Radiotherapy (CARO-SBRT), and the National Radiotherapy Implementation Group of the UK all agree that SBRT is a method of external beam radiotherapy (EBRT) that accurately delivers a high dose of irradiation in one or few treatment fractions to an extracranial target [114–117]. They have published historical background, simulation, immobilization, clinical requirements, treatment delivery details, and quality assurance details in task 101 to guide new starting institutes and set the standards of SBRT approach [114].

SBRT can be performed with traditional linear accelerators equipped with suitable image-guidance technology, accelerators specifically adapted for SBRT, or dedicated delivery systems with either photon or particle therapy. The most important part is to ensure more sophisticated QA procedures compared to conventional radiotherapy including system-specific end-to-end tests for both static and moving targets, in addition to the verification of the alignment of imaging and treatment isocenters on a daily basis. Heterogeneity correction is the most important part of treatment planning system. The AAPM report no. 85 on "Tissue Inhomogeneity Corrections for Megavoltage (MV) Beams" reports that 5 % change in dose may result in a 10–20 % change in tumor control probability. Low-density lung tissue surrounding tumor in the chest has effects on the accuracy of the dose distributions which can result in underdosage of the tumor [118, 119]. Therefore, the RTOG has implemented the obligation that algorithms using heterogeneity corrections be used for treatment planning in lung cancer [120].

Retrospective and prospective studies published since mid-1990 have established the feasibility, safety, and efficacy of SBRT in early-stage inoperable, refused surgery or medically inoperable patients using multiple different sets of dose regimens and technologies. Lung SBRT results demonstrate excellent, around 90 %, local control with little acute toxicity compared to historical controls of fractionated radiotherapy local control [120–122]. Onishi et al. analyzed 87 patients with stage I NSCLC who were medically operable but refused surgery. The SBRT total dose was 45–72.5 Gy at the isocenter which had been administered in three to ten fractions. During follow-up (median, 55 months), cumulative local control rates for T1 and T2 tumors at 5 years after SBRT were 92 % and 73 %, respectively, with 1.1 % grade 2 and above pulmonary complications [123].

The Fox Chase Cancer Center phase I dose escalation trial of SBRT for lung tumors has escalated total doses by 8 Gy (i.e., 2 Gy per fraction) increments from 40 to 56 Gy [124, 125] with the highest dose level biologically equivalent to 114 Gy. With a mean follow-up of 17 months, the 1-year local control rate was 97 % and 18 month local control rate was 93 % and no late pulmonary complications have been observed. No patient had a decrease in FEV1 or DLCO by 1 month after treatment [124, 125]. Literature showed an SBRT dose–response relationship for lung cancer. To achieve maximum control rates, SBRT doses are recommended to be a biologically equivalent dose of at least equivalent to 100 Gy10 which was depicted by Onishi et al. in their series of retrospectively analyzed 275 patients of early stage-lung cancer [56]. Mediastinal or hilar nodal failures appear to be ranging from 0 % to 10 % besides distant failure at the rate of 15–30 % which remains the predominant pattern of failure [126]. The Radiation Therapy Oncology Group (RTOG) phase I/II trial (RTOG 0236) in medically inoperable peripherally located early-stage NSCLC using a regimen of 60 Gy (54 Gy with heterogeneity correction) in three fractions with a rigid immobilization frame and abdominal pressure was promising for a 3-year primary tumor control rate of 97.6 % and a locoregional control rate of 87.2 %[127, 128]. Grade 3 or higher rates were reported to be less than 4 %, and the incidence of symptomatic radiation pneumonitis is very low, ranging from 0 % to 5 % in reported series [120]. Chest wall symptoms such as chest wall pain or rib fracture were reported in 5–15 % of patients with peripheral lesions influenced by primarily treatment dose, fractionation, and beam arrangement [129, 130]. Although there initially was a great anxiety to treat central tumors with SABR due to previous fatal complications with RTOG 0236 regimen of 60 Gy (54 Gy with heterogeneity correction) in three fractions [131], normal tissue dose-volume constraints for central and peripheral lesions are generally in common consensus to those treated with SABR [132, 133].

Although ongoing prospective trials are exploring dose and fractionation schedules in the inoperable population and are starting to explore the role of SBRT for the operable patient, SABR has already been reported to be feasible with no toxicity above grade 3 in a community cancer center setting [134, 135]. A recent important data regarding operable stage I NSCLC is the pooled analysis of two randomized, phase 3 trials of SABR (STARS and ROSEL) which were closed early due to slow accrual [135]. Estimated 3-year survival rates were 79 % in the surgery group and 95 % in the SABR group, while recurrence-free survival rates at 3 years were 80 % and 86 %, respectively [135]. None of the patients treated with SABR had high-grade toxicity. Most criticized part of this promising result is small sample size and limited follow-up time [135]. Two new randomized studies are expected to be opened: VALOR (veterans affairs lung cancer surgery or stereotactic radiotherapy trial), in the USA, and, in the UK, SABRtooth, a multicenter pilot study of SABR versus surgery in patients with peripheral stage I NSCLC considered at higher risk of complications from surgical resection.

As there is not a 100 % standardized SABR planning and delivery, each department should customize their approach with available guidelines. Along being an MD Anderson facility, our recommendation is to routinely use 4D-CT and ITV approach with heterogeneity correction-able software planning to deliver SABR with daily volumetric image guidance.

Conclusion

During the last decade, technology has provided remarkable improvements and accessibility to cutting-edge techniques in many departments. The major goal is set to improve quality of life and toxicity profiles of mediastinal treatments without compromising the local control and overall survival. Moving from 2D to 3D and 4D simulation has exposed the secrets of moving targets to individualize margins on specified targets and organs at risk, in addition to ensuring precision to minimize the interobserver variability in target delineation via incorporation of FDG-PET fusion in customization. Image-guided radiotherapy with either planar or volumetric imaging increased accurate and appropriate daily localization, promoting comfort to encourage dose escalation or respiratory phase-specific treatment strategies along with motion management in thoracic malignancies.

As randomized trials are lacking for many new technologies, knowledge-based tailoring and implementation of any site- and stage-specific requirement per patient have been a common practice in the recent years, such as SBRT, IMRT, VMAT, or protons.

References

1. Auperin A, Le Pechoux C, Rolland E, Curran WJ, Furuse K, Fournel P, Belderbos J, Clamon G, Ulutin HC, Paulus R, et al. Meta-analysis of concomitant versus sequential radiochemotherapy in locally advanced non-small-cell lung cancer. J Clin Oncol Off J Am Soc Clin Oncol. 2010;28(13):2181–90.
2. Christodoulou M, Bayman N, McCloskey P, Rowbottom C, Faivre-Finn C. New radiotherapy approaches in locally advanced non-small cell lung cancer. Eur J Cancer. 2014;50(3):525–34.
3. Selek U, Chang JY. Evolution of modern-era radiotherapy strategies for unresectable advanced non-small-cell lung cancer. Lung Cancer Manag. 2013;2(3):213–25.

4. Grant JD, Chang JY. Proton-based stereotactic ablative radiotherapy in early-stage non-small-cell lung cancer. BioMed Res Int. 2014;2014:389048.
5. Nguyen QN, Ly NB, Komaki R, Levy LB, Gomez DR, Chang JY, Allen PK, Mehran RJ, Lu C, Gillin M, et al. Long-term outcomes after proton therapy, with concurrent chemotherapy, for stage II-III inoperable non-small cell lung cancer. Radiother Oncol J Eur Soc Ther Radiol Oncol. 2015;115(3):367–72.
6. Li H, Zhang X, Park P, Liu W, Chang J, Liao Z, Frank S, Li Y, Poenisch F, Mohan R, et al. Robust optimization in intensity-modulated proton therapy to account for anatomy changes in lung cancer patients. Radiother Oncol J Eur Soc Ther Radiol Oncol. 2015;114(3): 367–72.
7. Selek U, Bolukbasi Y, Welsh JW, Topkan E. Intensity-modulated radiotherapy versus 3-dimensional conformal radiotherapy strategies for locally advanced non-small-cell lung cancer. Balkan Med J. 2014;31(4):286–94.
8. Glide-Hurst CK, Chetty IJ. Improving radiotherapy planning, delivery accuracy, and normal tissue sparing using cutting edge technologies. J Thorac Dis. 2014;6(4):303–18.
9. Zhu A, Marcus DM, Shu HK, Shim H. Application of metabolic PET imaging in radiation oncology. Radiat Res. 2012;177(4):436–48.
10. Chi A, Nguyen NP, Welsh JS, Tse W, Monga M, Oduntan O, Almubarak M, Rogers J, Remick SC, Gius D. Strategies of dose escalation in the treatment of locally advanced non-small cell lung cancer: image guidance and beyond. Front Oncol. 2014;4:156.
11. Gambhir SS, Czernin J, Schwimmer J, Silverman DH, Coleman RE, Phelps ME. A tabulated summary of the FDG PET literature. J Nucl Med Off Publ Soc Nucl Med. 2001;42(5 Suppl):1S–93.
12. Duan YL, Li JB, Zhang YJ, Wang W, Li FX, Sun XR, Guo YL, Shang DP. Comparison of primary target volumes delineated on four-dimensional CT and 18 F-FDG PET/CT of non-small-cell lung cancer. Radiat Oncol. 2014;9:182.
13. Belohlavek O, Carrio I, Danna M, Deniaud-Alexandre E, Inoue T. The role of PET/CT in radiation treatment planning for cancer patient treatment. International Atomic Energy Agency, Vienna; 2008.
14. Okubo M, Nishimura Y, Nakamatsu K, Okumura M, Shibata T, Kanamori S, Hanaoka K, Hosono M. Radiation treatment planning using positron emission and computed tomography for lung and pharyngeal cancers: a multiple-threshold method for [(18)F]fluoro-2-deoxyglucose activity. Int J Radiat Oncol Biol Phys. 2010;77(2):350–6.
15. Caldwell CB, Mah K, Skinner M, Danjoux CE. Can PET provide the 3D extent of tumor motion for individualized internal target volumes? A phantom study of the limitations of CT and the promise of PET. Int J Radiat Oncol Biol Phys. 2003;55(5):1381–93.
16. Bradley J, Thorstad WL, Mutic S, Miller TR, Dehdashti F, Siegel BA, Bosch W, Bertrand RJ. Impact of FDG-PET on radiation therapy volume delineation in non-small-cell lung cancer. Int J Radiat Oncol Biol Phys. 2004;59(1):78–86.
17. Vanuytsel LJ, Vansteenkiste JF, Stroobants SG, De Leyn PR, De Wever W, Verbeken EK, Gatti GG, Huyskens DP, Kutcher GJ. The impact of (18)F-fluoro-2-deoxy-D-glucose positron emission tomography (FDG-PET) lymph node staging on the radiation treatment volumes in patients with non-small cell lung cancer. Radiother Oncol J Eur Soc Ther Radiol Oncol. 2000;55(3):317–24.
18. Hanna GG, McAleese J, Carson KJ, Stewart DP, Cosgrove VP, Eakin RL, Zatari A, Lynch T, Jarritt PH, Young VA, et al. (18)F-FDG PET-CT simulation for non-small-cell lung cancer: effect in patients already staged by PET-CT. Int J Radiat Oncol Biol Phys. 2010;77(1):24–30.
19. Fox JL, Rengan R, O'Meara W, Yorke E, Erdi Y, Nehmeh S, Leibel SA, Rosenzweig KE. Does registration of PET and planning CT images decrease interobserver and intraobserver variation in delineating tumor volumes for non-small-cell lung cancer? Int J Radiat Oncol Biol Phys. 2005;62(1):70–5.
20. Ashamalla H, Rafla S, Parikh K, Mokhtar B, Goswami G, Kambam S, Abdel-Dayem H, Guirguis A, Ross P, Evola A. The contribution of integrated PET/CT to the evolving definition

of treatment volumes in radiation treatment planning in lung cancer. Int J Radiat Oncol Biol Phys. 2005;63(4):1016–23.
21. Shim SS, Lee KS, Kim BT, Chung MJ, Lee EJ, Han J, Choi JY, Kwon OJ, Shim YM, Kim S. Non-small cell lung cancer: prospective comparison of integrated FDG PET/CT and CT alone for preoperative staging. Radiology. 2005;236(3):1011–9.
22. De Ruysscher D, Wanders S, Minken A, Lumens A, Schiffelers J, Stultiens C, Halders S, Boersma L, Baardwijk A, Verschueren T, et al. Effects of radiotherapy planning with a dedicated combined PET-CT-simulator of patients with non-small cell lung cancer on dose limiting normal tissues and radiation dose-escalation: a planning study. Radiother Oncol J Eur Soc Ther Radiol Oncol. 2005;77(1):5–10.
23. Cole AJ, Hanna GG, Jain S, O'Sullivan JM. Motion management for radical radiotherapy in non-small cell lung cancer. Clin Oncol. 2014;26(2):67–80.
24. International Commission on Radiation Units & Measurements. Prescribing, recording and reporting photon beam therapy (Report 62). Bethesda; 2000.
25. Keall PJ, Mageras GS, Balter JM, Emery RS, Forster KM, Jiang SB, Kapatoes JM, Low DA, Murphy MJ, Murray BR, et al. The management of respiratory motion in radiation oncology report of AAPM Task Group 76. Med Phys. 2006;33(10):3874–900.
26. Korreman S, Persson G, Nygaard D, Brink C, Juhler-Nottrup T. Respiration-correlated image guidance is the most important radiotherapy motion management strategy for most lung cancer patients. Int J Radiat Oncol Biol Phys. 2012;83(4):1338–43.
27. Guckenberger M, Krieger T, Richter A, Baier K, Wilbert J, Sweeney RA, Flentje M. Potential of image-guidance, gating and real-time tracking to improve accuracy in pulmonary stereotactic body radiotherapy. Radiother Oncol J Eur Soc Ther Radiol Oncol. 2009;91(3):288–95.
28. Mageras GS, Pevsner A, Yorke ED, Rosenzweig KE, Ford EC, Hertanto A, Larson SM, Lovelock DM, Erdi YE, Nehmeh SA, et al. Measurement of lung tumor motion using respiration-correlated CT. Int J Radiat Oncol Biol Phys. 2004;60(3):933–41.
29. White BM, Zhao T, Lamb JM, Bradley JD, Low DA. Physiologically guided approach to characterizing respiratory motion. Med Phys. 2013;40(12):121723.
30. Hutchinson A, Bride P. 4DCT radiotherapy for NSCLC: a review of planning methods. J Radiother Pract. 2014;14(1):10.
31. Nygaard DE, Persson GF, Brink C, Specht L, Korreman SS. Evaluation of methods for selecting the midventilation bin in 4DCT scans of lung cancer patients. Acta Oncol. 2013;52(8):1715–22.
32. Liu HH, Balter P, Tutt T, Choi B, Zhang J, Wang C, Chi M, Luo D, Pan T, Hunjan S, et al. Assessing respiration-induced tumor motion and internal target volume using four-dimensional computed tomography for radiotherapy of lung cancer. Int J Radiat Oncol Biol Phys. 2007;68(2):531–40.
33. Pantarotto JR, Piet AH, Vincent A, van Sornsen de Koste JR, Senan S. Motion analysis of 100 mediastinal lymph nodes: potential pitfalls in treatment planning and adaptive strategies. Int J Radiat Oncol Biol Phys. 2009;74(4):1092–9.
34. Cole AJ, O'Hare JM, McMahon SJ, McGarry CK, Butterworth KT, McAleese J, Jain S, Hounsell AR, Prise KM, Hanna GG, et al. Investigating the potential impact of four-dimensional computed tomography (4DCT) on toxicity, outcomes and dose escalation for radical lung cancer radiotherapy. Clin Oncol. 2014;26(3):142–50.
35. Ruan D, Fessler JA, Balter JM, Berbeco RI, Nishioka S, Shirato H. Inference of hysteretic respiratory tumor motion from external surrogates: a state augmentation approach. Phys Med Biol. 2008;53(11):2923–36.
36. Seppenwoolde Y, Shirato H, Kitamura K, Shimizu S, van Herk M, Lebesque JV, Miyasaka K. Precise and real-time measurement of 3D tumor motion in lung due to breathing and heartbeat, measured during radiotherapy. Int J Radiat Oncol Biol Phys. 2002;53(4):822–34.
37. Yu ZH, Lin SH, Balter P, Zhang L, Dong L. A comparison of tumor motion characteristics between early stage and locally advanced stage lung cancers. Radiother Oncol J Eur Soc Ther Radiol Oncol. 2012;104(1):33–8.

38. Underberg RW, Lagerwaard FJ, Slotman BJ, Cuijpers JP, Senan S. Benefit of respiration-gated stereotactic radiotherapy for stage I lung cancer: an analysis of 4DCT datasets. Int J Radiat Oncol Biol Phys. 2005;62(2):554–60.
39. Lin H, Lu H, Shu L, Huang H, Chen H, Chen J, Cheng J, Pang Q, Peng L, Gu J, et al. Dosimetric study of a respiratory gating technique based on four-dimensional computed tomography in non-small-cell lung cancer. J Radiat Res. 2014;55(3):583–8.
40. Schmidt ML, Hoffmann L, Kandi M, Moller DS, Poulsen PR. Dosimetric impact of respiratory motion, interfraction baseline shifts, and anatomical changes in radiotherapy of non-small cell lung cancer. Acta Oncol. 2013;52(7):1490–6.
41. Spoelstra FO, van der Weide L, van Sornsen de Koste JR, Vincent A, Slotman BJ, Senan S. Feasibility of using anatomical surrogates for predicting the position of lung tumours. Radiother Oncol J Eur Soc Ther Radiol Oncol. 2012;102(2):287–9.
42. Liao ZX, Komaki RR, Thames Jr HD, Liu HH, Tucker SL, Mohan R, Martel MK, Wei X, Yang K, Kim ES, et al. Influence of technologic advances on outcomes in patients with unresectable, locally advanced non-small-cell lung cancer receiving concomitant chemoradiotherapy. Int J Radiat Oncol Biol Phys. 2010;76(3):775–81.
43. Josipovic M, Aznar MC, Persson GF. Deep inspiration breath hold radiotherapy of lung cancer: the good, the bad and the ugly case. Acta Oncol. 2014;53(10):1446–8.
44. Bolukbasi Y, Saglam Y, Selek U, Topkan E, Kataria A, Unal Z, Alpan V. Reproducible deep-inspiration breath-hold irradiation with forward intensity-modulated radiotherapy for left-sided breast cancer significantly reduces cardiac radiation exposure compared to inverse intensity-modulated radiotherapy. Tumori. 2014;100(2):169–78.
45. Hayden AJ, Rains M, Tiver K. Deep inspiration breath hold technique reduces heart dose from radiotherapy for left-sided breast cancer. J Med Imaging Radiat Oncol. 2012;56(4):464–72.
46. Yeung R, Conroy L, Long K, Walrath D, Li H, Smith W, Hudson A, Phan T. Cardiac dose reduction with deep inspiration breath hold for left-sided breast cancer radiotherapy patients with and without regional nodal irradiation. Radiat Oncol (London, England). 2015;10(1):200.
47. Berson AM, Emery R, Rodriguez L, Richards GM, Ng T, Sanghavi S, Barsa J. Clinical experience using respiratory gated radiation therapy: comparison of free-breathing and breath-hold techniques. Int J Radiat Oncol Biol Phys. 2004;60(2):419–26.
48. Scotti VML, Saieva C, Agresti B, Meattini I, Desideri I, Cecchini S, Bertocci S, Franzese C, De Luca Cardillo C, Zei G, Loi M, Greto D, Mangoni M, Bonomo P, Livi L, Biti GP. Impact of a breathing-control system on target margins and normal-tissue sparing in the treatment of lung cancer: experience at the radiotherapy unit of Florence University. Radiol Med. 2014;119:13–9.
49. Partridge M, Tree A, Brock J, McNair H, Fernandez E, Panakis N, Brada M. Improvement in tumour control probability with active breathing control and dose escalation: a modelling study. Radiother Oncol J Eur Soc Ther Radiol Oncol. 2009;91(3):325–9.
50. Gagel B, Demirel C, Kientopf A, Pinkawa M, Piroth M, Stanzel S, Breuer C, Asadpour B, Jansen T, Holy R, et al. Active breathing control (ABC): determination and reduction of breathing-induced organ motion in the chest. Int J Radiat Oncol Biol Phys. 2007;67(3):742–9.
51. Wilson EM, Williams FJ, Lyn BE, Wong JW, Aird EG. Validation of active breathing control in patients with non-small-cell lung cancer to be treated with CHARTWEL. Int J Radiat Oncol Biol Phys. 2003;57(3):864–74.
52. Smith RL, Yang D, Lee A, Mayse ML, Low DA, Parikh PJ. The correlation of tissue motion within the lung: implications on fiducial based treatments. Med Phys. 2011;38(11):5992–7.
53. Chi A, Nguyen NP, Komaki R. The potential role of respiratory motion management and image guidance in the reduction of severe toxicities following stereotactic ablative radiation therapy for patients with centrally located early stage non-small cell lung cancer or lung metastases. Front Oncol. 2014;4:151.
54. Heinzerling JH, Anderson JF, Papiez L, Boike T, Chien S, Zhang G, Abdulrahman R, Timmerman R. Four-dimensional computed tomography scan analysis of tumor and organ

motion at varying levels of abdominal compression during stereotactic treatment of lung and liver. Int J Radiat Oncol Biol Phys. 2008;70(5):1571–8.
55. Liu HH, Wang X, Dong L, Wu Q, Liao Z, Stevens CW, Guerrero TM, Komaki R, Cox JD, Mohan R. Feasibility of sparing lung and other thoracic structures with intensity-modulated radiotherapy for non-small-cell lung cancer. Int J Radiat Oncol Biol Phys. 2004;58(4):1268–79.
56. Onishi H, Shirato H, Nagata Y, Hiraoka M, Fujino M, Gomi K, Niibe Y, Karasawa K, Hayakawa K, Takai Y, et al. Hypofractionated stereotactic radiotherapy (HypoFXSRT) for stage I non-small cell lung cancer: updated results of 257 patients in a Japanese multi-institutional study. J Thorac Oncol Off Publ Int Assoc Stud Lung Cancer. 2007;2(7 Suppl 3):S94–100.
57. Bouilhol G, Ayadi M, Rit S, Thengumpallil S, Schaerer J, Vandemeulebroucke J, Claude L, Sarrut D. Is abdominal compression useful in lung stereotactic body radiation therapy? A 4DCT and dosimetric lobe-dependent study. Phys Med PM Int J Devoted Appl Phys Med Biol Off J Ital Assoc Biomed Phys. 2013;29(4):333–40.
58. Negoro Y, Nagata Y, Aoki T, Mizowaki T, Araki N, Takayama K, Kokubo M, Yano S, Koga S, Sasai K, et al. The effectiveness of an immobilization device in conformal radiotherapy for lung tumor: reduction of respiratory tumor movement and evaluation of the daily setup accuracy. Int J Radiat Oncol Biol Phys. 2001;50(4):889–98.
59. Bissonnette JP, Franks KN, Purdie TG, Moseley DJ, Sonke JJ, Jaffray DA, Dawson LA, Bezjak A. Quantifying interfraction and intrafraction tumor motion in lung stereotactic body radiotherapy using respiration-correlated cone beam computed tomography. Int J Radiat Oncol Biol Phys. 2009;75(3):688–95.
60. Mampuya WA, Matsuo Y, Ueki N, Nakamura M, Mukumoto N, Nakamura A, Iizuka Y, Kishi T, Mizowaki T, Hiraoka M. The impact of abdominal compression on outcome in patients treated with stereotactic body radiotherapy for primary lung cancer. J Radiat Res. 2014;55(5):934–9.
61. Zhang J, Yu XL, Zheng GF, Zhao F. Intensity-modulated radiotherapy and volumetric-modulated arc therapy have distinct clinical advantages in non-small cell lung cancer treatment. Med Oncol (Northwood, London, England). 2015;32(4):94.
62. Broderick M, Menezes G, Leech M, Coffey M, Appleyard R. A comparison of kilovoltage and megavoltage cone beam CT in radiotherapy. J Radiother Pract. 2007;6(03):173–8.
63. Korreman S, Rasch C, McNair H, Verellen D, Oelfke U, Maingon P, Mijnheer B, Khoo V. The European Society of Therapeutic Radiology and Oncology-European Institute of Radiotherapy (ESTRO-EIR) report on 3D CT-based in-room image guidance systems: a practical and technical review and guide. Radiother Oncol J Eur Soc Ther Radiol Oncol. 2010;94(2):129–44.
64. McAleese J, Baluch S, Drinkwater K. The quality of curative-intent radiotherapy for non-small cell lung cancer in the UK. Clin Oncol. 2015;27(9):498–504.
65. Chang J, Mageras GS, Yorke E, De Arruda F, Sillanpaa J, Rosenzweig KE, Hertanto A, Pham H, Seppi E, Pevsner A, et al. Observation of interfractional variations in lung tumor position using respiratory gated and ungated megavoltage cone-beam computed tomography. Int J Radiat Oncol Biol Phys. 2007;67(5):1548–58.
66. Juhler-Nottrup T, Korreman SS, Pedersen AN, Persson GF, Aarup LR, Nystrom H, Olsen M, Tarnavski N, Specht L. Interfractional changes in tumour volume and position during entire radiotherapy courses for lung cancer with respiratory gating and image guidance. Acta Oncol. 2008;47(7):1406–13.
67. Bissonnette JP, Purdie TG, Higgins JA, Li W, Bezjak A. Cone-beam computed tomographic image guidance for lung cancer radiation therapy. Int J Radiat Oncol Biol Phys. 2009;73(3):927–34.
68. Higgins J, Bezjak A, Hope A, Panzarella T, Li W, Cho JB, Craig T, Brade A, Sun A, Bissonnette JP. Effect of image-guidance frequency on geometric accuracy and setup margins in radiotherapy for locally advanced lung cancer. Int J Radiat Oncol Biol Phys. 2011;80(5):1330–7.

69. Nielsen TB, Hansen VN, Westberg J, Hansen O, Brink C. A dual centre study of setup accuracy for thoracic patients based on cone-beam CT data. Radiother Oncol J Eur Soc Ther Radiol Oncol. 2012;102(2):281–6.
70. Owen R, Kron T, Foroudi F, Milner A, Cox J, Duchesne G, Cleeve L, Zhu L, Cramb J, Sparks L, et al. Comparison of CT on rails with electronic portal imaging for positioning of prostate cancer patients with implanted fiducial markers. Int J Radiat Oncol Biol Phys. 2009;74(3):906–12.
71. Yin F, Wong J. The role of in-room kv x-ray imaging for patient setup and target localization: Report of Task group 104. College Park, M: AAPM; 2009.
72. Bayman N, Blackhall F, McCloskey P, Taylor P, Faivre-Finn C. How can we optimise concurrent chemoradiotherapy for inoperable stage III non-small cell lung cancer? Lung Cancer. 2014;83(2):117–25.
73. Chang JY. Intensity-modulated radiotherapy, not 3 dimensional conformal, is the preferred technique for treating locally advanced lung cancer. Semin Radiat Oncol. 2015;25(2):110–6.
74. Machtay M, Paulus R, Moughan J, Komaki R, Bradley JE, Choy H, Albain K, Movsas B, Sause WT, Curran WJ. Defining local-regional control and its importance in locally advanced non-small cell lung carcinoma. J Thorac Oncol Off Publ Int Assoc Stud Lung Cancer. 2012;7(4):716–22.
75. Bradley JD, Paulus R, Komaki R, Masters G, Blumenschein G, Schild S, Bogart J, Hu C, Forster K, Magliocco A, et al. Standard-dose versus high-dose conformal radiotherapy with concurrent and consolidation carboplatin plus paclitaxel with or without cetuximab for patients with stage IIIA or IIIB non-small-cell lung cancer (RTOG 0617): a randomised, two-by-two factorial phase 3 study. Lancet Oncol. 2015;16(2):187–99.
76. Chun SG, Hu C, Choy H, Komaki RU, Timmerman RD, Schild SE, Bogart JA, Dobelbower MC, Bosch WR, Galvin JM et al. Comparison of 3-D conformal and intensity modulated radiation therapy outcomes for locally advanced non-small cell lung cancer in NRG oncology/RTOG 0617. Int J Radiat Oncol Biol Phys. 2015;93(3):S1–2.
77. Grills IS, Yan D, Martinez AA, Vicini FA, Wong JW, Kestin LL. Potential for reduced toxicity and dose escalation in the treatment of inoperable non–small-cell lung cancer: a comparison of intensity-modulated radiation therapy (IMRT), 3D conformal radiation, and elective nodal irradiation. Int J Radiat Oncol Biol Phys. 2003;57(3):875–90.
78. Sura S, Gupta V, Yorke E, Jackson A, Amols H, Rosenzweig KE. Intensity-modulated radiation therapy (IMRT) for inoperable non-small cell lung cancer: the Memorial Sloan-Kettering Cancer Center (MSKCC) experience. Radiother Oncol J Eur Soc Ther Radiol Oncol. 2008;87(1):17–23.
79. Uyterlinde W, Belderbos J, Baas C, van Werkhoven E, Knegjens J, Baas P, Smit A, Rikers C, van den Heuvel M. Prediction of acute toxicity grade >/= 3 in patients with locally advanced non-small-cell lung cancer receiving intensity modulated radiotherapy and concurrent low-dose Cisplatin. Clin Lung Cancer. 2013;14(5):541–8.
80. Yom SS, Liao Z, Liu HH, Tucker SL, Hu CS, Wei X, Wang X, Wang S, Mohan R, Cox JD, et al. Initial evaluation of treatment-related pneumonitis in advanced-stage non-small-cell lung cancer patients treated with concurrent chemotherapy and intensity-modulated radiotherapy. Int J Radiat Oncol Biol Phys. 2007;68(1):94–102.
81. Shirvani SM, Juloori A, Allen PK, Komaki R, Liao Z, Gomez D, O'Reilly M, Welsh J, Papadimitrakopoulou V, Cox JD, et al. Comparison of 2 common radiation therapy techniques for definitive treatment of small cell lung cancer. Int J Radiat Oncol Biol Phys. 2013;87(1):139–47.
82. Movsas B, Hu C, Sloan J, Bradley JD, Kavadi VS, Narayan S, Robinson C, Johnson DW, Paulus R, Choy H. Quality of Life (QOL) Analysis of the Randomized Radiation (RT) Dose-Escalation NSCLC Trial (RTOG 0617): the rest of the story. Int J Radiat Oncol Biol Phys. 2013;87(2):S1–2.
83. Jiang X, Li T, Liu Y, Zhou L, Xu Y, Zhou X, Gong Y. Planning analysis for locally advanced lung cancer: dosimetric and efficiency comparisons between intensity-modulated radiotherapy (IMRT), single-arc/partial-arc volumetric modulated arc therapy (SA/PA-VMAT). Radiat Oncol. 2011;6:140.

84. Chan OS, Lee MC, Hung AW, Chang AT, Yeung RM, Lee AW. The superiority of hybrid-volumetric arc therapy (VMAT) technique over double arcs VMAT and 3D-conformal technique in the treatment of locally advanced non-small cell lung cancer – a planning study. Radiother Oncol J Eur Soc Ther Radiol Oncol. 2011;101(2):298–302.
85. Holt A, van Vliet-Vroegindeweij C, Mans A, Belderbos JS, Damen EM. Volumetric-modulated arc therapy for stereotactic body radiotherapy of lung tumors: a comparison with intensity-modulated radiotherapy techniques. Int J Radiat Oncol Biol Phys. 2011;81(5):1560–7.
86. Dickey M, Roa W, Drodge S, Ghosh S, Murray B, Scrimger R, Gabos Z. A planning comparison of 3-dimensional conformal multiple static field, conformal arc, and volumetric modulated arc therapy for the delivery of stereotactic body radiotherapy for early stage lung cancer. Med Dosim Off J Am Assoc Med Dosimet. 2015;40(4):347–51. Epub 2015/05/28.
87. McGrath SD, Matuszak MM, Yan D, Kestin LL, Martinez AA, Grills IS. Volumetric modulated arc therapy for delivery of hypofractionated stereotactic lung radiotherapy: a dosimetric and treatment efficiency analysis. Radiother Oncol J Eur Soc Ther Radiol Oncol. 2010;95(2):153–7.
88. Scorsetti M, Navarria P, Mancosu P, Alongi F, Castiglioni S, Cavina R, Cozzi L, Fogliata A, Pentimalli S, Tozzi A, et al. Large volume unresectable locally advanced non-small cell lung cancer: acute toxicity and initial outcome results with rapid arc. Radiat Oncol. 2010;5:94.
89. Song CH, Pyo H, Moon SH, Kim TH, Kim DW, Cho KH. Treatment-related pneumonitis and acute esophagitis in non-small-cell lung cancer patients treated with chemotherapy and helical tomotherapy. Int J Radiat Oncol Biol Phys. 2010;78(3):651–8.
90. Shi A, Zhu G, Wu H, Yu R, Li F, Xu B. Analysis of clinical and dosimetric factors associated with severe acute radiation pneumonitis in patients with locally advanced non-small cell lung cancer treated with concurrent chemotherapy and intensity-modulated radiotherapy. Radiat Oncol. 2010;5:35.
91. van Baardwijk A, Wanders S, Boersma L, Borger J, Ollers M, Dingemans AM, Bootsma G, Geraedts W, Pitz C, Lunde R, et al. Mature results of an individualized radiation dose prescription study based on normal tissue constraints in stages I to III non-small-cell lung cancer. J Clin Oncol Off J Am Soc Clin Oncol. 2010;28(8):1380–6.
92. Tvilum M, Khalil AA, Møller DS, Hoffmann L, Knap MM. Clinical outcome of image-guided adaptive radiotherapy in the treatment of lung cancer patients. Acta Oncol. 2015;54(9):1430–7. Epub 2015/07/24.
93. RTOG 1106/ACRIN 6697, Randomized phase II trial of individualized adaptive radiotherapy using during treatment FDG-PET/CT and modern technology in locally advanced Non-Small Cell Lung Cancer (NSCLC). [https://www.rtog.org/ClinicalTrials/ProtocolTable/StudyDetails.aspx?study=1106].
94. Wink KC, Roelofs E, Solberg T, Lin L, Simone 2nd CB, Jakobi A, Richter C, Lambin P, Troost EG. Particle therapy for non-small cell lung tumors: where do we stand? A systematic review of the literature. Front Oncol. 2014;4:292.
95. Berman AT, James SS, Rengan R. Proton beam therapy for non-small cell lung cancer: current clinical evidence and future directions. Cancers. 2015;7(3):1178–90.
96. Dowdell S, Grassberger C, Sharp GC, Paganetti H. Interplay effects in proton scanning for lung: a 4D Monte Carlo study assessing the impact of tumor and beam delivery parameters. Phys Med Biol. 2013;58(12):4137–56.
97. Gomez DR, Chang JY. Accelerated dose escalation with proton beam therapy for non-small cell lung cancer. J Thorac Dis. 2014;6(4):348–55.
98. Hoppe BS, Flampouri S, Henderson RH, Pham D, Bajwa AA, D'Agostino H, Huh SN, Li Z, Mendenhall NP, Nichols RC. Proton therapy with concurrent chemotherapy for non-small-cell lung cancer: technique and early results. Clin Lung Cancer. 2012;13(5):352–8.
99. Hoppe BS, Huh S, Flampouri S, Nichols RC, Oliver KR, Morris CG, Mendenhall NP, Li Z. Double-scattered proton-based stereotactic body radiotherapy for stage I lung cancer: a dosimetric comparison with photon-based stereotactic body radiotherapy. Radiother Oncol J Eur Soc Ther Radiol Oncol. 2010;97(3):425–30.

100. Kadoya N, Obata Y, Kato T, Kagiya M, Nakamura T, Tomoda T, Takada A, Takayama K, Fuwa N. Dose-volume comparison of proton radiotherapy and stereotactic body radiotherapy for non-small-cell lung cancer. Int J Radiat Oncol Biol Phys. 2011;79(4):1225–31.
101. Nakayama H, Satoh H, Sugahara S, Kurishima K, Tsuboi K, Sakurai H, Ishikawa S, Tokuuye K. Proton beam therapy of Stage II and III non-small-cell lung cancer. Int J Radiat Oncol Biol Phys. 2011;81(4):979–84.
102. Mohan R, Zhang X, Matney J, Bluett J, Dong L, Balter P, Engelsman M, Choi N, Komaki R, Liao Z. IMRT vs. Passively Scattered Proton Therapy (PSPT) for Locally Advanced Non-small Cell Lung CA (LA NSCLC) randomized trial – is there equipoise? Int J Radiat Oncol Biol Phys, 2010;78(3):S201–S202.
103. Grassberger C, Dowdell S, Sharp G, Paganetti H. Motion mitigation for lung cancer patients treated with active scanning proton therapy. Med Phys. 2015;42(5):2462–9.
104. Li Y, Kardar L, Li X, Li H, Cao W, Chang JY, Liao L, Zhu RX, Sahoo N, Gillin M, et al. On the interplay effects with proton scanning beams in stage III lung cancer. Med Phys. 2014;41(2):021721.
105. Grassberger C, Dowdell S, Lomax A, Sharp G, Shackleford J, Choi N, Willers H, Paganetti H. Motion interplay as a function of patient parameters and spot size in spot scanning proton therapy for lung cancer. Int J Radiat Oncol Biol Phys. 2013;86(2):380–6.
106. Dowdell S, Grassberger C, Paganetti H. Four-dimensional Monte Carlo simulations demonstrating how the extent of intensity-modulation impacts motion effects in proton therapy lung treatments. Med Phys. 2013;40(12):121713.
107. Stuschke M, Kaiser A, Pottgen C, Lubcke W, Farr J. Potentials of robust intensity modulated scanning proton plans for locally advanced lung cancer in comparison to intensity modulated photon plans. Radiother Oncol J Eur Soc Ther Radiol Oncol. 2012;104(1):45–51.
108. Zhu Z, Liu W, Gillin M, Gomez DR, Komaki R, Cox JD, Mohan R, Chang JY. Assessing the robustness of passive scattering proton therapy with regard to local recurrence in stage III non-small cell lung cancer: a secondary analysis of a phase II trial. Radiat Oncol. 2014;9:108.
109. Bush DA, Cheek G, Zaheer S, Wallen J, Mirshahidi H, Katerelos A, Grove R, Slater JD. High-dose hypofractionated proton beam radiation therapy is safe and effective for central and peripheral early-stage non-small cell lung cancer: results of a 12-year experience at Loma Linda University Medical Center. Int J Radiat Oncol Biol Phys. 2013;86(5):964–8.
110. Chang JY, Komaki R, Lu C, Wen HY, Allen PK, Tsao A, Gillin M, Mohan R, Cox JD. Phase 2 study of high-dose proton therapy with concurrent chemotherapy for unresectable stage III nonsmall cell lung cancer. Cancer. 2011;117(20):4707–13.
111. Oshiro Y, Mizumoto M, Okumura T, Hashimoto T, Fukumitsu N, Ohkawa A, Kanemoto A, Hashii H, Ohno T, Sakae T, et al. Results of proton beam therapy without concurrent chemotherapy for patients with unresectable stage III non-small cell lung cancer. J Thor Oncol Off Publ Int Assoc Stud Lung Cancer. 2012;7(2):370–5.
112. Sejpal S, Komaki R, Tsao A, Chang JY, Liao Z, Wei X, Allen PK, Lu C, Gillin M, Cox JD. Early findings on toxicity of proton beam therapy with concurrent chemotherapy for nonsmall cell lung cancer. Cancer. 2011;117(13):3004–13.
113. RTOG 1308, Phase III randomized trial comparing overall survival after photon versus proton chemoradiotherapy for inoperable stage II–IIIB NSCLC NCI/Local Protocol #: RTOG-1308/RTOG 1308.2015. In.
114. Benedict SH, Yenice KM, Followill D, Galvin JM, Hinson W, Kavanagh B, Keall P, Lovelock M, Meeks S, Papiez L, et al. Stereotactic body radiation therapy: the report of AAPM Task Group 101. Med Phys. 2010;37(8):4078–101.
115. Potters L, Kavanagh B, Galvin JM, Hevezi JM, Janjan NA, Larson DA, Mehta MP, Ryu S, Steinberg M, Timmerman R, et al. American Society for Therapeutic Radiology and Oncology (ASTRO) and American College of Radiology (ACR) practice guideline for the performance of stereotactic body radiation therapy. Int J Radiat Oncol Biol Phys. 2010;76(2):326–32.
116. Kirkbride P, Cooper T. Stereotactic body radiotherapy. Guidelines for commissioners, providers and clinicians: a national report. Clin Oncol. 2011;23(3):163–4.

117. Sahgal A, Roberge D, Schellenberg D, Purdie TG, Swaminath A, Pantarotto J, Filion E, Gabos Z, Butler J, Letourneau D, et al. The Canadian Association of Radiation Oncology scope of practice guidelines for lung, liver and spine stereotactic body radiotherapy. Clin Oncol. 2012;24(9):629–39.
118. Xiao Y, Papiez L, Paulus R, Timmerman R, Straube WL, Bosch WR, Michalski J, Galvin JM. Dosimetric evaluation of heterogeneity corrections for RTOG 0236: stereotactic body radiotherapy of inoperable stage I-II non-small-cell lung cancer. Int J Radiat Oncol Biol Phys. 2009;73(4):1235–42.
119. Chetty IJ, Curran B, Cygler JE, DeMarco JJ, Ezzell G, Faddegon BA, Kawrakow I, Keall PJ, Liu H, Ma CM, et al. Report of the AAPM Task Group No. 105: Issues associated with clinical implementation of Monte Carlo-based photon and electron external beam treatment planning. Med Phys. 2007;34(12):4818–53.
120. Rosenzweig KE, Chang JY, Chetty IJ, Decker RH, Ginsburg ME, Kestin LL, Kong FM, Lally BE, Langer CJ, Movsas B, et al. ACR appropriateness criteria nonsurgical treatment for non-small-cell lung cancer: poor performance status or palliative intent. J Am College Radiol JACR. 2013;10(9):654–64.
121. Baba F, Shibamoto Y, Tomita N, Ikeya-Hashizume C, Oda K, Ayakawa S, Ogino H, Sugie C. Stereotactic body radiotherapy for stage I lung cancer and small lung metastasis: evaluation of an immobilization system for suppression of respiratory tumor movement and preliminary results. Radiat Oncol. 2009;4:15.
122. Guckenberger M, Andratschke N, Alheit H, Holy R, Moustakis C, Nestle U, Sauer O. Deutschen Gesellschaft fur R: definition of stereotactic body radiotherapy: principles and practice for the treatment of stage I non-small cell lung cancer. Strahlenther Onkol Organ Dtsch Rontgengesellschaft. 2014;190(1):26–33.
123. Onishi H, Shirato H, Nagata Y, Hiraoka M, Fujino M, Gomi K, Karasawa K, Hayakawa K, Niibe Y, Takai Y et al. Stereotactic Body Radiotherapy (SBRT) for operable stage I non–small-cell lung cancer: can SBRT be comparable to surgery? Int J Radiat Oncol Biol Phys, 2007;81(5):1352–8.
124. Feigenberg SJ, Sharma N, Wang L, Cohen R, Buyyounouski M, Lally B, Movsas B. Phase I dose escalation trial of image guided stereotactic body radiotherapy for lung tumors. Int J Radiat Oncol Biol Phys, 2008;72(1):S114.
125. Sharma NK, Ruth K, Konski AA, Buyyounouski MK, Nicolaou N, Lally BE, Yu JQ, Langer CJ, Movsas B, Feigenberg SJ. Low morbidity and excellent local control using Image Guided Stereotactic Body Radiotherapy (IGSBRT) for lung tumors. Int J Radiat Oncol Biol Phys, 2008;72(1):S454.
126. ACR Appropriateness Criteria®; early-stage non-small-cell lung cancer [http://www.guideline.gov/content.aspx?id=47693].
127. Timmerman R, Paulus R, Galvin J, Michalski J, Straube W, Bradley J, Fakiris A, Bezjak A, Videtic G, Johnstone D, et al. Stereotactic body radiation therapy for inoperable early stage lung cancer. JAMA. 2010;303(11):1070–6.
128. Timmerman RD, Hu C, Michalski J, Straube W, Galvin J, Johnstone D, Bradley J, Barriger R, Bezjak A, Videtic GM, et al. Long-term Results of RTOG 0236: a phase II trial of Stereotactic Body Radiation Therapy (SBRT) in the treatment of patients with medically inoperable stage I non-small cell lung cancer. Int J Radiat Oncol Biol Phys. 2014;90(1):S30.
129. Mutter RW, Liu F, Abreu A, Yorke E, Jackson A, Rosenzweig KE. Dose–volume parameters predict for the development of chest wall pain after stereotactic body radiation for lung cancer. Int J Radiat Oncol Biol Phys, 2011;82(5):1783–90.
130. Dunlap NE, Cai J, Biedermann GB, Yang W, Benedict SH, Sheng K, Schefter TE, Kavanagh BD, Larner JM. Chest wall volume receiving >30 Gy predicts risk of severe pain and/or rib fracture after lung stereotactic body radiotherapy. Int J Radiat Oncol Biol Phys, 2008;76(3):796–801.
131. Timmerman R, McGarry R, Yiannoutsos C, Papiez L, Tudor K, DeLuca J, Ewing M, Abdulrahman R, DesRosiers C, Williams M, et al. Excessive toxicity when treating central

tumors in a phase II study of stereotactic body radiation therapy for medically inoperable early-stage lung cancer. J Clin Oncol Off J Am Soc Clin Oncol. 2006;24(30):4833–9.
132. Chang JY, Bezjak A, Mornex F. Stereotactic ablative radiotherapy for centrally located early stage non-small-cell lung cancer: what we have learned. J Thorac Oncol Off Publ Int Assoc Stud Lung Cancer. 2015;10(4):577–85.
133. Chang JY, Li QQ, Xu QY, Allen PK, Rebueno N, Gomez DR, Balter P, Komaki R, Mehran R, Swisher SG, et al. Stereotactic ablative radiation therapy for centrally located early stage or isolated parenchymal recurrences of non-small cell lung cancer: how to fly in a "no fly zone". Int J Radiat Oncol Biol Phys. 2014;88(5):1120–8.
134. Heal C, Ding W, Lamond J, Wong M, Lanciano R, Su S, Yang J, Feng J, Arrigo S, Markiewicz D, et al. Definitive treatment of early-stage non-small cell lung cancer with stereotactic ablative body radiotherapy in a community cancer center setting. Front Oncol. 2015;5.
135. Chang JY, Senan S, Paul MA, Mehran RJ, Louie AV, Balter P, Groen HJM, McRae SE, Widder J, Feng L et al. Stereotactic ablative radiotherapy versus lobectomy for operable stage I non-small-cell lung cancer: a pooled analysis of two randomised trials. Lancet Oncol, 2015;16(6):630–37.

Guidelines for the Delineation of Primary Tumor Target Volume in Lung Cancer

3

Gokhan Ozyigit, Melis Gultekin, Sezin Yuce Sari, Pervin Hurmuz, and Gozde Yazici

Introduction

The lungs are located bilaterally in the mediastinum. The apex of the lungs lies 2–3 cm above the clavicle and the base is situated on the diaphragm. The lungs have two surfaces; the costal surface lies along the chest wall, whereas the mediastinal surface covers other mediastinal structures such as the heart, trachea, and great vessels. The lungs are covered with a serous membrane called visceral pleura and the chest cavity is covered with parietal pleura. The pleural space between visceral and parietal pleurae is filled with fluid and has an important role in respiration.

The right lung has three lobes. The major fissure in the right lung divides the upper and lower lobes and lies between the level of the fifth thoracic vertebra and the diaphragm. The minor fissure divides the right lung into the upper and middle lobes. The left lung is divided into two lobes (i.e., upper and lower lobes) by an oblique fissure. The lingula which is located in the left upper lobe is homologous to the right middle lobe.

The trachea connects the larynx to the main bronchi. It is approximately 12 cm long in adults, and it starts from the level of the sixth cervical vertebra and ends at the level of the fourth to sixth thoracic vertebra. The posterior wall of the trachea is purely membranous, whereas other walls also contain muscular elements and a cartilaginous structure that is half ring shaped. The trachea is covered with ciliary epithelium which has a role in removing the foreign bodies in the air.

G. Ozyigit, MD • M. Gultekin, MD (✉) • S.Y. Sari, MD • P. Hurmuz, MD • G. Yazici, MD
Department of Radiation Oncology, Faculty of Medicine, Hacettepe University, Ankara, Turkey
e-mail: gozyigit@hacettepe.edu.tr; melisbahadir@yahoo.com; sezin_yuce@hotmail.com; phurmuz@yahoo.com; yazicig@hacettepe.edu.tr

G. Ozyigit et al. (eds.), *Principles and Practice of Radiotherapy Techniques in Thoracic Malignancies*, DOI 10.1007/978-3-319-28761-4_3

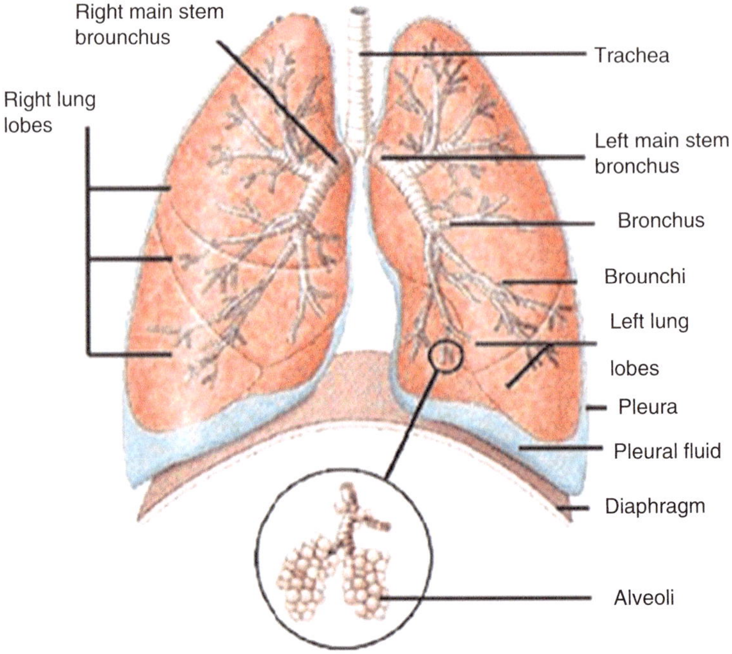

Fig. 3.1 Anatomy of the respiratory track and the lungs (With permission from Beyzadeoglu et al. [68])

The trachea bifurcates at the level of the carina and divides into right and left main bronchi. The right main bronchus is shorter and thicker than the left main bronchus and lies vertically, whereas the left main bronchus lies horizontally. Main bronchus in each lung is divided into lobar bronchi that supply each lobe of the lungs, and each lobar bronchus divides into smaller bronchi that end up at the bronchopulmonary segments which are the functional units of the lungs. The bronchi and arteries enter these segments from the central, whereas the veins and lymphatics leave from the peripheral. The structure that is the port to the vessels, nerves, and bronchi is called "the hilum." The lymphatic vessels eventually drain into the mediastinum. The bronchopulmonary segments divide further to form segmental bronchi, bronchioles, and finally alveoli in which the blood-gas exchange occurs. The proximal airways, including the trachea, comprise the non-respiratory unit of the lungs, whereas the terminal bronchioles that consist of respiratory bronchioles and alveolar ducts along with the alveolar sacs and alveoli constitute the respiratory unit. The anatomy of the respiratory track and lungs is shown in Fig. 3.1.

The basal membrane of the alveolar epithelium is covered with type I and type II cells. Type I cells do not contain organelles; however, they have cytoplasmic extensions that are responsible for the gas exchange. Type I cells do not have the ability to regenerate and they are replaced by type II cells in case of injury. Besides their differentiation potential to type I cells and regeneration, type II cells also secrete surfactant that reduces the surface tension and prevents atelectasis. They also have a role in conserving fluid balance in the alveolar space via sodium transportation.

Target Volume Delineation

Several studies have recommended that the treatment of lung cancers by RT should be individualized as the movement of the lesion during respiration is unique in every patient [1–3]. Based on these data, individualized computerized tomography (CT)-based treatment planning is being used as a standard for the delineation of target volumes and organs at risk (OAR) in patients with lung cancer. Locoregional treatment with three-dimensional conformal radiation therapy (3D CRT) and intensity-modulated radiation therapy (IMRT) requires accurate target and normal tissue delineation. For the CT simulation, most patients are immobilized using a wing board with a T- or U-grip handle in supine position. Patient positioning is shown in Fig. 3.2.

The patient undergoes CT simulation, and contrast injection is not necessary unless the tumor is adjacent to the mediastinum or hilum. To define the isocenter, three radiopaque pellet markers are placed at the anterior midline and at right and left lateral points on the skin. The CT scan is acquired in ≤5 mm slices from the level of the cricoid cartilage to the level of the second lumbar vertebra and should include both lungs [4]. If stereotactic ablative radiotherapy (SABR) is planned, slice thickness of 1–3 mm is recommended based on the American Association of Physicists in Medicine (AAPM) Group Report No. 101 [5]. The gross tumor volume (GTV), clinical target volume (CTV), internal target volume (ITV), and planning target volume (PTV) as well as OARs should be delineated separately in each slice based on the recommendations in International Commission on Radiation Units and Measurements (ICRU) reports 50 and 62 [6, 7].

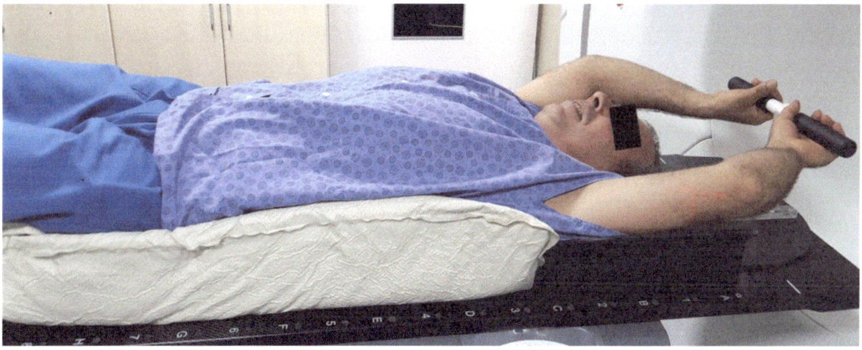

Fig. 3.2 Patient positioning during computed tomography simulation and radiotherapy treatment

Tracking Tumor Mobility

Assessment of respiratory motion is crucial for the treatment planning in order to prevent the distortion of CT scans and to delineate the tumor adequately [8]. In case of a tumor motion exceeding 5 mm, the AAPM Task Group Report No. 76 recommends considering motion assessment [8]. It was shown that in tumors located close to the diaphragm, the mean superior-inferior movement is 15 mm, and the movement can be as high as 52 mm [9, 10]. On the other hand, for the tumors located more superiorly, the superior-inferior movement is approximately 4 mm and the anterior-posterior movement is 2 mm. Respiratory motion tracking, therefore, is necessary particularly in the treatment of lower lobe tumors.

Fluoroscopy has been proposed to be used for motion assessment; however, it is not suitable for simultaneous use with CT simulation and can negatively affect the tumor visualization [1, 11]. The four-dimensional (4D) CT simulation is the optimal choice for detecting internal motion. This technique is performed by recording the respiratory waves simultaneously with CT scans and multiple slices are acquired for at least one full respiratory cycle. However, this technique is not suitable for lower lobe tumors which are highly mobile as it involves too much radiation to healthy tissue [12].

If 4D simulation is not available, a slow (i.e., 4 s per slice) helical CT scan or the fusion of CT images at maximal inspiration and expiration can be performed [2, 13, 14]. In the slow CT scan technique, centrally located target volumes are fused with target volumes from the CT scans performed during quiet respiration. The GTV is then formed with a 5 mm margin in order to take into account the factors that may change tumor mobility [15]. The fused image technique of inspiratory- and expiratory-phase CT scans results in decreased toxicity in OARs; however, it can overestimate the actual tumor volume owing to deep inspiration and expiration and its reproducibility is limited [16–18].

Respiratory gating is one of the frequently used techniques for assessing tumor motion. For this technique, both the CT and the linear accelerator should be equipped with the gating system. Prospective gating in which CT scans are respiration triggered is highly time consuming as one slice is acquired per one respiratory cycle and pre-scan preparation is needed to detect the correct time for scanning [19]. It can also lead to increased patient motion because of long scanning time. The disadvantages of this technique can be cleared by adapting 4D CT scans into "retrospective gating" [20].

Real-time tumor tracking can also be used to follow tumor motion during lung RT. In this technique radio-opaque markers are inserted inside or adjacent to the tumor prior to the treatment planning. At least four markers should be inserted in order to detect the variations in tumor location accurately; however, this is not possible in many patients [21]. The radiation beam turns on only when the location of the markers detected by fluoroscopy is in the correct position. The two major limitations in this technique are (1) the fiducial markers cannot always be accurately inserted in the tumor and (2) markers can only be inserted in peripheral lesions because of the early displacement problem in central tumors [22, 23].

There are several other techniques that can be used to spare normal lung volume. Deep-inspiration breath hold is performed by assisting the patient to hold breath at the end of inspiration in order to decrease tumor mobility [24, 25]. However, problems with patient coordination and tolerance limit the usage of this technique [24, 26, 27]. The active breathing control technique helps to obtain reproducible target volumes but does not generally lead to a decrease in PTVs owing to residual tumor mobility [28, 29]. In another technique called "self-breath-holding system," the patient controls own breathing according to the radiation beam-on and beam-off positions [30]. However, this technique requires at least three CT scans in order to obtain reproducible target volumes.

Gross Tumor Volume (GTV)

The GTV is the clinically macroscopic disease together with specular extensions detected by CT scan with contrast and/or [18F]-fluoro-deoxy-glucose (FDG) positron emission tomography/CT (PET/CT). The windowing of the CT has a great effect on the size of GTV. It was reported that the pulmonary nodules are best visualized with windowing width of 850 Hounsfield unit (HU) and windowing length of −750 HU [31]. This is called the "lung windowing" and should be used for the delineation of the primary lung tumor (Fig. 3.3).

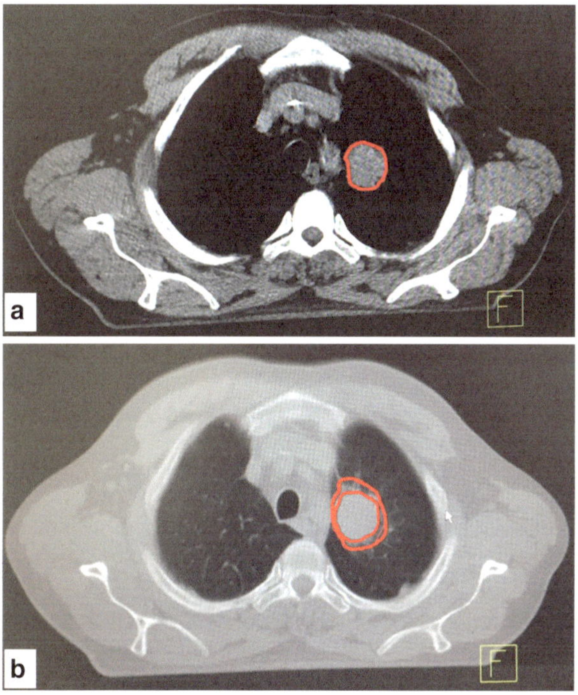

Fig. 3.3 (**a**) Primary lung tumor on a planning computed tomography (CT) image in "mediastinal windowing." (**b**) Same CT image of the primary lung tumor in "lung windowing." It can clearly be seen that the gross tumor volume (GTV) is enlarged by the addition of the specular extensions

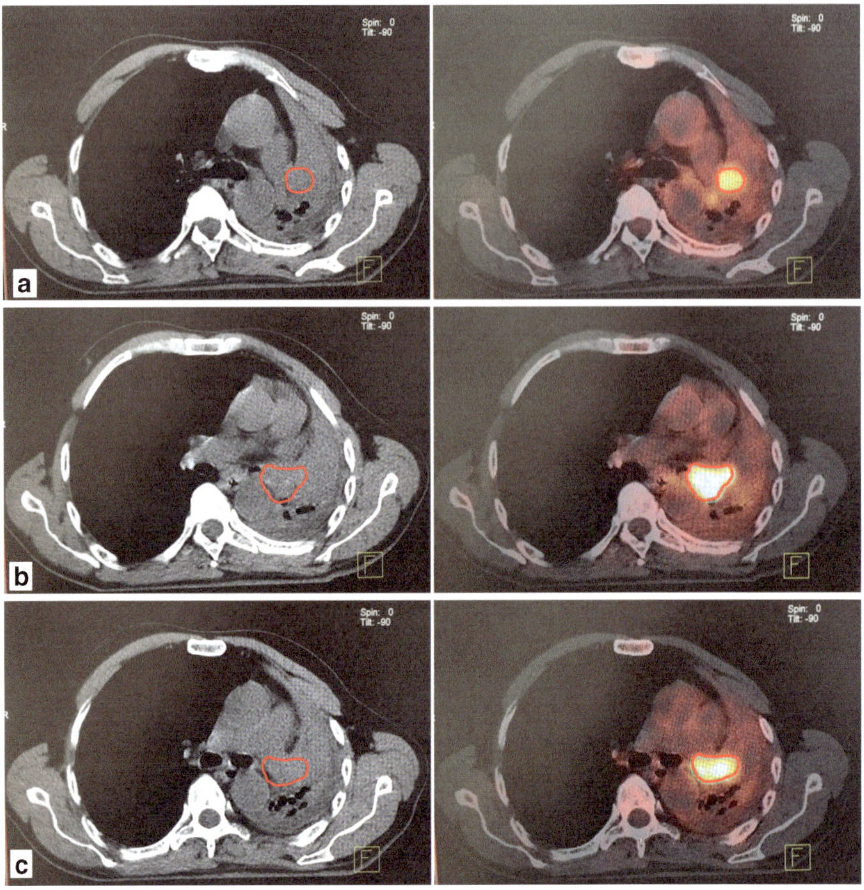

Fig. 3.4 The planning computed tomography (CT) images of a 62-year-old male with T4N2M0 squamous cell lung carcinoma. (**a**) Show the superior, (**b**) show the middle, and (**c**) show the inferior parts of the primary tumor. Prominent atelectasis is observed in the left lower lobe around the primary lung lesion. (**a–c**) Images on planning CT and the corresponding fusion images of planning CT and positron emission tomography (PET)/CT). Although the distinction between the primary tumor and atelectasia cannot be made on the prior figures, the tumor can be clearly identified from the atelectatic regions on the latter figures

The most important role of PET/CT is distinguishing atelectasis from tumor; however, there is no threshold for the exact determination of the margins of the primary tumor [32, 33] (Fig. 3.4). The sensitivity and specificity of FDG-PET/CT are higher than conventional CT in lung cancer and were reported to be 83 % and 91 %, respectively [34]. It should also be kept in mind that FDG uptake can increase in cases of infection, inflammation, and granulomatous disease, whereas it can decrease in necrotic or hypoxic tumor regions [35, 36]. It was shown that PET/CT-based delineation of GTV resulted in larger volumes compared to conventional CT-based delineations because of possible respiratory motion tracking [37]. However, there are also studies reporting that PET/CT-based delineation significantly decreases the target volume resulting in a decrease in toxicity [38, 39]. Several methods have been used for the delineation of the primary tumor using PET/CT; direct visualization of the tumor is the simplest method, threshold of standard uptake value $(SUV)_{max}$ of 2.5 can be used to delineate GTV, or a threshold of 35–50 % of SUV_{max} can be used to delineate ITV [40–43]. Although automatic contouring based on PET/CT resulted in reduced variations in the delineation of GTV between clinicians, it is not recommended to be used routinely, and the cooperation of the radiation oncologist with the nuclear medicine physicist should be preferred for the most accurate delineation of the primary tumor [44, 45].

The Radiation Therapy Oncology Group (RTOG) 1106 study has proposed a consensus guideline for the delineation of primary lung tumors in non-small-cell lung cancer (NSCLC) by the help of PET/CT [46]. The authors recommend delineating the primary tumor under a standard lung window level in CT slices, and in case that the tumor margins were not defined accurately, the radiation oncologist would decide for the final target volume. They defined PET-metabolic tumor volume (MTV) that is constituted by contouring a 1.2 cm diameter structure in the center of ascending aorta and transferring this structure to PET/CT image for the accurate fusion of the CT and PET/CT. The target is then checked using 1.5 times intensity of the mean aorta activity. The OARs are subsequently defined in related slices and the parts of OARs that are in the target volume are manually removed.

In patients with limited stage small-cell lung cancer (SCLC) induction chemotherapy can be administered in the presence of bulky disease at diagnosis. However, there are concerns whether pre- or post-chemotherapy volume should be delineated. In the study of South Western Oncology Group (SWOG), no difference in local recurrence was found between patients who received RT to the pre- and post-chemotherapy volume [47]. Several studies, mostly retrospective, also reported that most locoregional recurrences (LRRs) occurred in the post-chemotherapy volume [48–51]. On the other hand, Mira and Livingston stated that most of the recurrences in their patients occurred out of field [52]. Jenkins et al. reported that following induction chemotherapy, the GTV and PTV decreased by 37 % and 26 %, respectively [53]. When they delineated the post-chemotherapy volume, they detected a significant decrease in the irradiated lung volume receiving ≥20 Gy; however they also stated that irradiating post-chemotherapy tumor volume can result in increased marginal recurrence rate. Based on these findings, delineation of the post-chemotherapy volume of the primary tumor can be adequate for definitive treatment. However, in patients who responded less than partially to induction chemotherapy, particularly with small tumors, pre-chemotherapy volume can also be irradiated. No significant difference in toxicity was reported between pre- and post-chemotherapy volume treatment [47].

Postoperative RT to the primary tumor bed is indicated in patients with NSCLC in case of positive or close (≤5 mm) surgical margins after complete excision in order to increase survival and decrease LRR rate [54]. In this case, GTV is not applicable and there is no consensus guideline for the delineation of the tumor bed. However, as the peribronchial tumor extension has poorer prognosis, the bronchus stump is recommended to be delineated in patients with positive or close bronchial surgical margin, and concurrent chemotherapy is added in order to increase overall and disease-free survival rates [55–59].

For patients diagnosed with stage I (T1-2 N0 M0) or peripherally located stage II (T3 N0 M0) NSCLC who refuse surgery or are medically inoperable, SABR is the treatment of choice as the local control rates are significantly higher than conventional treatments [60]. As the margins for CTV and PTV are smaller in treatment with SABR, the tumor extension should be delineated accurately on imaging modalities.

Clinical Target Volume (CTV)

The CTV is the volume in which there is a high possibility of microscopic disease. It was reported that a 9 mm margin around the gross tumor is adequate to encompass the microscopic disease in 90 % of adenocarcinomas [61]. For NSCLC, Giraud et al. showed that the microscopic tumor extended 2.69 mm and 1.48 mm further from the gross tumor in adenocarcinoma and squamous cell carcinoma (SCC), respectively [62]. Based on this finding, the CTV for 3D CRT and IMRT is constituted by adding 6 and 8 mm margin to the GTV for SCC and adenocarcinoma, respectively, in order to encompass 95 % of the microscopic disease. For other histological types, they recommend a 5 mm margin. However, for tumors with unspecified histology, 8 mm margin is recommended to stay on the safe side.

In SCLC, there is no defined standard CTV margin. The ongoing Cancer and Leukemia Group B (CALGB) 30610/Radiation Therapy Oncology Group (RTOG) 0538 study recommends 0.5–1 cm margins for SCLC which will also be including the ipsilateral hilum.

The CTV should be restricted with anatomical structures such as the chest wall, vertebrae, and vessels.

Internal Target Volume (ITV)

The ITV is the volume that is enlarged in order to encompass the tumor with respect to physiologic movements, which here is respiration. According to the ICRU report 62, the ITV is recommended to be used if it positively affects the treatment planning and is not routinely contoured in every cancer treatment planning [7, 63]. The term "IGTV" represents the GTV together with the respiration effect and should be taken into account during the delineation of lung tumors [20]. After the respiratory motion is detected, the CTV is formed by adding adequate margins to the IGTV.

Planning Target Volume (PTV)

The PTV is constituted by adding a certain margin to the CTV by taking setup variability into account. The PTV margins vary based on the simulation technique; the prior 13 mm margin was reduced to 9 mm in patients immobilized with a stereotactic body frame and to 1–2 mm in patients positioned with cone beam CT [64]. If the respiratory motion is assessed either by 4D CT or cone beam CT, a 5–10 mm margin is adequate, whereas if both techniques are used, the margin can be decreased to 3 mm. A margin of 5 mm is adequate in patients who undergo 4D CT planning with daily kilo-voltage (kV) imaging during treatment. However, if the respiratory motion cannot be assessed, 10–15 mm margin should be added to the CTV to constitute the PTV [13]. For SABR and other image guided techniques, smaller margins of 3–6 mm are recommended [65–67].

Conclusion

Patient-based treatment planning has been the standard in lung cancer in recent years. 3D CRT and particularly IMRT offer better target coverage and decreased toxicity rates compared to conventional RT. Recommended simulation and delineation techniques are summarized in this chapter. If these recommendations are applied in clinical practice, the variations in the treatment techniques between institutions can be minimized.

References

1. Stevens CW, Munden RF, Forster KM, et al. Respiratory-driven lung tumor motion is independent of tumor size, tumor location, and pulmonary function. Int J Radiat Oncol Biol Phys. 2001;51:62–8.
2. van Sornsen de Koste JR, Lagerwaard FJ, Schuchhard-Schipper RH, et al. Dosimetric consequences of tumor mobility in radiotherapy of stage I non-small cell lung cancer – an analysis of data generated using 'slow' CT scans. Radiother Oncol. 2001;61:93–9.
3. Sixel KE, Ruschin M, Tirona R, Cheung PC. Digital fluoroscopy to quantify lung tumor motion: potential for patient-specific planning target volumes. Int J Radiat Oncol Biol Phys. 2003;57:717–23.
4. Senan S, De Ruysscher D, Giraud P, et al. Literature-based recommendations for treatment planning and execution in high-dose radiotherapy for lung cancer. Radiother Oncol. 2004;71:139–46.
5. Benedict SH, Yenice KM, Followill D, et al. Stereotactic body radiation therapy: the report of AAPM Task Group 101. Med Phys. 2010;37:4078–101.
6. International Commission on Radiation Units and Measurements. ICRU report 50: prescribing, recording, and reporting photon beam therapy. Bethesda: Maryland, USA. 1993.
7. International Commission on Radiation Units and Measurements. ICRU report 62: prescribing, recording and reporting photon beam therapy (supplement to ICRU report 50). Bethesda: Maryland, USA. 1999.
8. Keall PJ, Mageras GS, Balter JM, et al. The management of respiratory motion in radiation oncology report of AAPM Task Group 76. Med Phys. 2006;33:3874–900.
9. Van de Steene J, Van den Heuvel F, Bel A, et al. Electronic portal imaging with on-line correction of setup error in thoracic irradiation: clinical evaluation. Int J Radiat Oncol Biol Phys. 1998;40:967–76.
10. Giraud P, De Rycke Y, Dubray B, et al. Conformal radiotherapy (CRT) planning for lung cancer: analysis of intrathoracic organ motion during extreme phases of breathing. Int J Radiat Oncol Biol Phys. 2001;51:1081–92.
11. Halperin R, Pobinson D, Murray B, et al. Fluoroscopy for assessment of physiologic movement of lung tumors, a pitfall of clinical practice? Proceeding of Innovative Technology in Radiation Medicine Toronto, October 22–27. Radioth Oncol. 2002;65:s1. abstract 87.
12. Jouin A, Pourel N. Target volume margins for lung cancer: internal target volume/clinical target volume. Cancer Radiother. 2013;17:428–33.

13. Gomez DR, Liao Z. Non-small cell lung cancer (NSCLC) and small cell lung cancer (SCLC). In: Lee NY, Lu JJ, editors. Target volume delineation and field setup- a practical guide for conformal and intensity-modulated radiation therapy. 1st ed. Berlin: Springer; 2013. p. 87–103.
14. Lagerwaard FJ, Van Sornsen de Koste JR, Nijssen-Visser MR, et al. Multiple "slow" CT scans for incorporating lung tumor mobility in radiotherapy planning. Int J Radiat Oncol Biol Phys. 2001;51:932–7.
15. Van Sornsen de Koste JRLF, de Boer HC, et al. Are multiple CT scans required for planning curative radiotherapy in lung tumors of the lower lobe? Int J Radiat Oncol Biol Phys. 2003;55:1394–9.
16. Yamada K, Soejima T, Yoden E, et al. Improvement of three-dimensional treatment planning models of small lung targets using high-speed multi-slice computed tomographic imaging. Int J Radiat Oncol Biol Phys. 2002;54:1210–6.
17. Senan S, Lagerwaard FJ, Nijssen-Visser MR. Incorporating lung tumor mobility in radiotherapy planning. Int J Radiat Oncol Biol Phys. 2002;52:1142–3; author reply 1144.
18. Ozhasoglu C, Murphy MJ. Issues in respiratory motion compensation during external-beam radiotherapy. Int J Radiat Oncol Biol Phys. 2002;52:1389–99.
19. Ford EC, Mageras GS, Yorke E, et al. Evaluation of respiratory movement during gated radiotherapy using film and electronic portal imaging. Int J Radiat Oncol Biol Phys. 2002;52:522–31.
20. Vedam SS, Keall PJ, Kini VR, et al. Acquiring a four-dimensional computed tomography dataset using an external respiratory signal. Phys Med Biol. 2003;48:45–62.
21. Murphy MJ. Fiducial-based targeting accuracy for external-beam radiotherapy. Med Phys. 2002;29:334–44.
22. Shirato H, Harada T, Harabayashi T, et al. Feasibility of insertion/implantation of 2.0-mm-diameter gold internal fiducial markers for precise setup and real-time tumor tracking in radiotherapy. Int J Radiat Oncol Biol Phys. 2003;56:240–7.
23. Harada T, Shirato H, Ogura S, et al. Real-time tumor-tracking radiation therapy for lung carcinoma by the aid of insertion of a gold marker using bronchofiberscopy. Cancer. 2002;95:1720–7.
24. Murphy MJ, Martin D, Whyte R, et al. The effectiveness of breath-holding to stabilize lung and pancreas tumors during radiosurgery. Int J Radiat Oncol Biol Phys. 2002;53:475–82.
25. O'Dell WG, Schell MC, Reynolds D, Okunieff R. Dose broadening due to target position variability during fractionated breath-held radiation therapy. Med Phys. 2002;29:1430–7.
26. Hara R, Itami J, Kondo T, et al. Stereotactic single high dose irradiation of lung tumors under respiratory gating. Radiother Oncol. 2002;63:159–63.
27. Barnes EA, Murray BR, Robinson DM, et al. Dosimetric evaluation of lung tumor immobilization using breath hold at deep inspiration. Int J Radiat Oncol Biol Phys. 2001; 50:1091–8.
28. Wong JW, Sharpe MB, Jaffray DA, et al. The use of active breathing control (ABC) to reduce margin for breathing motion. Int J Radiat Oncol Biol Phys. 1999;44:911–9.
29. Cheung PC, Sixel KE, Tirona R, Ung YC. Reproducibility of lung tumor position and reduction of lung mass within the planning target volume using active breathing control (ABC). Int J Radiat Oncol Biol Phys. 2003;57:1437–42.
30. Onishi H, Kuriyama K, Komiyama T, et al. A new irradiation system for lung cancer combining linear accelerator, computed tomography, patient self-breath-holding, and patient-directed beam-control without respiratory monitoring devices. Int J Radiat Oncol Biol Phys. 2003; 56:14–20.
31. Harris KM, Adams H, Lloyd DC, Harvey DJ. The effect on apparent size of simulated pulmonary nodules of using three standard CT window settings. Clin Radiol. 1993;47:241–4.
32. Nestle U, Walter K, Schmidt S, et al. 18F-deoxyglucose positron emission tomography (FDG-PET) for the planning of radiotherapy in lung cancer: high impact in patients with atelectasis. Int J Radiat Oncol Biol Phys. 1999;44:593–7.
33. Caldwell CB, Mah K, Ung YC, et al. Observer variation in contouring gross tumor volume in patients with poorly defined non-small-cell lung tumors on CT: the impact of 18FDG-hybrid PET fusion. Int J Radiat Oncol Biol Phys. 2001;51:923–31.

34. Gambhir SS, Czernin J, Schwimmer J, et al. A tabulated summary of the FDG PET literature. J Nucl Med. 2001;42:1S–93.
35. Bakheet SM, Saleem M, Powe J, et al. F-18 fluorodeoxyglucose chest uptake in lung inflammation and infection. Clin Nucl Med. 2000;25:273–8.
36. Pitman AG, Hicks RJ, Binns DS, et al. Performance of sodium iodide based (18) F-fluorodeoxyglucose positron emission tomography in the characterization of indeterminate pulmonary nodules or masses. Br J Radiol. 2002;75:114–21.
37. Hanna GG, McAleese J, Carson KJ, et al. (18)F-FDG PET-CT simulation for non-small-cell lung cancer: effect in patients already staged by PET-CT. Int J Radiat Oncol Biol Phys. 2010;77:24–30.
38. De Ruysscher D, Wanders S, Minken A, et al. Effects of radiotherapy planning with a dedicated combined PET-CT-simulator of patients with non-small cell lung cancer on dose limiting normal tissues and radiation dose-escalation: a planning study. Radiother Oncol. 2005;77:5–10.
39. van Elmpt W, De Ruysscher D, van der Salm A, et al. The PET-boost randomised phase II dose-escalation trial in non-small cell lung cancer. Radiother Oncol. 2012;104:67–71.
40. Nestle U, Hellwig D, Schmidt S, et al. 2-Deoxy-2-[18F]fluoro-D-glucose positron emission tomography in target volume definition for radiotherapy of patients with non-small-cell lung cancer. Mol Imaging Biol. 2002;4:257–63.
41. Bradley J, Thorstad WL, Mutic S, et al. Impact of FDG-PET on radiation therapy volume delineation in non-small-cell lung cancer. Int J Radiat Oncol Biol Phys. 2004;59:78–86.
42. Paulino AC, Johnstone PA. FDG-PET in radiotherapy treatment planning: Pandora's box? Int J Radiat Oncol Biol Phys. 2004;59:4–5.
43. Erdi YE, Mawlawi O, Larson SM, et al. Segmentation of lung lesion volume by adaptive positron emission tomography image thresholding. Cancer. 1997;80:2505–9.
44. Zheng Y, Sun X, Wang J, et al. FDG-PET/CT imaging for tumor staging and definition of tumor volumes in radiation treatment planning in non-small cell lung cancer. Oncol Lett. 2014;7:1015–20.
45. Jin Z, Arimura H, Shioyama Y, et al. Computer-assisted delineation of lung tumor regions in treatment planning CT images with PET/CT image sets based on an optimum contour selection method. J Radiat Res. 2014;55:1153–62.
46. Kong FM XY, Machtay M, Werner-Wasik M, et al. Atlases for CT gross tumor volume (CTGTV) and PET metabolic tumor volume (PETMTV) for RTOG 1106. In: RTOG Lung Steering Committee and ATIC Committee.
47. Kies MS, Mira JG, Crowley JJ, et al. Multimodal therapy for limited small-cell lung cancer: a randomized study of induction combination chemotherapy with or without thoracic radiation in complete responders; and with wide-field versus reduced-field radiation in partial responders: a Southwest Oncology Group Study. J Clin Oncol. 1987;5:592–600.
48. Liengswangwong V, Bonner JA, Shaw EG, et al. Limited-stage small-cell lung cancer: patterns of intrathoracic recurrence and the implications for thoracic radiotherapy. J Clin Oncol. 1994;12:496–502.
49. Bonner JA, Sloan JA, Shanahan TG, et al. Phase III comparison of twice-daily split-course irradiation versus once-daily irradiation for patients with limited stage small-cell lung carcinoma. J Clin Oncol. 1999;17:2681–91.
50. Brodin O, Rikner G, Steinholtz L, Nou E. Local failure in patients treated with radiotherapy and multidrug chemotherapy for small cell lung cancer. Acta Oncol. 1990;29:739–46.
51. Arriagada R, Pellae-Cosset B, Ladron de Guevara JC, et al. Alternating radiotherapy and chemotherapy schedules in limited small cell lung cancer: analysis of local chest recurrences. Radiother Oncol. 1991;20:91–8.
52. Mira JG, Livingston RB. Evaluation and radiotherapy implications of chest relapse patterns in small cell lung carcinoma treated with radiotherapy-chemotherapy: study of 34 cases and review of the literature. Cancer. 1980;46:2557–65.
53. Jenkins P, Milliner R, Latimer P. Shrinkage of locally advanced non-small-cell lung cancers in response to induction chemotherapy: implications for radiotherapy treatment planning. Int J Radiat Oncol Biol Phys. 2007;69:993–1000.

54. Kara M, Sak SD, Orhan D, Yavuzer S. Changing patterns of lung cancer; (3/4 in.) 1.9 cm; still a safe length for bronchial resection margin? Lung Cancer. 2000;30:161–8.
55. Massard G, Doddoli C, Gasser B, et al. Prognostic implications of a positive bronchial resection margin. Eur J Cardiothorac Surg. 2000;17:557–65.
56. Snijder RJ, Brutel de la Riviere A, Elbers HJ, van den Bosch JM. Survival in resected stage I lung cancer with residual tumor at the bronchial resection margin. Ann Thorac Surg. 1998;65:212–6.
57. Soorae AS, Stevenson HM. Survival with residual tumor on the bronchial margin after resection for bronchogenic carcinoma. J Thorac Cardiovasc Surg. 1979;78:175–80.
58. Rosell R, Gomez-Codina J, Camps C, et al. Preresectional chemotherapy in stage IIIA non-small-cell lung cancer: a 7-year assessment of a randomized controlled trial. Lung Cancer. 1999;26:7–14.
59. Bradley JD, Paulus R, Graham MV, et al. Phase II trial of postoperative adjuvant paclitaxel/carboplatin and thoracic radiotherapy in resected stage II and IIIA non-small-cell lung cancer: promising long-term results of the Radiation Therapy Oncology Group – RTOG 9705. J Clin Oncol. 2005;23:3480–7.
60. Grutters JP, Kessels AG, Pijls-Johannesma M, et al. Comparison of the effectiveness of radiotherapy with photons, protons and carbon-ions for non-small cell lung cancer: a meta-analysis. Radiother Oncol. 2010;95:32–40.
61. Grills IS, Fitch DL, Goldstein NS, et al. Clinicopathologic analysis of microscopic extension in lung adenocarcinoma: defining clinical target volume for radiotherapy. Int J Radiat Oncol Biol Phys. 2007;69:334–41.
62. Giraud P, Antoine M, Larrouy A, et al. Evaluation of microscopic tumor extension in non-small-cell lung cancer for three-dimensional conformal radiotherapy planning. Int J Radiat Oncol Biol Phys. 2000;48:1015–24.
63. Craig T, Battista J, Moiseenko V, Van Dyk J. Considerations for the implementation of target volume protocols in radiation therapy. Int J Radiat Oncol Biol Phys. 2001;49:241–50.
64. Grills IS, Hugo G, Kestin LL, et al. Image-guided radiotherapy via daily online cone-beam CT substantially reduces margin requirements for stereotactic lung radiotherapy. Int J Radiat Oncol Biol Phys. 2008;70:1045–56.
65. Slotman BJ, Lagerwaard FJ, Senan S. 4D imaging for target definition in stereotactic radiotherapy for lung cancer. Acta Oncol. 2006;45:966–72.
66. Shah C, Grills IS, Kestin LL, et al. Intrafraction variation of mean tumor position during image-guided hypofractionated stereotactic body radiotherapy for lung cancer. Int J Radiat Oncol Biol Phys. 2012;82:1636–41.
67. Timmerman R, Abdulrahman R, Kavanagh BD, Meyer JL. Lung cancer: a model for implementing stereotactic body radiation therapy into practice. Front Radiat Ther Oncol. 2007;40:368–85.
68. Beyzadeoglu M, Ozyigit G, Ebruli C, editors. Basic radiation oncology. Berlin: Springer; 2010. p. 303–28.

Guidelines for the Delineation of Lymphatic Target Volumes in Lung Cancer

4

Gokhan Ozyigit, Melis Gultekin, Sezin Yuce Sari, Gozde Yazici, and Pervin Hurmuz

Introduction

Regional lymph node (LN) involvement is an important prognostic factor for locoregional recurrence (LRR), distant metastasis (DM), and overall survival (OS) in patients with lung cancer [1, 2]. According to the most recent Surveillance, Epidemiology, and End Results (SEER) data, 22 % of all patients with lung cancer have LN metastasis at the time of diagnosis [3]. The incidence of LN metastasis depends on the primary tumor size and tumor histology [4]. The most common LNs involved in patients with lung cancer are hilar and mediastinal LNs.

In 1929, Rouvière described the LNs that each lobe of the lungs drains into and acknowledged that predicting the route of lymphatic drainage was possible based on tumor location [5]. Patterns of lymphatic drainage in lung cancer were also investigated by other researchers later in the 1950s and 1960s [6–8]. These studies clearly revealed that tumors in the right upper lobe primarily drain into the right paratracheal region and tumors in the left upper lobe drain into the periaortic and subaortic regions, whereas tumors in the middle and lower lobes drain into the subcarinal and right paratracheal regions [9]. However, skip metastasis was shown in 7–26 % of lung cancer patients, particularly in the upper lobe tumors and adenocarcinoma histology [8, 10, 11]. The hilar LNs can be skipped, and the drainage can be directly into the mediastinal LNs in tumors located in the upper lobes.

Subsequently Cahan described the method of hilar and mediastinal LN dissection [12, 13]. Japanese surgeons started to perform this surgical method, and in 1967 the first mediastinal LN map was developed by Naruke in Japan. The map was

G. Ozyigit, MD (✉) • M. Gultekin, MD • S.Y. Sari, MD • G. Yazici, MD • P. Hurmuz, MD
Department of Radiation Oncology, Faculty of Medicine, Hacettepe University, Ankara, Turkey
e-mail: gozyigit@hacettepe.edu.tr; melisbahadir@yahoo.com; sezin_yuce@hotmail.com; yazicig@hacettepe.edu.tr; phurmuz@yahoo.com

G. Ozyigit et al. (eds.), *Principles and Practice of Radiotherapy Techniques in Thoracic Malignancies*, DOI 10.1007/978-3-319-28761-4_4

started to be used in Japan, North America, and Europe [14]. Consequently, the American Thoracic Society (ATS) and the American Joint Committee of Cancer (AJCC) adapted new maps based on the Naruke map. In 1996, the modified Mountain-Dressler ATS (MD-ATS) map was introduced as a unified map which was mainly accepted across North America; however, Japanese clinicians continued to use the Naruke map [15]. The main difference between these two maps was the definition of level 7 LN. In the Naruke map, level 7 included the hilar and subcarinal LNs. This led to significant difference in the diagnosis of N stage. Furthermore, level 1 LNs in the Naruke map corresponded to levels 1 and 2 in the MD-ATS map; and levels 2, 3, 4R, and 4L corresponded to levels 4R and 4L. To overcome this issue and with suggestions for further revisions by the European clinicians, the International Association for the Study of Lung Cancer (IASLC) proposed a revised map in 2009 [9]. This map clears the controversies in the anatomical descriptions, the boundary between right and left level 2 and 4 LNs and defined level 1 LNs which were not accepted as distinct LNs in previous maps.

The recently proposed LN delineation guideline by IASLC is composed of 14 LN levels. Levels 10–14 are called "hilar," and levels 1–9 are called "mediastinal" LNs. According to the consensus of IASLC and AJCC, at least six LNs (i.e., three from the mediastinum and three from the hilum) should be evaluated for the accurate staging of LN involvement [16]. However, the patient is accepted as pN0; even fewer LNs are evaluated in case all are negative [17]. There are ongoing studies to improve the correlation between staging and survival rates of patients more accurately, and these studies focus on grouping the LNs as "zones."

Treatment Strategies in Non-small Cell Lung Cancer

Surgery is the treatment of choice in patients with stage I–II and selected patents with stage III non-small cell lung cancer (NSCLC). However, LRR rates after surgery can be as high as 20 % in stage I disease and approximately 50 % in stage III disease [18, 19]. The surgical stump and mediastinal LNs are the most common regions of recurrence. Postoperative radiotherapy (RT) was shown to decrease local recurrence (LR) rates, particularly in stage II and IIIA disease [20]. A SEER analysis on patients with stage II–III NSCLC undergoing surgery reported that postoperative RT increased 5-year OS in patients with pN2 disease; however, OS rates in patients with pN0 and pN1 disease were significantly decreased [21]. The Adjuvant Navelbine International Trialist Association (ANITA) trial compared the results of adjuvant chemotherapy (CHT) to surgery alone [22]. Some centers in this trial also added RT (45–60 Gy) to the adjuvant treatment. Patients with pN1 disease benefited from postoperative RT alone; however, survival was lower after postoperative RT+CHT. On the other hand, survival was increased in patients with pN2 disease with both adjuvant CHT and RT+CHT. Based on these trials, postoperative RT is indicated in case of pN2 disease. The recent standard approach of adjuvant treatment is to start with CHT in patients with pN2 disease or extracapsular extension (ECE) and continue with mediastinal irradiation.

In patients with inoperable NSCLC, definitive CRT is the treatment of choice in order to decrease LRR and increase survival rates [1, 23]. In the two-dimensional (2D) treatment era, elective nodal irradiation was widely performed for advanced stage NSCLC. By the time that three-dimensional (3D) RT was introduced, involved-field RT (IFRT) gained popularity in order to increase RT dose to decrease toxicity rates. However, postsurgical data have shown that occult LN metastasis can be present in 10–35 % of patients with cN0 disease [24]. Nevertheless, the 2-year nodal control rates with IFRT were reported 88–92.4 % [25, 26]. These high rates of local control (LC) could be the result of an incidental dose received by the elective nodal areas [26]. In the only prospective trial comparing IFRT to elective nodal irradiation, there was a significant increase in LC and OS rates in the IFRT arm [27]. However, this study has limitations; RT dose was higher in the IFRT arm (68–74 Gy vs 60–64 Gy), and the lung volume that received at least 20 Gy (V_{20}) was lower. Fernandes et al. reported similar results with IFRT compared to extended-field RT with lower toxicity rates [28]. These data show that IFRT provides satisfying survival and disease control rates with lower toxicity in patients with NSCLC.

Treatment Strategies in Small Cell Lung Cancer

Surgery can be a potential treatment of choice in patients with T1-2N0M0 small cell lung cancer (SCLC). However, the most common type of failure after surgery in SCLC is DM [29]. Due to increased LC and OS rates, concurrent CRT is the treatment of choice for patients with limited stage SCLC (other than T1-2N0 disease) [30, 31]. Unfortunately, patients with SCLC frequently present with advanced disease and CHT is used to increase disease control. In selected cases with good response to CHT, consolidative RT can be administered [32]. Adjuvant and definitive RT indications in SCLC are similar to the ones for NSCLC.

Target Volume Delineation

The simulation process and techniques for tracking respiratory motion are discussed deeply in Chap. 1. Unless there is a contraindication, intravenous contrast is administered during simulation to better visualize the nodal disease. Lymph nodes with ≥1-cm diameter in the short axis on computerized tomography (CT) are generally considered positive [33]. The size of nonmetastatic LNs varies according to the LN level. Lower paratracheal and subcarinal LNs' diameter can physiologically be 11 mm; upper paratracheal LNs are generally smaller in size and are usually around 7 mm. Right hilar, left hilar, and paraesophageal LNs can be 10 mm, 7 mm, and 7–10 mm in size, respectively. Comparison studies to evaluate for new or enlarging LNs (even if they are <1 cm) are helpful in defining the metastatic LNs. [^{18}F]-fluorodeoxy-glucose (FDG) positron emission tomography (PET)/CT can give more accurate information about LN involvement as its sensitivity and specificity are higher than CT alone, which are 81 % and 90 % for PET/CT and 59 % and 79 % for

CT, respectively [34–36]. However, pathological evaluation of the mediastinal LNs is highly recommended as the false negativity of PET/CT in detecting mediastinal LNs <1 cm is approximately 25 % [37].

Level 1 (Low Cervical/Supraclavicular LNs)

Level 1 LNs are divided into 1R (right) and 1L (left) by the midline of the trachea which also constitutes the medial border of 1R and 1L LNs. It starts from the inferior border of the cricoid cartilage (approximately at the inferior border of the fourth cervical vertebra) superiorly and ends at the level of the thoracic inlet. The LNs in level 1 can be sampled by endobronchial ultrasound (EBUS), endoscopic ultrasound (EUS), and percutaneous fine-needle aspiration. If ipsilateral level 1 LN is positive, the patient is staged as N2, and if contralateral or bilateral level 1 LNs are positive, the patient is staged as N3.

Level 2 (Upper Paratracheal LNs)

Level 2 LNs are divided into 2R and 2L by the left lateral border of the trachea. The superior border is the level of the thoracic inlet. The inferior border of 2R is the intersection of the inferior border of the left innominate vein with the trachea. The inferior border of 2L is the superior border of the aortic arch. Level 2R can be sampled by cervical mediastinoscopy, electromagnetic navigation bronchoscopy (EMNB), EBUS, extended mediastinoscopy, transcervical extended mediastinal lymphadenectomy (TEMLA), video-assisted mediastinoscopic lymphadenectomy (VAMLA), and right video-assisted thoracoscopic surgery (VATS). Level 2L can be sampled by all techniques mentioned for 2R except VATS, and it can additionally be sampled by EUS. If ipsilateral level 2 LN is positive, the patient is staged as N2, and if contralateral or bilateral level 2 LNs are positive, the patient is staged as N3.

Level 3A (Prevascular LNs)

Level 3A is not divided into two by IASLC; however, it would be easier to evaluate the N stage if it is separated into 3AR and 3AL by the midline of the trachea. The superior border is the thoracic inlet and the inferior border is the level of the carina. These LNs, together with level 6 LNs, are called the "anterior mediastinal LNs" and initially drain into the right and left bronchomediastinal trunks and then into the right lymphatic duct, into the thoracic duct, or independently into the jugulo-subclavian venous confluence. Level 3A LNs can be sampled by TEMLA, VATS, and transthoracic needle aspiration (TTNA). If it is positive unilaterally, the lymphatic stage is N2, and if it is positive bilaterally or contralaterally, the lymphatic stage is N3.

Level 3P (Retrotracheal LNs)

Level 3P starts from the thoracic inlet and ends at the level of the carina. The anterior border is the posterior aspect of the trachea. It can be sampled by EMNB, EBUS, EUS, TEMLA, and right VATS. If it is positive in a patient with right lung cancer, the stage is N2; however, if it is positive in left lung cancer, the stage becomes N3.

Level 4 (Lower Paratracheal LNs)

Level 4 is divided into 4R and 4L by the left lateral border of the trachea. Level 4R starts from the intersection of the inferior border of the left innominate vein with the trachea and ends at the level of the right tracheobronchial angle. The superior border of 4L is the superior border of the aortic arch, and the inferior border is the superior border of the left main pulmonary artery. Level 4R can be sampled by cervical mediastinoscopy, EBUS, EMNB, extended mediastinoscopy, right VATS, TEMLA, and VAMLA. Level 4L can be sampled by all techniques mentioned for 4R except right VATS; it can be sampled by left VATS and additionally by EUS. If it is positive unilaterally, the lymphatic stage is N2, and if it is positive bilaterally or contralaterally, the stage becomes N3.

Level 5 (Subaortic/AP Window LNs)

Level 5 is located lateral to the ligamentum arteriosum. The superior border is the inferior border of the aortic arch, and the inferior border is the superior border of the left main pulmonary artery. Level 5 LNs can be sampled by Chamberlain procedure, extended mediastinoscopy, TEMLA, TTNA, and left VATS. The N stage is N2 if positive in left-sided disease and N3 if positive in right lung cancer.

Level 6 (Para-aortic LNs)

Level 6 includes the LNs anterior and lateral to the ascending aorta and the aortic arch. It starts superiorly from an imaginary line tangential to the superior border of the aortic arch and ends at the inferior border of the same structure. It can be sampled by Chamberlain procedure, extended mediastinoscopy, TEMLA, TTNA, and left VATS. In case of a positive level 6 LN, the patient is diagnosed with N2 disease if the primary disease is in the left lung and with N3 disease if the primary disease is in the right lung.

Level 7 (Subcarinal LNs)

Level 7 starts from the level of the carina and ends at the inferior border of the intermediate bronchus on the right side and the superior border of the left lower lobe bronchus on the left side. It can be sampled by cervical mediastinoscopy (only LNs in the anterior location), EMNB, EBUS, EUS, extended mediastinoscopy, TEMLA, VAMLA, and left or right VATS. If it is positive, the patient is staged as N2 whether it is a right or left lung cancer.

Level 8 (Paraesophageal LNs)

The IASLC does not divide level 8 into two; however, distinguishing 8R from 8L by the midline of the esophagus makes the diagnosis of N stage easier. Level 8 is constituted by the LNs lying adjacent to the wall of the esophagus (excluding subcarinal LNs). It starts from the inferior border of the intermediate bronchus on the right side and the superior border of the left lower lobe on the left side. Level 8 and 9 LNs are called "posterior mediastinal LNs" together and drain into the tracheobronchial group, mainly subcarinal, the thoracic duct, and subdiaphragmatic para-aortic/celiac nodes. Level 8 LNs can be sampled by EUS, TEMLA, VAMLA, and left or right VATS. If it is unilaterally positive, the stage is N2, and if bilaterally or contralaterally positive, the stage becomes N3.

Level 9 (Pulmonary Ligament LNs)

Level 9 is divided into 9R and 9L. Level 9R LNs lie within the right pulmonary artery. They start from the level of the right inferior pulmonary vein and ends at the diaphragm. They can be sampled by EUS, TEMLA, and right VATS. N2 and N3 disease is diagnosed if it is positive in right and left lung cancer, respectively. Level 9L LNs lie within the left pulmonary artery. Level 9L starts from the level of the left pulmonary vein and ends at the diaphragm. It can be sampled by EUS, TEMLA, and left VATS. N2 and N3 disease is diagnosed if it is positive in the left and right lung, respectively.

Level 10–14 LNs

Levels 10, 11, 12, 13, and 14 include hilar and perihilar, interlobar, lobar, segmental, and subsegmental LNs, respectively. They are all subdivided into right and left parts. Level 11 LNs are also divided into 11 s (LNs between the upper lobe bronchus and bronchus intermedius on the right) and 11i (LNs between the middle and lower lobe bronchi on the right). Although level 10–14 LNs are named separately, they are delineated together starting from the level of the right and left tracheobronchial angles to the level that bilateral main bronchi divide. Lobar LNs initially drain into interlobar and hilar LNs and then into subcarinal LNs or directly into level 4 LNs. They can be sampled by EMNB, EBUS, and right and left VATS. Level 10 can also be sampled by cervical mediastinoscopy and TEMLA. If levels 10–14 are positive ipsilaterally, the stage is N1, and if positive contralaterally or bilaterally, the stage becomes N3.

Boundaries for all the LN levels mentioned above are shown in Table 4.1. A detailed atlas for the delineation of all mediastinal lymph nodes are depicted in Fig. 4.1.

Certain anatomical structures can be contoured as LN regions by mistake. Pericardial recesses and sinuses are often mistaken for LNs; superior aortic recess is often confused with paratracheal, para-aortic, prevascular, or subaortic LNs. The oblique sinus is often mistaken for subcarinal LNs, and the pulmonary venous recesses are often confused with pulmonary LNs.

The right upper lobe drains into the ipsilateral mediastinum (levels 10, 11–14, 4, and 3), the left upper lobe drains into the ipsilateral and contralateral mediastinum (levels 10, 11–14, 5, and 6), and the right lower lobe drains into the subcarinal region and into the right upper and lower mediastinum (levels 10, 11–14, 7, and 4), whereas the left lower lobe drains into the subcarinal region and then into the right or left upper and lower mediastinum (levels 10, 11–14, 7, 5, and 6). Left lower lobe tumors are the most common site for contralateral mediastinal LN metastasis. Feng et al. reported that the most common site of LN failure is 2R, followed by 10R, 4R, and 7 in right-sided disease, and 4R, followed by 7, 4L, 6, 10L, and 5 in left lung cancers (10). Based on these anatomical and clinical data, for tumors located in the right lung levels 2R, 4R, 7, 8, and 9 and for tumors in the left lung levels 4L, 5, 6, 7, 8, and 9 should be sampled during surgery for accurate LN staging (11). Sampling adequate number of LNs is extremely important as IFRT is now preferred over elective nodal irradiation.

Clinical Target Volume and Planning Target Volume

The involved LNs constitute the gross tumor volume (GTV). It was reported that in LNs smaller than 2 cm, a 3-mm margin around LN-GTV will encompass 95 % of the microscopic nodal disease [38]. For larger LNs, although there is no consensus, larger margins should be preferred. It was reported that an 8-mm margin would be more adequate to cover the 95 % of the microscopic nodal disease for LNs with a diameter of ≥2 cm [38]. The details about the internal target volume (ITV) and planning target volume (PTV) can be found in Chap. 3.

Table 4.1 Boundaries for the mediastinal and hilar lymph node levels

LN levels	Boundaries of LN levels					
	Superior	Inferior	Medial	Lateral	Anterior	Posterior
1R	Cricoid cartilage	Thoracic inlet	Midline of the trachea	Body of the R clavicle	Head of the R clavicle	Vertebral body
1L	Cricoid cartilage	Thoracic inlet	Midline of the trachea	Body of the L clavicle	Head of the L clavicle	Vertebral body
2R	Thoracic inlet (sup. border of the manubrium)	Int. of sup. border of LIV with the trachea	L lat. border of the trachea	R lung parenchyma	Ant. border of the innominate artery	Post. border of the trachea
2L	Thoracic inlet	Sup. border of the aortic arch	L lat. border of the trachea	Med. border of the LSA	Post. border of the innominate artery	Post. border of the trachea
3A	Thoracic inlet	Carina	Lung parenchyma	Lung parenchyma	Post. of the manubrium sterni	Ant. border of VCS on the R, L carotid artery on the L
3P	Thoracic inlet	Carina	Esophagus	R lung parenchyma	Post. border of the trachea	Vertebral body
4R	Int. of sup. border of LIV with the trachea	R tracheobronchial angle	L lat. border of the trachea	R lung parenchyma	Post. border of the LIV and VCS confluence	Post./Ant. border of the trachea
4L	Sup. border of the aortic arch	Sup. border of the LMPA	L lat. border of the trachea	Aortic arch	Aortic arch	Esophagus
5	Inf. border of the aortic arch	Sup. border of the LMPA	Ligamentum arteriosum	L lung parenchyma	Line tangential to the sup. border of the aortic arch	
6	Line tangential to the sup. border of the aortic arch	Inf. border of the aortic arch	Ascending aorta and aortic arch	L lung parenchyma	Ant. border of the aortic arch	Ascending aorta and aortic arch

7	Carina	Inf. border of IB on the R/sup. border of the LLLB on the L	[a]	[a]	Post. border of the RMPA	Post. border of the esophagus
8	Inf. border of IB on the R/sup. border of the LLLB on the L	Diaphragm	L lat. border of the thoracic duct	Descending aorta	Esophagus	Vertebral body
9	RIPV on the R/LIPV on the L	Diaphragm	Lat. borders of the esophagus	R lung parenchyma on the R/L lung parenchyma on the L	Post. aspect of the pericardium	R lung parenchyma on the R/Ant. border of the descending aorta on the L
10R	R tracheobronchial angle	Interlobar region				
10L	L tracheobronchial angle	Interlobar region				

LN lymph node, *int*. intersection, *sup*. superior, *LIV* left innominate vein, *lat*. lateral, *ant*. anterior, *post*. posterior, *med*. medial, *VCS* vena cava superior, *LSA* left subclavian artery, *LMPA* left main pulmonary artery, *inf*. inferior, *IB* intermediate bronchus, *LLLB* left lower lobe bronchus, *RMPA* right main pulmonary artery, *RIPV* right inferior pulmonary vein, *LIPV* left inferior pulmonary vein, *R* right, *L* left

[a]Lies between right and left main bronchi

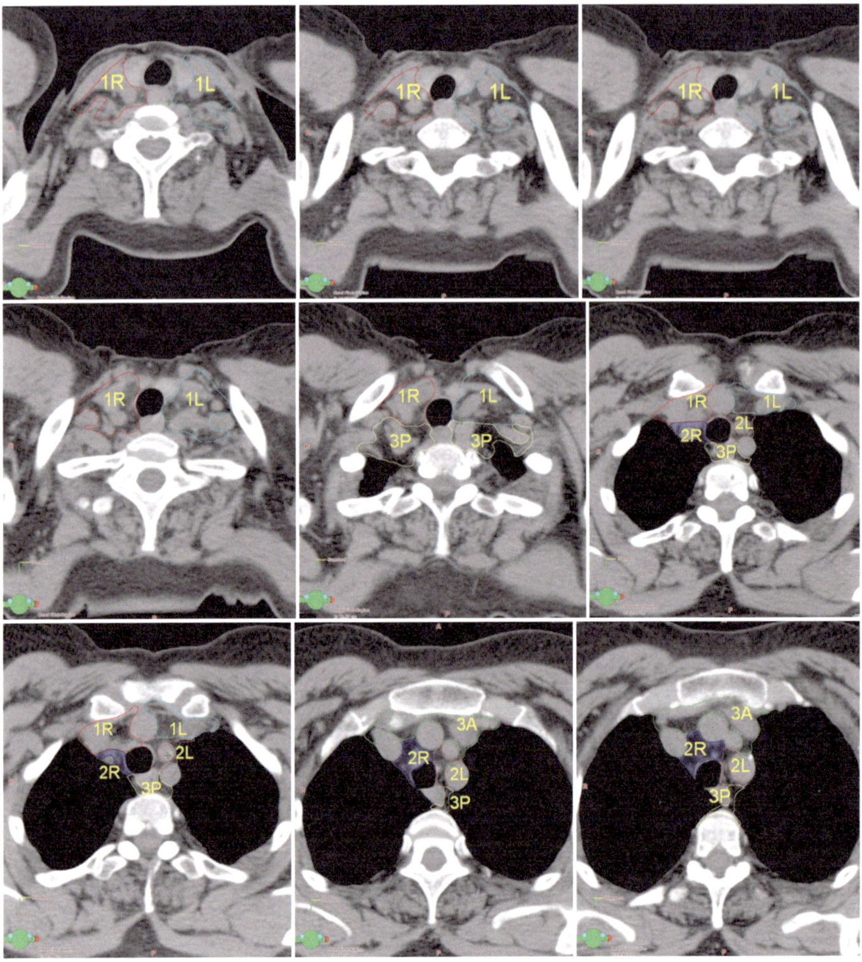

Fig. 4.1 Atlas for the delineation of lymph nodes for lung cancers

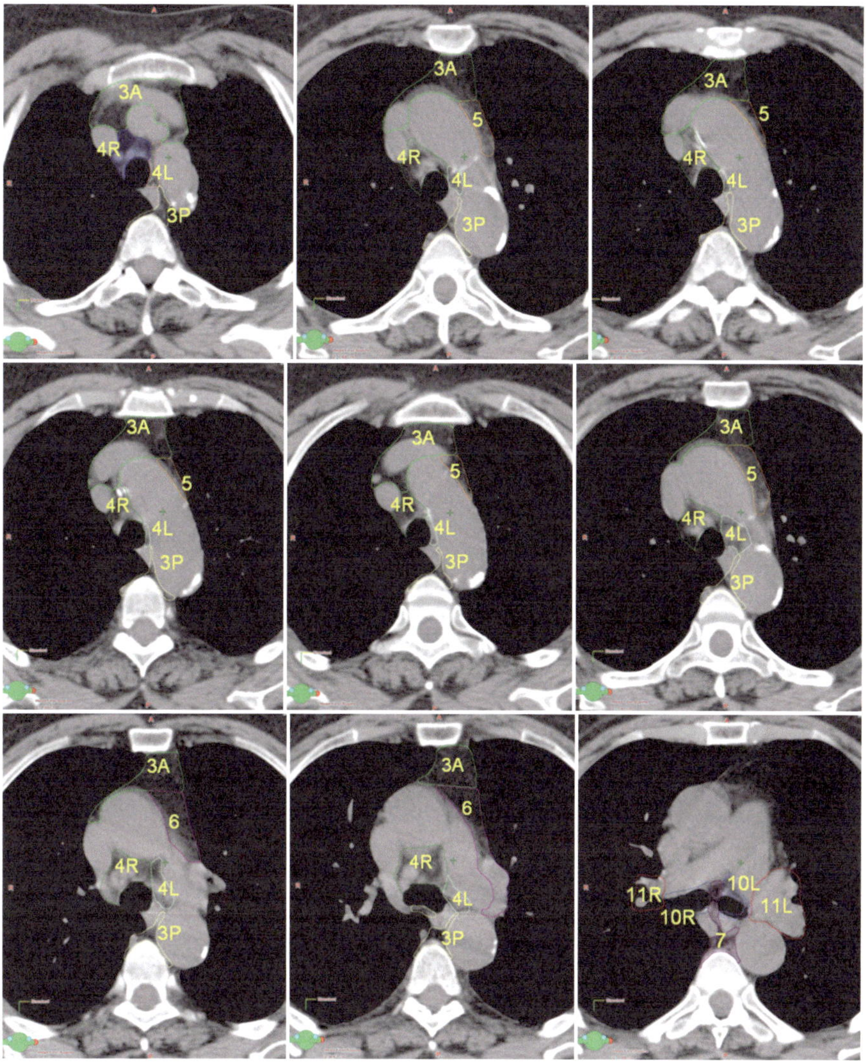

Fig. 4.1 (continued)

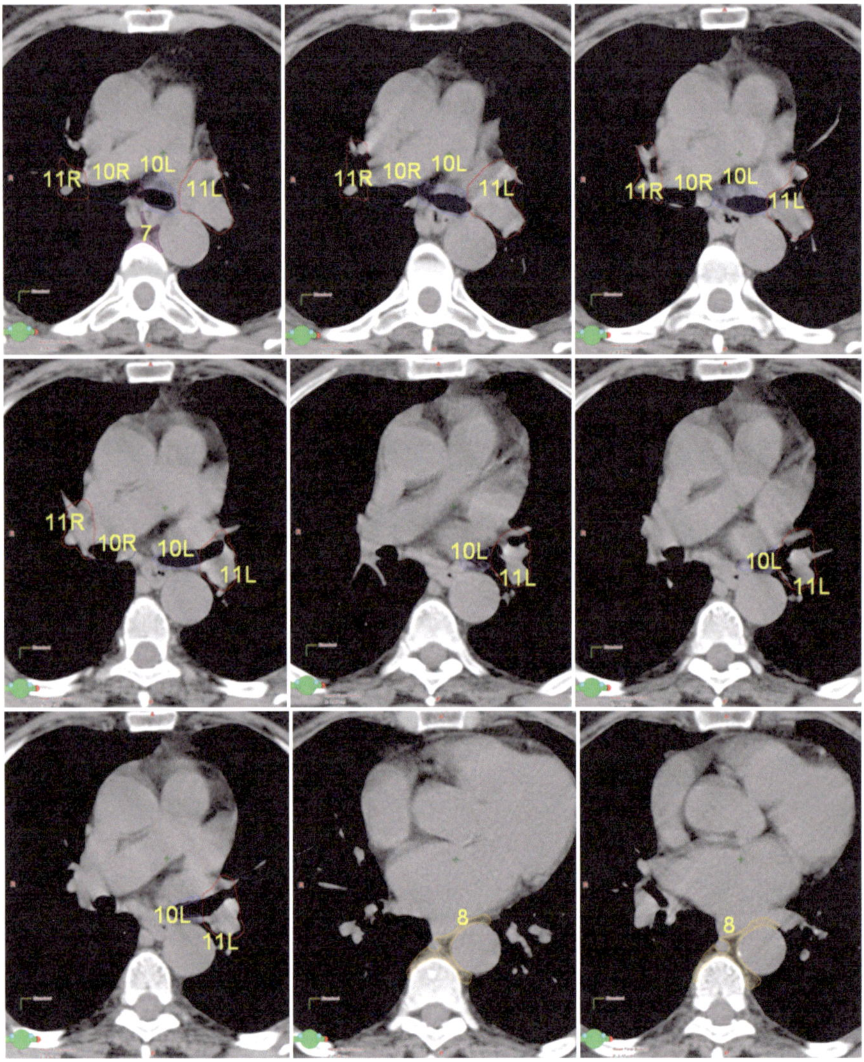

Fig. 4.1 (continued)

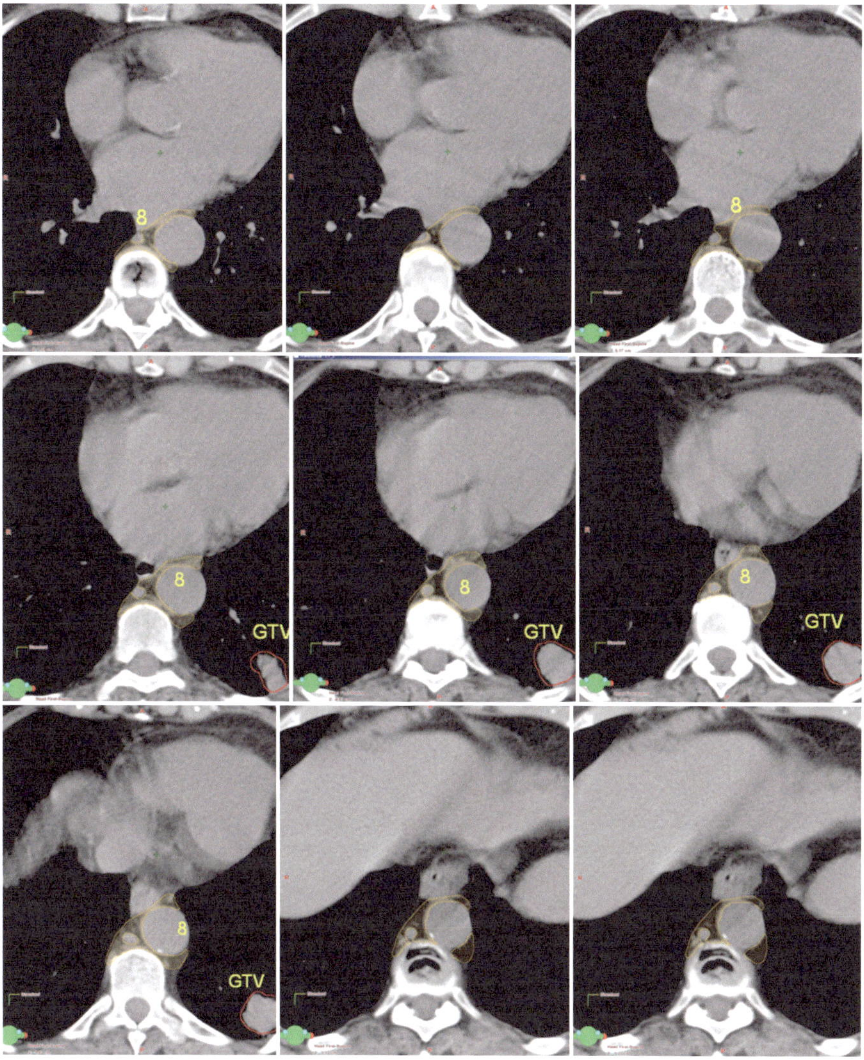

Fig. 4.1 (continued)

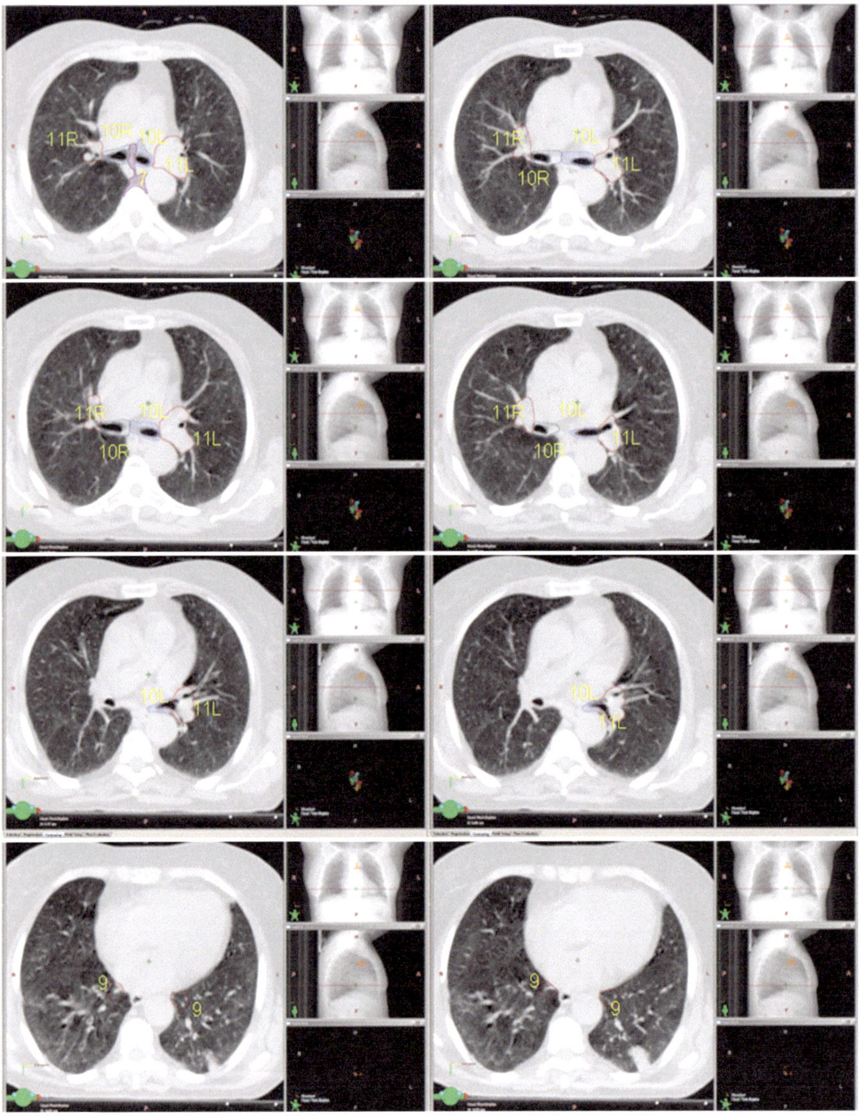

Fig. 4.1 (continued)

Conclusion

Elective nodal irradiation is the standard treatment of care in patients with lung cancer who undergo RT. The recommended delineation guidelines of the mediastinal and hilar LNs are summarized in this chapter. The variations in contouring the LNs between the institutions can be minimized if these recommendations are applied in clinical practice.

References

1. Schaake-Koning C, van den Bogaert W, Dalesio O, et al. Effects of concomitant cisplatin and radiotherapy on inoperable non-small-cell lung cancer. N Engl J Med. 1992;326:524–30.
2. Malissard L, Nguyen TD, Jung GM, et al. Localized adenocarcinoma of the lung: a retrospective study of 186 non-metastatic patients from the French Federation of Cancer Institutes – the Radiotherapy Cooperative Group. Int J Radiat Oncol Biol Phys. 1991;21:369–73.
3. Howlader NNA, Krapcho M, et al. SEER stat fact sheets: lung and bronchus. Bethesda: National Cancer Institute; 2011.
4. Line DH, Deeley TJ. The necropsy findings in carcinoma of the bronchus. Br J Dis Chest. 1971;65:238–42.
5. Rouvière H. Les vaisseaux lymphatiques des poumons et les ganglions visceraux intrathoraciques. Ann Anat Pathol. 1929;6:113–58.
6. Nohl HC. An investigation into the lymphatic and vascular spread of carcinoma of the bronchus. Thorax. 1956;11:172–85.
7. Pennell TC. Anatomical study of the peripheral pulmonary lymphatics. J Thorac Cardiovasc Surg. 1966;52:629–34.
8. Riquet M, Hidden G, Debesse B. Direct lymphatic drainage of lung segments to the mediastinal nodes. An anatomic study on 260 adults. J Thorac Cardiovasc Surg. 1989;97:623–32.
9. Rusch VW, Asamura H, Watanabe H, et al. The IASLC lung cancer staging project: a proposal for a new international lymph node map in the forthcoming seventh edition of the TNM classification for lung cancer. J Thorac Oncol. 2009;4:568–77.
10. Riquet M, Manac'h D, Saab M, et al. Factors determining survival in resected N2 lung cancer. Eur J Cardiothorac Surg. 1995;9:300–4.
11. Libshitz HI, McKenna Jr RJ, Mountain CF. Patterns of mediastinal metastases in bronchogenic carcinoma. Chest. 1986;90:229–32.
12. Cahan WG. Radical lobectomy. J Thorac Cardiovasc Surg. 1960;39:555–72.
13. Cahan WG, Watson WL, Pool JL. Radical pneumonectomy. J Thorac Surg. 1951;22:449–73.
14. Naruke T, Suemasu K, Ishikawa S. Lymph node mapping and curability at various levels of metastasis in resected lung cancer. J Thorac Cardiovasc Surg. 1978;76:832–9.
15. Mountain CF, Dresler CM. Regional lymph node classification for lung cancer staging. Chest. 1997;111:1718–23.
16. Darling GE, Allen MS, Decker PA, et al. Randomized trial of mediastinal lymph node sampling versus complete lymphadenectomy during pulmonary resection in the patient with N0 or N1 (less than hilar) non-small cell carcinoma: results of the American College of Surgery Oncology Group Z0030 Trial. J Thorac Cardiovasc Surg. 2011;141:662–70.
17. Edge SB, AJCoC. AJCC cancer staging manual. New York: Springer; 2010.
18. Harpole Jr DH, Herndon 2nd JE, Young Jr WG, et al. Stage I nonsmall cell lung cancer. A multivariate analysis of treatment methods and patterns of recurrence. Cancer. 1995;76:787–96.
19. Trodella L, Granone P, Valente S, et al. Adjuvant radiotherapy in non-small cell lung cancer with pathological stage I: definitive results of a phase III randomized trial. Radiother Oncol. 2002;62:11–9.

20. Logan DM, Lochrin CA, Darling G, et al. Adjuvant radiotherapy and chemotherapy for stage II or IIIA non-small-cell lung cancer after complete resection. Provincial Lung Cancer Disease Site Group. Cancer Prev Control. 1997;1:366–78.
21. Lally BE, Zelterman D, Colasanto JM, et al. Postoperative radiotherapy for stage II or III non-small-cell lung cancer using the surveillance, epidemiology, and end results database. J Clin Oncol. 2006;24:2998–3006.
22. Douillard JY, Rosell R, De Lena M, et al. Impact of postoperative radiation therapy on survival in patients with complete resection and stage I, II, or IIIA non-small-cell lung cancer treated with adjuvant chemotherapy: the adjuvant Navelbine International Trialist Association (ANITA) Randomized Trial. Int J Radiat Oncol Biol Phys. 2008;72:695–701.
23. O'Rourke N, Roque IFM, Farre Bernado N, Macbeth F. Concurrent chemoradiotherapy in non-small cell lung cancer. Cochrane Database Syst Rev. 2010;(6):CD002140.
24. Timmerman R, Paulus R, Galvin J, et al. Stereotactic body radiation therapy for inoperable early stage lung cancer. JAMA. 2010;303:1070–6.
25. Rosenzweig KE, Sura S, Jackson A, Yorke E. Involved-field radiation therapy for inoperable non small-cell lung cancer. J Clin Oncol. 2007;25:5557–61.
26. Kepka L, Bujko K, Zolciak-Siwinska A, Garmol D. Incidental irradiation of mediastinal and hilar lymph node stations during 3D-conformal radiotherapy for non-small cell lung cancer. Acta Oncol. 2008;47:954–61.
27. Yuan S, Sun X, Li M, et al. A randomized study of involved-field irradiation versus elective nodal irradiation in combination with concurrent chemotherapy for inoperable stage III nonsmall cell lung cancer. Am J Clin Oncol. 2007;30:239–44.
28. Fernandes AT, Shen J, Finlay J, et al. Elective nodal irradiation (ENI) vs. involved field radiotherapy (IFRT) for locally advanced non-small cell lung cancer (NSCLC): a comparative analysis of toxicities and clinical outcomes. Radiother Oncol. 2010;95:178–84.
29. Yu JB, Decker RH, Detterbeck FC, Wilson LD. Surveillance epidemiology and end results evaluation of the role of surgery for stage I small cell lung cancer. J Thorac Oncol. 2010;5:215–9.
30. Arriagada R, Pignon JP, Ihde DC, et al. Effect of thoracic radiotherapy on mortality in limited small cell lung cancer. A meta-analysis of 13 randomized trials among 2,140 patients. Anticancer Res. 1994;14:333–5.
31. Warde P, Payne D. Does thoracic irradiation improve survival and local control in limited-stage small-cell carcinoma of the lung? A meta-analysis. J Clin Oncol. 1992;10:890–5.
32. Jeremic B, Shibamoto Y, Nikolic N, et al. Role of radiation therapy in the combined-modality treatment of patients with extensive disease small-cell lung cancer: a randomized study. J Clin Oncol. 1999;17:2092–9.
33. Glazer GM, Gross BH, Quint LE, et al. Normal mediastinal lymph nodes: number and size according to American Thoracic Society mapping. AJR Am J Roentgenol. 1985;144:261–5.
34. De Ruysscher D, Wanders S, van Haren E, et al. Selective mediastinal node irradiation based on FDG-PET scan data in patients with non-small-cell lung cancer: a prospective clinical study. Int J Radiat Oncol Biol Phys. 2005;62:988–94.
35. Belderbos JS, Heemsbergen WD, De Jaeger K, et al. Final results of a phase I/II dose escalation trial in non-small-cell lung cancer using three-dimensional conformal radiotherapy. Int J Radiat Oncol Biol Phys. 2006;66:126–34.
36. Dwamena BA, Sonnad SS, Angobaldo JO, Wahl RL. Metastases from non-small cell lung cancer: mediastinal staging in the 1990s – meta-analytic comparison of PET and CT. Radiology. 1999;213:530–6.
37. Gould MK, Kuschner WG, Rydzak CE, et al. Test performance of positron emission tomography and computed tomography for mediastinal staging in patients with non-small-cell lung cancer: a meta-analysis. Ann Intern Med. 2003;139:879–92.
38. Yuan S, Meng X, Yu J, et al. Determining optimal clinical target volume margins on the basis of microscopic extracapsular extension of metastatic nodes in patients with non-small-cell lung cancer. Int J Radiat Oncol Biol Phys. 2007;67:727–34.

Stereotactic Ablative Radiotherapy for Lung Cancers

5

Gokhan Ozyigit, Sezin Yuce Sari, Gozde Yazici, Pervin Hurmuz, and Melis Gultekin

Introduction

The standard treatment for early-stage non-small cell lung cancer (NSCLC) is surgery, and the preferred surgical technique is lobectomy with mediastinal lymph node (LN) dissection. The reported 5-year survival rates for early-stage lung cancer patients treated with surgery range between 60 % and 80 % [1]. The American College of Chest Physicians (ACCP) recommends that all patients should undergo preoperative evaluation for pulmonary reserve [2]. If the predicted forced expiratory volume in 1 s (FEV1) or diffusion capacity for carbon monoxide (DLCO) is <40 %, the risk of postoperative complications increases. Lobectomy is contraindicated in patients with FEV1 <30 %, and sublobar resection is an option for this group. On the other hand, radiotherapy (RT) is a remarkable alternative for patients who are medically inoperable or who refuse surgery [3].

The reported overall survival (OS) rates with conventionally fractionated RT alone are not satisfactory (6–45 %), and the primary reason for decreased survival is local failure (LF) [3–5]. In patients who were medically inoperable and were treated with conventionally fractionated RT to a median dose of 66 Gy, the local control (LC) rates were significantly inferior to surgical series, and 85 % of the patients died of lung cancer in 5 years [4–6]. Although dose-escalation studies resulted in increased LC and OS with conventionally fractionated doses of ≥70 Gy, LC rates were 60 % at most with 5-year OS rates of 6–32 % even with a total dose of 80 Gy [7–9]. On the other hand, the Radiation Therapy Oncology Group (RTOG) 9311 trial showed no further improvement in LC rates with doses higher than 77 Gy [10]. Increased toxicity with increased total doses and accelerated repopulation due

G. Ozyigit, MD (✉) • S.Y. Sari, MD • G. Yazici, MD • P. Hurmuz, MD • M. Gultekin, MD
Department of Radiation Oncology, Faculty of Medicine, Hacettepe University, Ankara, Turkey
e-mail: gozyigit@hacettepe.edu.tr; sezin_yuce@hotmail.com; yazicig@hacettepe.edu.tr; phurmuz@yahoo.com; melisbahadir@yahoo.com

G. Ozyigit et al. (eds.), *Principles and Practice of Radiotherapy Techniques in Thoracic Malignancies*, DOI 10.1007/978-3-319-28761-4_5

to prolonged treatment time are the major limitations of conventionally fractionated RT [11]. For every extra day of RT after 6 weeks of treatment, the LC decreases by 1.6 % due to the repopulation of tumor cells [12]. The only way to overcome these issues is the administration of stereotactic ablative RT (SABR) which gives a higher and more homogeneous dose to the target while decreasing the dose to normal tissues by highly developed techniques of immobilization and tumor tracking.

SABR in Inoperable Early-Stage Non-small Cell Lung Cancer

The first method of SABR for extracranial targets was described by Lax and Blomgren [13]. They administered 30 Gy in three fractions with 2–3 days between fractions. After a phase I trial revealed satisfactory results with 60–66 Gy in three fractions in early-stage NSCLC, several prospective studies emerged reporting 79–97 % LC rates [14–19] (Table 5.1). In the RTOG 0236 trial, where a scheme of 54 Gy in three fractions was used in 59 patients with peripheral tumors smaller than 5 cm, the 3-year OS and disease-free survival (DFS) rates were 56 % and 48 %, respectively [20]. In this study only one patient had LF; the main reason for treatment failure was distant metastasis (DM). Timmerman et al. stated that in order to achieve an LC rate of 85 %, the biologically equivalent dose (BED) should be ≥100 (with $\alpha/\beta = 10$) for lung tumors [21]. They also reported that BED_{10} should be <210 Gy in order to reduce the treatment-related mortality rate by 75 %. In a meta-analysis by Koshy et al., it was suggested that BED_{10} should be >150 Gy for T2 lesions in order to increase OS [22]. Kong et al. proposed a new model in a review

Table 5.1 Prospective studies of SABR in early-stage NSCLC

Trial	N of patients	Tumor location, size	Dose (Gy)/N of fractions	Median follow-up (months)	3-year OS (%)/CSS (%)	3-year DFS (%)/PFS (%)	3-year LC (%)	Grade >2 toxicity (%)
McGarry et al. [14]	47	?, ≤7 cm	24–72/3	27.4 (T1) 19.1 (T2)	–/–	–/–	79	?
Nagata et al. [15]	45	?, ≤4 cm	48/4	30	92 (IA), 82 (IB)/–	83 (IA), 72(IB)/–	98	4
Xia et al. [16]	43	P and C, ≤7 cm	50/5	54	78/–	–/–	95	8.9
Lagerwaard et al. [17]	206	P and C, ≤6 cm	60/3-5-8	?	2y 64/–	2y 68/–	97	3
Baumann et al. [18]	57	P, ≤5 cm	45/3	35	60/88	–/52	92	28
Fakiris et al. [19]	70	P and C, ≤7 cm	60–66/3	50.2	42.7/81.7	–/–	88.1	37.7

SABR stereotactic ablative radiotherapy, *NSCLC* non-small cell lung cancer, *N* number, *3y* 3-year, *2y* 2-year, *OS* overall survival, *CSS* cause-specific survival, *DFS* disease-free survival, *PFS* progression-free survival, *LC* local control, *P* peripheral, *C* central

Table 5.2 Results of different fractionation schemes of SABR for early-stage NSCLC

Trial	N of patients	Tumor location, size	Dose (Gy)/N of fractions	Median follow-up (months)	3-year OS (%)/ CSS (%)	3-year DFS (%)/ PFS (%)	3-year LC (%)	Grade >2 toxicity
Timmerman et al. [21]	37	P and C, ≤7 cm	24–42/3	15.2	64/–	50/–	87	5.4
Nakagawa et al. [25]	10	?, ≤5 cm	19–26/1	14.9	2y 64/–	–/–	80	0
Uematsu et al. [26]	50	P and C, ≤ cm	50–60/ 5–10	36	66/88	–/–	94	0

SABR stereotactic ablative radiotherapy, *NSCLC* non-small cell lung cancer, *N* number, *3y* 3-year, *2y* 2-year, *OS* overall survival, *CSS* cause-specific survival, *DFS* disease-free survival, *PFS* progression-free survival, *LC* local control, *P* peripheral, *C* central

and claimed that total dose (D) x fraction dose (d) yields better prediction of LC compared to BED_{10}; however, this method has not been accepted widely [23].

In a study on the data from Surveillance, Epidemiology, and End Results (SEER), 367 patients ≥67 years old with stage I NSCLC that received SABR were compared to 711 patients who underwent surgery [24]. It was observed that although acute toxicity rate was higher in the surgery arm, toxicity rates were similar in both arms at 2 years. On the other hand, the mortality rate was significantly lower in the SABR arm at 3 months, but 2-year mortality rate was significantly lower in the surgery arm. There was no difference in mortality rates between the two arms in patients with short (<5 years) life expectancies; however, surgery yielded better results in patients with long life expectancies, and the authors concluded that surgery should be preferred over SABR in these particular patients.

Reported LC rates in NSCLC for different fractionation schemes of SABR are between 80 % and 94 % [21, 25, 26] (Table 5.2). In medically inoperable stage IA and IB (tumor <4 cm) NSCLC patients, the OS rates were 87 % and 80 %, respectively, with a scheme of 48 Gy in four fractions (BED_{10} of 88 Gy) in 2 weeks [27]. In a retrospective analysis of 241 patients from 13 Japanese institutions, the LF and 3-year OS rates were 20 % and 42 %, respectively, when BED10 was <100 Gy [28]. In patients treated with a dose of BED10 >100 Gy, the LF rate was 6.5 % and OS rate was 46 %.

Onishi et al. published their multi-institutional results in 245 patients with stage IA and IB NSCLC and stated that inoperable patients had significantly lower survival rates [29]. The 5-year survival rate of patients irradiated with BED_{10} ≥100 Gy and <100 Gy was 90 % and 84 %, respectively, which are comparable to surgery results. Wulf et al. reported their results in 92 lung tumors (36 primary, 56 metastatic) which were treated with different SABR regimens [30]. The reported 2-year LC rates were 100 % for 1×26 Gy, 92 % for 3×12.5 Gy, and 71 % for 3×10 Gy, respectively, and the only significant predictor for LC in multivariate analysis was the BED at the planning target volume (PTV) margin. McGarry et al. reported that doses >16 Gy/fraction resulted in better LC in stage IA and IB NSCLC patients treated in three fractions, and the maximum tolerated dose for tumors >5 cm was 72 Gy [14]. Grills et al. found a

2-year LF rate of 4 % for $BED_{10} \geq 105$ Gy, whereas it was 15 % for $BED_{10} < 105$ in T1-3 tumors [31]. Le et al. reported that 1-year LC rate was 91 % and 54 % in NSCLC patients treated with a single fraction of >20 Gy and <20 Gy, respectively [32]. Nuyttens et al. reported 85 % of a 2-year LC rate in patients with central lung tumors treated to a dose of 60 Gy in five fractions ($BED_{10} > 100$ Gy) and 60 % for 45–50 Gy in five fractions ($BED_{10} \leq 100$ Gy) [33]. van der Voort van Zyp et al. reported that the LC rate was 95 % for 60 Gy in three fractions and 78 % for 45 Gy in three fractions in patients with stage I tumor [34]. In RTOG 0236, 60 Gy in three fractions (BED10 = 180 Gy) was administered to 55 patients with peripheral stage IA (80 % of patients) and IB NSCLC. They reported 3-year primary tumor LC, in-lobe LC, regional (LN) control, distant control, and OS rates as 97.6 %, 90.6 %, 87.2 %, 77.9 %, and 55.8 %, respectively. Seventeen percent of the patients had grade ≥3 pulmonary toxicity; however, the majority of them already had chronic obstructive pulmonary disease prior to treatment. The very high LC rate in this study caused a discussion whether the dose was redundantly high [35]. The RTOG 0915 trial, comparing 34 Gy in a single fraction to 48 Gy in four fractions in peripheral tumors, is closed to accrual and the final results are awaited. The preliminary results revealed 1-year OS, LC, and toxicity rates of 85.4 %, 97.1 %, and 9.8 % for 34 Gy and 91.1 %, 97.6 %, and 13.3 % for 48 Gy, respectively. Kelley et al. treated 67 patients with peripheral NSCLC with a median dose of 48 Gy in four fractions (median BED10 = 105.6 Gy) and reported 1-year LC and OS rates of 81.8 % and 86.2 %, respectively. They also concluded that none of the patients with LF survived 1 year [36].

The ideal fractionation scheme in inoperable early-stage NSCLC patients is not available yet. The final results of RTOG trials 0813 for central and 0915 for peripheral tumors are awaited [17, 37]. The superior arm in 0915 will be compared to 54 Gy in three fractions which was the dose in RTOG 0236 [38].

Patient Preparation, Simulation, and Treatment for CyberKnife™

A more detailed preparation before the treatment is required in order to achieve accurate target recognition by SBRT devices. Immobilization is extremely important for patients treated with SBRT. Besides, extra caution is necessary when treating tumors in the thorax or abdomen due to respiratory motion. Not only immobilization but also tracking the tumor in accordance with the respiration is required when treating lung tumors. To accurately track the tumor, at least three fiducial markers, usually made of gold, which have a diameter of 0.7–1.2 mm and a length of 3–6 mm are inserted into the tumor by interventional techniques before the simulation process (Fig. 5.1). To minimize the errors, the ideal number of the fiducials to be inserted is four to six. The distance and angle between each fiducial should be at least 15 mm and 15^0, respectively, and the maximum distance between the fiducial and the tumor should not be further than 50–60 mm. In order to restrict the motion of the fiducials, the planning CT should be delayed for approximately 1 week to allow the development of fibrosis around the fiducials.

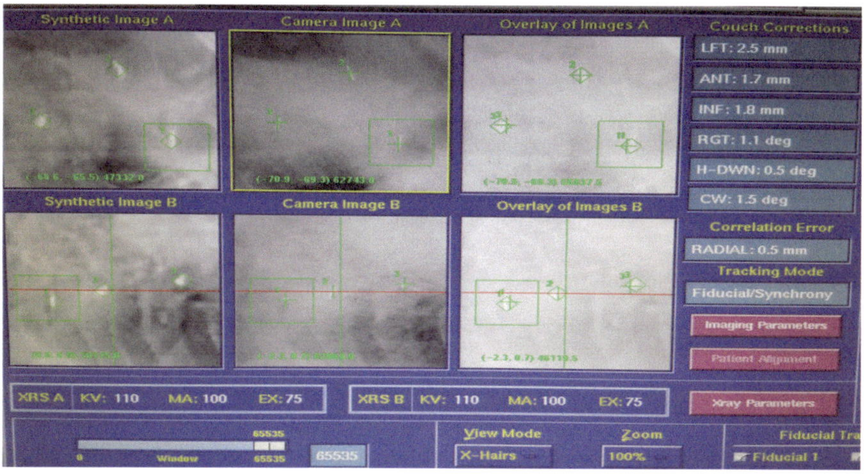

Fig. 5.1 *Gold* fiducials seen prior to set-up for CyberKnife™ (Courtesy of Hacettepe University)

The patient undergoes CT simulation without contrast injection wearing a synchrony vest, and the arms are parallel to the body in contrast to 3D simulation (Fig. 5.2). The CT scan is acquired in 1–3 mm slices from the level of the cricoid cartilage to the level of the second lumbar vertebra and includes both lungs. The gross tumor volume (GTV), clinical target volume (CTV), internal target volume (ITV), planning target volume (PTV), and OARs should be delineated separately in each slice (Fig. 5.3).

During the treatment, the respiratory motion is tracked by three light-emitting diodes (LED) and a camera with the help of the infrared LEDs on the synchrony vest (Fig. 5.4). These devices acquire the information of tumor location during the whole respiratory cycle, and the robotic head corrects the target deviations due to respiratory or patient's motion during the treatment (Fig. 5.5).

If the tumor is in close proximity to the spine and is >15 mm on all dimensions, X-sight tracking by the help of bony structures of the vertebrae can be used for tracking. Tracking is made by the help of contrast difference between the tumor and the lung. This technique only calculates the planar movement but not rotations.

The final CyberKnife plan approved by physician is usually delivered in three to four fractions in consecutive days (Fig. 5.6).

Treatment According to Tumor Localization

The localization of the tumor is important for SABR treatment as the toxicity rates and the organs at risk (OAR) differ with different tumor locations. Centrally located lung tumors are reported to have an increased risk for toxicity. Timmerman et al. found that the 2-year grade ≥3 toxicity rate was 46 % in patients with central tumors treated to a total dose of 60–66 Gy in three fractions, whereas the toxicity rate was

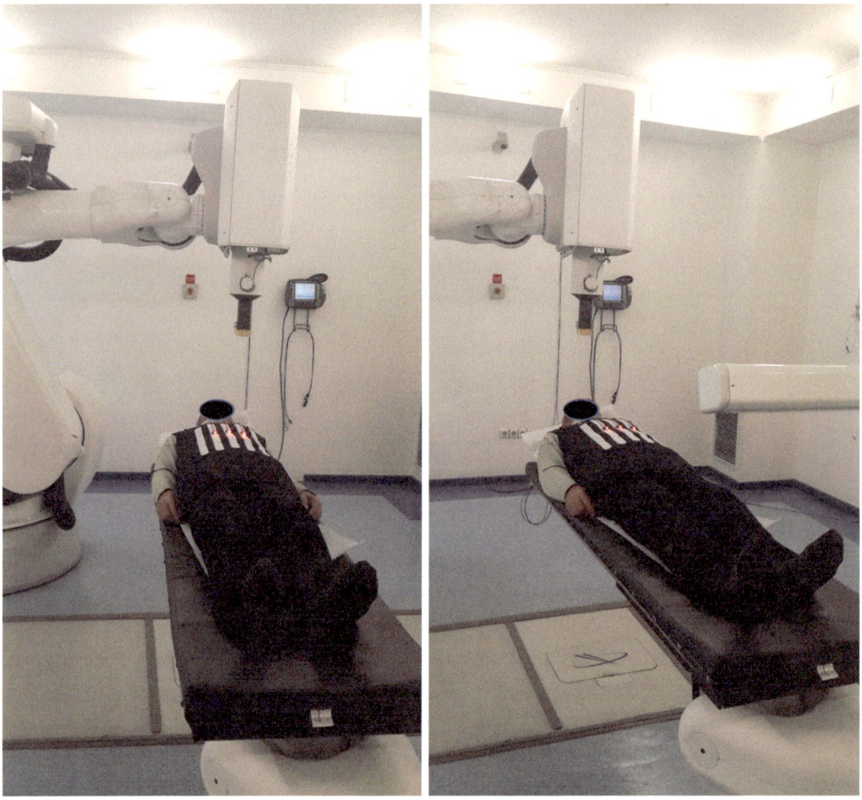

Fig. 5.2 Patient undergoes CT simulation without contrast injection wearing a synchrony vest, and the arms are parallel to the body in contrast to 3D simulation for CyberKnife™ (Courtesy of Hacettepe University)

only 17 % for peripheral tumors [20]. In RTOG 0236, Timmerman et al. described the tumors as central if they were located inside the first 2 cm of the trachea and proximal bronchial tree ("no-fly zone") [38]. On the other hand, in the RTOG 0813 trial, tumors with a PTV in intersection with mediastinal structures are also regarded as central [17].

The RTOG 0813 trial is a dose-escalation study for central lung tumors where a total dose of 50–60 Gy is given in five fractions [17]. This study is closed for accrual and the final results are awaited. It is important to remind that a tumor with a PTV in contact with mediastinal or pericardial pleura is also considered central in this trial. For centrally located tumors, more protracted regimens can be safer [16, 39]. The treatment of endobronchial tumors is extremely risky due to increased rate of grade 5 toxicity such as fistula formation and bronchial stricture [40, 41]. Nishimura et al. reported fatal hemoptysis in 2 patients out of 133 with central tumors treated

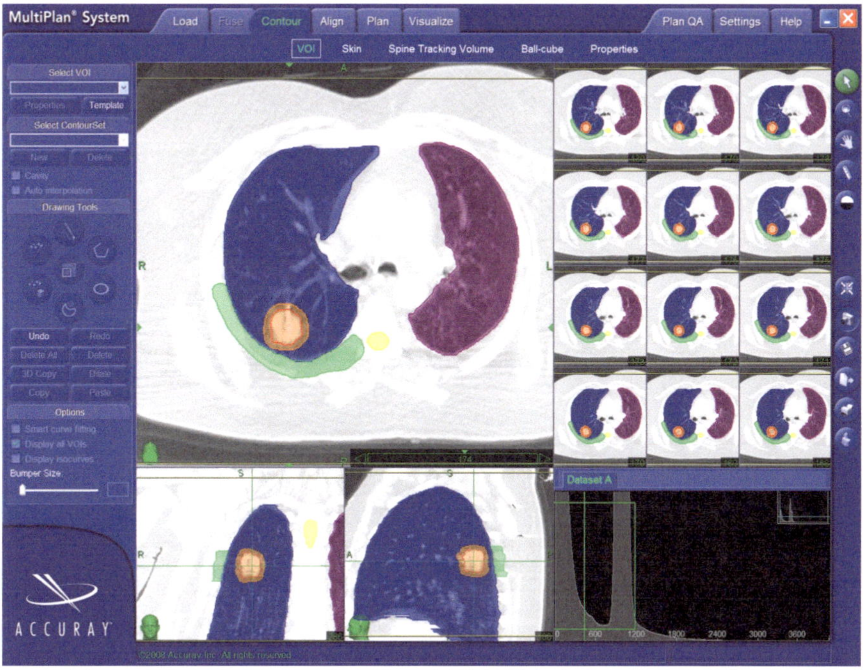

Fig. 5.3 CT scan is acquired in 1–3 mm slices from the level of the cricoid cartilage to the level of the second lumbar vertebra. The gross tumor volume (GTV), clinical target volume (CTV), internal target volume (ITV), planning target volume (PTV), and OARs should be delineated separately in each slice for CyberKnife™ (Courtesy of Hacettepe University)

with 40–60 Gy in five fractions [42]. On the other hand, Robertson et al. found no statistically significant difference in grade ≥2 pulmonary or cardiovascular toxicity in 17-month follow-up between 110 central and 119 peripheral NSCLC lesions treated with 48–60 Gy in four to five fractions [43]. Chang et al. reported the results of 100 patients with T1-2 central tumors treated with 50 Gy in four fractions [44]. They switched the scheme to 70 Gy in ten fractions (BED_{10} = 119 Gy) in patients whose target dose requirements were not met and found no difference in OS, LC, or toxicity rates between the two treatment arms.

Treatment of Larger Tumors with SABR

In a retrospective study of 138 patients, Baumann et al. found that LF after SABR was significantly higher in T2 tumors compared to T1 tumors [45]. Onishi et al. reported higher LF rates in stage IB tumors compared to IA in patients who received doses with BED_{10} <100 Gy [29]. Similarly, Chi et al. observed lower LC rates in tumors >5 cm with BED_{10} <120 Gy [46]. Davis et al. reported that the LC rate was

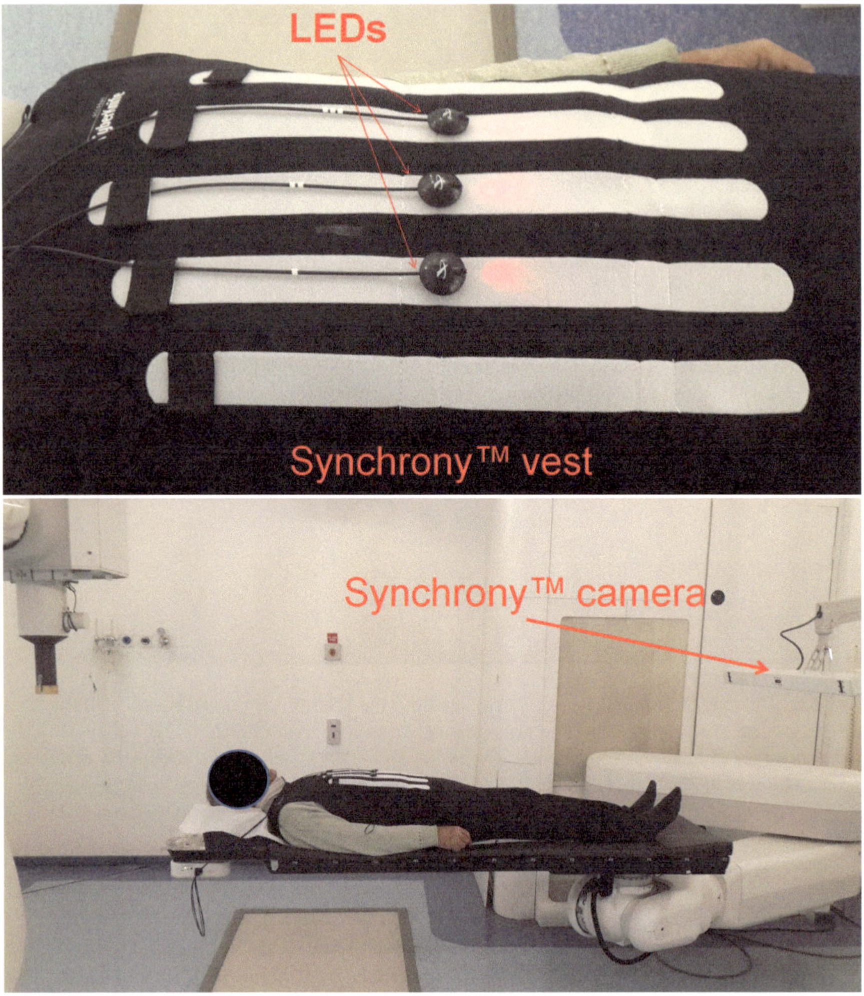

Fig. 5.4 During the treatment the respiratory motion is tracked by three light-emitting diodes (LED) and a camera with the help of the infrared LEDs on the synchrony vest

95 % with BED_{10} ≥105 Gy and was significantly higher compared to 43 % with BED_{10} <105 Gy in T2 tumors in 17 months of follow-up [47]. On the contrary, Allibhai et al. found no correlation between the tumor size and LF, OS, and DM rates after SABR in 185 patients [48].

It was reported that grade 3–5 toxicity increases in tumors with >10 mL volume when treated with SABR [14]. The RTOG trials exclude tumors >5 cm out of SABR studies. However, treatment of tumors >5 cm is claimed to be safe if strict constraints are followed [49]. If this is not possible, more protracted regimens can be administered [50].

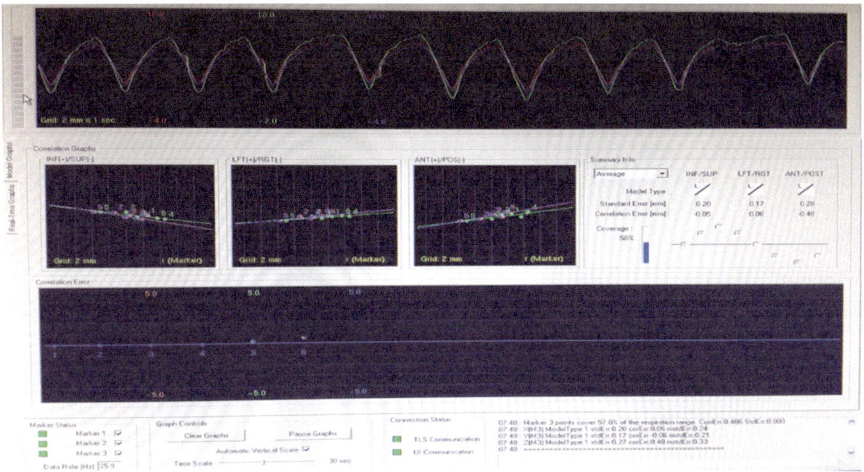

Fig. 5.5 Synchrony™ acquires the information of tumor location during the whole respiratory cycle, and the robotic head corrects the target deviations due to respiratory or patient's motion during the treatment by a specific model

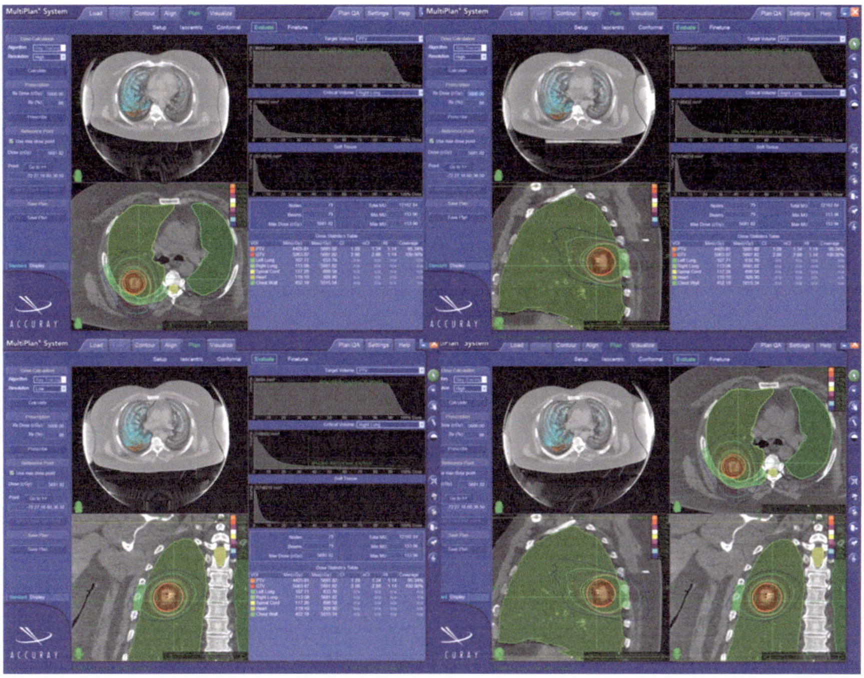

Fig. 5.6 A CyberKnife plan in a patient with T1N0M0 non-small cell lung cancer for a peripheral lesion. The usual dosing schedule is 60 Gy in three fractions. However, 50 Gy in four fractions was delivered due to the close proximity to the chest wall and ribs

SABR in Operable Lung Cancer Patients

Despite all innovations in the field of RT and satisfactory results with SABR, surgery is still the treatment of choice in stage I–II NSCLC patients. The National Comprehensive Cancer Network guidelines recommend surgery for every operable lung cancer patient.

Onishi et al. reported 5-year LC and OS rates of 92 % and 72 % for T1 and 73 % and 62 % for T2 tumors, respectively, in 87 operable patients with stage I NSCLC who were treated with SABR [51]. Lagerwaard et al. reported 3-year LC and OS rates of 93 % and 85 % with SABR in patients who were suitable for surgery [52]. The RTOG 0618 trial in which 60 Gy in three fractions of SABR was administered to patients with operable T1 and T2 peripheral tumors is closed to accrual. Initial results revealed 2-year LC, OS, and progression-free survival (PFS) rates of 92.3 %, 65.4 %, and 84.4 %, respectively, with a conclusion that surgery is not essential in patients with early-stage peripheral lung cancer. However, this is yet an early conclusion for the sufficiency of SABR as the number of patients and the duration of follow-up are limited in studies. Surgery also yields the chance for the evaluation of mediastinal and hilar LNs. Although positron emission tomography/computed tomography (PET/CT) has high sensitivity and specificity for LN involvement, false negativity rate for mediastinal LNs smaller than 1 cm is approximately 25 % [53]. Besides, it was shown that the rate of pathological N2 disease was 3 % in patients with clinical N0 disease. Interestingly, patients treated with SABR had only 4–10 % failure rates in LNs even they are only staged with PET/CT [54]. Based on these data, it is appropriate to rely on PET/CT in patients who will be treated with SABR.

A Dutch study recommended SABR in patients whose surgical mortality rate is expected to be over 4 % [55]. Three phase 3 studies comparing sublobar resection to SABR in patients with high surgical risk (ROSEL trial, STARS trial, and American College of Surgeons Oncology Group [ACOSOG]/RTOG 0870/Cancer and Leukemia Group B [CALGB] 140503 trial) were closed early due to poor accrual. In a meta-analysis which compared the results of SABR (4,850 patients) and surgery (7,071 patients) in stage I NSCLC patients, OS and DFS rates were lower but LC rates higher in the SABR arm [56]. However, when only operable patients in the SABR arm were evaluated, OS was not different between the two arms. Until there is more evidence, SABR is the treatment of choice for patients with early-stage NSCLC who are not suitable for or who refuse surgery [52, 57].

Is There Any Contraindication for Lung SABR?

All patients with early-stage lung cancer can be safely treated with SABR. There is no contraindication owing to age, prior treatment, or comorbidities. It was shown that older age can increase toxicity; however, no grade ≥3 toxicity was observed in elderly patients except the ones who already had lung disease [58, 59]. Patients with prior surgery can undergo SABR without additional risk of toxicity. Pulmonary function test results should not affect the decision of SABR because it does not predict survival or toxicity [60, 61]. Patients with active interstitial lung disease (ILD) should be evaluated more carefully prior to SABR as increased rates of fatal radiation pneumonitis were reported [62]. As the rates were not higher than the ones reported with other treatment modalities such as surgery or chemotherapy, SABR is a safe modality also in patients with ILD [63, 64].

Following Tumor Response After Lung SABR

Treatment with SABR generally leads to lung injury (i.e., pneumonitis and fibrosis) which is observed as increased density and opacity on CT and an increased uptake on PET/CT [65]. As the PTV, radiation dose, and duration from the end of the treatment increase, these changes are more commonly encountered [66]. However, the majority of patients stay asymptomatic. It was reported that SABR-related lung injury can be observed in CT images up to 2 years and in PET/CT up to 1 year in approximately 90 % of the patients [66, 67]. The lung injury related to conventional RT is observed at the edges of treatment portals; however, after SABR the changes are observed as a mass-like image on CT and can easily be misdiagnosed with recurrence [68].

There is controversy about the threshold maximum standardized uptake value (SUVmax) in PET/CT for the distinction of recurrence from lung injury. It was reported that lung injury following SABR can lead to SUVmax as high as 7; on the other hand, SUVmax above 5 was stated as the marker for recurrence in a systematic review [69, 70]. Enlargement after 12 months or in subsequent CT studies, particularly in craniocaudal axis, growing opacity, disappearance of linear margin or bulging margin, and loss of air bronchogram are high risk factors for recurrence, and diagnostic confirmation is required [71].

Conclusion

Surgery is the treatment of choice in patients with early-stage NSCLC. In patients who are medically inoperable or who refuse surgery, SABR is the alternative treatment with comparable LC rates. However, OS rates are inferior to surgery which probably is the result of poor performance status or pulmonary function in inoperable patients. Different regimens of SABR lead to similar disease control rates; however, it is crucial to administer a dose with $BED_{10} \geq 100$ Gy in order to achieve satisfactory results.

References

1. Goldstraw P, Crowley J, Chansky K, et al. The IASLC Lung Cancer Staging Project: proposals for the revision of the TNM stage groupings in the forthcoming (seventh) edition of the TNM classification of malignant tumours. J Thorac Oncol. 2007;2:706–14.
2. Colice GL, Shafazand S, Griffin JP, et al. Physiologic evaluation of the patient with lung cancer being considered for resectional surgery: ACCP evidenced-based clinical practice guidelines (2nd edition). Chest. 2007;132:161S–77.

3. Jeremic B, Classen J, Bamberg M. Radiotherapy alone in technically operable, medically inoperable, early-stage (I/II) non-small-cell lung cancer. Int J Radiat Oncol Biol Phys. 2002;54:119–30.
4. Sibley GS. Radiotherapy for patients with medically inoperable stage I nonsmall cell lung carcinoma: smaller volumes and higher doses – a review. Cancer. 1998;82:433–8.
5. Sibley GS, Jamieson TA, Marks LB, et al. Radiotherapy alone for medically inoperable stage I non-small-cell lung cancer: the Duke experience. Int J Radiat Oncol Biol Phys. 1998;40:149–54.
6. Lagerwaard FJ, Senan S, van Meerbeeck JP, et al. Has 3-D conformal radiotherapy (3D CRT) improved the local tumour control for stage I non-small cell lung cancer? Radiother Oncol. 2002;63:151–7.
7. Willner J, Baier K, Caragiani E, et al. Dose, volume, and tumor control prediction in primary radiotherapy of non-small-cell lung cancer. Int J Radiat Oncol Biol Phys. 2002;52:382–9.
8. Martel MK, Ten Haken RK, Hazuka MB, et al. Estimation of tumor control probability model parameters from 3-D dose distributions of non-small cell lung cancer patients. Lung Cancer. 1999;24:31–7.
9. Qiao X, Tullgren O, Lax I, et al. The role of radiotherapy in treatment of stage I non-small cell lung cancer. Lung Cancer. 2003;41:1–11.
10. Bradley J, Graham MV, Winter K, et al. Toxicity and outcome results of RTOG 9311: a phase I-II dose-escalation study using three-dimensional conformal radiotherapy in patients with inoperable non-small-cell lung carcinoma. Int J Radiat Oncol Biol Phys. 2005;61:318–28.
11. Wulf J, Haedinger U, Oppitz U, et al. Stereotactic radiotherapy for primary lung cancer and pulmonary metastases: a noninvasive treatment approach in medically inoperable patients. Int J Radiat Oncol Biol Phys. 2004;60:186–96.
12. Mehta M, Scrimger R, Mackie R, et al. A new approach to dose escalation in non-small-cell lung cancer. Int J Radiat Oncol Biol Phys. 2001;49:23–33.
13. Blomgren H, Lax I, Naslund I, Svanstrom R. Stereotactic high dose fraction radiation therapy of extracranial tumors using an accelerator. Clinical experience of the first thirty-one patients. Acta Oncol. 1995;34:861–70.
14. McGarry RC, Papiez L, Williams M, et al. Stereotactic body radiation therapy of early-stage non-small-cell lung carcinoma: phase I study. Int J Radiat Oncol Biol Phys. 2005;63:1010–5.
15. Nagata Y, Takayama K, Matsuo Y, et al. Clinical outcomes of a phase I/II study of 48 Gy of stereotactic body radiotherapy in 4 fractions for primary lung cancer using a stereotactic body frame. Int J Radiat Oncol Biol Phys. 2005;63:1427–31.
16. Xia T, Li H, Sun Q, et al. Promising clinical outcome of stereotactic body radiation therapy for patients with inoperable Stage I/II non-small-cell lung cancer. Int J Radiat Oncol Biol Phys. 2006;66:117–25.
17. Lagerwaard FJ, Haasbeek CJ, Smit EF, et al. Outcomes of risk-adapted fractionated stereotactic radiotherapy for stage I non-small-cell lung cancer. Int J Radiat Oncol Biol Phys. 2008; 70:685–92.
18. Baumann P, Nyman J, Hoyer M, et al. Outcome in a prospective phase II trial of medically inoperable stage I non-small-cell lung cancer patients treated with stereotactic body radiotherapy. J Clin Oncol. 2009;27:3290–6.
19. Fakiris AJ, McGarry RC, Yiannoutsos CT, et al. Stereotactic body radiation therapy for early-stage non-small-cell lung carcinoma: four-year results of a prospective phase II study. Int J Radiat Oncol Biol Phys. 2009;75:677–82.
20. Timmerman R, McGarry R, Yiannoutsos C, et al. Excessive toxicity when treating central tumors in a phase II study of stereotactic body radiation therapy for medically inoperable early-stage lung cancer. J Clin Oncol. 2006;24:4833–9.
21. Timmerman R, Papiez L, McGarry R, et al. Extracranial stereotactic radioablation: results of a phase I study in medically inoperable stage I non-small cell lung cancer. Chest. 2003;124:1946–55.
22. Koshy M, Malik R, Weichselbaum RR, Sher DJ. Increasing radiation therapy dose is associated with improved survival in patients undergoing stereotactic body radiation therapy for stage I non-small-cell lung cancer. Int J Radiat Oncol Biol Phys. 2015;91:344–50.

23. Kong C, Guo WJ, Zha WW, et al. A new index comparable to BED for evaluating the biological efficacy of hypofractionated radiotherapy schemes on early stage non-small cell lung cancer: analysis of data from the literature. Lung Cancer. 2014;84:7–12.
24. Yu JB, Soulos PR, Cramer LD, et al. Comparative effectiveness of surgery and radiosurgery for stage I non-small cell lung cancer. Cancer. 2015;121:2341–9.
25. Nakagawa K, Aoki Y, Tago M, et al. Megavoltage CT-assisted stereotactic radiosurgery for thoracic tumors: original research in the treatment of thoracic neoplasms. Int J Radiat Oncol Biol Phys. 2000;48:449–57.
26. Uematsu M, Shioda A, Tahara K, et al. Focal, high dose, and fractionated modified stereotactic radiation therapy for lung carcinoma patients: a preliminary experience. Cancer. 1998;82:1062–70.
27. Hiraoka M, Nagata Y. Stereotactic body radiation therapy for early-stage non-small-cell lung cancer: the Japanese experience. Int J Clin Oncol. 2004;9:352–5.
28. Nagata Y, Negoro Y, Aoki T, et al. Clinical outcomes of 3D conformal hypofractionated single high-dose radiotherapy for one or two lung tumors using a stereotactic body frame. Int J Radiat Oncol Biol Phys. 2002;52:1041–6.
29. Onishi H, Araki T, Shirato H, et al. Stereotactic hypofractionated high-dose irradiation for stage I nonsmall cell lung carcinoma: clinical outcomes in 245 subjects in a Japanese multiinstitutional study. Cancer. 2004;101:1623–31.
30. Wulf J, Baier K, Mueller G, Flentje MP. Dose-response in stereotactic irradiation of lung tumors. Radiother Oncol. 2005;77:83–7.
31. Grills IS, Hope AJ, Guckenberger M, et al. A collaborative analysis of stereotactic lung radiotherapy outcomes for early-stage non-small-cell lung cancer using daily online cone-beam computed tomography image-guided radiotherapy. J Thorac Oncol. 2012;7:1382–93.
32. Le QT, Loo BW, Ho A, et al. Results of a phase I dose-escalation study using single-fraction stereotactic radiotherapy for lung tumors. J Thorac Oncol. 2006;1:802–9.
33. Nuyttens JJ, van der Voort van Zyp NC, Praag J, et al. Outcome of four-dimensional stereotactic radiotherapy for centrally located lung tumors. Radiother Oncol. 2012;102:383–7.
34. van der Voort van Zyp NC, Prevost JB, Hoogeman MS, et al. Stereotactic radiotherapy with real-time tumor tracking for non-small cell lung cancer: clinical outcome. Radiother Oncol. 2009;91:296–300.
35. Palma D, Lagerwaard F, Rodrigues G, et al. Curative treatment of Stage I non-small-cell lung cancer in patients with severe COPD: stereotactic radiotherapy outcomes and systematic review. Int J Radiat Oncol Biol Phys. 2012;82:1149–56.
36. Kelley KD, Benninghoff DL, Stein JS, et al. Medically inoperable peripheral lung cancer treated with stereotactic body radiation therapy. Radiat Oncol. 2015;10:120.
37. Videtic GM, Hu C, Singh A, et al. Radiation Therapy Oncology Group (RTOG) protocol 0915: a randomized phase 2 study comparing 2 Stereotactic Body Radiation Therapy (SBRT) schedules for medically inoperable patients with stage I peripheral non-small cell lung cancer. Int J Radiat Oncol Biol Phys. 2013;87:3.
38. Timmerman R, Paulus R, Galvin J, et al. Stereotactic body radiation therapy for inoperable early stage lung cancer. JAMA. 2010;303:1070–6.
39. Haasbeek CJ, Lagerwaard FJ, Slotman BJ, Senan S. Outcomes of stereotactic ablative radiotherapy for centrally located early-stage lung cancer. J Thorac Oncol. 2011;6:2036–43.
40. Unger K, Ju A, Oermann E, et al. CyberKnife for hilar lung tumors: report of clinical response and toxicity. J Hematol Oncol. 2010;3:39.
41. Song SY, Choi W, Shin SS, et al. Fractionated stereotactic body radiation therapy for medically inoperable stage I lung cancer adjacent to central large bronchus. Lung Cancer. 2009;66:89–93.
42. Nishimura S, Takeda A, Sanuki N, et al. Toxicities of organs at risk in the mediastinal and hilar regions following stereotactic body radiotherapy for centrally located lung tumors. J Thorac Oncol. 2014;9:1370–6.
43. Mangona VS, Aneese AM, Marina O, et al. Toxicity after central versus peripheral lung stereotactic body radiation therapy: a propensity score matched-pair analysis. Int J Radiat Oncol Biol Phys. 2015;91:124–32.

44. Chang JY, Li QQ, Xu QY, et al. Stereotactic ablative radiation therapy for centrally located early stage or isolated parenchymal recurrences of non-small cell lung cancer: how to fly in a "no fly zone". Int J Radiat Oncol Biol Phys. 2014;88:1120–8.
45. Baumann P, Nyman J, Lax I, et al. Factors important for efficacy of stereotactic body radiotherapy of medically inoperable stage I lung cancer. A retrospective analysis of patients treated in the Nordic countries. Acta Oncol. 2006;45:787–95.
46. Chi A, Liao Z, Nguyen NP, et al. Systemic review of the patterns of failure following stereotactic body radiation therapy in early-stage non-small-cell lung cancer: clinical implications. Radiother Oncol. 2010;94:1–11.
47. Davis JN, Medbery 3rd C, Sharma S, et al. Stereotactic body radiotherapy for early-stage non-small cell lung cancer: clinical outcomes from a National Patient Registry. J Radiat Oncol. 2015;4:55–63.
48. Allibhai Z, Taremi M, Bezjak A, et al. The impact of tumor size on outcomes after stereotactic body radiation therapy for medically inoperable early-stage non-small cell lung cancer. Int J Radiat Oncol Biol Phys. 2013;87:1064–70.
49. Timmerman RD. An overview of hypofractionation and introduction to this issue of seminars in radiation oncology. Semin Radiat Oncol. 2008;18:215–22.
50. Shultz DB, Diehn M, Loo Jr BW. To SABR or not to SABR? Indications and contraindications for stereotactic ablative radiotherapy in the treatment of early-stage, oligometastatic, or oligoprogressive non-small cell lung cancer. Semin Radiat Oncol. 2015;25:78–86.
51. Onishi H, Shirato H, Nagata Y, et al. Stereotactic body radiotherapy (SBRT) for operable stage I non-small-cell lung cancer: can SBRT be comparable to surgery? Int J Radiat Oncol Biol Phys. 2011;81:1352–8.
52. Lagerwaard FJ, Verstegen NE, Haasbeek CJ, et al. Outcomes of stereotactic ablative radiotherapy in patients with potentially operable stage I non-small cell lung cancer. Int J Radiat Oncol Biol Phys. 2012;83:348–53.
53. Gould MK, Kuschner WG, Rydzak CE, et al. Test performance of positron emission tomography and computed tomography for mediastinal staging in patients with non-small-cell lung cancer: a meta-analysis. Ann Intern Med. 2003;139:879–92.
54. Reed CE, Harpole DH, Posther KE, et al. Results of the American College of Surgeons Oncology Group Z0050 trial: the utility of positron emission tomography in staging potentially operable non-small cell lung cancer. J Thorac Cardiovasc Surg. 2003;126:1943–51.
55. van der Voort van Zyp NC, Prevost JB, van der Holt B, et al. Quality of life after stereotactic radiotherapy for stage I non-small-cell lung cancer. Int J Radiat Oncol Biol Phys. 2010;77:31–7.
56. Zheng X, Schipper M, Kidwell K, et al. Survival outcome after stereotactic body radiation therapy and surgery for stage I non-small cell lung cancer: a meta-analysis. Int J Radiat Oncol Biol Phys. 2014;90:603–11.
57. Hurkmans CW, Cuijpers JP, Lagerwaard FJ, et al. Recommendations for implementing stereotactic radiotherapy in peripheral stage IA non-small cell lung cancer: report from the Quality Assurance Working Party of the randomised phase III ROSEL study. Radiat Oncol. 2009;4:1.
58. Takeda A, Sanuki N, Eriguchi T, et al. Stereotactic ablative body radiation therapy for octogenarians with non-small cell lung cancer. Int J Radiat Oncol Biol Phys. 2013;86:257–63.
59. Hayashi S, Tanaka H, Kajiura Y, et al. Stereotactic body radiotherapy for very elderly patients (age, greater than or equal to 85 years) with stage I non-small cell lung cancer. Radiat Oncol. 2014;9:138.
60. Thompson R, Giuliani M, Yap ML, et al. Stereotactic body radiotherapy in patients with previous pneumonectomy: safety and efficacy. J Thorac Oncol. 2014;9:843–7.
61. Stanic S, Paulus R, Timmerman RD, et al. No clinically significant changes in pulmonary function following stereotactic body radiation therapy for early- stage peripheral non-small cell lung cancer: an analysis of RTOG 0236. Int J Radiat Oncol Biol Phys. 2014;88:1092–9.
62. Yamaguchi S, Ohguri T, Ide S, et al. Stereotactic body radiotherapy for lung tumors in patients with subclinical interstitial lung disease: the potential risk of extensive radiation pneumonitis. Lung Cancer. 2013;82:260–5.

63. Voltolini L, Bongiolatti S, Luzzi L, et al. Impact of interstitial lung disease on short-term and long-term survival of patients undergoing surgery for non-small-cell lung cancer: analysis of risk factors. Eur J Cardiothorac Surg. 2013;43:e17–23.
64. Kato M, Shukuya T, Takahashi F, et al. Pemetrexed for advanced non-small cell lung cancer patients with interstitial lung disease. BMC Cancer. 2014;14:508.
65. Huang K, Dahele M, Senan S, et al. Radiographic changes after lung stereotactic ablative radiotherapy (SABR) – can we distinguish recurrence from fibrosis? A systematic review of the literature. Radiother Oncol. 2012;102:335–42.
66. Palma DA, van Sornsen de Koste J, Verbakel WF, et al. Lung density changes after stereotactic radiotherapy: a quantitative analysis in 50 patients. Int J Radiat Oncol Biol Phys. 2011; 81:974–8.
67. Pastis Jr NJ, Greer TJ, Tanner NT, et al. Assessing the usefulness of 18F-fluorodeoxyglucose PET-CT scan after stereotactic body radiotherapy for early-stage non-small cell lung cancer. Chest. 2014;146:406–11.
68. Takeda A, Kunieda E, Takeda T, et al. Possible misinterpretation of demarcated solid patterns of radiation fibrosis on CT scans as tumor recurrence in patients receiving hypofractionated stereotactic radiotherapy for lung cancer. Int J Radiat Oncol Biol Phys. 2008;70:1057–65.
69. Singhvi M, Lee P. Illustrative cases of false positive biopsies after stereotactic body radiation therapy for lung cancer based on abnormal FDG-PET-CT imaging. BMJ Case Rep. 2013. doi:10.1136/bcr-2012-007967.
70. Bollineni VR, Widder J, Pruim J, et al. Residual (1)(8)F-FDG-PET uptake 12 weeks after stereotactic ablative radiotherapy for stage I non-small-cell lung cancer predicts local control. Int J Radiat Oncol Biol Phys. 2012;83:e551–5.
71. Huang K, Senthi S, Palma DA, et al. High-risk CT features for detection of local recurrence after stereotactic ablative radiotherapy for lung cancer. Radiother Oncol. 2013;109:51–7.

Radiochemotherapy and Fractionation in Locally Advanced Non-small-cell Lung Cancer

6

Erkan Topkan, Ozan Cem Guler, and Ugur Selek

Introduction

Worldwide, accounting for more than 1.4 million deaths per year, lung cancer (LC) is the leading cause of cancer-related mortality [1]. LC has customarily been classified into two main histological types: small-cell LC (SCLC) and non-small-cell LC (NSCLC). Previously called oat cell carcinoma, SCLC accounts for approximately 15 % all LC, while the more common NSCLC constitutes the remaining 85 % of which 40 % are adenocarcinoma (AC), 25–30 % are squamous cell carcinoma (SCC), and 10–15 % are large cell carcinomas [2, 3].

The most important behavioral risk factor is tobacco abuse which directly relates with more than 85 % of all cases of LC [2, 4]. The casual relationship between smoking and LC is well established without any doubt since the middle of the twentieth century [5, 6]. An extensive number of studies have demonstrated that smokers have a relative 15- to 30-fold increased risk for LC compared with nonsmokers [6]. Despite the positive trend of a reduction in smoking habits in the general population as a result of smoking cessation programs, it is estimated that LC will keep on being a major health problem for the next 40–50 years [2]. There is likewise satisfactory confirmation to reason that exposure to "passive smoking" can cause LC. Supporting

E. Topkan, MD (✉) • O.C.Guler
Department of Radiation Oncology, Faculty of Medicine, Baskent University, Adana, Turkey
e-mail: docdretopkan@gmail.com; ocgule@gmail.com

U. Selek, MD
Department of Radiation Oncology, Faculty of Medicine, Koc University, Istanbul, Turkey

Department of Radiation Oncology, The University of Texas MD Anderson Cancer Center, Houston, TX, USA

G. Ozyigit et al. (eds.), *Principles and Practice of Radiotherapy Techniques in Thoracic Malignancies*, DOI 10.1007/978-3-319-28761-4_6

this, the number of never-smoker LC cases has increased lately which might either be an aftereffect of passive smoking, exposure to other air pollutants, or both or unidentified carcinogenic agents [4]. Regardless of the exact causative, it is clear that any increment in cessation of smoking habits in general community will undoubtedly translate into reduced rates of LC in passive smokers as well.

Lung Cancer Screening

Screening for breast, colon, stomach, and prostate cancers has a long history, while LC screening has only recently been implemented into the radiologic and clinical practice of most health-care centers with the advent of low-dose computed tomography (LDCT). The expanded enthusiasm for performing LC screening with LDCT is in large part based on the outcomes of the National Lung Screening Trial (NLST), which exhibited reduced mortality from LC in high-risk patients screened with serial LDCT examinations [7]. As a consequence, the National Comprehensive Cancer Network (NCCN), the American Lung Association, the American College of Chest Physicians with the American Society for Clinical Oncology, and the American Association for Thoracic Surgery have all published recommendations regarding the screening of high-risk individuals. These societies recommend that screening with LDCT be considered for the individuals meeting the following criteria: (a) 55–74 years of age and (b) current and former smokers with a smoking history of 30 pack-years. The NCCN guidelines suggest that screening should also be considered for individuals who are 50 years of age with a 20-pack-year smoking history and at least one additional risk factor including the chronic obstructive pulmonary disease, pulmonary fibrosis, radon or occupational exposure, personal history of cancer, or family history of LC. The American Association for Thoracic Surgery has recommended screening for all LC survivors as well.

As a result of LC screening with LDCT, it is rational to anticipate that the percentage of early-stage LC will increase likewise the stage migration experienced in prostate cancer patients with the routine use of prostate-specific antigen. This may also translate into a relative increase in LC survivors and willingly reduced LC-related mortality rates in the near future.

Biology of Lung Cancer

Albeit any comprehensive discussion of biologic changes in LC cells is beyond the scope of this manuscript, a short introductory summary will be presented owing to its strong impact on oncological practice. The application of advanced molecular biology techniques to LC research has led to the recognition of LC as a molecularly diverse set of tumor types [8, 9]. The unique commonality of these tumors is their origination in the lung. Classification of LC is significantly more complex than the shortsighted gathering into SCLC and NSCLC variants that was once thought to speak to a homogeneous tumor population with an equivalent outcome when treated in a comparative manner [10]. Although the light microscopy-based subdivision of LC may distinguish the biologic behavior of a clinically indolent pure-type bronchoalveolar carcinoma from the highly invasive and rapidly progressing AC or an exceedingly aggressive and dedifferentiated sarcomatoid variant of NSCLC with high accuracy, yet the light microscopy uses only one of numerous phenotypic manifestations of the underlying genetic changes. Like other cancers, LC development is a consequential result of a multistep malignant transformation of normal respiratory epithelium either on account of genetic susceptibility or following exposure to carcinogens, such as tobacco smoke, or both. In this regard, the Noguchi classification of lung AC represents an honorable effort by relating the tumor histology with radiologic and clinical characteristics [10], which resulted in identification of atypical adenomatous hyperplasia and AC in situ as preinvasive neoplastic lung lesions that serve as precursors to invasive AC (A, B, and C types) with excellent survival outcomes at the one end of the malignant transformation spectrum and highly aggressive solid type AC (D, E, and F types) with a well-recognized poor prognosis at the other end.

Staging of NSCLC

The updated American Joint Committee on Cancer seventh edition [11] tumor-node-metastasis (TNM) staging manual for NSCLC was published in early 2010 and recommended for clinical use (Table 6.1). The new staging system incorporates major changes that allows for an improved stratification capacity in prognostic gathering of NSCLC patients. The "T" status of tumors has been categorized into less than 2 cm (T1a), 2–3 cm (T1b), 3–5 cm (T2a), 5–7 cm (T2b), and greater than 7 cm (T3), while no change in the "N" descriptors has been made in the new staging system. Based on the absence (M1a) or presence (M1b) of extrathoracic disease, the "M" status has been redefined by dividing into two descriptors. Because of its poorer prognosis compared with the rest of the T4 descriptors, the presence of malignant pleural effusion has been upstaged to M1a. Another major change is the redefinition of additional nodules in the same lobe (T3) and other ipsilateral lobes (T4).

Recent advances in procedures like computerized tomography (CT), 18 F-fluorodeoxyglucose positron emission tomography-CT (FDG-PET/CT), magnetic resonance imaging (MRI), endobronchial ultrasound-guided fine-needle aspiration, and mediastinoscopy have increased the accuracy of clinical staging of NSCLC. Although the accuracy of staging is vital in deciding appropriate treatment, it is problematic that the execution of diverse imaging tools varies significantly. Typically, CT is used to assess the anatomic extent of the primary tumor and lymph nodes and define borders of the critical organs, while FDG-PET improves the detection of nodal and extrathoracic metastatic disease and discrimination between collapsed lung segments from the solid tumor component which may alter treatment decisions or radiation fields. Similarly, MRI imaging can demonstrate valuably in assessing the tumor extension into the chest wall, vertebral bodies, spinal canal, brachial plexus, esophagus, and heart and in detecting brain metastasis [12]. Albeit every imaging methodology has its pros and cons, use of appropriately selected

Table 6.1 Staging of non-small-cell lung carcinoma according to AJCC 7th edition [11]

Primary tumor (T)	
TX	Primary tumor cannot be assessed or tumor proven by the presence of malignant cells in sputum or bronchial washings but not visualized by imaging or bronchoscopy
T0	No evidence of primary tumor
Tis	Carcinoma in situ
T1	Tumor 3 cm or less in greatest dimension, surrounded by the lung or visceral pleura, without bronchoscopic evidence of invasion more proximal than the lobar bronchus (e.g., not in the main bronchus)[a]
T1a	Tumor 2 cm or less in greatest dimension
T1b	Tumor more than 2 cm but 3 cm or less in greatest dimension
T2	Tumor more than 3 cm but 7 cm or less or tumor with any of the following features (T2 tumors with these features are classified T2a if 5 cm or less): involves main bronchus, 2 cm or more distal to the carina; invades visceral pleura (PL1 or PL2); associated with atelectasis or obstructive pneumonitis that extends to the hilar region but does not involve the entire lung
T2a	Tumor more than 3 cm but 5 cm or less in greatest dimension
T2b	Tumor more than 5 cm but 7 cm or less in greatest dimension
T3	Tumor more than 7 cm or one that directly invades any of the following: parietal pleural (PL3), chest wall (including superior sulcus tumors), diaphragm, phrenic nerve, mediastinal pleura, parietal pericardium; or tumor in the main bronchus less than 2 cm distal to the carina1 but without involvement of the carina; or associated atelectasis or obstructive pneumonitis of the entire lung or separate tumor nodule(s) in the same lobe
T4	Tumor of any size that invades any of the following: the mediastinum, heart, great vessels, trachea, recurrent laryngeal nerve, esophagus, vertebral body, carina, separate tumor nodule(s) in a different ipsilateral lobe
Regional lymph nodes (N)	
NX	Regional lymph nodes cannot be assessed
N0	No regional lymph node metastases
N1	Metastasis in ipsilateral peribronchial and/or ipsilateral hilar lymph nodes and intrapulmonary nodes, including involvement by direct extension
N2	Metastasis in ipsilateral mediastinal and/or subcarinal lymph node(s)
N3	Metastasis in contralateral mediastinal, contralateral hilar, ipsilateral or contralateral scalene, or supraclavicular lymph node(s)
Distant metastasis (M)	
M0	No distant metastasis
M1	Distant metastasis
M1a	Separate tumor nodule(s) in a contralateral lobe, tumor with pleural nodules or malignant pleural (or pericardial) effusion[b]
M1b	Distant metastasis in extrathoracic organs
Anatomic stage/prognostic groups	
Occult carcinoma	TX N0 M0
Stage 0	Tis N0 M0

Table 6.1 (continued)

Stage IA	T1a N0 M0
	T1b N0 M0
Stage IB	T2a N0 M0
Stage IIA	T2b N0M0
	T1a N1 M0
	T1b N1 M0
	T2a N1 M0
Stage IIB	T2b N1 M0
	T3 N0 M0
Stage IIIA	T1a N2 M0
	T1b N2 M0
	T2a N2 M0
	T2b N2 M0
	T3 N1 M0
	T3 N2 M0
	T4 N0 M0
	T4 N1 M0
Stage IIIB	T1a N3 M0
	T1b N3 M0
	T2a N3 M0
	T2b N3 M0
	T3 N3 M0
	T4 N2 M0
	T4 N3 M0
Stage IV	Any T any N M1a
	Any T any N M1b

[a]The uncommon superficial spreading tumor of any size with its invasive component limited to the bronchial wall, which may extend proximally to the main bronchus, is also classified as T1a

[b]Most pleural (and pericardial) effusions with lung cancer are due to tumor. In a few patients, however, multiple cytopathologic examinations of pleural (pericardial) fluid are negative for tumor, and the fluid is nonbloody and is not an exudate. Where these elements and clinical judgment dictate that the effusion is not related to the tumor, the effusion should be excluded as a staging element and the patient should be classified as M0

multiple imaging modalities in conjunction with minimally invasive procedures may prove beneficial in minimizing the inherent inferiorities of each modality and may allow better staging of the disease.

Prognostic Factors

A prognostic factor (PF) is defined as a variable independent of the treatment that will be assessed before any treatment and correlated to an evaluation end point that is valuable in estimating the patient's future. The role of therapeutic variables may

Table 6.2 Prognostic factors for non-small-cell lung carcinomas

Biologic variables	Patient's characteristics	Tumor characteristics	Treatment parameters
Calcium levels	Weight loss	Histological grade	Adjuvant chemotherapy to surgery
Lactate dehydrogenase alkaline phosphatase leukocytosis	Comorbidity	Metastasis status	Type of chemotherapy
Neutrophil count	Smoking status	Number of metastatic sites	Concurrent chemoradiotherapy
Hemoglobin level	Body mass index	Cancer-related symptoms	Overall treatment interval for radiotherapy
	Ethnicity	Vascular or local invasion, malignant pleural effusion	Objective response to treatment
		Primary tumor site	Expertise of the medical team
		Tumor size	
		Lymph node status	
		Laterality of involved nodes	
		Bulk of involved nodes	
		Number of involved nodal stations	
		Number of involved nodes	

also be analyzed by extension [13]. Disease stage, with its prognostic and operational values, is of now the strongest PF in patients with NSCLC for the definitive objective of survival. Other commonly reported PFs include gender, age, performance status, weight loss prior to or during treatment, histology, hemoglobin level, some primary tumor characteristics such as tumor size and local extension, hilar or mediastinal neoplastic infiltration, and number and bulk of involved lymph nodes [13, 14]. Some other variables have also been suggested less frequently as PFs in NSCLC but their true value are still debated as reported outcomes vary between studies. Clearly confirmed and limitedly suggested but not proven yet PFs of NSCLC can be systematically assigned to four separate groups as summarized in Table 6.2.

Locally advanced NSCLC (stage IIIA/B) is diagnosed in a highly heterogeneous group of patients for which multimodality treatment approach is usually recommended as the standard treatment. However, there are extensive inconsistencies in the therapeutics that can be proposed, while some patients are receiving surgery as a part of the treatment others are treated with induction protocols or definitive concurrent chemoradiotherapy (C-CRT), and a few receiving either only palliative TRT or chemotherapy or both. There is strong enthusiasm for discovering strong PFs in LA-NSCLC in order to accumulate patients into more homogeneous gatherings of individuals with similar outcomes, permitting a fitting comparison among studies and eventually selecting those patients at higher risk and in need of more intensive therapy.

In a recent literature review by Berghmans et al. [13], prognostic worthiness of conventional, metabolic, and biologic variables in stage III patients was assessed. The authors reviewed the literature on this topic and separated the available information into three groups: conventional PFs, metabolic criteria (standardized uptake value [SUV] measured on 18F-FDG-PET), and new biomarkers. Outcomes of this review demonstrated that the subgroup of stage (IIIA vs. B), high performance status, young age, female gender, and absence of weight loss appeared to be the most prominent determinants on survival outcomes in patients treated with any treatment modality, while in surgical series, patients presenting with a TN or a mediastinal downstaging, an objective response after induction chemotherapy (ICT), or a complete tumoral resection had an improved survival with a specific emphasis on clinical or pathological positive N2 status being associated with poorer prognosis. Overall among all evaluated conventional PFs, the disease substage and performance status were reported to be the principal factors associated with survival. Metabolically, although higher average SUV (SUVavg) and SUVmax values were reported to be associated with poorer survival outcomes, considering the availability of only limited number of studies particularly addressing the impact of PET-based measurements in LA-NSCLC patients, the authors impacted the need for further confirmatory evidence. Regarding the novel biologic markers, the authors suggested a potential prognostic value for p53, Bcl-2, the apoptotic index, hMSH2, cyclin D1, and DR5 receptor of the rhTRAIL [13].

Although no specific emphasis was made in the abovementioned review, another strong PF is the anaplastic lymphoma kinase (ALK) gene rearrangements. First discovered by Soda et al. in 2007 [15], ALK rearrangements are either inversions or translocations of the ALK-tyrosine kinase (-TK) receptor gene with other fusion partners, whose product invariably consists of a constitutively activated receptor TK with pro-oncogenic effects [16]. As a consequence, tumors with ALK rearrangements are addicted to ALK signaling, thus being effectively inhibited by small molecules ALK-TK inhibitors [17]. Approximately 4–5 % of all NSCLC cases are ALK-rearranged (ALK+) and this is, apart from rare exceptions, mutually exclusive with other oncogenic drivers (e.g., EGFR and KRAS mutations) [18].

In addition, although the incidence of ALK+ NSCLC is much higher in patients with certain clinicopathologic characteristics such as never/light smoking history, young age (median age of onset 52 years), and AC histology (commonly showing distinct solid or acinar growth patterns with or without signet-ring cell histology), it is not possible to rule out the possibility of an ALK rearrangement solely on the basis of the aforementioned features [18, 19]. Therefore, it can be expected that also SCCs could be considered for ALK testing, as recently acknowledged by NCCN guidelines, particularly in patients with a never/light smoking history, small biopsy specimens or mixed histology.

In retrospective clinical studies, the ALK inhibitor crizotinib has been reported to be effective in advanced NSCLC patients. However its efficacy compared with the standard chemotherapy as first-line treatment for advanced ALK+ NSCLC was not known until recently. The PROFILE 1014 study was an open-label phase 3 trial comparing first-line platinum/pemetrexed chemotherapy versus crizotinib in 343 patients with ALK+ advanced non-SCC NSCLC and showed that crizotinib significantly improved progression-free survival (PFS) and overall response rate (ORR) with an acceptable safety profile, thus establishing crizotinib as standard of care for patients with previously untreated ALK+ disease [20].

Treatment of LA-NSCLC

Since stage III disease represents more than 35 % of all newly diagnosed cases of NSCLC, improving outcomes for these patients has been an area of active research. Despite the fact that gains have been made in the workup, staging, and treatment, yet, critical clinical difficulties still remain to be solved. Development of a "class solution" for all stage III patients is virtually impossible because of significant heterogeneities within stage and patients groups which significantly contribute to clinical outcomes, such as the baseline pulmonary function status, the extent of nodal involvement (single vs. multistation disease), invasion of vital organs, and coexisting comorbidities.

A significant proportion of NSCLC is diagnosed confined to the thorax and not amenable to potentially curative resection because of invasion of adjacent structures and/or LN metastases. By definition of AJCC (7th ed.) staging system, these patients have stage III disease and the optimal management of this large and heterogeneous population remains controversial. Another ongoing controversy is associated with the 15 % of all stage III NSCLC patients who are initially considered as suitable candidates for surgery. For patients with stage IIIA (N2) tumors, Detterbeck reported that a substantial proportion of patients judged to be resectable end up undergoing an R1,2 resection, which calls into question both the accuracy and exact definition of the term "resectable" [21]. This data also underscores the vitality of accurate preoperative staging of mediastinal LNs in patients with potentially resectable NSCLC for prevention of unnecessary surgery and related potential complications.

Radiotherapy Alone

Due to its favorable characteristics such as relative well tolerance and ability to offer satisfactory symptom palliation, thoracic radiotherapy (TRT) has been utilized for decades in management of LA-NSCLC patients. In 1968, the Veterans' Affairs group reported the outcomes of their study comparing TRT with best supportive care in LA-NSCLC, in which TRT was demonstrated to improve median OS time [22]. Similarly, another randomized study by Reinfuss et al. [23] confirmed that the

2-year OS was superior with immediate 50 Gy TRT than with observation and late palliative TRT when severe local symptoms developed (18 % vs. 0 %). Based on these results, TRT gained wide acceptance as the mainstay of LA-NSCLC treatment during this time period.

In the benchmark RTOG 73-01 trial, continuous course of 50 or 60 Gy TRT was compared with either 40 Gy split-course or continuous-course TRT and its results demonstrated that continuous-course 60 Gy TRT arm had the lowest 3-year thoracic recurrence rates compared to 50 Gy or 40 Gy split-/continuous-course TRT (33 % vs. 42 % vs. 52 %/44 %; $p=0.02$) [24]. After the publication of these results, continuous-course 60 Gy TRT has then been adopted as the standard RT schedule all over the world. However, despite of this improvement in outcomes, yet the reported respective median and 5-year OS rates were unacceptably low being only 9–10 months and 3–6 % in prospective randomized trials TRT [24–26]. Additionally, the unacceptable high rates of locoregional and distant failures led to conduction of further studies to enhance thoracic and distant control rates with different TRT strategies and addition of systemic chemotherapy [24–26]. Considering the TRT, various altered fractionation regimens have been implemented to improve thoracic control rates [27–29]. The RTOG 83-11 trial has investigated the impact of hyperfractionated RT (HFRT; 1.2 Gy b.i.d.) and reported that the survival of a subgroup of patients with favorable PFs who received HFRT ≥69.6 Gy was superior than those treated with conventionally fractionated 60 Gy [29]. Later, continuous hyperfractionated accelerated RT (CHART) was tested against standard fractionation in LA-NSCLC patients and showed better outcomes with this novel approach [30]. Because this treatment design was extremely complicated for daily clinical practice, several studies attempted to modify this regimen either by omitting weekend days or by adding neoadjuvant chemotherapy to original regime. However, considering that the underlying radiobiologic principle of CHART was acceleration of TRT to combat with accelerated tumor repopulation, such efforts clearly destructed this principle. Resultantly, it was not surprising that the CHART weekend-less (CHARTWEL) trial which compared 66 Gy in 33 daily fractions with 60 Gy in 40 fractions in 18 treatment days (t.i.d.) was not able to demonstrate a survival advantage favoring CHARTWEL [31].

Evidence coming from altered fractionated TRT alone studies reconfirmed that both the locoregional and distant control rates were far lower than the acceptable limits and stressed the need for implementation of chemotherapy into the treatment protocols in order to enhance both locoregional control and combat possible distant (microscopic) spread which is not addressed by the TRT. The outcomes of initial investigations designed with that goal were frustrating as they were not different than those obtained with TRT alone. However, chemotherapy was usually administrated adjuvantly when RT-induced fibrotic changes in lungs prevented successful blood/drug perfusion and consisted of less effective non-platinum-based drugs in these first trials [32, 33]. As a consequential result of such unsuccessful attempts, paradigm changed in favor of platinum-based chemotherapies either neoadjuvant to or concurrent with TRT.

Induction (Neoadjuvant) Chemotherapy Followed by TRT

ICT strategies mainly aims (1) to decrease tumor burden to permit reduced volume TRT, (2) to eradicate distant micrometastatic disease which may probably be present before initiation of intended treatment, (3) to increase drug delivery to the tumor delivery before the settlement of fibrotic lung changes, and (4) to achieve this latter aim with lessened rates of severe toxicities, particularly the pneumonitis and esophagitis. Because of these theoretic advantages and unacceptably higher rates of locoregional and/or distant failures with TRT alone, several RCTs of ICT followed by TRT versus TRT alone were conducted and demonstrated a survival benefit favoring ICT regimens over TRT alone.

The Cancer and Leukemia Group B 8433 trial was the landmark RCT which compared ICT and TRT combination versus TRT alone in 155 LA-NSCLC patients with good performance status and minimal weight loss [34]. ICT consisted two cycles of cisplatin and vinblastine combination. TRT to a total dose of 60 Gy (2 Gy/day) was received by the both arms and began on day 50 in the ICT plus TRT arm. Although the addition of chemotherapy did not impair the ability to deliver TRT and there were no toxic deaths on either arm, the addition of ICT increased the number of hospital admissions for vomiting (5 % vs. 0 %) and infection (7 % vs. 3 %). The CALGB authors reported significantly improved median (13.8 vs. 9.7 months, $p=0.0066$) and 3-year (23 % vs. 11 %) OS rates with ICT in the initial report [34], which was later confirmed with the updated 7-year outcomes [35].

The RTOG/ECOG intergroup trial randomized 458 LA-NSCLC patients with favorable prognosis (Karnofsky performance status of ≥70 and weight loss less than 5 %) to one of (1) standard 60 Gy TRT (2 Gy day), (2) two cycles of ICT followed by standard 60 Gy TRT (2 Gy day), and (3) twice-daily 69.6 Gy TRT (1.2 Gy, b.i.d.) arms. The median OS was statistically superior in the ICT plus TRT arm than both the standard 60 Gy TRT and twice-daily 69.6 Gy TRT arms (13.8 vs. 11.4 vs. 12.3 months; $p=0.03$), respectively [36]. But, long-term OS rate was unfortunately less than 10 % at an update report [37].

In a French phase III trial, Le Chevalier et al. [38] reported the comparative results of 353 LA-NSCLC enrolled on to TRT alone (65 Gy in 2.5 Gy/day) or 3-monthly cycles of cisplatin-based chemotherapy followed by the same TRT and followed again by the same chemotherapy. The distant metastasis rate was significantly lower in the ICT group ($p<0.001$) with significantly increased median (12 vs. 10 months; $P=0.02$) and 2-year OS (21 % vs. 14 %) rates. But unfortunately, long-term results demonstrated that the local control rate was only 8 % at 5 years with only 6 % (ICT plus TRT) and 3 % (TRT alone) survivors [39], pointing out the vital importance of successful locoregional control in achievement of prolonged survival. A later randomized phase III study by Medical Research Council enrolling 447 LA-NSCLC patients also confirmed the superiority of cisplatin-based ICT followed by TRT over TRT alone (13.0 vs. 9.9 months, $p=0.056$) strategy [40], despite of the fact that the TRT dose was minimal (50 Gy) compared to the currently practiced range: 60–74 Gy.

A new method of ICT for stage LA-NSCLC, constituting intratumoral chemotherapy with paclitaxel liposome combined with systemic chemotherapy combination of carboplatin and gemcitabine, was just recently reported by Lu et al. [41]. In this study, paclitaxel liposome was injected at 1–3 mg/ml concentration into the tumor lesion and proven involved lymph nodes of 48 patients by CT-guided percutaneous fine-needle intratumoral injection on days 1 and 8. Patients were also given three cycles of systemic carboplatin and gemcitabine. The overall objective response rate was 81 % with 36 (75 %) partial and 2 (4.2 %) complete responders. However, the observed 16.5 and 23.2 months of median PFS and OS times were not superior than the range recently reported with C-CRT.

Superiority of ICT followed by TRT over TRT alone is also supported by the evidence provided three large meta-analyses. The authors of Non-small Cell Lung Cancer Collaborative Group meta-analysis [42] reported a 13 % reduction in overall mortality with implementation of ICT to TRT which translated into 4 % absolute survival benefit at 2 years. In another meta-analysis by Marino et al. [43], a 30 % reduction in 2-year mortality rates (HR: 0.70) was reported for ICT. Similarly, in meta-analysis of Pritchard and Anthony [44], ICT reduced overall mortality by 13 % (HR 0.87).

Concurrent Chemoradiotherapy

As detailed in the above sections, several phase III trials and meta-analyses have demonstrated a survival benefit for ICT and preferably induction C-CRT. However these strategies are also associated with potential disadvantages including (1) excessive chemotherapy-induced toxicity preventing or delaying the delivery of full TRT dose; (2) prolonged overall treatment time; (3) chemotherapy-induced tumor cell resistance which may potentially result in reduced TRT efficacy; (4) accelerated tumor cell repopulation, expected also to occur during the chemotherapy phase of the combined treatment; (5) potential for technically more difficult and complicated surgery; and (6) potentially less effective TRT due to the time gap between two courses of irradiation, namely, split-course TRT, if R0 resection cannot be achieved.

Although induction strategies proved beneficial compared to TRT alone, reports of locoregional failure rates up to 85 % were unacceptable. Therefore, this has raised the question as to whether delivering full-dose TRT and chemotherapy concurrently and in a definitive manner without surgical attempts could improve outcomes by reducing both local and distal failures. In this respect two benchmark RCTs have compared definitive C-CRT with induction protocols in LA-NSCLC patients [45, 46].

In RTOG-9410 trial, a total of 610 patients were randomly assigned to two concurrent regimens and one sequential chemotherapy and TRT regimen in a three-arm phase III trial [45]. The induction arm included cisplatin at 100 mg/m^2 on days 1 and 29 and vinblastine at 5 mg/m^2 per week for 5 weeks with 63 Gy TRT delivered as once-daily fractions beginning on day 50. Arm 2 used the same chemotherapy regimen as arm 1 with 63 Gy TRT delivered as once-daily fractions beginning on day 1.

Arm 3 used cisplatin at 50 mg/m^2 on days 1, 8, 29, and 36 with oral etoposide at 50 mg twice daily for 10 weeks on days 1, 2, 5, and 6 with 69.6 Gy delivered as 1.2 Gy twice-daily fractions beginning on day 1. The OS outcome was significantly improved in the concurrent arm with once-daily radiation to 60 Gy when compared with the induction arm with regard to median survival time (17.0 vs. 14.6 months; $p=0.046$), 4-year survival (17 % vs. 12 %), and local control (65.6 % vs. 59.2 %) rates. Although late toxicity was similar in all groups at median 6 years, this clinical advantage was achieved at cost of increased rates of acute grade ≥3 toxicities: 30 % in the induction, 48 % in the daily C-CRT, and 62 % in the hyperfractionated C-CRT arms, respectively.

West Japan Lung Cancer Group (WJLCG) performed a phase III study to determine whether concurrent or sequential treatment improves survival in 320 unresectable stage III NSCLC patients [46]. Patients were enrolled on one of the two treatment arms: In the concurrent arm, chemotherapy consisted of cisplatin (80 mg/m^2 on days 1 and 29), vindesine (3 mg/m^2 on days 1, 8, 29, and 36), and mitomycin (8 mg/m^2 on days 1 and 29). TRT began on day 2 at a dose of 28 Gy (2 Gy per fraction) followed by a rest period of 10 days, and then the same schedule was repeated. In the induction arm, the same chemotherapy was given, but TRT was initiated after completing chemotherapy and consisted of 56 Gy (2 Gy per fraction). The overall objective response rate (84.0 % vs. 66 %; $p=0.0002$) and the median OS duration (16.5 vs. 13.3 months; $p=0.03998$) were significantly better in the C-CRT arm. Confirming the long-term superiority of the C-CRT over the induction protocol, at 5 years the percentage of survivors were comparatively almost doubled in the C-CRT arm (15.8 % vs. 8.9 %) which was possibly associated with improved locoregional thoracic disease control (50 % vs. 35 %). However, this survival advantage was achieved again at the cost of increased rates of acute toxicity.

Recently, Yamamoto et al. [47] presented the data from a phase III trial of C-CRT (WJTOG0105) which was conducted to compare third- with second-generation chemotherapy in patients with unresectable stage III NSCLC. Eligible patients received the following treatments: (A) (control) four cycles of mitomycin (8 mg/m^2 on day 1)/vindesine (3 mg/m^2 on days 1, 8)/cisplatin (80 mg/m^2 on day 1) plus TRT 60 Gy (1-week treatment break); (B) weekly irinotecan (20 mg/m^2)/carboplatin (AUC=2) for 6 weeks plus TRT 60 Gy, followed by two courses of irinotecan (50 mg/m^2 on days 1, 8)/carboplatin (AUC = 5 on day 1); and (C) weekly paclitaxel (40 mg/m^2)/carboplatin (AUC = 2) for 6 weeks plus TRT 60 Gy, followed by two courses of paclitaxel (200 mg/m^2 on day 1)/carboplatin (AUC = 5 on day 1). The median OS time and 5-year survival rates were 20.5, 19.8, and 22.0 months and 17.5, 17.8, and 19.8 % in arms A–C, respectively. While no significant differences in OS times were apparent among the treatment arms, noninferiority of the experimental arms was not achieved. This study confirmed effectiveness of third-generation chemotherapy and concurrent TRT in the setting of unresectable stage III NSCLC.

Segawa et al. [48] in a similar study reported on a phase III trial comparing docetaxel and cisplatin combination with mitomycin, vindesine, and cisplatin combination chemotherapy with C-CRT in LA-NSCLC. Patients ($n=200$) were randomly assigned to two arms consisting of docetaxel 40 mg/m^2 and cisplatin 40 mg/m^2 on days 1, 8, 29, and 36 or mitomycin, vindesine, and cisplatin chemotherapy with concurrent TRT. The 2-year OS (60.3 % vs. 48.1 %) was favorable in the docetaxel and cisplatin arm ($p=0.059$) with strong trend approaching statistical significance. Moreover, grade 3 febrile neutropenia (22 % vs.39 %; $p=0.012$) occurred less often in the docetaxel and cisplatin arm in cost of a nonsignificant trend for higher grade 3–4 radiation-induced esophagitis incidence (14 %vs. 6 %; $p=0.056$). Therefore, docetaxel and cisplatin combination appears to be a good alternative for mitomycin, vindesine, and cisplatin combination.

In the meta-analysis by O'Rourke et al. [49], the authors identified 19 randomized studies including 2,728 patients enrolled on C-CRT versus TRT alone and reported that C-CRT significantly reduced overall risk of death by 29 % (HR: 0.71) and improved PFS by 31 % (HR: 0.69). C-CRT improved OS by 26 % compared to induction chemotherapy followed by TRT which corresponds to a 10 % absolute survival benefit at 2 years. However, there was increased severe esophagitis with C-CRT (RR: 4.96).

In another meta-analysis, Liang et al. [50] systematically reviewed 11 trials ($N=2,043$ patients; C-CRT = 1,019, ICT = 1,024) that compared C-CRT with ICT followed by TRT. Results confirmed that C-CRT was associated with statistically significant increase in median OS (16.3 vs.13.9 months; OR: 1.17), response rate (64.0 % vs. 56.3 %; OR: 1.38), and tumor-relapse control (OR: 0.82), Again these gains were attained at the expense of increased hematologic (neutropenia and thrombocytopenia) and non-hematologic toxicities (nausea, vomiting, stomatitis, and esophagitis).

The final meta-analysis on this issue was reported by Aupérin et al. [51] utilizing updated individual patient data. Combined results of the included trials were obtained using the stratified log-rank test in order to calculate pooled HRs. Of seven eligible trials, data from six trials including 1,205 patients were received which corresponds to 92 % of all randomly assigned patients to date. Similar to previous meta-analyses, the results favored the C-CRT over the induction strategies in terms of OS (HR: 0.84; $p=0.004$), with an absolute 5.7 % increment at 3 years (23.8 % vs. 18.1 %) and 4.5 % at 5 years. There was a strong trend favoring C-CRT for PFS (HR: 0.90; $p=0.07$). C-CRT reduced locoregional progression (HR: 0.77; $p=0.01$) with no beneficial impact on distant failures (HR = 1.04; $p=0.69$).C-CRT again increased acute grade 3–4 esophageal toxicity (18 % vs. 4 %; RR: 4.9; $p<0.001$), but no significant difference regarding acute pulmonary toxicity was observed. The results of this meta-analysis clearly demonstrated that compared to ICT plus TRT the C-CRT improved survival of LA-NSCLC patients, mainly because of a superior locoregional control in absence of any benefit at distant sites, underlining the need for more efficacious systemic therapeutics.

Although many concerns remain to be investigated, such as the determination of best drug combination, optimal fractionation of TRT, utility of targeted agents during the C-CRT course, conjugation of novel immunotherapies, etc., available evidence from landmark phase III RCTs and their combined analyses in large meta-analyses clearly set the C-CRT as the current best treatment option for patients with unresectable stage IIIA-B NSCLC. However, because all enrolled patients had to be medically well conditioned according to the predefined eligibility criteria, these results also suggest that intensified therapies remain suitable for select fit patients, rather than being a common strategy for all LA-NSCLC patients regardless of their overall health status. Therefore, choosing the best regimen for patients with a less favorable health profile remains an open question. In this respect, the results of a South West Oncology Group phase II trial investigating comparing concurrent administration of carboplatin and etoposide during TRT in performance scores 0–1 versus 2 LA-NSCLC patients demonstrated equivalent toxicity and survival outcomes between two groups, suggesting that medically frail patients may be treated with acceptable success rates similar their well-conditioned counterparts [52].

In conclusion, based on the results of two benchmark phase III RCTs and three meta-analyses, C-CRT with administration of full-dose chemotherapy and 60–66 Gy TRT is the current standard form of therapy for medically fit inoperable LA-NSCLC patients. Therefore ICT protocols or less intense C-CRT regimes should be reserved only for medically frail patients and those patients with heavy primary and/or mediastinal tumor load not permitting standard C-CRT because of excess severe toxicity risk.

Preoperative Chemoradiotherapy for Stage IIIA-N2 Patients

There is no consensus on the optimal treatment strategy of stage IIIA-N2 NSCLC and the outcomes are quite poor with surgery or TRT alone [53, 54]. Because the 5-year OS rates are essentially under 10 % with either modality, pre- and postoperative chemotherapy and TRT have been incorporated to enhance poor rates. Induction therapies prior to surgery have the potential theoretical benefits such as (1) in vivo assessment of tumor responsiveness to classical chemotherapeutics and targeted agents, (2) higher likelihood of patients to tolerate intended chemotherapy and TRT doses, (3) improved resectability chance due to potential to downsizing or downstaging of the tumor, (4) improved chance for R0 resection due to early intervention against occult microscopic tumor aggregates at the periphery of the primary tumor, (5) increased potential to achieve pN0, and (6) early intervention against occult systemic dissemination, if systemic chemotherapy and/or targeted therapy utilized. Conversely, disadvantages include (1) delayed surgery in nonresponders of selected induction strategy, (2) possibility of lesser benefit for patients with bulkier disease, (3) risk for disease progression and loss of resectability chance, and (4) potential for increased rates of morbidity and mortality if surgical resection requires pneumonectomy, including empyema, fistula, neutropenia, esophagitis, tracheal stump leakage, wound infection, delayed wound recovery, and death.

Several small phase III trials randomized stage IIIA NSCLC patients either to surgery or three cycles of preoperative ICT and demonstrated improved clinical response, median, and overall survival rates with ICT and TRT of postoperative 50 Gy [55, 56]. In a large multicenter European trial constituting 355 resectable stage I (except T1N0), II, and IIIA NSCLC, patients evaluated whether preoperative ICT could improve survival. Patients were randomized to receive either of surgery alone or two cycles pre- and postoperative mitomycin-C, ifosfamide, and cisplatin [54]. In both arms, patients with pT3 or pN2 disease received 50 Gy TRT. Overall response to ICT was 64 %. There were two preoperative toxic deaths. Postoperative mortality was 6.7 % in the ICT arm and 4.5 % in the non-ICT arm (p=0.38). A nonstatistically significant increase in median OS (37 vs. 26 months; p=0.15) and a statistically significant improvement in DFS (26.7 vs. 12.9; p=0.033 months) favored the ICT arm. A quantitative interaction between N status and treatment was observed, with benefit confined to N0–1 patients (RR: 0.68; p=0.027) with a statistically nonsignificant excess risk of death in stage IIIA patients. The more recent phase III randomized intergroup trial (Southwest Oncology Group Trial S9900) also compared the surgery alone with three cycles of induction carboplatin and paclitaxel followed by surgery [57]. The trial was closed early with 354 patients after reports of a survival benefit for postoperative chemotherapy in other studies. The median PFS (33 vs. 20 months; p=0.10) and OS (62 vs. 41 months; p=0.11) were numerically superior in ICT arm than the surgery-alone arm but this superiority could not reach statistically significance. Therefore, unfortunately again no demonstrable significant survival advantage was achieved with addition of ICT to surgery.

Feasibility of induction C-CRT for stage IIIA disease has also been investigated. Southwest Oncology Group Trial 8805 included 126 patients with stage IIIA BNSCLC [58]. Patients were treated with two cycles of induction cisplatin and etoposide concurrent with TRT of 45 Gy before surgery. Surgery was attempted in patients with any objective response or stable disease. A C-CRT boost was given if either unresectable disease or positive margins or nodes was found. Although toxicity was relatively low, and a majority of patients were able to undergo surgery, there was no significant difference in survival between the IIIA and IIIB patients, and the 3-year OS rate was 26 % which is not better than the currently reported rates with definitive C-CRT. Importantly, the strongest predictor of long-term survival after thoracotomy was absence of tumor in the mediastinal nodes at surgery (median OS = 30 vs. 10 months; p=0.0005 and 3-year OS = 44 % vs. 18 %).

Interestingly, because the 3-year survival rate of 26 % after trimodality treatment was found to be encouraging by the investigators a subsequent phase III trial was conducted by the RTOG team to further test this protocol in a randomized manner [59]. In this trial induction, C-CRT followed by surgery was compared with immediate definitive C-CRT in 202 patients with IIIA NSCLC. Patients were randomly assigned in a 1:1 ratio either to concurrent ICT (two cycles of cisplatin and etoposide) administered concurrent with 45 Gy TRT followed by surgery if no progression reported or definitive 61 Gy C-CRT groups, respectively. The primary end point was OS. Although the PFS was significantly improved for patients who underwent surgery (12.8 vs. 10.5 months; p=0.017), there were no significant differences in median- (23.6 vs. 22.2 months; p=0.24) and 5-year OS rates (27 % vs. 20 %; p=0.10). Treatment-related deaths were more common in the induction C-CRT (8 % vs. 2 %) than in definitive C-CRT group. Moreover, perioperative mortality

(30 days of postoperative period) rate for patients who underwent a pneumonectomy (26 %) and particularly a right pneumonectomy (38 %) was unacceptably high. Respiratory and cardiac causes including acute respiratory distress syndrome appeared as the major causes of the higher than expected rates of postoperative mortality among pneumonectomy patients in an exploratory subgroup analysis. Matched patients analysis according to age, sex, performance status, and clinical T-stage suggested that patients undergoing pneumonectomy fared poorly when compared with the matched cohort of definitive C-CRT patients and patients who underwent a lobectomy fared better than those treated with definitive C-CRT. However the results of this unplanned and post hoc analysis should only be viewed as purely hypothesis generating rather than a treatment shaping recommendation. Therefore, the main conclusion of this study should be perceived in the way that that trimodality therapy has no superiority over definitive C-CRT in unselected stage IIIA patients.

The EORTC conducted a trial in which selected patients with histologically or cytologically proven stage IIIA-N2 NSCLC were given three cycles of platinum-based ICT. Responding patients were subsequently randomly assigned to surgical resection or 60 Gy of TRT [60]. A total of 167 patients were allocated to resection and 165 to TRT. Postoperative TRT was administered to 62 (40 %) patients in the surgery arm. There was no difference in median OS (16.4 vs. 17.5 months; HR: 1.06) or PFS (9 vs. 11.3 months; HR: 1.06) between the TRT and surgery arms, respectively. In view of its lower morbidity and mortality, TRT was recommended as the preferred locoregional treatment for these patients by the authors.

In a recent meta-analysis of six trials (four ICT and four induction CRT) consisting 868 patients with N2 disease, McElnay et al. [61] reported that the patients randomized to surgery after induction CRT (HR = 0.87) had better OS rates than those patients randomized to surgery after ICT (HR: 1.01).This finding suggests the use of C-CRT rather than chemotherapy as an induction measure, if insisted on induction methods as a treatment strategy.

Considering the fact that NSCLC cells are relatively resistant to conventional 45–50 Gy even in the microscopic setting, Bharadwaj et al. [62] reviewed their experience in clinical stage IIIA (N2) NSCLC patients ($N=52$) treated with trimodality therapy involving two radiation strategies to determine the response rates, operative results, recurrence patterns, and long-term survival. Eighteen patients were treated to doses of ≥60 Gy and 34 to lower doses (45, 50, or 54 Gy). There were significantly more postoperative complications in the high-dose group ($p<0.001$). Pathological complete response (50 % vs. 15 %, $p=0.016$) and mediastinal nodal clearance (75 % vs. 42 %, $p=0.254$) rates were also higher in the high-dose group. That did not, however, translate into better DFS and OS rates. Importantly, long-term noncancer mortality was significantly higher after higher dose preoperative TRT.

In summary, based on the results of two benchmark phase III RCTs, there appears no survival benefit of surgery in the management of unselected N2 patients [59, 60]. However, if surgery is considered in a subset with the hope of benefit from resection, then lobectomy should be the procedure of choice.

Management of Elderly LA-NSCLC Patients

In the last decade, the incidence and mortality rates of NSCLC have decreased among individuals younger than 50 years, but have increased in those older than ≥70 [63]. Surveillance, Epidemiology and End Results registry (SEER) data exhibited that the median age at diagnosis in NSCLC was 69 years [64], clearly demonstrating that 47 % of all NSCLC patients are ≥70 years at initial diagnosis [63, 64]. Moreover, this trend together with population aging suggests that the increase in relative percentage and absolute numbers of geriatric NSCLC will continue.

As mentioned before, two landmark studies have clearly shown that C-CRT improves survival in medically fit patients with LA-NSCLC [45, 46]. However, in these and other studies on C-CRT, the mean ages of the patients ranged from 54 to 63 years [65, 66]. Thus, these studies on C-CRT may have excluded or underrepresented elderly patients [67]. This may reflect under-treatment of these patients because of a general hesitation in performing radical C-CRT on senior patients. Although this hesitation may relate partly to the presence of comorbidities, significant weight loss, or low performance status (PS) in some patients, it may also reflect the unsubstantiated belief that elderly patients are inherently more vulnerable to C-CRT-associated toxicities even if they are medically fit.

To date the feasibility of C-CRT with full-dose multi-agent chemotherapy in medically fit patients with LA-NSCLC has never been investigated in a prospective single-arm study or RCT. Several studies on C-CRT in elderly patients with LA-NSCLC have yielded conflicting outcomes [68–70], while elderly patients were poorly represented in large benchmark trials on C-CRT in LA-NSCLC [71–73]. Although a phase III randomized trial by the Japan Clinical Oncology Group (JCOG-0301) in >70-year-old patients with stage III NSCLC revealed that C-CRT significantly improved survival compared to RT alone (22.4 vs. 16.9 months; $p=0.0179$) [74], low-dose carboplatin was used rather than the full-dose cisplatin doublet.

The unique study addressing the toxicity and efficacy of full-dose C-RCT in elderly patients has been reported by Topkan et al. [75]. This retrospective analysis included 89 medically fit, stage IIIB NSCLC septuagenarians. TRT to a total dose of 66 Gy in 2 Gy fractions was delivered concurrently with one to two cycles of full-dose cisplatin-based doublet chemotherapy. Overall the treatment was relatively well tolerated with no grade 4/5 acute toxicities. Acute grade 3 hematologic and non-hematologic toxicity rates were reported to be 55.1 % and 39.3 %, respectively. Only 3 of the 89 patients (3.4 %) experienced grade 3 late toxicities: esophagitis ($n=2$) and peripheral neuropathy ($n=1$). At median 21.7 months of follow-up, median OS, local-regional-PFS, and PFS were 17.7, 10.5, and 7.8 months, respectively. On multivariate analyses the number of chemotherapy cycles received concurrently with TRT ($p<0.001$) and absence of weight loss during the course of C-CRT ($p<0.001$) were identified as the independent factors to significantly associate with longer survival times. Considering the relatively acceptable toxicity profile of the protocol and promising median OS duration of 17.7 months, the authors recommended C-CRT for highly selected medically fit septuagenarians with

LA-NSCLC in order to improve survival outcomes. The results of this study are also supported by the age-based subgroup analyses of 4 benchmark studies [45, 71–73] and a meta-analysis [76] of C-RCT that failed to identify age as a negative prognosticator.

A major concern of C-CRT, particularly in elderly patients with LA-NSCLC, is the dose-limiting acute and late toxicity. However, tolerability analyses have yielded inconsistent results: two reported excessive toxicity and lack of survival benefit [77, 78], one found that C-CRT was both feasible and effective [71], and still another reported increased toxicity but survival rates that were equivalent to those of younger individuals [72]. The C-CRT trials [71–73] consistently reported that although patients with LA-NSCLC who were aged >70 and ≤70 years had equivalent survival rates, albeit older patients had experienced higher rates of grade ≥3 acute toxicities. However, the two groups did not differ markedly in late toxicity. Interestingly, the acute ≥grade 3 toxicity rates of the elderly subgroups of these benchmark studies were much higher (ranging from 81 % to 92 %) than the rates of elderly specific and retrospective age-based comparison studies [68, 69, 75]. One of these, a phase II study [68] of hyperfractionated C-CRT with carboplatin/etoposide in septuagenarians, did not detect any grade 4–5 toxicity and reported excellent grade 3 esophageal and pulmonary toxicity rates of 7 % and 4 %, respectively. Moreover, another retrospective analysis [69] reported that the median survival of ≥75-year-old patients with an ECOG PS of 0–1 rose from 7.8 months with another treatment protocol to 19.9 months with C-CRT and that this was not associated with a significant rise in toxicity rates. These observations point out that C-CRT in carefully selected elderly patients with LA-NSCLC could yield outcomes similar to C-CRT in their younger counterparts without adding toxicity.

Although randomized phase III evidence is needed before concluding in a solid manner on optimal treatment of elderly LA-NSCLC patients, available data suggests that chronological age should not shape the treatment options of carefully selected elderly patients with LA-NSCLC who have a good performance status, minor/no weight loss, and no comorbidity; instead, like younger patients, they should be offered radical C-CRT as the standard of care.

Radiotherapy Techniques in NSCLCs

The main objective of sophisticated RT practice is to deliver the prescribed therapeutic dose to the target (TV) volume in a precise and accurate manner and simultaneously minimize dose to surrounding normal tissues and organs at risk (OARs) in order to increase the therapeutic ratio. As expected, this vital and multistep objective became achievable by the aid of rapid and significant advances in anatomic and metabolic definition of local and regional tumor burden and neighboring critical structures and the technology of RT planning (RTP) and delivery including the verification methods over the past 30 years. During this time period, the RT technology improved step by step from two-dimensional RT (2D-RT) to three-dimensional conformal RT (3D-CRT) and lastly to intensity-modulated radiation therapy (IMRT) together with daily image guidance and four-dimensional (4D) image-based motion management (4D-IGRT). Additionally, the old but highly conformal techniques such as proton therapy and carbon-ion therapy regained interest in the last decade because of technologic advances in hadron therapy planning and delivery methods.

Radiotherapy Planning (RTP)

Three-Dimensional Conformal Radiotherapy (3D-CRT)

RT planning is simply the process of arrangement of beams to irradiate a defined target volume to the prescribed dose. According to this simple definition, there is a predetermined TV that is to be encompassed with appropriately designed radiation beams. Considering the 2D-RT, this definition is satisfactory as the unique aim is the coverage of empirically determined (by experience) TV by the prescribed dose with little or no respect to the neighboring tissues in absence of image-based TV delineation. Such a treatment plan may theoretically cover the TV adequately with the prescribed dose but is usually handicapped by various factors such as the following: (1) TV may be larger than the original one and may carry excessive risk of unnecessary but potentially debilitating acute or late toxicity; (2) TV may be larger than the determined one and may carry risk of undercoverage of the real TV and therefore decreased chance for cure or palliation; (3) because usually opposing fields or bony landmark-based box/diamond fields are used, large fields receive high doses unnecessarily which increases the risk of radiation-induced second cancers as the possibility of stochastic effects of radiation increases with doses in the therapeutic range, even not toxic in clinical terms. Because of these disadvantages and improvements in accurate TV and OAR definitions with the implementation of computerized image-based RTP and resultant patient-specific 3D calculations in 1980s, the 2D-RT has almost been abandoned in LA-NSCLC alike with the other tumor sites. Therefore, since then the 3D-CRT became the minimum standard of care in this patient group.

Treatment planning of LA-NSCLC is complicated by the number of dose-limiting OARs such as the spinal cord, uninvolved lung(s), esophagus, heart, large vessels, and brachial plexus. In this respect, 3D-CRTproves beneficial in reducing the volumes of unavoidably irradiated normal tissues on the way of radiation beams via designing field shapes with the guidance of beam's eye view (BEV) and use of multiple noncoplanar beam arrangements [79]. Moreover, 3D-CRT RTP allows volumetric evaluation of the dose distributions throughout the tumor, OARs, and even the entire patient by use of dose-volume histograms (DVH) and therefore facilitates the chance for achieving intended optimal plan by appropriate rearrangements of the beam angles and weights whenever necessitated.

The vital steps of a typical 3D-CRT of LA-NSCLC are as follows:

Immobilization

For an optimal 3D-CRT plan, the imaging data set should be obtained with the patient set in the simulation/treatment position. During the imaging procedure, the patient should lay on a support table in the position that mimics the treatment setup

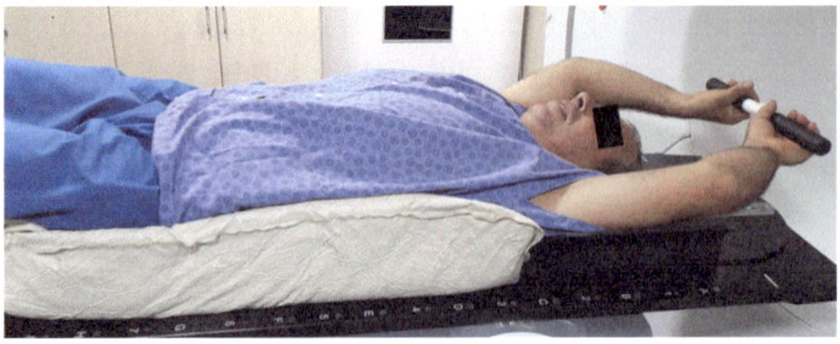

Fig. 6.1 Patient immobilization and positioning during imaging procedure with use of alpha cradle and T-bar accessories

after being immobilized with commercially available custom devices such as commonly used foam cradles. In effort to prevent passage of radiation beams through the arms and likewise not to restrict the liberty of beam angle selection, the arms should optimally be positioned above their head with use of available accessory devices, like T-bars (Fig. 6.1).

Imaging

Imaging is the first crucial step of target and OAR volume definition which will guide the whole remaining RT, simulation, treatment, and quality assurance procedures. Although additional MRI data may prove beneficial in particular cases, CT and PET-CT are the commonly used imaging tools, with CT being commonest one. CT and PET-CT are both useful for tumor volume definitions, while CT is the preferred imaging method for accurate definition of the exact borders of the OARs because of metabolic PET's limited anatomic resolution capacity.

Target Volume Definition

In order to promote the use of universal terminology and systematic TV definitions through the whole radiation oncology community, the International Commission on Radiation Units and Measurements (ICRU) has published nomenclature and guidelines in 1993 and 1999. For TV delineation procedure, three interconnected volumes have been defined: in case of lung cancers, (a) gross tumor volume (GTV) represents for the visible extent of tumor mass on imaging studies, including any involved nodes, (b) clinical target volume (CTV) is defined as the volume constructed by addition of a margin around the GTV to account for invisible but potentially involved microscopic or subclinical tumor extensions at the periphery of primary tumor or regional nodes, and (c) planning target volume (PTV) is the expansion around the CTV that accounts for the uncertainties of the geographic position of the CTV between fractions, intrafraction tumor motion, organ movements, and setup uncertainties. Although the GTV and CTV are constructed for biologic considerations and therefore represent for biologic volumes, PTV is constructed for nonbiologic but mostly mechanical considerations such as physiologic organ motions and setup problems (Figs. 6.2 and 6.3).

GTV Delineation

The parenchymal and the hilar/mediastinal extent of NSCLC should be delineated using pulmonary and mediastinal window, respectively (Fig. 6.2). The best

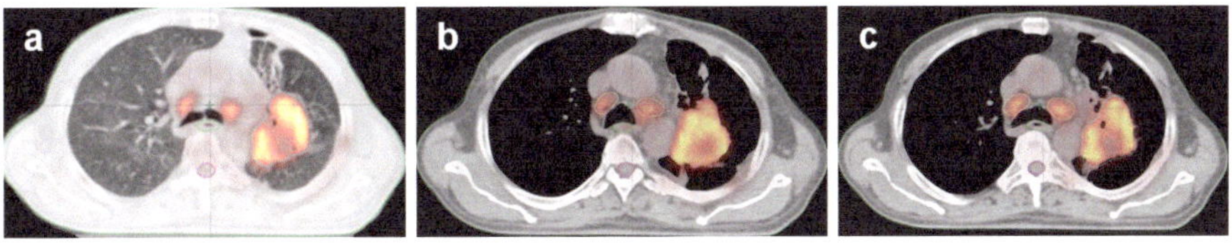

Fig. 6.2 Gross tumor volume (GTV) contouring: (**a**) parenchymal GTV contoured by setting the window width 1,600 and level −600; (**b**) regional nodal GTV contoured by setting the window width 400 and level of 20; (**c**) total GTV = parenchymal GTV + nodal GTV

concordance between the CT image and the actual dimensions of the parenchymal tumor has been established at the window width 1,600 and level −600. For lymph nodes and centrally located parenchymal lesions, it is useful to use mediastinal window setting with recommended window width of 400 and level of 20 [80]. Of note, as calibration of CT may differ between centers, "in-house" measurements of appropriate window settings are strongly recommended for each department. The contrast-enhanced CT may be useful in tumors localized in the hilar region for the purpose of distinguishing of vessels in this area. The bronchoscopy findings should be considered for central locations of tumor with endobronchial component, because even high-resolution CT does not visualize this component and the estimated sensitivity and specificity of FDG-PET are 73 % and 85 %, respectively [81]. If RTP is based on the CT only data, then the usual policy would be to consider all hilar and mediastinal lymph nodes with a diameter at short axis of higher than 10 mm as tumor positive and include in the GTV, because the risk is >15 % for tumor cell positivity. However, if RTP utilizes co-registered FDG-PET-CT data, it is well known that for FDG-PET-negative lymph nodes of 10–15 mm, the probability of metastatic involvement is <5 %; therefore these metabolically uninvolved lymph nodes should safely be ignored. This is mainly based on the fact that PET-CT improves the mediastinal staging in comparison with CT alone, although it is far from being perfect. Supporting this, an overview done by Silvestri et al. [82] demonstrated that the sensitivity of PET scanning was significantly superior than the CT scanning (74 % vs. 51 %) in mediastinal staging of NSCLC patients. FDG-PET-CT has a particular importance for RTP of stage III patients as it may prove beneficial in discriminating tumor tissue from the benign but collapsed parenchyme and in categorization of suspected hilar/mediastinal enlarge lymph nodes. Because the probability of metastatic involvement is 21 % for any FDG-PET-negative lymph nodes measuring >15 mm in short axis, such lymph nodes should be included in the GTV or should undergo pathologic confirmation if granulomatous diseases are suspected [83]. Although various algorithms are used to define involved primary and nodal GTVs (e.g., SUVmax >2.5), RTOG-11-06 protocol recommends the use of the PET intensity of a 1 cm^3 volume contoured in the aortic arch. According to this protocol definition, any primary or nodal disease on PET with an intensity ≥1.5 times the mean of the aortic arch intensity should be included in the GTV.

In cases initially treated with ICT and demonstrated tumor regression, it is questionable whether the GTV should be created according to the pre- or

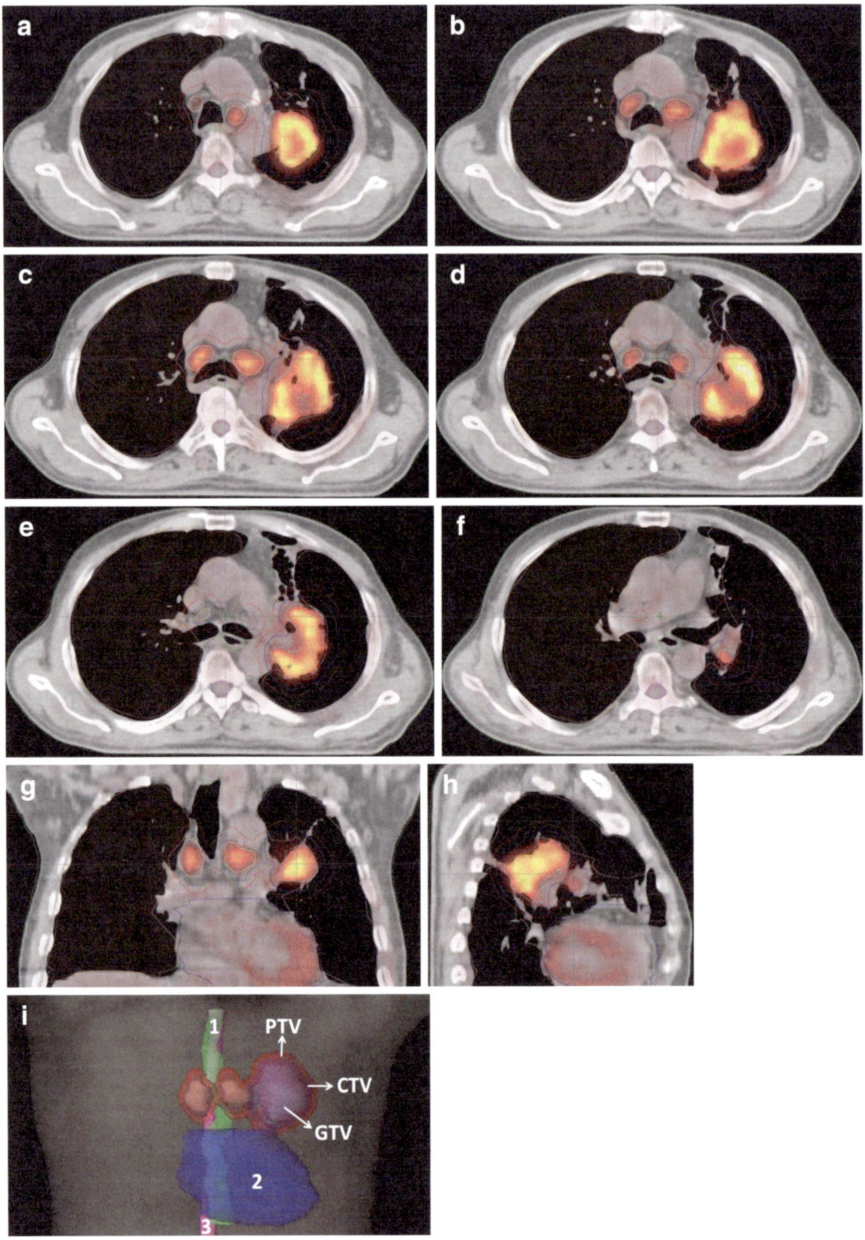

Fig. 6.3 (**a**–**i**) Target volume and organs at risk contouring: *GTV* gross tumor volume, *CTV* clinical target volume, *PTV* planning target volume, *1* esophagus; *2* heart; *3* spinal cord

post-chemotherapy tumor volumes. Although there is no strict recommendation and the clinical practice varies widely among centers and even between the clinicians of the same institution, pre-chemotherapy volumes have almost exclusively been utilized for GTV definition in all aforementioned phase III RCTs. Therefore, except for the patients in whom pre-chemotherapy volumes may lead to an unacceptable risk of radiation-induced pulmonary toxicity, it may be more appropriate to construct GTVs according to the pre-chemotherapy volumes. Such an approach may potentially be more toxic but is oncologically safer considering the fact that the radiologic negativity may not mean microscopic negativity in every patients demonstrating objective response after ICT.

CTV Delineation

CTV margin represents the effort to cover microscopic disease spread in the absence of imaging studies capable of detecting it. Therefore, CTV margins are created mainly on the basis of the correlation of imaging with pathologic data. For TRT of NSCLC, there are three distinct types of CTV margins which are sources of separate problems. These are (a) margin for pulmonary parenchyma, (b) margin for endobronchial spread, and (c) margin for extracapsular extension in mediastinal and/or hilar lymph nodes.

In the seminal work by Giraud et al. [84], the authors investigated the extent of microscopic disease spread of NSCLC within the pulmonary parenchyma by correlating the pathologic findings with preoperative CT images. The authors reported that a margin of 8 and 6 mm around pulmonary GTV was needed to encompass 95 % of microscopic disease for AC and SCC, respectively. Furthermore, the authors reported that although the empirical 5 mm margin was able to satisfactorily cover 91 % of SCC, but this rate decreased to 80 % in AC histology. Another seminal work evaluating the margins for adequate coverage of microscopic spread in 35 AC patients demonstrated that 9 mm was required for covering 90 % of cases if appropriate pulmonary window was used for GTV definition [85]. The authors also noted that compared to its high-grade counterpart, low-grade AC was found to be associated with significantly larger microscopic disease extension which may be related with the presence of relatively increased frequency of bronchioalveolar histology in low-grade AC.

Microscopic tumor spread along the bronchi may be mucosal, submucosal, intraparietal, or mix type. The endobronchial tumor spread has been extensively addressed in surgical and brachytherapy series, but interestingly, although data of central tumors demonstrated that the proximal microscopic tumor extension occurs in 30 % of all NSCLC with a mean dimension of about 10 mm [86], yet there is no clear recommendation for this issue in the external-beam RT literature. Surgical specimen studies suggest 15–20 mm as the appropriate and safe proximal margin from the visible tumor on the bronchial level [87]. Therefore, in the absence of exclusive RT data, it is reasonable to recommend 15–20 mm safety margin along the bronchotracheal tract for of CTV creation in tumors extending to or residing within the bronchial tract.

The extent of CTV margin around involved lymph nodes has been limitedly studied compared to the margin around the primary parenchymal tumor mass. Although

Yuan et al. [88] determined the adequate margin at 3 mm for lymph nodes of size up to 20 mm, the authors also reported that the extracapsular microscopic extension might reach 12 mm in lymph nodes between 21 and 30 mm, with no specific comment on lymph nodes >30 mm. In the absence of evidence-based recommendations, different measures are taken to overcome this problem such as inclusion of the whole lymph node station that contains the involved lymph node (s) in the CTV [80, 89]. However, this approach is questionable in the era of "omission of elective irradiation of uninvolved lymph nodes." Therefore, the current common practice is to expand the involved lymph nodes with a margin similar to the primary parenchymal tumor that is 8 and 6 mm for AC and SCC histologies, respectively.

Of note, it is clear that the expansions around the primary tumor and involved lymph nodes should not necessarily be applied uniformly along all axes and should always be individualized respecting their locations and the neighboring OARs. As rule of thumb, the CTV of the primary tumor should not extend into the mediastinum in the absence of radiographic proof of invasion. Likewise, in the absence of evidence of CT- and/or MRI-confirmed invasion, CTV expansions of involved lymph nodes should not extend into the lungs, major airways, chest wall, esophagus, heart, or vertebral bodies.

PTV Delineation

PTV is the margin around the CTV that accounts for the interfraction setup inaccuracies and intrafraction physiologic organ motions. Setup uncertainties should be determined on the institutional premise as it may vary widely depending on the technique being used and expertise of the team on NSCLC treatment. However, if immobilized appropriately by use of commercially available Vac-Lok bag and T-bar and if weekly port film is used, then an empirical 7 mm along all axes of the CTV will usually be satisfactory to overcome setup errors in more than 95 % cases. This margin may securely be reduced to 5 mm or even to as low as 3 mm if daily kV image or on board image check with utilization of cone-beam CT or CT on rails, respectively. Additionally, as the tumor motion due to physiologic movements of the lung may cause significant alterations in exact location of the tumor during the irradiation procedure, considerations for compensatory margins may be commanded. The magnitude of the tumor motion may vary significantly relying upon its location and size, which mandates the addition of "tumor movement margin" to the CTV expansion and setup uncertainties [90]. Division of each lung into four quadrants may serve beneficial for determination of adequate margins. A 6 mm margin may be satisfactory for upper lobe lesions regardless of the tumor size and middle-lobe lesions <50 mm. A tumor movement margin of 13 mm may be adequate in most cases with tumors <50 mm in size and located in the middle two quadrants of the involved lung or lowest quadrant tumors of 50–80 mm. For lowest quadrant tumors <50 mm, an 18 mm margin will usually be adequate to compensate tumor movement problems. Although most tumors move superior/inferior direction impacting the need for specific care at this direction, yet the best solution to overcome movement problems is its individualized measurement at all dimensions and determination of appropriate margins for each case with use of specific imaging tools such as regular X-ray fluoroscopy.

Internal Target Volume (ITV) Delineation

An internal margin (IM) must be added to the CTV to adjust for physiologic varieties in size, shape, and position of the CTV during treatment in connection to a predetermined reference point and the related coordinate system. The commonly asymmetric IM around the CTV compensates for movements and variations in site, size, and shape of the tissues which contain or are neighboring to the CTV, coming about because of respiration and heart beats in an account of lung cancers. To address this issue, the ICRU-62 Report proposed the notion of ITV which is the volume encompassing the CTV by taking into account the fact that the CTV varies in position, shape, and size. The ITV is defined by the individually measured IM, as described above, and is referred to the patient coordinate system.

The importance of tumor movement and need for ITV have been investigated by various authors. In one of the notable studies, Liu et al. [90] analyzed the 3D-respiration-induced tumor motion and related ITV in 166 tumors from 152 lung cancer patients. All patients underwent 4D-CT during normal breathing TRT. The expiratory phase of 4D-CT images was used as the reference set to GTVs. The GTV on other respiratory phases and resulting ITVs were determined using rigid-body registration of 4D-CT images. Analysis demonstrated that the proportions of tumors that moved >5 mm along the superior-inferior (SI), lateral, and anterior-posterior (AP) axes during normal breathing were 39.2 %, 1.8 %, and 5.4 %, respectively. The magnitude of motion was less than 13.4 mm, 4 mm, and 5.9 mm along the SI, lateral, and AP directions for 95 % of the tumors. The principal component of tumor motion was in the SI direction, with only 10.8 % of tumors moving >10 mm. The tumor movement was discovered to be connected with diaphragm motion, the SI tumor location in the lung, size of the GTV, and disease T-stage. On the grounds of these outcomes, the authors concluded that the tumor movement was principally determined by diaphragm motion, and the motion of lung tumors was unlikely to surpass 10 mm during quiet normal breathing except for small lesions located in the lower half of the lung.

It is presently conceivable to image patients as they breathe in real time and to evaluate organ motion utilizing 4D-CT with the advent of multislice detectors and faster image reconstruction methods. Although 4D-CT-based ITV methodology may serve helpful in any patients with lung cancer, contingent upon the accessibility of essential supplies, assisted breath-hold or respiratory gating or tumor tracking techniques might likewise be utilized as alternative options to minimize tumor movements during TRT.

Delineation of OAR Volumes

The major critical organs include the lungs, heart, esophagus, spinal cord, and brachial plexus (Fig. 6.3).Contouring of the lungs, spinal cord, esophagus, heart and pericardium, and brachial plexus should be performed by utilizing the published atlas on OAR that is available on the RTOG website, http://www.rtog.org/CoreLab/ContouringAtlases.aspx. The following recommendations should be considered during OAR contouring:

Lungs: Both lungs should be contoured using pulmonary windows. The right and left lungs can be contoured separately, but they should be considered as one structure for lung dosimetry. All inflated and collapsed, fibrotic, and emphysematic lungs should be contoured; small vessels extending beyond the hilar regions should be included; however, hilars and trachea/main bronchus should not be included in this structure. Total lung volume should be calculated for metric measurements with the formula below:

$$\text{Total lung volume} = (\text{Right lung volume} + \text{left lung volume}) \quad \text{GTV}$$

Heart: The heart will be contoured along with the pericardial sac. The superior aspect (or base) will begin at the level of the inferior aspect of the pulmonary artery passing the midline and extend inferiorly to the apex of the heart.

Esophagus: The esophagus should be contoured from the beginning at the level just below the cricoid to its entrance to the stomach at GE junction. The esophagus will be contoured using mediastinal window/level on CT to correspond to the mucosal, submucosa, and all muscular layers out to the fatty adventitia.

Spinal cord: The spinal cord will be contoured based on the bony limits of the spinal canal. The spinal cord should be contoured starting at the level just below cricoid (base of skull for apex tumors) and continuing on every CT slice to the bottom of L2. Neural foramens should not be included.

Brachial plexus: The contouring of brachial plexus is only required for patients with tumors of upper lobes. Only the ipsilateral brachial plexus is required. This will include the spinal nerves exiting the neuroforamens from top of C5 to top of T2. In contrast to prior RTOG lung studies of contouring the major trunks of the brachial plexus with inclusion of subclavian and axillary vessels, this trial requests contouring the nerves according to the CT anatomy on every other CT slice. The structure should extend at least 3 cm above the PTV.

Pericardium: The structure of pericardium includes pericardial fatty tissue, part of great vessels, normal recesses, pericardial effusion (if applicable), and heart chambers. Pericardium starts at one slice above the top of the aortic arch and ends at the last slice of the heart apex at the diaphragm. Pericardium includes the heart.

Role of Elective Nodal Irradiation

Terminologically elective nodal irradiation (ENI) represents for inclusion of any of the uninvolved areas of the hilum, mediastinum, and occasionally supraclavicular region(s) in CTV and therefore its extension PTV. For decades, the standard TRT for LA-NSCLC patients was delivered in two steps. In the first step, conventionally fractionated 40–50 Gy was traditionally delivered to the primary parenchymal lesion and the regional lymph nodes including the ipsi- and contralateral hilar, mediastinal, and supraclavicular (in certain cases) with no evidence of tumoral involvement. In the second step, a conventionally fractionated boost dose of 20 Gy was delivered to the primary tumor region in the form of reduced fields designed to spare the spinal cord. ENI protocols are based on the rationale that adequate coverage of the elective nodes may result in eradication of probable regional micrometastases which may translate into superior disease control and therefore survival outcomes. For several decades, the RTOG 73-01 trial has been accepted as the proof of ENI as the authors reported statistically insignificant ($p=0.35$) but numerically superior survival rates in patients with no protocol variations and adequate hilar and mediastinal coverage [91]. However, it is obvious that the ENI volume could appear as a barrier against achieving clinically efficient TRT doses to eradicate both microscopic and gross tumor foci because of the potential for increased toxicity rates and protocol compliance problems.

The opponents of ENI argue that the large field irradiation is irrational considering the high rates of local disease recurrences within the previous radiation portal, high risk of distant relapses, and volume-associated increase in toxicity rates. Additionally, if the gross locoregional tumor cannot be controlled, it is not logical to enlarge radiation ports for a theoretically increased chance of controlling microscopic disease foci at the cost of increased rates of toxic events. This argument is justified by the retrospective series reporting 5–9 % risk of isolated nodal failures [80] and the planning studies [85] suggesting reductions in rates of severe pulmonary and esophageal toxicities as a benefit of omission of ENI. Additional support for omission of ENI comes from the randomized study by Yuan et al. [92], in which the patients receiving involved field C-CRT had significantly less radiation-induced pneumonitis (17 % vs. 29 %; $p=0.04$) than patients treated with ENI. Similar trends appeared in the radiation-induced esophagitis and pericarditis between the ENI and involved field arms. In a retrospective comparative analysis of 108 NSCLC patients, Fernandes et al. [93] demonstrated that esophageal toxicity was significantly reduced with use of involved field TRT (OR: 0.31; $p=0.036$).

The impact of omission of ENI on regional tumor control rates and survival outcomes are strongly debated as to date only one RCT addressed this issue in the literature. In general retrospective analyses report similar tumor control and survival rates for ENI and involved field TRT. In the study of Fernandes et al. [93], the 2-year local control (39.2 % vs. 59.6 %), elective nodal control (84.3 % vs. 84.3 %), distant control (47.7 % vs. 52.7 %), and OS (40.1 % vs. 43.7 %) rates were reported to be statistically similar. In a larger analysis of 524 NSCLC patients from Memorial Sloan-Kettering Cancer Center, Rosenzweig et al. [94] reported only 6.1 % isolated elective nodal failure rate with a 92.4 % primary tumor control rate utilizing escalated doses of TRT. Therefore, the authors recommended involved field TRT as an acceptable treatment method that allows for dose escalation while minimizing toxicity.

In the unique RCT specifically addressing this issue by Yuan et al. [92], a total of 200 eligible patients with inoperable stage III NSCLC were treated with C-CRT and randomized into either an involved field or ENI arm. A total of four to six cycles of cisplatin-based chemotherapy were delivered, and concurrent TRT was started after the second cycle of chemotherapy. 3D-CRT was delivered in once-daily fractions of 1.8–2 Gy to 68–74 Gy for involved field or 60–64 Gy for ENI arms. Patients in the involved field arm achieved better overall response rate (90 % vs. 79 %, $p=0.032$)

and better 5-year local control rate (51 % vs. 36 %, $p=0.032$) than those in the ENI arm. The 1-, 2-, and 5-year survival rates were 60.4 %, 25.6 %, and 18.3 % for the ENI and 69.9 %, 39.4 %, and 25.1 % for the involved field arms, respectively. However, only the 2-year survival rates favored involved field TRT arm in a statistically significant manner ($p=0.048$).

Use of co-registered PET-CT improved the accuracy of both the staging and determination of target volumes of LA-NSCLC patients. A study of 118 NSCLC patients staged with FDG-PET by Sulman et al. [95] demonstrated that total and isolated nodal failures in the unirradiated elective nodal regions were only 4.3 % and 1.7 %, respectively. Therefore, for patients with LA-NSCLC, it is critical to deliver adequate doses of TRT to gross primary and apparently involved nodal areas rather than the theoretically positive elective nodal regions. In summary, based on the available literature, ENI appears to be unnecessary and toxic particularly in patients staged with modern sophisticated imaging methods which are also utilized in delineation of TVs.

Thoracic Radiotherapy Doses

The initial landmark study that investigated the optimal dose of TRT with standard fractionation was the RTOG 73-01 [53]. In this study LA-NSCLC patients were randomly assigned to one of four treatment arms. Three of these arms involved standard fractionation (2 Gy/day given 5 days/week) to total doses of 40 Gy, 50 Gy, and 60, while the fourth arm involved split-course hypofractionation given to a total dose of 40 Gy in 5 weeks (4 Gy/day, 20 Gy, followed by a 3-week rest and a second course of 4 Gy/day, 20 Gy). The authors of RTOG reported that the conventionally fractionated 60 Gy dose arm had the best survival rates, which was achieved at the cost of a relative increase in toxicity rates. After the publication of this RCT conventionally fractionated continuous course, 60 Gy has then been adopted as the standard TRT regimen all over the world. However, locoregional and distant failures were quite high with 60 Gy which led to search for more effective regimens in the forms of dose escalation, C-CRT, or both.

Escalated doses of TRT, in the absence or presence of concurrent chemotherapy, have been extensively studied in an effort to enhance locoregional control rates of LA-NSCLC patients. In 1990 the results of the randomized phase I/II RTOG 8311 trial which tested multiple total dose targets using a 1.2 Gy twice-daily regimen with 4–8 h between fractions in 848 patients were published by Cox et al. [96]. In this study total doses of 60, 64.8, 69.6, 74.5, and 79.2 Gy were tested. No significant differences in survival among the three highest doses were reported, but survival with in the 69.6 Gy group was significantly better than the 60 and 64.8 Gy groups. Following this study and the introduction of 3D-CRT to routine clinical practice in the 1990s, further early-phase trials assessed the tolerability of dose escalation in NSCLC.

The randomized phase II CALGB 30105 trial randomized stage IIIA/B NSCLC patients into ICT with either carboplatin (AUC = 6; days 1 and 22) with paclitaxel (225 mg/m^2; days 1 and 22; arm A) or carboplatin (AUC = 5; days 1 and 22) with gemcitabine (1,000 mg/m^2; days 1, 8, 22, and 29; arm B). On day 43, arm A received weekly carboplatin (AUC = 2) and paclitaxel (45 mg/m^2) while arm B received biweekly gemcitabine (35 mg/m^2) both delivered concurrently with 74 Gy of TRT utilizing 3D-RTP. The primary end point was OS at 18 months. Arm B was closed prematurely due to a high rate of grade 4–5 pulmonary toxicity attributed to the radiosensitizing effect of gemcitabine. However the carboplatin/paclitaxel arm demonstrated 66.6 % overall response rate with a median survival of 24 months and a 12 % rate of grade 3 or higher pulmonary toxicity [97, 98]. This compared favorably to the historical standard C-CRT doses of 60–66 Gy and formed the basis for the experimental arm in the recently reported phase III RTOG 0617 trial [99]. In this 2×2 factorial design trial, patients with stage III NSCLC were treated with weekly carboplatin–paclitaxel chemotherapy and concurrent TRT. Patients were randomized to receive 60 Gy or 74 Gy (2 Gy per fraction for each) TRT with or without cetuximab. After TRT, all patients received additional two cycles of chemotherapy, with/without cetuximab. High-dose TRT arm was closed prematurely when a planned interim analysis after 85 documented events demonstrated a non-superior median OS and indicated a low likelihood of achieving a survival benefit with high-dose TRT [99]. Sadly, the median OS was significantly longer in the standard dose than the high-dose TRT (28.7 vs. 20.3 months; $p=0.004$). Subsequent updated analysis after 207 events demonstrated that, although the numerically higher treatment-related deaths in the high-dose arms (10 vs. 2) could not reach statistical significance, 37 % (HR = 1.37; $p=0.0319$) and 56 % (HR = 1.56; $p=0.0007$) increased risks of local failures and deaths in the high-dose arms were significant.

The assumption that radiotherapy dose escalation using conventional dose fractionation regimens with concurrent chemotherapy will improve outcome in stage III NSCLC has been challenged because of the poorer outcomes observed in high-dose arms of the RTOG 0617 trial. Although the exact causatives of poorer survival in the high-dose arms are not clarified yet, hypothetically these poor results can be attributed to the effect of accelerated repopulation due to longer overall treatment times, increased reported protocol deviations in the high-dose arms, underreporting of lung and cardiac treatment-related death inpatients who received excessive radiation dose to the heart and lung, and a possible negative interaction between cetuximab and high-dose TRT.

Altered Fractionation and Isotoxic TRT

As underlined above dose escalation with conventional fractionation which results in a longer overall treatment time may be one possible explanation for the poor outcomes observed in the high-dose arms of the RTOG 0617 [99]. In the absence of compensatory measures for longer overall treatment times, the potential advantage of a higher overall treatment dose might disappear and may further negate the outcomes, considering the well-recognized accelerated repopulation of tumor cells as a consequence of prolonged treatments [100]. In this manner CHART or similarly designed shorter TRT regimens may overcome the accelerated repopulation effect and, as has been demonstrated previously, may result in a significant survival benefit compared to conventional regimens [101]. An individual patient data meta-analysis of ten randomized trials with enrolled 2,000 patients has confirmed that hyperfractionated and/or accelerated TRT increased 5-year OS rates by 3 % compared to conventional fractionation (HR = 0.88; $p=0.0009$) [102].

Dose escalation TRT approach is limited by the dose received by the OARs. The majority of available dose escalation trials, such as the RTOG 0617, have employed a fixed treatment dose while mandating dose constraints for OAR, and as a consequence, only selected patients were eligible to higher TRT doses. In contrast, isotoxic dose escalation defines the treatment dose by the maximum dose by accounting for the highest possible BED achievable with keeping dose to OARs within predefined safe limits. INDAR (individualized accelerated radiotherapy) is such strategy which aims to reduce the impact of accelerated repopulation. In a recent phase II trial, van Baardwijk et al. [103] treated 137 stage IIINSCLC patients fit for C-CRT with INDAR. An individualized prescribed TRT dose based on normal tissue dose constraints was applied: mean lung dose (MLD) 19 Gy, spinal cord 54 Gy, brachial plexus 66 Gy, and central structures 74 Gy. A total dose between 51 and 69 Gy was delivered in 1.5 Gy b.i.d. up to 45 Gy, followed by 2 Gy QD. TRT was started at the second or third course of chemotherapy. Primary end point was OS. The median dose was 65.0 ± 6.0 Gy delivered in 35 ± 5.7 days. With a median follow-up of 30.9 months, the median and 2-year OS were 25.0 months and 52.4 %, respectively. Grade ≥3 acute toxicity was reported in 35.8 % patients, mainly in the form of grade 3 dysphagia during TRT (25.5 %). Grade ≥3 late toxicity was observed in ten patients (7.3 %).

In summary, although efforts are ongoing to improve outcomes, available literature suggests the conventionally fractionated 60–66 Gy as the currently recommended TRT dose for LA-NSCLC patients treated with C-CRT. In this respect carefully planned hyperfractionated regimes may also be beneficial on the basis of reported 3 % survival benefit at 5 years [102]. However, it is vital to complete overall C-CRT course in the shortest possible time to enhance the tumor control and survival outcomes by mitigating the negative impact of long-treatment course-related accelerated tumor repopulation.

IMRT in LA-NSCLC

3D-CRT typically utilizes 3–4 unmodulated fields, while IMRT utilizes optimized 6–12 modulated fields or arc rotations such as volumetric-modulated arc therapy (VMAT) designed to deliver dose directly to the targets (Fig. 6.1). RTPs generated with IMRT technique can deliver prescribed high doses to the targets and spare OARs more efficiently than that can be achieved with 3D-CRT. This is possible with IMRT, because of the capability of the technique to optimize the shapes and intensities of each field by means of computer algorithms to conform the dose to the targets and spare the neighboring OARs. VMAT delivers the intended dose by rotating the gantry through one or more arcs, whereas the radiation beam remains on while changing rotation speed, shape of the treatment aperture, and delivery dose rate (Fig. 6.1). By this way VMAT can deliver highly conformal dose distributions and improve treatment efficiency by reducing the delivery time by up to 50 %. Additionally, IMRT and VMAT can improve the physical and biologic dose conformity and allow integrated dose escalation and dose "painting" within the PTV that collectively lead to the delivery of higher doses to high-risk areas of the tumor such as GTV, hypoxic areas, or areas showing high SUV on PET-CT with no increments in the number of treatment fractions and while minimizing dose exposure to OARs.

No prospective RCT results have been published comparing the efficacy and toxicity of 3D-CRT versus IMRT for lung tumors. However, retrospective clinical reviews from MD Anderson demonstrated the capability of IMRT in reducing the incidence and severity of pneumonitis and esophagitis in LA-NSCLC patients undergoing C-CRT [104, 105]. Additionally, IMRT was suggested to potentially improve the survival in LA-NSCLC patients [106]. A comparison of outcomes for patients treated before and after the implementation of IMRT showed no differences in out-of-field, elective nodal, or in-field recurrences [24]. Indeed, even with propensity score-matched analyses, no significant differences were found in local-regional relapse, distant metastasis, DFS, or OS between treatment groups. Patients treated with IMRT tend to experience fewer severe acute esophagitis requiring a feeding tube. Sura et al. [107] retrospectively analyzed clinical outcomes of NSCLC patients after IMRT with escalated doses up to. Even though IMRT tended to be used for larger tumors and tumors close to critical organs, IMRT produced favorable local control and survival rates without increasing toxicity. Together, these findings suggest that the theoretical concerns regarding the use of IMRT for lung cancer do not affect clinical outcomes, provided that strict quality assurance and compensation for respiratory motion are rigorously applied.

Another form of comparison comes from the results of aforementioned RTOG 0617 trial in which about half of all patients received IMRT and the other half received 3D-CRT. The two groups were well balanced in terms of patient characteristics except that the IMRT group tended to have larger tumors. Representing the first prospective findings to support the idea that IMRT can reduce treatment toxicity and improve quality of life measures, preliminary analysis of patient-reported quality of life from that RTOG 0617 suggested that the quality of life was better after IMRT than after 3D-CRT.

Other important concerns about the IMRT use in LA-NSCLC include the increased risk for pulmonary toxicity by exposing large amounts of lung to "low-dose baths," increased regional lymph node recurrences because of reduced incidental doses, or reduced overall locoregional control because of lower dose rates. However, no data has been reported to support these negative concerns in any of the clinical studies published to date. Based on the available RTP and clinical outcome data, the benefits of IMRT/IGRT can be summarized as follows [108]:

- With appropriate motion management and plan optimization, IMRT and VMAT can provide more conformal thoracic radiotherapy and can spare more critical structures than can 3DCRT. IMRT or VMAT does not increase lung low-dose exposure of the lung relative to 3DCRT when lung sparing has been taken into consideration
- Motion management techniques and fractionated regimens can be used to minimize the interplay effects of IMRT and VMAT.
- IGRT and adaptive replanning may minimize target miss and the risk of overdosing OARs in selected cases in which tumor motion or size or patient anatomy changes substantially over the treatment course.
- Locoregional control is not compromised with IMRT if the PTV doses are kept in similar to those used in 3D-CRT.
- Minimization of treatment-related toxicities with IMRT appears to improve quality of life of NSCLC patients.
- Further dose escalation with integrated boost techniques may be possible by use of IMRT/VMAT/IGRT within the PTV based on anatomic, biologic, and molecular information without prolonging treatment time.

Treatment Plan Evaluation

Radiotherapy Dose, Target Volume Coverage, and Organ at Risk Dose Limits

Based on the aforementioned literature, the currently recommended TRT dose is conventionally fractionated (1.8–2 Gy daily fractions) total dose of 60–66 Gy administered concurrently with platinum-based chemotherapy. Hyperfractionated schemes can be utilized with a moderate but significant survival gain at cost of increased toxicity rates, particularly the esophagitis. Based on the unfavorable outcomes of RTOG 617 trial, despite of hypothetic radiobiological advantage, escalated doses are currently not recommended outside the clinical trial settings until the emergence of novel supportive evidence.

For 3D-CRT (Figs. 6.4 and 6.5), basically the prescribed dose should encompass the defined PTV with isodose lines not 'cooler' than 95 % and not 'hotter' than 107 % with respecting the OAR limits depicted in Table 6.3. For a typical IMRT plan (Figs. 6.6 and 6.7), Table 6.3 can be utilized for target volume coverage, likewise respecting the OAR limits given in Table 6.4.

Treatment for Intrathoracic Recurrences

Locoregional failures local and/or regional recurrences in or at the margins of the previous RT field are reported in 31–48 % of all LA-NSCLC patients [45, 46, 109, 110] and remain to be a medical challenge regarding its negative impacts on patients' survival outcomes and quality of life measures. As recurrences may appear either in

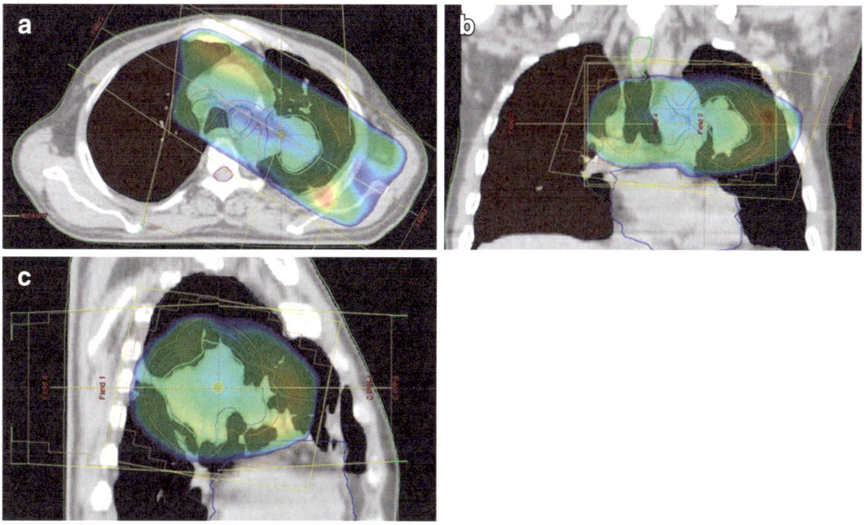

Fig. 6.4 Typical 3D conformal radiation therapy plans: (**a**) axial; (**b**) coronal; (**c**) sagittal view

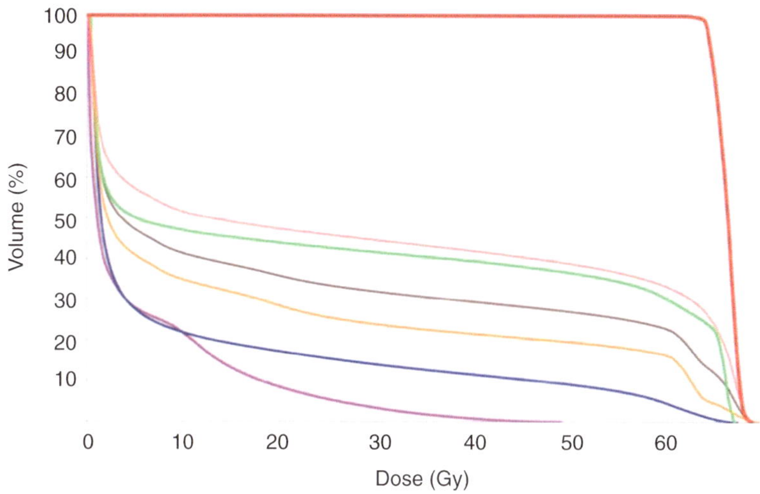

Structure	Min. dose (Gy)	Max. dose (Gy)	Mean dose (Gy)
PTV 66	61.1	68.9	66.0
Total Lung	0.1	69.6	22.0
Right Lung	0.1	69.6	17.1
Left Lung	0.2	69.5	29.5
Esophagus	0.4	67.1	27.1
Heart	0.3	67.4	10.2
Spinal Cord	0.1	49.0	5.5

Fig. 6.5 Dose-volume histogram and related evaluation metrics table for a typical 3D conformal radiation therapy plan

Table 6.3 Typical IMRT plan assessment specifications

PTV	No variation	Minor variation
PTV_{66}	95 % of any PTV_{66} is at or above 66 Gy	95 % of PTV_{66} is at or above 66 Gy
	99 % of PTV_{66} is at or above 61.4 Gy	97 % of PTV_{66} is at or above 61.4 Gy
	No more than 20 % of PTV_{66} is at or above 72.6 Gy	No more than 40 % of PTV_{66} is at or above 72.6 Gy
	No more than 5 % of PTV_{66} is at or above 76 Gy	No more than 20 % of PTV_{66} is at or above 76 Gy
	Mean dose ≤70 Gy	Mean dose ≤72 Gy

IMRT intensity-modulated radiation therapy, *PTV* planning target volume (subscript denotes for prescribed dose)

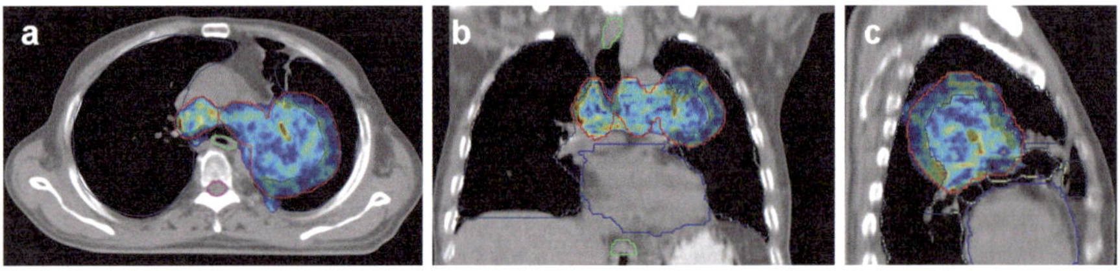

Fig. 6.6 Typical seven-field intensity-modulated radiation therapy plans: (**a**) axial; (**b**) coronal; (**b**) sagittal view; and related dose-volume histogram

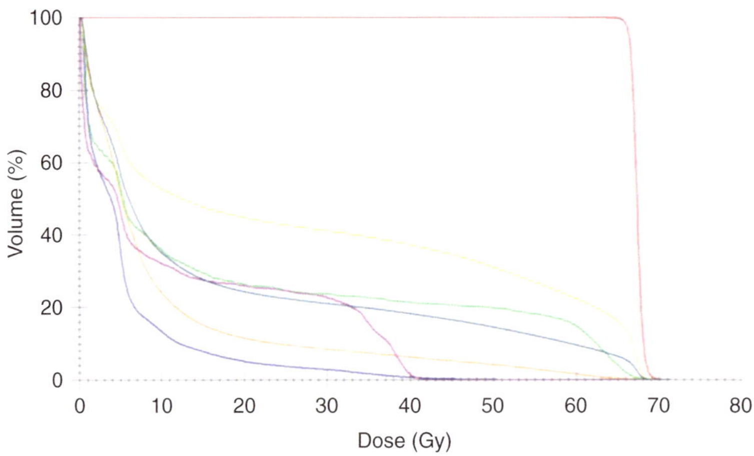

Structure	Min. dose (Gy)	Max. dose (Gy)	Mean dose (Gy)
PTV 66	62.713	71.073	67.273
Total Lung	0.116	70.237	16.390
Right Lung	0.116	70.030	9.630
Left Lung	0.137	70.237	27.195
Esophagus	0.325	68.318	17.549
Heart	0.307	56.626	5.409
Spinal Cord	0.054	42.525	11.496

Fig. 6.7 Dose-volume histogram and related evaluation metrics table for a typical seven-field intensity-modulated radiation therapy plan

Table 6.4 Recommended critical organ dose limits for concurrent chemoradiotherapy

Critical organ	Description	Metric	Per protocol	Variation acceptable	Variation unacceptable
Lungs[a]	Lungs minus GTV	Max dose (0.03 cc)	≤110 % PD	>110 % but ≤113 % PD	>113 % PD
		Mean dose	≤20 Gy	>20 Gy but ≤21 Gy	>21 Gy
		Vol >10 Gy	≤45 %	>45 Gy but ≤50 Gy	>50 Gy
		Vol >20 Gy	≤35 %	>35 % but ≤36 %	>36 %
		Vol >5 Gy	≤65 %	>65 % but ≤75 %	>75 %
Heart	Heart/pericardium	Max dose (0.03 cc)	≤70 Gy	>70 Gy but ≤75 Gy	>75 %
		Mean dose	≤30 Gy	>30 Gy but ≤31 Gy	>31 Gy
		Vol >30 Gy	≤50 %	>50 % but ≤55 %	>55 %
		Vol >40 Gy	≤35 %	>35 % but ≤40 %	>40 %
Esophagus	Esophagus	Max dose (0.03 cc)	≤74 Gy	>74 Gy but ≤76 Gy	>76 Gy
		Mean dose	≤34 Gy	>34 Gy but ≤35 Gy	>35 Gy
		Vol >70 Gy	≤20 %	>20 % but ≤25 %	>25 %
		Vol >50 Gy	≤40 %	>40 % but ≤45 %	>50 %
Spinal canal	Spinal cord	Max dose (0.03 cc)	≤50 Gy	>50 Gy but ≤52 Gy	>52 Gy
Brachial plexus	Brachial plexus	Max dose (0.03 cc)	≤63 Gy	>63 Gy but ≤65 Gy	>65 Gy
Midline structures	Non-PTV	Max hotspot (1 cc)	≤105 % PD	>105 % but ≤110 % PD	>110 % PD

GTV gross tumor volume, *Max* maximum, *PD* prescribed dose
[a]For patients who undergo pneumonectomy before TRT or C-CRT, the recommended doses are mean lung dose = 8 Gy, V20 >10 %, and V5 <60 %

lymph node regions or ipsi-/contralateral lung parenchyma alone or both, it is vital to discriminate the metachronous second primary NSCLC from true recurrences as their treatment options may differ significantly. According to Martini and Melamed [111], a metachronous second primary NSCLC can be defined as a tumor that appears after the initial treatment of the primary NSCLC and shares the following criteria: (I) with different histology or (II) with the same histology as NSCLC but if (a) at least 2 years of free interval between the presentations of two tumors, (b) second cancer originating on the carcinoma in situ ground, or (c) second cancer located in a lobe different than the first cancer or contralateral lung with neither cancer in lymphatics common to both cancers nor extrapulmonary metastases present at diagnosis.

Reports on the reirradiation of thoracic recurrences exist in the literature, but the actual proportion of patients undergoing reirradiation following local/regional recurrences is unknown. However, considering the in-field failure incidences of 31–48 % in published reports of C-CRT [14, 45, 46, 109], the reirradiation rate of only 1.5–6.4 % [110, 112] is quite low and reflects the strong hesitation of clinicians to perform reirradiation in this setting because of a partially mistaken belief that the lung has lower tolerance to reirradiation rather than an evidence-based approach. This is particularly true in the era of sophisticated 3D-CRT, IMRT, and stereotactic radiosurgery era. The feasibility and efficacy of reirradiation were clearly documented in several early reports on treatment of recurrent lung cancer [113–115]. These studies were retrospective and included a heterogeneous group of patients with postsurgical relapses, postoperatively irradiated patients, and those with metastasis and second primary NSCLC. TRT dose ranges were 25–80 Gy for initial and 6–70 Gy for reirradiation with a cumulative dose range of 43–150 Gy.

Recent studies utilizing modern RT techniques proved the safety and efficacy of thoracic reirradiation. In a study by [116], the authors retreated 34 patients with local recurrences by utilizing external-beam TRT. Reirradiation was performed radically in 18 and palliatively in other 16 patients, respectively, with a median interval of 23 months between the two TRT courses. The initial, reirradiation, and cumulative doses were in the ranges of 30–80 Gy (median: 60 Gy; 1.5–2.0-Gy per fraction), 10–70 Gy (median: 50 Gy; 1.8–3.0-Gy per fraction), and 56.5–150 Gy (median: 110 Gy). An objective response was observed in 14 out of 18 radically reirradiated patients (77.8 %). The median OS after radical reirradiation was 15 months with six survivors living beyond 20 months. In the absence of radiation-induced myelopathy, 19 and 6 patients were reported to experience symptomatic radiation-induced pneumonitis and esophagitis, respectively.

Griffoen et al. [117] retrospectively investigated the efficacy of high-dose conventional thoracic reirradiation in NSCLC patients with locoregional recurrences and new primary tumors. Of 24 patients, 54 % had a locoregional recurrence and 46 % a new primary tumor. The 63 % had stage III NSCLC at both initial and second treatments; median intervals between treatments and follow-up after reirradiation were 51 months and 19.3 months, respectively. Median OS after reirradiation was 13.5 months, with 1-year survival 51 %. Except for three deaths due to possible grade 5 bleeding, the treatment protocol was reported to be well tolerated. Notably PTV at reirradiation was found to be the most important prognostic factor; PTV <300 versus ≥300 cm^3 was significantly associated with median OS (17.4 vs. 8.2 months, $p=0.03$).

In a relatively larger study including 102 patients from the University of Texas MD Anderson Cancer Center, McAvoy et al. [118] reported their thoracic reirradiation experience using IMRT and proton beam therapy, focusing on patterns of failure, criteria for patient selection, and predictors of toxicity. All doses were recalculated to an equivalent dose in 2-Gy fractions (EQD2). All patients had received TRT for NSCLC (median initial dose: 70 EQD2 Gy), with median interval to reirradiation of 17 months and median reirradiation dose of 60.48 EQD2 Gy. Ninety-nine patients (97 %) completed reirradiation with a median follow-up time of 6.5 months. Median local failure-free survival and OS times were 11.4 and 14.7 months, respectively. Toxicity was acceptable, with respective grade 3 esophageal and pulmonary toxicity rates of 7 % and 10 %. Of the patients who developed local failure after reirradiation, 88 % had failure in either the original or the reirradiation field. Poor local control was associated with T4 disease, squamous histology, and ECOG PS >1. Higher T status, Eastern Cooperative Oncology Group performance status >1, squamous histology, and larger reirradiation target volumes were found to be associated with worse OS, while receipt of concurrent chemotherapy and higher EQD2 were associated with improved OS.

In summary, although further confirmatory studies are needed to establish both the efficacy and tolerability of thoracic reirradiation, available results suggest that external-beam reirradiation can achieve satisfactory tumor control and survival rates for local recurrence of NSCLC provided that attention is paid to the possible hazards. In this respect IMRT and proton beam therapy appear to be encouraging treatment techniques. However, rates of locoregional recurrence and distant metastasis are still high, and patients should be selected carefully to maximize the benefit of additional aggressive local therapy while minimizing the risk of adverse side effects.

Recommended Treatment Algorithm for LA-NSCLC

An algorithm for treatment of LA-NSCLC is as presented in Fig. 6.8.

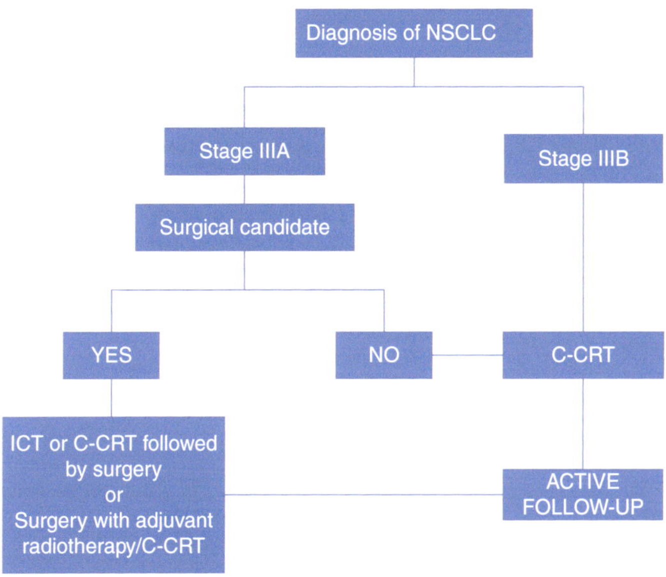

Fig. 6.8 Our institutional treatment algorithm for LA-NSCLC patients; *C-CRT* concurrent chemoradiotherapy, *ICT* induction chemotherapy, *NSCLC* non-small-cell lung cancer

Conclusion

Based on the results of two landmark phase III randomized controlled trials (RCT), the standard of care for unresectable LA- NSCLC is definitive C-CRT with utilizing platinum-based doublets in order to offer these patients the highest chance for prolonged DFS and overall survival (OS) [45, 46]. Hyperfractionated radiotherapy may provide a further 3 % survival gain at long term, but in cost of increased acute toxicity rates. However, even with such an aggressive approach, the outcome of these patients still remains poor with median OS of only 15.3–21.7 months, impacting the need for novel treatment strategies.

Although randomized phase III evidence is needed before concluding in a solid manner on optimal management of elderly LA-NSCLC patients, available data suggests that chronological age should not shape the treatment options of carefully selected elderly patients with LA-NSCLC who have a good performance status, minor/no weight loss, and no comorbidity; instead, like younger patients, they should be offered radical C-CRT as the standard of care.

Likewise, although further confirmatory studies are needed to establish both the efficacy and tolerability of thoracic reirradiation, available results suggest that external-beam reirradiation can achieve satisfactory tumor control and survival rates for local recurrence of NSCLC provided that attention is paid to the possible hazards. In this respect novel TRT technologies such as IMRT may serve beneficial by permitting dose escalation with no excess risk of toxicity.

References

1. Jemal A, Center MM, Desantis C, Ward EM. Global patterns of cancer incidence and mortality rates and trends. Cancer Epidemiol Biomarkers Prev. 2010;19:1893–907.
2. Ramalingam SS, Owonikoko TK, Khuri FR. Lung cancer: new biological insights and recent therapeutic advances. CA Cancer J Clin. 2011;61(2):91–112.
3. Novaes FT, Cataneo DC, Ruiz Junior RL, et al. Lung cancer: histology, staging, treatment and survival. J Bras Pneumol. 2008;34(8):595–600.
4. Wakelee HA, Chang ET, Gomez SL, et al. Lung cancer incidence in never smokers. J Clin Oncol. 2007;25:472–8.
5. Haussmann HJ. Smoking and lung cancer: future research directions. Int J Toxicol. 2007;26(4):353–64.
6. Sasco AJ, Secretan MB, Straif K. Tobacco smoking and cancer: a brief review of recent epidemiological evidence. Lung Cancer. 2004;45 Suppl 2:3–9.
7. Aberle DR, Adams AM, Berg CD, National Lung Screening Trial Research Team, et al. Reduced lung-cancer mortality with low-dose computed tomographic screening. N Engl J Med. 2011;365:395–409.
8. Fujii T, Dracheva T, Player A, et al. A preliminary transcriptome map of non-small cell lung cancer. Cancer Res. 2002;62:3340–6.
9. Garber ME, Troyanskaya OG, Schluens K, et al. Diversity of gene expression in adenocarcinoma of the lung. Proc Natl Acad Sci U S A. 2001;98:13784–9.
10. Noguchi M. Stepwise progression of pulmonary adenocarcinoma–clinical and molecular implications. Cancer Metastasis Rev. 2010;29:15–21.
11. Edge SB, Byrd DR, Compton CC, et al. AJCC cancer staging manual. 7th ed. New York: Springer; 2010. ISBN 0387884408.

12. Koyama H, Ohno Y, Seki S, et al. Magnetic resonance imaging for lung cancer. J Thorac Imaging. 2013;28(3):138–50.
13. Berghmans T, Paesmans M, Sculier JP. Prognostic factors in stage III non-small cell lung cancer: a review of conventional, metabolic and new biological variables. Ther Adv Med Oncol. 2011;3(3):127–38.
14. Topkan E, Parlak C, Selek U. Impact of weight change during the course of concurrent chemoradiation therapy on outcomes in stage IIIB non-small cell lung cancer patients: retrospective analysis of 425 patients. Int J Radiat Oncol Biol Phys. 2013;87(4):697–704.
15. Soda M, Choi YL, Enomoto M, et al. Identification of the transforming EML4-ALK fusion gene in non-small-cell lung cancer. Nature. 2007;448:561–6.
16. Kerr KM. ALK testing in non-small cell lung carcinoma: what now? J Thorac Oncol. 2014;9(5):593–5.
17. Koivunen JP, Mermel C, Zejnullahu K, et al. EML4-ALK fusion gene and efficacy of an ALK kinase inhibitor in lung cancer. Clin Cancer Res. 2008;14(13):4275–83.
18. Gainor JF, Varghese AM, Ou SH, et al. ALK rearrangements are mutually exclusive with mutations in EGFR or KRAS: an analysis of 1,683 patients with non-small cell lung cancer. Clin Cancer Res. 2013;19(15):4273–81.
19. Shaw AT, Yeap BY, Mino-Kenudson M, et al. Clinical features and outcome of patients with non-small-cell lung cancer who harbor EML4-ALK. J Clin Oncol. 2009;27(26):4247–53.
20. Solomon BJ, Mok T, Kim DW, et al. First-line crizotinib versus chemotherapy in ALK-positive lung cancer. N Engl J Med. 2014;371(23):2167–77.
21. Detterbeck F. What to do with "Surprise" N2?: intraoperative management of patients with non-small cell lung cancer. J Thorac Oncol. 2008;3(3):289–302.
22. Roswit B, Patno ME, Rapp R, et al. The survival of patients with inoperable lung cancer: a large-scale randomized study of radiation therapy versus placebo. Radiology. 1968;90(4):688–97.
23. Reinfuss M, Glinski B, Kowalska T, et al. Radiotherapy for stage III, inoperable, asymptomatic small cell lung cancer. Final results of a prospective randomized study (240 patients). Cancer Radiother. 1999;3(6):475–9.
24. Perez CA, Bauer M, Edelstein S, Gillespie BW, Birch R. Impact of tumor control on survival in carcinoma of the lung treated with irradiation. Int J Radiat Oncol Biol Phys. 1986;12(4):539–47.
25. Petrovich Z, Stanley K, Cox JD, Paig C. Radiotherapy in the management of locally advanced lung cancer of all cell types: final report of randomized trial. Cancer. 1981;48(6):1335–40.
26. Perez CA, Pajak TF, Rubin P, et al. Long-term observations of the patterns of failure in patients with unresectable non-oat cell carcinoma of the lung treated with definitive radiotherapy. Report by the Radiation Therapy Oncology Group. Cancer. 1987;59(11):1874–81.
27. Saunders MI, Dische S. Continuous, hyperfractionated, accelerated radiotherapy (CHART) in non-small cell carcinoma of the bronchus. Int J Radiat Oncol Biol Phys. 1990; 19(5):1211–5.
28. Byhardt RW, Pajak TF, Emami B, et al. A phase I/II study to evaluate accelerated fractionation via concomitant boost for squamous, adeno, and large cell carcinoma of the lung: report of Radiation Therapy Oncology Group 84-07. Int J Radiat Oncol Biol Phys. 1993;26(3):459–68.
29. Cox JD, Pajak TF, Asbell S, et al. Interruptions of high-dose radiation therapy decrease long-term survival of favorable patients with unresectable non-small cell carcinoma of the lung: analysis of 1244 cases from 3 Radiation Therapy Oncology Group (RTOG) trials. Int J Radiat Oncol Biol Phys. 1993;27(3):493–8.
30. Saunders M, Dische S, Barrett A, et al. Continuous, hyperfractionated, accelerated radiotherapy (CHART) versus conventional radiotherapy in non-small cell lung cancer: mature data from the randomised multicentre trial. CHART Steering committee. Radiother Oncol. 1999;52(2):137–48.
31. Baumann M, Herrmann T, Koch R, et al. Final results of the randomized phase III CHARTWEL-trial (ARO 97-1) comparing hyperfractionated-accelerated versus conventionally fractionated radiotherapy in non-small cell lung cancer (NSCLC). Radiother Oncol. 2011;100(1):76–85.

32. Reynolds RD, O'Dell S. Combination modality therapy in lung cancer: a survival study showing beneficial results of AMCOF (adriamycin, methotrexate, cyclophosphamide, oncovin and 5-fluorouracil). Cancer. 1978;42(2):385–9.
33. White JE, Chen T, Reed R, et al. Limited squamous cell carcinoma of the lung: a Southwest Oncology Group randomized study of radiation with or without doxorubicin chemotherapy and with or without levamisole immunotherapy. Cancer Treat Rep. 1982;66(5):1113–20.
34. Dillman RO, Seagren SL, Propert KJ, et al. A randomized trial of induction chemotherapy plus high-dose radiation versus radiation alone in stage III non-small-cell lung cancer. N Engl J Med. 1990;323(14):940–5.
35. Dillman RO, Herndon J, Seagren SL, Eaton Jr WL, Green MR. Improved survival in stage III non-small-cell lung cancer: seven-year follow-up of cancer and leukemia group B (CALGB) 8433 trial. J Natl Cancer Inst. 1996;88(17):1210–5.
36. Sause WT, Scott C, Taylor S, et al. Radiation Therapy Oncology Group (RTOG) 88-08 and Eastern Cooperative Oncology Group (ECOG) 4588: preliminary results of a phase III trial in regionally advanced, unresectable non-small-cell lung cancer. J Natl Cancer Inst. 1995;87(3):198–205.
37. Sause W, Kolesar P, Taylor IV S, et al. Final results of phase III trial in regionally advanced unresectable non-small cell lung cancer: Radiation Therapy Oncology Group, Eastern Cooperative Oncology Group, and Southwest Oncology Group. Chest. 2000;117(2):358–64.
38. Le Chevalier T, Arriagada R, Quoix E, et al. Radiotherapy alone versus combined chemotherapy and radiotherapy in nonresectable non-small-cell lung cancer: first analysis of a randomized trial in 353 patients. J Natl Cancer Inst. 1991;83(6):417–23.
39. Arriagada R, Le Chevalier T, Rekacewicz C, et al. Cisplatin based chemotherapy (CT) in patients with locally advanced non-small cell lung cancer (NSCLC): late analysis of a French randomized trial. Proc Am Soc Clin Oncol. 1997;16:16 (abstract).
40. Cullen MH, Billingham LJ, Woodroffe CM, et al. Mitomycin, ifosfamide and cisplatin (MIC) in nonsmall cell lung cancer (NSCLC): 1. Results of a randomized trial in patients with localised, inoperable disease. Lung Cancer. 1997;18 Suppl 1:5 (abstract 10).
41. Lu B, Sun L, Yan X, Ai Z, Xu J. Intratumoral chemotherapy with paclitaxel liposome combined with systemic chemotherapy: a new method of neoadjuvant chemotherapy for stage III unresectable non-small cell lung cancer. Med Oncol. 2015;32(1):345.
42. Non-small Cell Lung Cancer Collaborative Group. Chemotherapy in non-small cell lung cancer: a meta-analysis using updated data on individual patients from 52 randomised clinical trials. BMJ. 1995;311(7010):899–909.
43. Marino P, Preatoni A, Cantoni A. Randomized trials of radiotherapy alone versus combined chemotherapy and radiotherapy in stages IIIa and IIIb nonsmall cell lung cancer. A meta-analysis. Cancer. 1995;76(4):593–601.
44. Pritchard RS, Anthony SP. Chemotherapy plus radiotherapy compared with radiotherapy alone in the treatment of locally advanced, unresectable, non-small-cell lung cancer. A meta-analysis. Ann Intern Med. 1996;125(9):723–9.
45. Curran Jr WJ, Paulus R, Langer CJ, et al. Sequential vs. concurrent chemoradiation for stage III non-small-cell lung cancer: randomized phase III trial RTOG 9410. J Natl Cancer Inst. 2011;103:1452–60.
46. Furuse K, Fukuoka M, Kawahara M, et al. Phase III study of concurrent versus sequential thoracic radiotherapy in combination with mitomycin, vindesine, and cisplatin in unresectable stage III non-small-cell lung cancer. J Clin Oncol. 1999;17(9):2692–9.
47. Yamamoto N, Nakagawa K, Nishimura Y, et al. Phase III study comparing second- and third-generation regimens with concurrent thoracic radiotherapy in patients with unresectable stage III non-small-cell lung cancer: West Japan Thoracic Oncology Group WJTOG0105. J Clin Oncol. 2010;28(23):3739–45.
48. Segawa Y, Kiura K, Takigawa N, et al. Phase III trial comparing docetaxel and cisplatin combination chemotherapy with mitomycin, vindesine, and cisplatin combination chemotherapy with concurrent thoracic radiotherapy in locally advanced non-small-cell lung cancer: OLCSG 0007. J Clin Oncol. 2010;28(20):3299–306.

49. O'Rourke N, Roqué I, Figuls M, Farré Bernadó N, Macbeth F. Concurrent chemoradiotherapy in non-small cell lung cancer. Cochrane Database Syst Rev. 2010;6:CD002140.
50. Liang HY, Zhou H, Li XL, et al. Chemo-radiotherapy for advanced non-small cell lung cancer: concurrent or sequential? It's no longer the question: a systematic review. Int J Cancer. 2010;127(3):718–28.
51. Aupérin A, Le Péchoux C, Rolland E, et al. Meta-analysis of concomitant versus sequential radiochemotherapy in locally advanced non-small-cell lung cancer. J Clin Oncol. 2010;28(13):2181–90.
52. Lau DH, Crowley JJ, Gandara DR, et al. Southwest Oncology Group phase II trial of concurrent carboplatin, etoposide, and radiation for poor-risk stage III non-small-cell lung cancer. J Clin Oncol. 1998;16(9):3078–81.
53. Perez CA, Stanley K, Rubin P, et al. A prospective randomized study of various irradiation doses and fractionation schedules in the treatment of inoperable non-oat-cell carcinoma of the lung. Preliminary report by the Radiation Therapy Oncology Group. Cancer. 1980; 45(11):2744–53.
54. Depierre A, Milleron B, Moro-Sibilot D, et al. Preoperative chemotherapy followed by surgery compared with primary surgery in resectable stage I (except T1N0), II, and IIIa non–small-cell lung cancer. J Clin Oncol. 2002;20:247–53.
55. Rosell R, Gomez-Codina J, Camps C, et al. A randomized trial comparing perioperative chemotherapy plus surgery with surgery alone in patients with non-small cell lung cancer. N Engl J Med. 1994;330:153–8.
56. Roth JA, Fosella F, Komaki R, et al. A randomized trial comparing perioperative chemotherapy and surgery with surgery alone in resectable stage IIIa non-small cell lung cancer. J Natl Cancer Inst. 1994;86:673–80.
57. Pisters KM, Vallières E, Crowley JJ, et al. Surgery with or without preoperative paclitaxel and carboplatin in early-stage non-small-cell lung cancer: Southwest Oncology Group Trial S9900, an intergroup, randomized, phase III trial. J Clin Oncol. 2010;28(11):1843–9.
58. Albain KS, Rusch VW, Crowley JJ, et al. Concurrent cisplatin/etoposide plus chest radiotherapy followed by surgery for stages IIIA (N2) and IIIB non-small-cell lung cancer: mature results of Southwest Oncology Group phase II study 8805. J Clin Oncol. 1995; 13(8):1880–92.
59. Albain KS, Swann RS, Rusch VW, et al. Radiotherapy plus chemotherapy with or without surgical resection for stage III non-small-cell lung cancer: a phase III randomised controlled trial. Lancet. 2009;374(9687):379–86.
60. Van Meerbeeck JP, Kramer GW, Van Schil PE, et al. Randomized controlled trial of resection versus radiotherapy after induction chemotherapy in stage IIIA-N2 non-small-cell lung cancer. J Natl Cancer Inst. 2007;99(6):442–550.
61. McElnay PJ, Choong A, Jordan E, Song F, Lim E. Outcome of surgery versus radiotherapy after induction treatment in patients with N2 disease: systematic review and meta-analysis of randomised trials. Thorax. 2015;70(8):764–8.
62. Bharadwaj SC, Vallières E, Wilshire CL, et al. Higher versus standard preoperative radiation in the trimodality treatment of stage IIIa lung cancer. Ann Thorac Surg. 2015;100(1): 207–14.
63. Wingo PA, Cardinez CJ, Landis SH, et al. Long-term trends in cancer mortality in the United States, 1930–1998. Cancer. 2003;97:3133–275.
64. Owonikoko TK, Ragin CC, Belani CP, et al. Lung cancer in elderly patients: an analysis of the surveillance, epidemiology, and end results database. J Clin Oncol. 2007;25:5570–7.
65. Cox JD, Le Chevalier T, Arriagada R, et al. Management of unresectable non-small cell carcinoma of the lung (NSCLC). Lung Cancer. 2003;42 Suppl 1:S15–6.
66. Semrau S, Klautke G, Virchow JC, Kundt G, Fietkau R. Impact of comorbidity and age on the outcome of patients with inoperable NSCLC treated with concurrent chemoradiotherapy. Respir Med. 2008;102:210–8.
67. Fentiman IS, Tirelli U, Monfardini S, et al. Cancer in the elderly: why so badly treated? Lancet. 1990;335:1020–2.

68. Jeremic B, Shibamoto Y, Milicic B, et al. A phase II study of concurrent accelerated hyperfractionated radiotherapy and carboplatin/oral etoposide for elderly patients with stage III non-small-cell lung cancer. Int J Radiat Oncol Biol Phys. 1999;44:343–8.
69. Paripati HR, Karlin NJ, Schild SE, et al. Multimodality therapy improves survival in elderly patients with locally advanced non-small cell lung cancer—a retrospective analysis. J Geriatr Oncol. 2012;3:104–10.
70. Atagi S, Kawahara M, Tamura T, et al. Standard thoracic radiotherapy with or without concurrent daily low-dose carboplatin in elderly patients with locally advanced nonsmall cell lung cancer: a phase III trial of the Japan Clinical Oncology Group (JCOG9812). Jpn J Clin Oncol. 2005;35:195–201.
71. Langer CJ, Hsu C, Curran WJ et al. Elderly patients with locally advanced non-small cell lung cancer benefit from combined modality therapy: secondary analysis of Radiation Therapy Oncology Group (RTOG 9410). Proc Am Soc Clin Oncol. 2002;21:[abstract 1193].
72. Schild SE, Stella PJ, Geyer SM, et al. The outcome of combined-modality therapy for stage III non-small-cell lung cancer in the elderly. J Clin Oncol. 2003;21:3201–6.
73. Rocha Lima CM, Herndon 2nd JE, Kosty M, Clamon G, Green MR. Therapy choices among older patients with lung carcinoma: an evaluation of two trials of the Cancer and Leukemia Group B. Cancer. 2002;94:181–7.
74. Atagi S, Kawahara M, Yokoyama A, et al. Thoracic radiotherapy with or without daily low-dose carboplatin in elderly patients with non-small-cell lung cancer: a randomised, controlled, phase 3 trial by the Japan Clinical Oncology Group (JCOG0301). Lancet Oncol. 2012;13(7):671–8.
75. Topkan E, Parlak C, Topuk S, Guler OC, Selek U. Outcomes of aggressive concurrent radiochemotherapy in highly selected septuagenarians with stage IIIB non-small cell lung carcinoma: retrospective analysis of 89 patients. Lung Cancer. 2013;81(2):226–30.
76. Auperin A, Le Pechoux C, Pignon JP, et al. Concomitant radio-chemotherapy based on platin compounds in patients with locally advanced non-small cell lung cancer (NSCLC): a meta-analysis of individual data from 1764 patients. Ann Oncol. 2006;17:473–83.
77. Movsas B, Scott C, Sause W, et al. The benefit of treatment intensification is age and histology-dependent in patients with locally advanced non-small cell lung cancer (NSCLC): a quality-adjusted survival analysis of radiation therapy oncology group (RTOG) chemoradiation studies. Int J Radiat Oncol Biol Phys. 1999;45:1143–9.
78. Werner-Wasik M, Scott C, Cox JD, et al. Recursive partitioning analysis of 1999 Radiation Therapy Oncology Group (RTOG) patients with locally-advanced nonsmall-cell lung cancer (LA-NSCLC): identification of five groups with different survival. Int J Radiat Oncol Biol Phys. 2000;48:1475–82.
79. McShan DL, Fraass BA, Lichter AS. Full integration of the beam's eye view concept into computerized treatment planning. Int J Radiat Oncol Biol Phys. 1990;18(6):1485–94.
80. De Ruysscher D, Faivre-Finn C, Nestle U, et al. European Organisation for Research and Treatment of Cancer recommendations for planning and delivery of high-dose, high-precision radiotherapy for lung cancer. J Clin Oncol. 2010;28(36):5301–10.
81. Pasic A, Brokx HA, Comans EF, et al. Detection and staging of preinvasive lesions and occult lung cancer in the central airways with 18F-fluorodeoxyglucose positron emission tomography: a pilot study. Clin Cancer Res. 2005;11(17):6186–9.
82. Silvestri GA, Gould MK, Margolis ML, et al. Noninvasive staging of non-small cell lung cancer: ACCP evidenced-based clinical practice guidelines (2nd edition). Chest. 2007;132 (3 Suppl):178S–201.
83. De Langen AJ, Raijmakers P, Riphagen I, Paul MA, Hoekstra OS. The size of mediastinal lymph nodes and its relation with metastatic involvement: a meta-analysis. Eur J Cardiothorac Surg. 2006;29(1):26–9.
84. Giraud P, Antoine M, Larrouy A, et al. Evaluation of microscopic tumor extension in non-small-cell lung cancer for three-dimensional conformal radiotherapy planning. Int J Radiat Oncol Biol Phys. 2000;48:1015–24.
85. Grills IS, Fitch DL, Goldstein NS, et al. Clinicopathologic analysis of microscopic extension in lung adenocarcinoma: defining clinical target volume for radiotherapy. Int J Radiat Oncol Biol Phys. 2007;69:334–41.

86. Kara M, Dizbay Sak S, Orhan D, et al. Proximal bronchial extension with special reference to tumor localization in non-small cell lung cancer. Eur J Cardiothorac Surg. 2001;20:350–5.
87. Kara M, Dizbay Sak S, Orhan D, et al. Changing patterns of lung cancer; (3/4 in.) 1.9 cm; still a safe length for bronchial resection margin? Lung Cancer. 2000;30:161–8.
88. Yuan S, Meng X, Yu J, et al. Determining optimal clinical target volume margins on the basis of microscopic extracapsular extension of metastatic nodes in patients with non-small-cell lung cancer. Int J Radiat Oncol Biol Phys. 2007;67:727–34.
89. Kepka L, Tatro D, Moran JM, et al. Designing targets for elective nodal irradiation in lung cancer radiotherapy: a planning study. Int J Radiat Oncol Biol Phys. 2009;73:1397–403.
90. Liu HH, Balter P, Tutt T, et al. Assessing respiration induced tumor motion and internal target volume using four-dimensional computed tomography for radiotherapy of lung cancer. Int J Radiat Oncol Biol Phys. 2007;68:531–40.
91. Perez CA, Stanley K, Grundy G, et al. Impact of irradiation technique and tumor extent in tumor control and survival of patients with unresectable non-oat cell carcinoma of the lung: report by the Radiation Therapy Oncology Group. Cancer. 1982;50(6):1091–9.
92. Yuan S, Sun X, Li M, et al. A randomized study of involved-field irradiation versus elective nodal irradiation in combination with concurrent chemotherapy for inoperable stage III nonsmall cell lung cancer. Am J Clin Oncol. 2007;30(3):239–44.
93. Fernandes AT, Shen J, Finlay J, et al. Elective nodal irradiation (ENI) vs. involved field radiotherapy (IFRT) for locally advanced non-small cell lung cancer (NSCLC): a comparative analysis of toxicities and clinical outcomes. Radiother Oncol. 2010;95(2):178–84.
94. Rosenzweig KE, Sura S, Jackson A, Yorke E. Involved-field radiation therapy for inoperable non small-cell lung cancer. J Clin Oncol. 2007;25(35):5557–61.
95. Sulman EP, Komaki R, Klopp AH, Cox JD, Chang JY. Exclusion of elective nodal irradiation is associated with minimal elective nodal failure in non-small cell lung cancer. Radiat Oncol. 2009;4:5.
96. Cox JD, Azarnia N, Byhardt RW, et al. A randomized phase I/II trial of hyperfractionated radiation therapy with total doses of 60.0 Gy to 79.2 Gy: possible survival benefit with greater than or equal to 69.6 Gy in favorable patients with Radiation Therapy Oncology Group stage III non-small-cell lung carcinoma: report of Radiation Therapy Oncology Group 83-11. J Clin Oncol. 1990;8(9):1543–55.
97. Socinski MA, Blackstock AW, Bogart JA, et al. Randomized phase II trial of induction chemotherapy followed by concurrent chemotherapy and dose-escalated thoracic conformal radiotherapy (74 Gy) in stage III non-small-cell lung cancer: CALGB 30105. J Clin Oncol. 2008;26(15):2457–63.
98. Salama JK, Stinchcombe TE, Gu L, et al. Pulmonary toxicity in Stage III non-small cell lung cancer patients treated with high-dose (74 Gy) 3-dimensional conformal thoracic radiotherapy and concurrent chemotherapy following induction chemotherapy: a secondary analysis of Cancer and Leukemia Group B (CALGB) trial 30105. Int J Radiat Oncol Biol Phys. 2011;81(4):269–74.
99. Bradley JD, Paulus R, Komaki R, et al. Standard-dose versus high-dose conformal radiotherapy with concurrent and consolidation carboplatin plus paclitaxel with or without cetuximab for patients with stage IIIA or IIIB non-small-cell lung cancer (RTOG 0617): a randomised, two-by-two factorial phase 3 study. Lancet Oncol. 2015;16(2):187–99.
100. Withers HR, Taylor JM, Maciejewski B. The hazard of accelerated tumor clonogen repopulation during radiotherapy. Acta Oncol. 1988;27(2):131–46.
101. Saunders M, Dische S, Barrett A, et al. Continuous hyperfractionated accelerated radiotherapy (CHART) versus conventional radiotherapy in non-small-cell lung cancer: a randomised multicentre trial. CHART Steering Committee. Lancet. 1997;350(9072):161–5.
102. Mauguen A, Le Péchoux C, Saunders MI, et al. Hyperfractionated or accelerated radiotherapy in lung cancer: an individual patient data meta-analysis. J Clin Oncol. 2012;30(22):2788–97.
103. Van Baardwijk A, Reymen B, Wanders S. Mature results of a phase II trial on individualised accelerated radiotherapy based on normal tissue constraints in concurrent chemo-radiation for stage III non-small cell lung cancer. Eur J Cancer. 2012;48(15):2339–46.

104. Yom SS, Liao Z, Liu HH, et al. Initial evaluation of treatment-related pneumonitis in advanced-stage non-small-cell lung cancer patients treated with concurrent chemotherapy and intensity-modulated radiotherapy. Int J Radiat Oncol Biol Phys. 2007;68(1):94–102.
105. Shirvani SM, Juloori A, Allen PK, et al. Comparison of 2 common radiation therapy techniques for definitive treatment of small cell lung cancer. Int J Radiat Oncol Biol Phys. 2013;87(1):139–47.
106. Liao ZX, Komaki RR, Thames Jr HD, et al. Influence of technologic advances on outcomes in patients with unresectable, locally advanced non-small-cell lung cancer receiving concomitant chemoradiotherapy. Int J Radiat Oncol Biol Phys. 2010;76(3):775–81.
107. Sura S, Gupta V, Yorke E, et al. Intensity-modulated radiation therapy (IMRT) for inoperable non-small cell lung cancer: the Memorial Sloan Kettering Cancer Center (MSKCC) experience. Radiother Oncol. 2008;87(1):17–23.
108. Chang JY. Intensity-modulated radiotherapy, not 3 dimensional conformal, is the preferred technique for treating locally advanced lung cancer. Semin Radiat Oncol. 2015;25(2):110–6.
109. Maguire J, Khan I, McMenemin R, et al. SOCCAR: a randomized phase II trial comparing sequential versus concurrent chemotherapy and radical hypofractionated radiotherapy in patients with inoperable stage III non-small cell lung cancer and good performance status. Eur J Cancer. 2014;50(17):2939–49.
110. Topkan E, Yildirim BA, Guler OC, et al. Safety and palliative efficacy of single-dose 8-Gy reirradiation for painful local failure in patients with stage IV non-small cell lung cancer previously treated with radical chemoradiation therapy. Int J Radiat Oncol Biol Phys. 2015;91(4):774–80.
111. Martini N, Melamed MR. Multiple primary lung cancers. J Thorac Cardiovasc Surg. 1975;70(4):606–12.
112. Gressen EL, Werner-Wasik M, Cohn J, et al. Thoracic reirradiation for symptomatic relief after prior radiotherapeutic management for lung cancer. Am J Clin Oncol. 2000;23(2):160–3.
113. Green N, Melbye RW. Lung cancer: retreatment of local recurrence after definitive irradiation. Cancer. 1982;49(5):865–8.
114. Jackson MA, Ball DL. Palliative retreatment of locally-recurrent lung cancer after radical radiotherapy. Med J Aust. 1987;147(8):391–4.
115. Montebello JF, Aron BS, Manatunga AK, Horvath JL, Peyton FW. The reirradiation of recurrent bronchogenic carcinoma with external beam irradiation. Am J Clin Oncol. 1993;16(6):482–8.
116. Okamoto Y, Murakami M, Yoden E, et al. Reirradiation for locally recurrent lung cancer previously treated with radiation therapy. Int J Radiat Oncol Biol Phys. 2002;52(2):390–6.
117. Griffioen GH, Dahele M, de Haan PF, et al. High-dose, conventionally fractionated thoracic reirradiation for lung tumors. Lung Cancer. 2014;83(3):356–62.
118. McAvoy S, Ciura K, Wei C, et al. Definitive reirradiation for locoregionally recurrent non-small cell lung cancer with proton beam therapy or intensity modulated radiation therapy: predictors of high-grade toxicity and survival outcomes. Int J Radiat Oncol Biol Phys. 2014;90(4):819–27.

Stereotactic Cranial Radiosurgery for Metastatic Non-small-cell Lung Carcinoma

7

Erkan Topkan, Yurday Ozdemir, and Ugur Selek

Introduction

Non-small-cell lung cancer (NSCLC) accounts for 85 % of all lung cancers (LC), which is the current leading cause of cancer-related deaths worldwide [1, 2]. Brain metastasis (BM), one of the most common and dismal complications of NSCLC, is either present at the initial presentation or emerges somewhere during the treatment course in up to 64 % patients [3, 4]. Moreover, as a result of improved survival times, this incidence rate tends to further increase in near future.

Although almost half of all NSCLC BM manifest as single metastasis at presentation, yet NSCLC is the most common type of cancer with the highest propensity to develop BM at multiple intracranial sites, excluding the malignant melanoma [5, 6]. Approximately 80 % of all BM of NSCL Care diagnosed in the cerebral hemispheres that are followed by cerebellum (15 %) and brainstem (5 %), respectively [7]. The presenting symptoms may vary in a wide range depending on the localization, number, and volume of BM as well as the presence of accompanying edema, intratumoral hemorrhage, or both [6]. Nevertheless, headache, nausea, vomiting, seizures, motor weakness, confusion, ataxia, visual defects, and cranial nerve palsies constitute the most common symptom types.

E. Topkan, MD (✉) • Y. Ozdemir
Department of Radiation Oncology, Faculty of Medicine,
Baskent University, Adana, Turkey
e-mail: docdretopkan@gmail.com;
yurdayozdemir@gmail.com

U. Selek, MD
Department of Radiation Oncology, Faculty of Medicine,
Koc University, Istanbul, Turkey

Department of Radiation Oncology, The University of Texas, MD Anderson Cancer Center,
Houston, TX, USA
e-mail: uselek@ku.edu.tr; ugurselek@yahoo.com

G. Ozyigit et al. (eds.), *Principles and Practice of Radiotherapy Techniques in Thoracic Malignancies*, DOI 10.1007/978-3-319-28761-4_7

Prognosis of patients with BM is extremely poor with expected median survival times between 1 and 2 months without any intervention or steroid administration [8]. Diagnosis and treatment of BM have evolved to a significant extent in the last decades, but starkly contrasting with this evolution, prognosis of such patients remained unacceptably poor with only a limited enhancement in the median survival times that is currently in the range of 4–7 months with addition of whole brain radiation therapy (WBRT) [9].

The standard treatment method and the priority of the available methods are not clear for NSCLC patients with BM. In general such patients are managed with either one of the neurosurgery, WBRT, stereotactic radiosurgery (SRS), or any combinations of them. The priority of the single- or combination-treatment modality is usually decided in view of the information about the patient's performance status, extracranial disease status, number, size, total volume, and localization of the BM.

Biology of Brain Metastasis

Tumor metastasis is a complicated multistep procedure which simply begins with detachment of individual tumor cells from the primary tumor and ends up with settlement of the metastatic cells at distant tissues and their adaptation to this new microenvironment [10]. Under normal conditions healthy epithelial cells are connected to each other tightly by adhesion proteins which provide the structural integrity and stabilization of the tissue. In contrast, it has been demonstrated that these adhesion proteins are downregulated in malignant tumors with resultant loss of intercellular tight connections and overtly increased tendency of metastasis to distant organs including the brain [11]. In malignant tissues the basal membrane is invaded and broken down by tumor cells and their secretions, namely, the proteolytic enzymes [12]. After the destruction of this critical barrier, tumor cells reach to systemic circulation through blood or lymphatic vessels. Although many other factors may have further roles, the proven presence of relatively higher direct connections between the primary LC cells and the arterial circulation may be one explanation for the relatively higher incidence of BM in LC than most of other tumor types. Additionally, the usual localization of the capillary beds at the intersection between the gray and white matters of brain may explain the higher propensity of BM to emerge particularly emerge at this zone [13]. The vascular migration of tumor cells may either be in the form of single cell body, cellular emboli, or cellular clots which are accompanied with aggregates of platelets and/or neutrophils. Withholding of tumor cells in brain vasculature may lead to development of tumor emboli, while tumor-induced proteolysis of the vascular wall creates the passage for tumor cell into the brain parenchyma, where the single tumor cell will proliferate and produce colonies of various sizes visible on imaging studies [11].

Prognostic Factors

Prognosis of NSCLC patients presenting with BM is extremely poor with an expected median survival of 4–7 months from the time of BM diagnosis [14]. Although most patients die because of widespread systemic disease, yet the life quality of such patients may be improved by radiotherapeutic interventions which effectively mitigate neurocognitive complications of BM [15]. There is also a subgroup of BM patients who may survive considerably longer than the usual expectations. These patients are potential candidates for more aggressive and potentially less neurotoxic treatment strategies like neurosurgery, SRS, or longer courses of standard radiotherapy schedules with lower per fraction but higher total doses [16].

A prognostic factor (PF) is defined as a variable independent of the treatment that will be assessed before any treatment and correlated to an evaluation end point that is valuable in estimating the patient's future [17]. Based on this definition, accurate definition of PFs in NSCLC patients with BM is of paramount importance not for only the determination of optimal management that fits best for the individual patient but also for stratification of patients for avoidance of unnecessary and futile treatments.

As presented in Table 7.1, to date various patient and tumor-related factors have been identified as PFs including the performance status, age at presentation, the status of primary tumor, the presence/absence of extracranial metastases, and the number and size of BM [18–21]. Different scoring systems aiming to accurately anticipate survival outcomes have been proposed by various investigators for patients with BM treated with WBRT [22]. In 1997, utilizing the recursive partitioning analysis (RPA) methodology and the data of 1,200 patients enrolled on previously reported three RTOG studies [23–25] who were treated by WBRT for BM, Gaspar et al. [26] published the most frequently referred scoring system which identified the KPS, age, primary tumor control status, and the status of extracranial metastases among a total of 21 analyzable factors (Table 7.2). According to this classification, patients with KPS ≥70, age <65 years, controlled primary, and no

Table 7.1 Prognostic factors in patients with brain metastases

Performance status
RPA
Age and sex
Number of brain metastases
Size and tumor volume
Period from primary diagnosis
to diagnosis of BM
Tumor location (especially effects to treatment modality and dose of SRS)
Neurologic deficits
Extracranial disease status
Tumor histology

RPA recursive partitioning analysis, *SRS* stereotactic radiosurgery

Table 7.2 Recursive partitioning analysis (RPA) grouping of the Radiation Therapy Oncology Group for patients with brain metastases

RPA class	Characteristics
RPA class 1	Patients <65 years old
	Karnofsky performance score ≥70
	Controlled primary disease
	No extracranial metastases
RPA class 2	Patients between classes 1 and 2
RPA class 3	Patients >65 years old
	Karnofsky performance score <70
	Active primary disease

Table 7.3 Score index for stereotactic radiosurgery (SIR) for brain metastases

Parameters	Score 0	Score 1	Score 2
Age	≥60	51–59	≤50
KPS	≤50	60–70	80–100
Systemic disease	Uncontrolled	Controlled	CR or NED
Lesions (n)	≥3	2	1
Target volume (cm^3)	13	5–13	<5

KPS Karnofsky performance status, *CR* complete response, *NED* nonevidence of disease, *n* number

extracranial systemic metastasis were included in RPA class I and had the best prognosis (median: 7.1 months). All patients with KPS <70 were classified as class III with worst survival (median: 2.3 months) and all remaining patients were classified as RPA II with intermediate survival rates (median: 4.2 months). Despite of its universal usage, RPA classification has certain limitations like the settlement of lower bound of KPS at 70, large variations between the trials in terms of WBRT doses, and exclusion of the number of BM from analysis [22]. Moreover, accumulation of majority of patients in the RPA class II, with a so-called intermediate survival outcome, may create inconveniences regarding the feasibility of RPA grouping in routine clinical practice [27]. Similarly, although the disease characteristics and outcomes of such patients may vary widely, all patients with KPS <70 were included in RPA class III irrespective of the other potential factors which may alter survival times in a significant manner. Supporting these adverse comments by analyzing the outcomes of 113 patients, Nieder et al. [28] reported that there was no survival difference between patients in classes II and III (3.6 vs. 4.2 months) after 30 Gy WBRT.

Another prognostic scoring system, score index for radiosurgery (SIR), includes the number of BM, volume of the largest BM, location of BM, and post radiosurgery WBRT in addition to the variables of RPA (Table 7.3) [21]. The SIR was suggested by the authors to be more reliable than RPA in predicting survival after SRS, which was later validated with further studies in patients subjected to surgery, WBRT with/without. Of note, SIR may potentially be less representative for the majority of BM patients as it was generated by depending on the data of only 65 patients who underwent SRS [29]. Currently the SIR is limitedly used in clinics because of the need for detailed workup for assessment of the systemic disease.

In 2004, Lorenzoni et al. [30] proposed a new scoring system, Basic Score for Brain Metastases (BSBM), that compared RPA with SIR (Table 7.4). This novel scoring system included only three factors: KPS, control of primary tumor, and the presence of extracranial disease, in order to keep the scoring simple. The analysis of 110 BM patients treated with SRS revealed a good correlation between the BSBM and SIR inaccurate prognostic stratification of patients. Further evaluation of BSBM in patients receiving WBRT plus surgery and WBRT with/without SRS landed confirmatory outcomes for Lorenzoni's findings [19, 31]. Therefore, BSBM was advocated as a reliable and easy to use prognostic index that has same definition of extracranial disease as the RPA. However, this scoring system is also limited by the fact that evidence is based on only 110 patients, which may be problematic because of large confidence intervals when it is applied to smaller cohorts [29].

The number of BM was demonstrated to be a significant prognosticator by RTOG 9508 investigators, in which patients with one to three BM were randomized to WBRT with or without SRS boost arms [32]. However, the number of BM was not included in the prognostic score by the previously reported RPA, BSBM, and Rotterdam scores [22]. Therefore, in 2007, another prognostic index called "Graded Prognostic Assessment (GPA)(Table 7.5)" was proposed which incorporated age, KPS, extracranial metastases (ECM), and number of BM in the scoring system by analyzing the outcomes of 1960 patients treated with WBRT alone, WBRT plus radiosensitizers, or WBRT plus SRS in the five RTOG trials (RTOG 7916, 8528, 8905, 9104, and 9508) [33]. Each factor was given a score of 0, 0.5, or 1.0 and GPA was calculated a sum score of all four factors with resultant four groups (Table 7.5). According to this novel prognostic index, patients with the best prognosis had GPA 4. Median survival was 2.6 months in GPA 0–1, 3.8 months in GPA 1.5–2.5, 6.9 months in GPA 3, and 11 months in GPA 3.5–4 score. The authors concluded that the GPA was least subjective, most quantitative, and easiest to use of the four indices (RPA, SIR, BSBM, and GPA) analyzed. Following this publication, various studies have confirmed the validity of the GPA [34–36], and therefore, GPA has

Table 7.4 Basic score for brain metastases (BSBM)

Parameters	Score 0	Score 1
Karnofsky performance status	50–70	>70
Extracranial metastases	Yes	No
Primary disease control	No	Yes

Table 7.5 Graded prognostic assessment (GPA)

Characteristics	Score 0	Score 1	Score 2
Karnofsky performance status	<70	70–80	>80
Extracranial metastases	Present	–	None
Number of lesions	>3	2–3	1
Age	>60	50–59	<50

Table 7.6 Comparison of commonly used prognostic indices for brain metastases

Parameters	RPA	GPA	SIR	ds-GPA	Rotterdam score	BSBM
Patients (n)	1,200	1,960	65	4,259	1,292	110
Performance status	KPS	KPS	KPS	KPS	ECOG	KPS
Primary control	+	–	+	–	–	+
Age	+	+	+	+	–	–
ECM	+	+	+	+	+	+
Volume of lesion	–	–	+	–	–	–
Number of lesion	–	+	+	+	–	–
Steroid response	–	–	–	–	+	–
Number of parameters	3	4	3	4	3	4

RPA recursive partitioning analysis, *GPA* graded prognostic assessment, *SIR* score index for radiosurgery, *ds-GPA* disease-specific graded prognostic assessment, *BSBM* basic score for brain metastases, *KPS* Karnofsky performance status, *ECOG* eastern cooperative oncology group, *ECM* extracranial metastases, (+) included, (−) not included

become one of the most commonly used prognostic indices for prognostic stratification of patients with BM.

As mentioned above and summarized in Table 7.6, all the indices invariably include KPS and ECM and differ by other factors such as age, number and volume of BM, control of primary tumor, and response to steroids. One important limitation of almost all prognostic systems is inclusion of relatively more favorable patients which makes it difficult to decide the best fit treatment for patients with comparably unfavorable prognostic features. Another common limitation is that all factors are derived to anticipate survival and there is no score that addresses end points other than survival. Therefore, future investigations should aim to develop novel prognostic models that can provide estimates of time to neurologic progression or decline, rather than uniquely focusing on survival outcomes. Additionally, such indices should be developed with the capability to discriminate deaths directly related with BM-associated neurologic decline from those emerging as a consequence of systemic disease progression.

Treatment

Simply the BM management strategies can be divided into two: symptomatic and therapeutic. Symptomatic treatment usually aims to reduce the intracranial pressure produced by the peritumoral edema and to prevent recurrent seizures. Steroids are effective for the former aim while anticonvulsants are used for seizure control. In addition, there is increasing data to suggest that medications such as methylphenidate and donepezil may be beneficial in improvement of neurocognitive functions, mood, and quality of life (QOL) measures in this patient group [37, 38].

Therapeutic strategies include chemotherapy, surgery, WBRT, SRS, or different combinations of them. The management decisions take into account PFs such as patient age, functional status, primary tumor histology, intracranial extent of BM, size and location of BM, total volume of BM, symptomatic status of patient, resectability of BM, status of the primary tumor site, number of extracranial tumor sites, prior therapies, comorbid conditions, and technical opportunities and qualifications of the cancer center. Because the chemotherapy, WBRT, and neurosurgery are beyond the scope of this chapter, from there on the remainder of the chapter will specifically focus on the outcomes of SRS only applications, its combinations with other treatment modalities, and SRS techniques.

Stereotactic Radiosurgery

Radiobiology of SRS

The term "SRS" was first suggested by Lars Leksellin 1951 with the purpose of treating of benign intracranial lesions with a noninvasive ablative method [39]. Contrasting with the conformal RT techniques which aim to irradiate target tumor volumes to a specified prescription dose while sparing neighboring healthy tissues, the unique aim of the SRS is to destruct all the tissues residing in the target volume irrespective of their malignancy or health status.

The major differences between the conventional RT and SRS are the size of treated volume and the dose applied during the treatment. In SRS the target volume (TV) is usually smaller than the volumes treated by conventional or even more sophisticated radiotherapy techniques such as IMRT, and the dose is in general a single fraction high dose while other radiotherapy techniques utilize smaller doses per fraction (1.5–4 Gy) and multi-fractionated regimes (5–40 fractions). Tumor volume is crucial in SRS applications, because the primary goal for the best radiobiological effect is to target the TV precisely by one shot of ionizing radiation with the neurosurgeon's ingenuity in excising tumor volumes with his knife. Fractionated RT is effective in management of relatively large targets with a better complication profile; however this advantage comes at the cost of decreased chance for escalating the RT doses up to tumoricidal levels which may be particularly essential in some certain relatively radioresistant tumor types. In this setting, SRS with its abrupt dose fall-off properties beyond the TV allows the radiation oncologist to achieve ultrahigh doses and to a large extent resolves the radioresistance problem [40].

Classical radiobiology evidence clearly states the hypoxic regions in the tumor volume as one source of radioresistance, which usually reside at the center of the mass. One important benefit of fractionated RT is its ability to overcome this hypoxia problem by destructing the surrounding normally oxygenated tissue around these regions which brings the hypoxic cells closer to more oxygenated regions. As a consequence of this process, hypoxic cells turn to be radiosensitive favoring multi-fractionated RT regimes over single fractionation. This basic radiobiologic advantage, namely, reoxygenation, disappears with single-fraction SRS. Another radiobiological basic issue that fails in SRS is the redistribution of cells in different phases of the cell cycle. Tumor cells demonstrate different radiosensitiveness through the phases of cell cycle with mitosis (M) phase being the most radiosensitive phase which is followed by gap-2 (G_2) phase. In this sense, redistribution of tumor cells into more radiosensitive phases by use of multi-fractionated RT may provide a therapeutic advantage over single-fraction regimes.

The aforementioned radiobiological disadvantages cause difficulties in explanation of the tumor ablation provided by SRS. However, this issue has been excellently reviewed previously by Brown et al. [41]. According to this review, the potential mechanisms underlying the lethal effects of SRS on tumor tissues and its advantages over multi-fractionated RT protocols are as follows:

- The benefit of reoxygenation may become negligible or even totally disappear because many tumors may not be hypoxic.
- In addition to loss of reproductive ability caused by double-strand DNA breaks, there are further antitumoral effects of single-fraction high-dose regimes which are not predicted by classic radiobiology, such as endothelial injury and enhanced antitumor immunity.
- The linear-quadratic model may be insufficient or even inaccurate for predicting cell killing in the SRS dose range. Assumedly this model may overpredict cell killing at high doses, and therefore, the damage to the late-responding tissues may be less than the calculated values, which may allow use of higher doses with a potential increase in chance of better tumor control rates.
- Advanced image guidance technologies enable application of larger doses with smaller safety margins by reducing the dosimetric uncertainties which increases the tumor control rates in the absence of excess toxicity.

Comparative Clinical Outcomes of SRS

SRS is a high-precision conformal RT administering a large-dose RT in a single session as a noninvasive alternative to neurosurgery for single BM. SRS has been used either as an adjunct to neurosurgery in the form of tumor bed SRS or WBRT or as the sole treatment option with various outcomes.

Multiple potential benefits are associated with the use of neurosurgery for BM. Neurosurgery is of value when the diagnosis is unknown or unclear which is of particular importance when a patient has no known primary tumor or has a primary cancer histology that is unlikely to metastasize to the brain or a brain lesion that appears several years after the initial primary tumor. It ought to be remembered that, even in patients with a known primary, a newly diagnosed brain mass can end up being a primary brain tumor or other nonmetastatic disease in about 9 % of cases [42]. Additionally, removal of a BM can lead to immediate elimination of life-threatening or symptom-generating mass effect and elimination of the source of perifocal edema, as well as reducing the requirement for and duration of steroid therapy.

Neurosurgery can also provide a survival and disease control benefit, as evidenced by two prospective phase III studies. In these studies, OS in patients with single BM undergoing neurosurgery and WBRT was improved from 4 to 6 months to 10 months when compared with WBRT alone [42, 43].

Limited comparative studies suggest similar outcomes for patients with a single BM undergoing surgery or SRS. The only randomized trial comparing the SRS against neurosurgery was closed early due to poor accrual [44]. In this study, patients with single BM that is <3 cm in diameter, KPS ≥ 70, and controlled primary were randomized to surgery plus WBRT versus Gamma Knife SRS alone. The outcomes of eligible 64 patients demonstrated no difference between two modalities with regard to OS ($p=0.8$), neurologic deaths ($p=0.3$), and local recurrence-free survival ($p=0.06$). The patients in SRS arm had more distant brain recurrences ($p=0.04$); but after the salvage SRS applications, this significance disappeared ($p=0.4$). SRS was reported to relate with shorter steroid usage, less hospitalization duration, and less grade 1–2 complications ($p=0.001$). The neurocognitive function tests assessing quality of life at 6 weeks were improved better with SRS ($p<0.05$) but which disappeared at 6 months. The strongest evidence suggesting similar clinical outcomes with neurosurgery and SRS comes from the recently published systemic review by Qin et al. [45]. In this study 713 patients enrolled on 18 trials were included. The authors reported that there was no significant difference between the neurosurgery and SRS in median (12.7 vs. 14.85 months) or 1-year (59 % vs. 62 %), 2-year (33 % vs. 33 %), and 5-year OS (19 % vs. 14 %) times.

Considering that the SRS and neurosurgery are almost clinically equal in terms of disease control and survival rates, noninvasive SRS appears to be the choice of treatment as it is additionally more cost-effective than neurosurgery [46, 47]. However, if the patient is neurologically symptomatic because of the mass effect of a larger BM (>8–10 cm^3), the tumor should be removed with a neurosurgical intervention for achieving immediate symptom control in the absence of further contraindications; otherwise WBRT should be the choice of treatment for such patients.

For decades, WBRT has been the standard treatment option for BM in most centers. However, SRS alone has gained significant popularity because of the concerns regarding the adverse effects of WBRT on QOL and neurocognitive functions [48]. Additionally, neither of the available RCTs could demonstrate a survival benefit favoring addition of WBRT to SRS in patients with up to four BM. Considering the negative impacts of WBRT on neurocognitive functions, it should be recognized that some patients might have already been affected before initiation of WBRT. Supporting this, the outcomes of a prospective trial reported that 90.5 % of the patients had failure in one or more neurologic function tests at baseline, and moreover, 42.5 % of them failed in four or more tests [49]. On the other hand, also the omission of WBRT does not mean that all risks for neurocognitive impairments were discarded at all. In this respect the outcomes of a small study of 36 BM patients who were treated by SRS alone at Kentucky are demonstrative [50]. Of the 36 patients, 17 (47 %) experienced recurrences in the brain, and 12 (70.6 %) and 10 (58.8 %) of them were symptomatic recurrences and with neurologic deficits, respectively. This study is a good representative for demonstration of aggravated neurologic functional abnormalities in recurrent cases even when the WBRT is totally omitted from the treatment schedule.

Various studies have been conducted to perform comparisons between SRS alone and WBRT plus SRS combination. In the trial by Aoyama et al. [51], 132 patients with one to four BM were randomly assigned to WBRT plus SRS or SRS alone. Only the patients with KPS >60 and BM not exceeding 3 cm were included.

The dose of WBRT was 3 Gy/30 Gy and the doses of SRS were 22–25 and 18–20 Gy for tumors ≤2 cm and 2.1–3 cm, respectively. Patients in SRS group were more likely to be in good KPS (90–100; 66 % vs. 52 %). There was no significant median OS difference (8 vs. 7.5 months; $p=0.42$) and neurologic cause death (19.3 % vs. 22.3 %, $p=0.64$) for SRS alone and WBRT plus SRS arms, respectively. One-year survival was quantitatively 36 % superior in the combined modality arm although this difference did not reach statistical significance. For this trial, Patchell reported that it was underpowered to statistically discriminate the OS outcomes of two groups [52]. WBRT increased the actuarial overall control rate at 1 year (53.2 % vs. 23.6 %; $p<0.001$). The patients in SRS arm needed more salvage treatments (43 % vs. 15 %; $p<0.001$). Distant brain recurrences were higher in the SRS arm (64 % vs. 42 %; $p=0.003$). Serious late complications were not significantly different between the arms.

In EORTC 22952-26001 trial [15], 359 patients with one to three BM and controlled primary disease were treated with surgery or SRS and randomly assigned to WBRT or observation arms. Although OS was not different (10.9 vs. 10.7 months, $p=0.89$), neurologic deaths were more common in observation arm (44 % vs. 28 %, $p=0.002$). The 2-year relapse rates at both the initial sites (surgery: 59–27 %; $p<0.001$; SRS: 31–19 %; $p=0.040$) and at new sites (surgery: 42 % vs. 23 %, $p=0.008$; SRS: 48 % vs. 33 %, $p=0.023$) were reduced by WBRT. Additionally, the need for salvage therapies was more common in the single-modality treatments than their combinations with WBRT. Similarly, in a recent retrospective review from Columbia University, patients with either single or multiple BM were treated with GK-SRS alone, GK-SRS plus WBRT, GK-SRS plus surgery, or GK-SRS plus WBRT plus surgery. Irrespective of the number of BM, the results significantly favored the multimodality treatments over GK-SRS alone in terms of OS [53].

In summary, enlightened with the available literature on the subject, it is clear that SRS alone is satisfactorily effective in irradiated tumor volumes but the distant BM recurrences are comparatively higher than the SRS plus WBRT strategies. Probably because of the aggressive nature of the tumors at extracranial destinations, this better in-brain control rates with the addition of WBRT did not translate into any survival benefit, suggesting that WBRT may safely be omitted in certain patients. However, acknowledging the fact that the brain is a sanctuary site for the vast majority of the accessible chemotherapeutics, it is critical to call attention to that WBRT may recapture extraordinary interest when more viable systemic chemotherapy agents get to be accessible in the future.

SRS for Multiple BM

In spite of the fact that the proof for more than three BM is not sufficiently adequate to achieve a dependable conclusion, various authors reported that even more than 30 BM can be viably and generally securely treated in a single session with GK-SRS and four to five BM with LINAC-based SRS [54]. In most of such patients, the lesions are usually small and asymptomatic. Thusly, in these patients instead of the quantity of BM, the aggregate tumor volume gains pivotal importance on prognosis,

Table 7.7 National Health Service commissioning criteria for stereotactic radiosurgery and stereotactic radiotherapy for brain metastases [89]

Criteria	Recommendation
Patient selection	Patients should be selected by local multidisciplinary team with understanding of the systemic and neurologic disease processes and neurosurgical options, as well as discussion by the specialist stereotactic radiosurgery multidisciplinary team
Performance status	Karnofsky performance score ≥70
Cancer diagnosis	Established
Primary disease	Absent or controllable
Life expectancy	≥6 months from extracranial disease
Total tumor volume	≤20 cm^3

which has been expressed among other inclusion criteria for SRS qualifications by the National Health Service commissioning criteria, as depicted in Table 7.7 [55, 56].

In the joined series of Serizawa and Yamamoto, 1,508 patients treated by GK-SRS were evaluated with no notable survival distinction between the patients with two to four and five to ten BM, respectively [57]. In another study from Yonsei University College of Medicine, Seoul, 323 BM patients were treated by GK-SRS and categorized into four groups per the number of BM: respective median OS times for patients with 1–5, 6–10, 11–15, and >15 BM were 10, 13, 10, and 8 months ($p > 0.05$) [58].

The MD Anderson Cancer Center GK-SRS alone series including 251 patients exhibited that the number of BM was not predictive of distant brain failure, local control, and OS [59]. Likewise, in the Stanford University School of Medicine retrospective post-WBRT GK-SRS series ($n = 310$), following exclusion of the patients with single BM, the investigators was not able to show any association between the number of BM and OS outcomes [60].

Available data suggests almost equal effectiveness of SRS in ≤3 versus >3 BM situations. Therefore, in lack of any documented evidence suggesting inefficacy of SRS in patients with >3 BM, in the absence of a more effective treatment option, it is reasonable to offer SRS for suitable patients in order to not miss the chance for a better tumor control, even if it may contradict with the traditional practice.

SRS for Large BM

The current standard treatment for patients presenting with large BM and mass-related significant neurologic symptoms is neurosurgery which is based on the results of RCTs demonstrating superior OS times and functional stability with neurosurgery than long-course fractionated WBRT [42, 61]. Alike with WBRT, SRS is also usually not recommended for BM of >3–4 cm because of higher likelihood of irradiation-induced edema progression. But, in some particular cases, tumor size may surpass these typically expressed cutoff points because of cyst formation. For such BM, although upfront SRS may be risky in terms of acute and particularly late toxicities, yet pre-SRS cyst aspiration may allow relatively safer utilization of SRS. In literature, LC represents the most common cancer type that presents with cystic BM and compression-related serious neurologic deficits [62]. In addition to the higher risk for SRS-related complications, the reported local control rates of BM with a cystic component larger than 10 ml are less favorable with SRS alone. Therefore, aspiration of the cystic regions before SRS should be an invariable component of such patients' management algorithm in order to both increase the tumor control probability and reduce radionecrosis risk [63, 64].

In RTOG 90-05, patients with BM <4 cm (regardless of the cystic component) were enrolled on the study and 15 Gy was determined to be the maximum tolerated dose of SRS for lesions sized 3.1–4 cm [65]. In this group severe neurologic complications were 16 times higher than the patients with BM <2 cm with the same dose of 15 Gy. The authors of this benchmark trial subsequently suggested the hypofractionated multifraction dose schedules as a potentially effective and safe treatment method [65]. Affirming proof for this suggestion has recently been reported by Murai et al. [66]. In this study 61 large BM (≥2.5 cm in maximum diameter) of a total of 102 in 54 patients were treated with fractionated stereotactic RT (FSRT) as a first-line therapy. Neurologic symptoms were observed in 47 of the 54 patients before FSRT. Three fractions were applied to tumors with a maximum diameter ≥2.5 cm and <4 cm, and five fractions were used for BM ≥4 cm. With the highest dose levels of 27–30 Gy/three fractions and 31–35 Gy/five fractions, local tumor control rates of the 61 large BM were 77 % and 69 % at 6 and 12 months, respectively, with no report of ≥ grade 3 toxicities.

SRS for Tumor Bed

SRS as a sole modality provides excellent local control rates in small BM [15, 67], but in certain cases neurosurgery is advantageous. Neurosurgery can provide histopathologic information, more rapid symptomatic relief, emergency decompression, and better local control in larger lesions [68]. Nonetheless, the rate of local failure following neurosurgery alone is 46–59 %, prompting the routine use of adjuvant WBRT following neurosurgery [15] Considerations for WBRT toxicity led to increased interest in combining the reduced complication and increased local control profile of SRS in patients who have undergone a resection for BM, namely, tumor bed SRS for (TB-SRS) [69–71].

TB-SRS is a relatively new treatment approach with no randomized data published to date, and only limited prospective data are available. Therefore, the majority of published data comes from single-institutional retrospective analyses. Currently, various ways of TB-SRS are now under investigation including adjuvant to neurosurgery, postsurgical boost to WBRT, and neoadjuvant SRS to the lesion that is planned to resection and as salvage SRS for patients who have recurred after previous resection and WBRT [68].

Roberge et al. investigated TB-SRS with WBRT in 27patients and later 44 patients with high performance status and good RPA classifications [70]. Most patients received 30 Gy (3 Gy per day) and 10 Gy of TB-SRS boost. Treatment was well tolerated with 1-year actuarial local control and crude rates of BM were 90 % and 13 %, respectively. TB-SRS may also be utilized as a salvage strategy after

WBRT failure. Kim et al. [72] reported the outcomes of 79 patients treated with resection and SRS following previous WBRT failure. The median GK-SRS dose, median OS, crude local recurrence, and radionecrosis requiring surgical intervention rates were 18 Gy, 17 months, 5.1 %, and 3.8 %, respectively.

TB-SRS to a resection cavity without WBRT is the most reported approach of tumor bed-directed SRS as a sole adjuvant to neurosurgery. Brennan et al. recently reported one of the limitedly available results of TB-SRS experience in this setting [73]. In this phase II trial, the role of TB-SRS for resected BM was investigated. Forty-nine patients with RPA class I (24 %) or II (76 %) and had one to two BM that were treated. Actuarial local failure and regional failure rates at 12 months were 22 % and 42 %, respectively. Tumors >3 cm with superficial dura or pial involvement had the highest risk of local failure with a local control rate of <50 %, while no failures were observed in patients with deeply located and sized <3 cm tumors. Despite the fact that the rate of pathologically confirmed radionecrosis was high (17.5 %), no noteworthy clinical or dosimetric factors were identifiable which may have potentially conceivably added to this rate.

A rarely applied but new and promising concept is performing SRS before BM as opposed to as TB-SRS. It has been suggested by some authors that such a neoadjuvant strategy allows for a vascular-mediated effect with resultant potential for enhanced clinical outcomes. Furthermore, conveying the SRS before resection takes into consideration a clearer delineation of the target and a hypothetically decreased risk of intraoperative tumor spread. In a recently reported study, Asher et al. [74] shared their institutional experience with neoadjuvant SRS followed by surgical resection in consecutively treated 47 patients with one to three BM and controlled systemic disease. The median dose was 14 Gy (range 11.6–18 Gy) and the planning target volume (PTV) was defined as the grossly visible tumor volume on imaging studies. Outcomes were encouraging with actuarial 6-, 12- and 24-month local control rates of 97.8 %, 85.6 %, and 71.8 %, respectively. However, despite of the potential advantages, SRS before BM also suffers from potential problems. First, Patchell et al. reported a rate of 11 % nonmetastatic histology for such patients [75]; therefore, this strategy is threatened with a significant risk of unnecessary irradiation of patients who have either primary brain neoplasms or nonmalignant pathology in the absence of pathologic confirmation. Second, the surgical resection may be complicated by an SRS-induced transient increase in tumor size and associated additional mass effect. And third, delivery of additional radiotherapy may turn to be difficult after a sub-total resection, which may alter tumor control rates in a negative manner.

In summary, the concept of tumor bed SRS is new and the evidence is gradually growing. Although the available data on use of TB-SRS is encouraging, yet much is still unknown about SRS when no true tumor is available: including the optimal doses, treatment modalities, and margins. Appropriately designed future studies, like the ongoing trials from Maria Sklodowska-Curie Memorial Cancer Center (NCT01535209), the MD Anderson Cancer Center (NCT00950001), and the Intergroup N107C trial, will most likely provide level 1 evidence in clearing some uncertainties and setting the optimal treatment decisions.

SRS for Recurrent Lesions

Local or distant in-brain recurrences of BM occur in a significant percentage of patients treated with either WBRT, surgery, or combined. Furthermore, these failures appear to be the cause of death in as high as 31–49 % instances despite the favorable control rates of WBRT or the combined multimodality treatments such as SRS or surgery following WBRT [76, 77]. Reirradiation with WBRT is usually ineffective and inacceptable because of insignificant local control rates as well as higher risk for radiation-induced neurotoxicities [78, 79]. These inconveniences render SRS as the most suitable or even the sole treatment alternative for such patients [79].

In a retrospective analysis by Kurtz et al. [80], 279 recurrent BM of WBRT in 106 patients were treated with GK-SRS. Utilizing a median dose of 21 Gy (range, 12–24), the authors reported 82.8 %, 60.1 %, and 46.8 % local control rates at 6 months, 1 year, and 3 years, respectively. Median OS was 11.7 months from salvage SRS. Young age, control of extracranial disease, and the interval between the initial RT and salvage SRS of at least 265 days were found to be significant associates of longer OS.

They were treated with salvage SRS [81]. Median interval between the end of WBRT and SRS was 9 months (range: 2–70 median interval between the end of WBRT and SRS was 9 months (range: 2–70). At a median follow-up of 9 months (1–57 months), BM recurrences were reported in 5 (5.2 %) individuals with a median GK-SRS dose of 16.2 Gy (11.8–23 Gy). One- and 2-year control rates were 91.3 % and 84 % for locally treated lesions 65 % and 57 % for the whole brain, respectively, with 1- and 2-year OS rates of 31 % and 28 %. Side effects were minimal with only two cases of grade 2 alopecia. On multivariate analysis, RPA was an independent variable of OS and brain free-disease survival, while the longer interval (14 months) between WBRT and SRS was associated with longer brain free-disease survival. Salvage SRS for limited brain recurrences ends up with 1- and 2-year local control rates of 70–90 % and 60–84 %, respectively, but reirradiation with SRS is roughly connected with 50 % radionecrosis risk [4]. Therefore, even for this sophisticated salvage technique, it is mandatory to carefully select suitable candidates in order to minimize the risk of severe and usually irreversible complications. Additionally, a certain group of patients with WBRT failure may present with poor performance status and uncontrolled primary and/or distant sites. As the normal survival length anticipation is restricted to just a couple of weeks to months, salvage SRS may be unnecessary for such patients, leaving the re-WBRT or best supportive care as appropriate palliative alternatives.

Complications of SRS

Acute Complications

Early complications occur within the first 3 months of SRS and usually include headache, nausea, vomiting, seizures, transient neurologic symptom deterioration, vertigo, regional alopecia, and fatigue. Although the majority of such complications are temporary and self-limiting, seizures may be problematic with an incidence range of 2–6 % which tends to further increase in patients undergoing SRS for cortical lesions [8, 82]. Peritumoral edema is usually associated with SRS of larger lesions or excessive doses beyond the target volume. Although corticosteroids may effectively manage edema in most cases, careful patient selection and tighter coverage of target volumes may further minimize the symptomatic edema development risk. Limiting the dose received by area postrema and antiemetic usage are the effective maneuvers for prevention and treatment of SRS-induced nausea and vomiting [83].

Late Complications

Radiation necrosis (RN) is the most frustrating chronic toxicity, and its incidence increases with higher radiation doses, prior RT history, and irradiation of larger and/or multiple tumor volumes. Despite the fact that it may exhibit from months to years, the incidence peak more or less lies between 12 and 15 months of the treatment. Patients' neurologic status may be significantly deteriorated by RN which may be difficult to discriminate from tumor recurrences even with the currently available imaging techniques and may mandate surgery [8]. The most commonly accused and also easily manageable two parameters for RN occurrence are the prescribed dose lesion size. Accordingly, appropriate selection of prescription doses and avoidance of large volume SRS may minimize the occurrence of this severe complication, if not obviate all.

RTOG-9005 was the first benchmark SRS trial which determined the maximum tolerated doses (MTD) of single-fraction SRS in patients with previously irradiated recurrent primary brain tumors or as an adjunct to WBRT for BM [65]. Patients were randomized to one of the three arms according to the size of lesion: ≤20 mm, 21–30 mm, and 31–40 mm. The initial SRS dose was determined as 18 Gy, 15 Gy, and 12 Gy, respectively. Then the dose was gradually escalated in 3 Gy increments by paying attention to the severe acute side effects. The MTD were determined as 24 Gy, 18 Gy, and 15 Gy for tumors ≤20 mm, 21–30 mm, and 31–40 mm, respectively. The actual rates of RN were 5 %, 8 %, 9 %, and 11 % at 6, 12, 18, and 24 months after SRS, respectively, and were found to be more prevalent in patients with larger tumors.

In another study Valery et al. [84] aimed to determine if the risk of RN after SRS was related to the normal tissue included in the prescription volume. The authors included 377 patients with 760 lesions. Median tumor volume was 4.9 cm^3 and the median peripheral dose (70 %) was 15.6 Gy. In multivariate analysis KPS, disease control and number of lesions were found to be the only parameters significantly influencing survival (median 8.6 months), while disease-free survival was correlated with the number of isocenters. The only reported parameter influencing the risk of RN was the conformity index ($p = 0.001$), emphasizing the importance of reducing falsely irradiated normal tissue during SRS as a measure for prevention of RN.

Quality of Life

WBRT has been shown to improve intracranial disease control, but this is of uncertain clinical value in the absence of any enhancement on survival outcomes and may unnecessarily affect patients' QOL measures in a negative manner [15, 51, 85, 86]. WBRT negatively alters health-related QOL scales particularly due to fatigue and hair loss and causes cognitive dysfunction immediately after the beginning of radiotherapy, and subacute radiation effects on verbal memory function are observed both after therapeutic and prophylactic cranial irradiation which is more pronounced in patients with better baseline performance [87, 88].

High-quality comparative data on neurocognitive functions are lacking, and available results are conflicting. Outcomes of a phase III trial by Aoyama et al. suggested a neurocognitive benefit from the addition of WBRT to SRS using the mini-mental state examination [89]. But the results of this study should be interpreted with caution as mini-mental state examination has a poor discriminatory power in assessment of such patients. QUARTZ was a randomized, noninferiority, phase III trial comparing optimal supportive care (OSC) plus WBRT against OSC in patients with inoperable BMs from NSCLC. The primary end point was quality-adjusted life years (QALY). Interim outcomes of this study indicated no significant differences between two groups in terms of QOL, OS, or QALY for patients allocated to OSC alone [90]. On the other hand, a small randomized trial noted higher risk of a decline in learning and memory functions by 4 months with addition of WBRT to SRS using more sensitive measures, although differences in OS between the arms may confound this interpretation [48]. The results of this study were interpreted as level I evidence to support the use of SRS alone. The recently published larger ($n = 359$) prospective randomized EORTC phase III trial by Soffietti et al. demonstrated that WBRT after neurosurgery or SRS of BM negatively impacted the health-related QOL [86].

Late significant nervous system toxicity as late as 6 years following fractionated cranial radiotherapy is a well-demonstrated phenomenon [91]. In a small prospective study after Gamma Knife treatment for BM, Dibiaase et al. reported that QOL parameters remained either unchanged or improved in patients who had no evidence of intracranial or extracranial tumor progression [92]. In RTOG 95-08, statistically significant improvements in performance status and lessened steroid need at 6-month time point were demonstrated in the SRS boost group compared to fractionated radiation [32]. Based on the available literature, it appears to be quite difficult to reach conclusive recommendations regarding the comparative neurocognitive toxicity profiles of WBRT, SRS, and WBRT plus SRS, but present evidence suggests better early and late neurologic functions with SRS alone compared to WBRT alone or combined with SRS, which may be of paramount importance in patients with longer survival expectations.

SRS Techniques

As defined by Larsson, the term SRS communicates any way of execution of ionizing radiation with the end goal of destruction of an objective volume absolutely and totally without evident toxicities to nearby typical tissues [4]. This ionizing radiation can be achieved either from the radioisotope sources or from X-ray-generating machines such as cobalt-60 or linear accelerators (LINAC), respectively. Ionizing radiation can be accomplished either from the radioisotope sources or from X-ray-generating machines, for example, cobalt-60 or linear accelerators (LINAC). Positively charged protons are likewise utilized for SRS which can be acquired from particle accelerators, such as cyclotrons and synchrotrons [93].

A modern GK unit incorporates 201 radioisotopes of ^{60}Co in a hemispherical array that converges and focuses on the target volume at a source to target distance of about 40 cm. The intended therapeutic dose is achieved by focusing many beamlines simultaneously on the target volume, while the dose derived from each source is clinically insignificant. Use of multiple sources with individual insignificant dosimetric value brings the benefit of satisfactory sparing of surrounding normal tissues [94]. The novel GK Perfexion uses multiple isocenters, created by numerous collimated beams of different sizes, coming from 192 individual ^{60}Co sources converging to a single point, called the isocenter.

In LINAC-based SRS, the radiation beam is shaped by a bunch of leaves defined as multi-leaf collimator which is usually made of a tungsten alloy. Although various LINAC systems are capable of performing SRS, they in common use isocentric, fixed intensity, and modulated or dynamically shaped arc beams to deliver intensity-modulated radiotherapy (DMLC IMRT). In these systems the dose is conformed to target volume by the computer-aided movements of each leaf. The robot-controlled CyberKnife is a variant of 6-MV LINAC which is mounted on a robotic arm with non-isocentric cone beams. Simply the CyberKnife utilizes the same principles of SRS alike with other LINACS. CyberKnife allows more choices in selection of the beam angles because of the continuous image guidance and its frameless usage, yet the long treatment time is one of the drawbacks of CyberKnife compared to GK and isocentric LINAC systems.

Although various systems are commercially available for SRS applications, they all utilize the same fundamentals regardless of the treatment device.

The fundamentals of SRS procedure are mentioned below regardless of the treatment device [8]:

- Stereotactic brain imaging using an MRI, a CT scan, and/or an angiogram
- Quality assurance of images
- Definition of target volumes
- Conformal SRS dose planning
- Quality assurance of treatment plans
- Periodic quality assurance of the devices

Most of the SRS planning techniques take their roots from the so-called "sphere packing" method initially described by Lars Leksell. This technique aims to direct a set of beams to a focus that resides at a pre-specified point in space, namely, the isocenter. The selected beams reach the isocenter through unique paths, giving both a geometric conformity and a high-dose gradient. Therefore, the capabilities of SRS devices are specified by their accuracy in conveying the beams to this particular point. Regardless of the device in use, the final dose distribution should emulate the shape of the target volume in order to represent a feasible treatment plan [8].

Patient Immobilization and Setup

The primary objective of SRS is to shape high-dose conformity and steep-dose gradients around the target volume that reduces the dose to surrounding healthy tissues by utilizing multiple and non-coplanar beams [54]. One of the essential strides in accomplishing this accuracy and precision on the target is immobilization of the patient. The likelihood of intra- and interfraction patient movements can be restricted with fixed-type invasive neurosurgical frames [95] or with a less precise mask-based immobilization that is consolidated with on-treatment imaging. In invasive immobilization techniques, the head is fixed by a frame attached to the patient's skull with four metal screws (Fig. 7.1). A fiducial reference box is likewise mounted during the imaging procedure for determination of the stereotactic coordinates of the target volume.

There are also noninvasive methods for immobilization, including the use of thermoplastic mask systems, bite blocks, and image guidance like orthogonal X-ray techniques and cone beam computed tomography (CT) [4]. Inter- and intrafraction motion constitutes the two imperative components of patient movement. The intrafraction errors have been exhibited to range between 1.6 and 3.9 mm with use

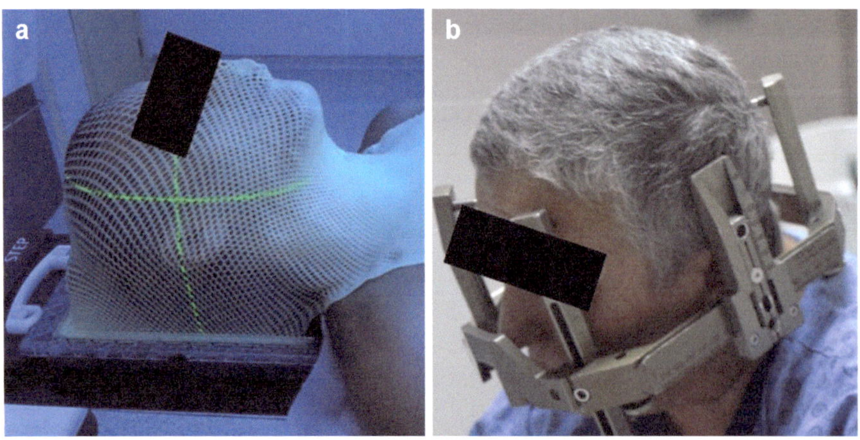

Fig. 7.1 Patient immobilization and positioning for SRS: (**a**) LINAC, (**b**) Gamma Knife based

of thermoplastic masks systems. Guckenberger reported the image guidance as the best method in minimizing the interfraction motion errors which was reduced from 3.9 to 0.9 mm [96, 97] where a residual deviation of 0.9 mm was caused by the intrafractional motion.

According to the report by Ramakrishna et al. [98], there were no noteworthy differences in either of inter- and intrafraction motion between frame-based and frameless image-guided SRS strategies. Thusly, if frameless SRS is arranged, a highly accurate treatment delivery can only be achieved with the image guidance; otherwise frame-based techniques should be preferred.

As a result, SRS can be performed with high accuracy only if image guidance is utilized combined with a frameless mask.

Imaging

Following the patient immobilization, the next fundamental step of SRS is imaging. The precision of this stride is just a key for each remaining strides of the SRS planning and treatment conveyance, including the delineation of the target volume and critical organs, guidance in simulation, setup, treatment, and quality assurance procedures. In this respect thin-sliced (≤2 mm) MRI is an excellent tool for imaging the tumor, soft tissues, and the entire intracranial structures. Fusion of MRI with CT may be valuable in discrimination of bony involvements and minimizing of the dose heterogeneities during the dose calculation process.

Delineation of Target Volume

The axial fusion images of CT and MRI are used for the delineation of the gross total volume (GTV) or organs at risk (OAR) (Fig. 7.2). The MRI should include T1- and T2-weighted and fluid-attenuated inversion recovery (FLAIR) sequences. Axial, sagittal, and coronal axis views should be available in order to increase the accuracy of three-dimensional volumetric delineation of the target volumes and OAR. The slice thickness of CT and MRI should not exceed 3 mm. Delineation process should start following a through revision of the CT and MRI fusion precision. GTV should include only the visible contrast-enhanced tumor volume on MRI without encompassing the surrounding edema. If neurosurgical frame-based SRS techniques are preferred, additional margins are not necessary for the creation of clinical target volume (CTV) or planning target volume (PTV). In this manner, GTV is equivalent to CTV and PTV in the frame-based SRS applications, yet a margin of 1–2 mm could possibly be added to GTV for definition of PTV if frameless SRS is arranged. For TB-SRS a 2 mm margin encompassing the surgical cavity at all dimensions should be considered for minimizing the marginal misses. In this appreciation, Choi et al. reported that such a margin was significantly effective in reducing the local recurrences without any augmentation in toxicity rates [99].

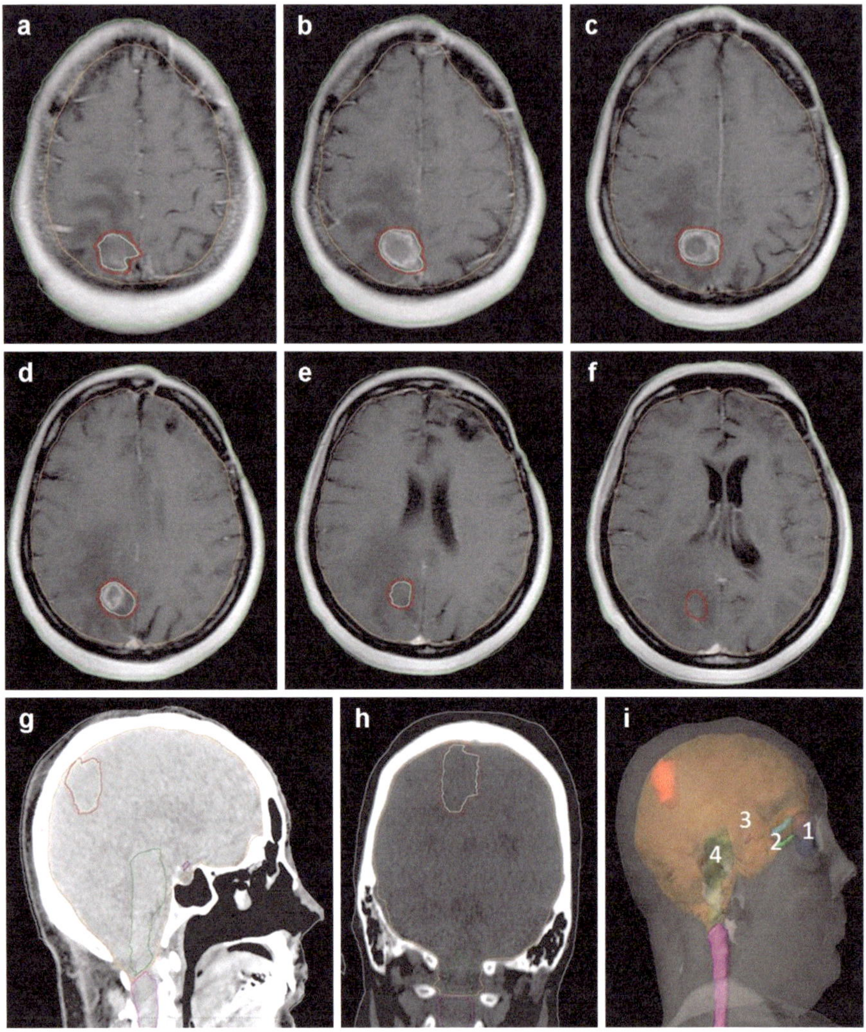

Fig. 7.2 (**a**–**i**) Target volume and organs at risk contouring: *GTV* gross tumor volume, *PTV* planning target volume, (*1*) globes, (*2*) optic nerves, (*3*) optic chiasm, (*4*) brainstem

Delineation of OAR Volumes

For a typical SRS of BM, the OARs include the brain, brainstem, optic chiasm, optic nerves, and cochlea. The following recommendations should be considered during OAR contouring:

Brain: Brain represents for the entire structures those that reside in the bony skull from the vertex to the lower border of foramen magnum or alternatively the upper border of the first cervical vertebrae.

Brainstem: Craniocaudally the brainstem is composed of the midbrain, pons, and medulla oblongata. Anatomically the brainstem starts from the level of superior border of the posterior clinoids and reclines down to the inferior border of the foramen magnum which corresponds to the superior border of the first cervical vertebrae. The midbrain is inferior to the third ventricle and is about 20 mm in length. Mammillary bodies comprise the anterior limit of the midbrain. The pons is the thickest portion of the brainstem that bulges anteriorly between the midbrain and medulla and is approximately 25–30 mm in length. The pons is separated from the midbrain and medulla by the superior and inferior pontine sulci, respectively, and is covered by the cerebellum posteriorly. The medulla oblongata is the lowest part of the brainstem and continues caudally with the spinal cord at the level of inferior border of the foramen magnum or the uppermost border of the first cervical vertebrae [100]. Simultaneous use of the axial and sagittal plane MRI images may be helpful in accurate delineation of the brainstem.

Optic chiasm: The optic chiasm is an X-shaped space, located in the forebrain, directly in front of the hypothalamus. Crucial to vision, the left and right optic nerves intersect at the chiasm, thus creating the hallmark X-shape. The optic chiasm has a transverse diameter of 10–20 mm, an anteroposterior width of 4–13 mm, and thickness of 3–5 mm. The optic chiasm is in direct contact with cerebrospinal fluid anteriorly within the subarachnoid space and posteriorly within the third ventricle. Inferiorly, the optic chiasm lies over the body of the sphenoid bone, typically above the diaphragma sellae and (paradoxically) only rarely within the sulcus chiasmatis. During the delineation procedure, it is critical to be aware of the fact that the relative position of the chiasm over the sella turcica is variable. The chiasm is (a) above the tuberculum sellae in 12 %, (b) above the diaphragm sellae in 79 %, and (c) above the dorsum sellae in 4 % of cases [101].

Optic Nerves: The optic nerves are mainly comprised of four segments: (a) intraocular segment lies within the posterior retina and emerges through a scleral opening (lamina cribrosa), (b) intraorbital segment passes posteriorly and centrally within the orbit, (c) intracanalicular segment constitutes the portion where the optic nerves exit through the tendinous ring and optic canal (optic foramen) inferior to the ophthalmic artery, and (d) intracranial or cisternal segment enters the middle cranial fossa and passes within the suprasellar cistern with the anterior cerebral artery at its superolateral aspect to join the contralateral optic nerve at the optic chiasm. The intracranial portion of the optic nerve is approximately 17 ± 2.4 mm in length [102].

Cochlea: The cochlea is a shell-shaped spiral that turns between two-and-a-half and two-and-three-quarters times around the modiolus (a central column of bone). The cochlea resides in a bony cavity in the petrous portion of the temporal bone. Its base lies against the lateral end of the internal acoustic meatus, its basal coil forms the promontory of the middle ear, and its apex is directed anterolaterally. A bony core, the modiolus, transmits the cochlear nerve and contains the spiral ganglion, the sensory ganglion for this nerve. The external diameter of the cochlea varies from approximately 9 mm at its base to approximately 5 mm at its apex. Although the cochlea is not directly visible on CT scan due to its small size and its deep location in the temporal bone, its volume can be defined on CT images as the bone cavity where it lies [101, 103].

Target Dose Selection

Principally the SRS dose is determined according to the size and location of BM and the neighboring normal tissues. The widely accepted MTD for BM were determined by the RTOG 90-05 dose escalation trial. According to this trial's outcomes, 24, 18, and 15 Gy were settled as the standard dose recommendations for lesions sized ≤20, 21–30, and 31–40, respectively [65]. However, a subsequent retrospective analysis by Shehata et al. evaluating the optimal SRS dose in patients with 468 BM sized ≤20 mm demonstrated that increasing the SRS dose beyond 20 Gy was connected with a trend of a higher rate of grade 3–4 neurotoxicity (5.9 % vs. 1.9 %, $p=0.078$) with no positive impact on tumor control rates [104]. Accordingly, at present a prescription dose of 20 Gy seems, by all accounts, to be satisfactory and more rational than 24 Gy in context of the severe toxicities.

FSRT is an option for larger BM or those in eloquent locations like brainstem or thalamus. Prospective and retrospective series reported similar outcomes for SRS and FSRT utilizing doses in the range of 24–30 Gy in three fractions, 30–35 Gy in four to five fractions, and 35–40 Gy in seven to ten fractions [54].

Another controversial issue is the adjuvant treatment of tumor bed as abovementioned. Although there is no standard of care in the management of BM following surgical excision, the conventional treatment is WBRT but some investigators has interested to search the outcomes of treating only the tumor bed with SRS. In the application of the SRS treatment, the optimal dose for cavity is unknown as well as the margin that is required. In a study, 37 patients with BM were performed three 8 Gy fractions of SRS with 2–3 mm margins around the cavity following resection and the local control rate was reported as 80 % [100]. The results of 101 patients with single BM were reported in a study of Minniti and colleagues in which the patients received three 9 Gy fractions of SRS for the cavities larger than 3 cm with a 2 mm margin. Local control was 93 % at 1 year and 84 % at 2 years [105]. Therefore, appreciating the available literature, it is reasonable to recommend 24–27 Gy in three fractions for patients undergoing TB-SRS that is prescribed to a volume encompassing the resection cavity by 2–3 mm.

Defining the Dose Prescription Isodose Lines

The dosimetric characteristics of the treatment plans are different according to each SRS device. Utilizing multiple isocenters for the treatments with Gamma Knife and LINAC-based SRS means that multiple spherical isodose distributions accumulate in the target. Inevitable coincidence of such high-dose spheres cause to occur high non-uniform dose in the target [8]. In the current era, mono-isocentric plans are also available and more commonly used in modern LINAC-based SRS applications. In general, for LINAC-based SRS, the dose is prescribed to 70–80 % (may be higher) isodose line encompassing the target volume implying that the peripheral dose is 70–80 % of the maximum dose in the target. In GK-SRS, the dose is usually prescribed to the 50–80 % isodose line which explains the cause of greater dose inhomogeneity in the target volume and an immediate initial dose fall-off outside the prescription isodose. The conventional limitations on dose uniformity are not applicable for SRS as the cardinal aim of the treatment plan is to spare the OAR satisfactorily rather than creating maximum dose uniformity [8].

The Assessment of Treatment Plan

The most commonly used and imperative tool for assessing the treatment plan is dose-volume histogram (DVH) which provides necessary metric data in analyzing the plots of the volume covered by each dose level (Figs. 7.3, 7.4, 7.5, and 7.6). The uniformity of the plan, coverage levels of the target volume(s), and doses received by the particular volumes of interested organs at risk (OAR) can be easily and objectively surveyed by DVH analysis. The comparison of different plans is also possible by evaluation of the related DVHs on the same plot. In spite of the fact that the DVH quantitatively allow detection of the hot or cold spots in a treatment plan, they do not give any hint about the exact three-dimensional localization of these points. However, this paucity can easily be overcome by slice by slice evaluation of the dosimetric plan [8].

In addition to this basic evaluation method, there are also more complicated tools for assessing the quality of treatment plan such as conformity index, Paddick conformity index, homogeneity index, selectivity, and gradient index (Table 7.8) [4].

RTOG Indices

The RTOG proposed three widely used metrics that can be employed to describe the quality of SRS plans [106].

The first metric is the conformity index, CIRTOG, which was defined as the volume of prescription isodose line divided by the target volume [8, 106]. This

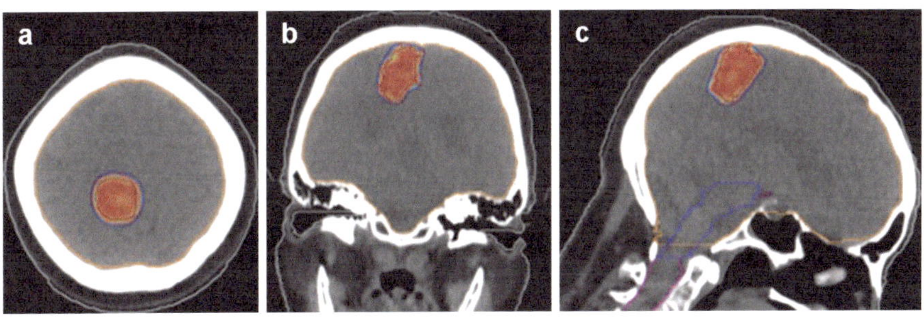

Fig. 7.3 A typical LINAC-based SRS plan: (**a**) axial, (**b**) coronal, (**c**) sagittal view

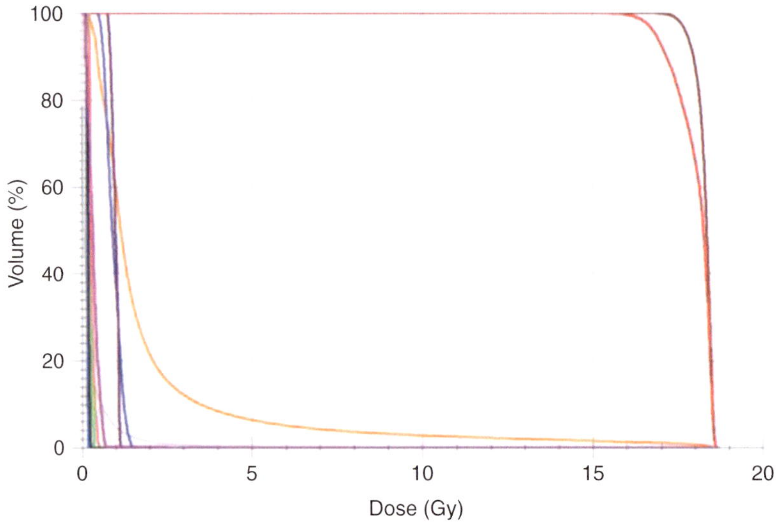

Structure	Min. dose (Gy)	Max. dose (Gy)	Mean dose (Gy)
PTV	15.33	18.68	18.01
CTV	16.81	18.68	18.28
Brainstem	0.47	1.55	0.93
Brain	0.21	18.68	1.91
Optic Chiasm	0.79	1.12	0.99
Right Optic Nerve	0.22	0.49	0.28
Left Optic Nerve	0.23	0.33	0.27
Right Lens	0.14	0.16	0.15
Left Lens	0.12	0.16	0.14

Fig. 7.4 Dose-volume histogram and related evaluation metrics for LINAC-based SRS

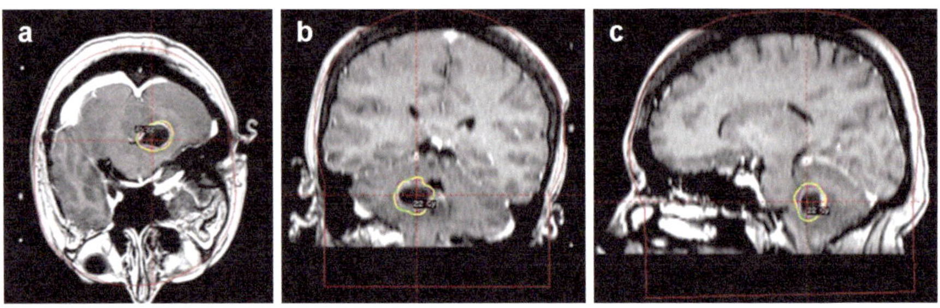

Fig. 7.5 A typical Gamma Knife SRS plan: (**a**) axial, (**b**) coronal, (**c**) sagittal view

simple parameter is a distinct measure of how well the prescribed dose conforms and covers the target volume [107] and however sadly does not give any information about the distinctive levels of dose received by the surrounding healthy tissue volumes. The ideal CI value is 1, meaning that the prescription isodose line matches

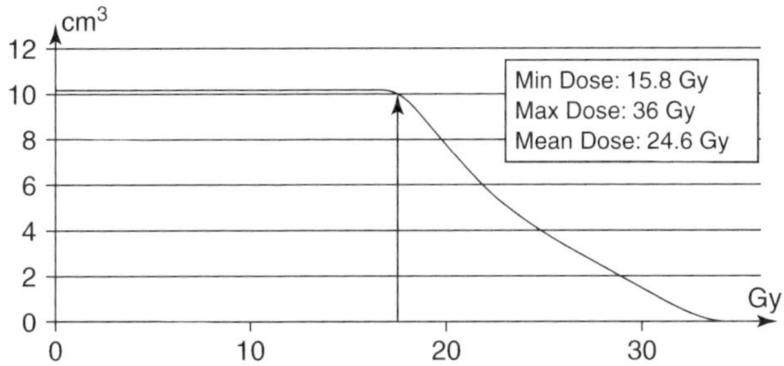

Fig. 7.6 Dose-volume histogram and related evaluation metrics for a typical Gamma Knife SRS plan

Table 7.8 Commonly used indices in evaluation of SRS

Dose plan indices	Formula	Acceptable value
Conformity index (CI)	PIV/TV	1–2 (0.9–3.5)
Paddick conformity index (PCI)	TV_{PIV}^2/TVxPIV	1
Selectivity index (SI)	TV_{PIV}/PIV	1
Gradient index (GI)	$PIV_{X\%}/PIV_{(X/2)\%}$	<3
Homogeneity index (HI)	D_{max}/PD	1 (1.1–2.5)
Coverage (Q)	D_{min}/PD	0.9–1
CI_{Lomax}	TV_{PIV}/TV	0–1

TV target volume, *PIV* volume of prescription isodose, *TVPIV* volume of prescription isodose in the target, *Dmax* maximum dose point in the treatment volume, *PD* prescription dose, *X* isodose which carries the prescription isodose, *X/2* isodose which carries half of the prescription isodose, *Dmin* minimum dose point in the treatment volume

exactly with the target volume with no spread-out prescription dose beyond the target volume. Therefore, CI values above 1 refer to over-coverage of the target volume with unnecessary high-dose regions beyond the intended target. Similarly, a CI value <1 indicates inadequate coverage of the target by the isodose which is undoubtedly unacceptable. The RTOG defines three categories of CI protocol compliance. Plans with a CI value between 1.0 and 2.0 are classified as not deviating from RTOG protocol; plans with a CI value between 2.0 and 2.5 or between 0.9 and 1.0 are classified as having minor deviations; plans with a CI value >2.5 or <0.9 are classified as having major deviations.

The second metric developed by the RTOG to evaluate SRS plans is quality of coverage, Q. This value is found by the calculation of the ratio of minimum dose in the target volume and the prescription isodose [108]. Plans where the 90 % isodose covers the target volume do not deviate from protocol, plans where the 80 % isodose covers the target volume are classified as having a minor deviation, and plans where the 80 % isodose line does not fully cover the target are classified as having a major deviation and therefore unacceptable.

The third metric proposed by the RTOG to evaluate SRS plan quality is the homogeneity index, HI [108]. This index is calculated by dividing the maximum point dose in the target volume to the prescription isodose line. Plans with a HI less than or equal to 2 are said to not deviate from protocol. Minor deviations result when the HI is between 2 and 2.5, and major deviations result when the value is >2.5.

Alternative Conformity Indices

In 2000 Paddick [109] proposed an alternative CI with the goal of providing an objective method for comparing plan quality and eliminating "false scores" provided by the CIRTOG. The proposed index builds on the criticism of the CIRTOG index that the overlap of the volume receiving the prescription isodose and the target volume is not accounted for. This new CI, Paddick CI is calculated as $CI_{Paddick} = TV^2_{PIV}/(TV^2 \times V_{PD})$, where TV is the target volume, TV_{PIV} is the target volume covered by the prescription isodose, and V_{PD} is the total volume covered by the prescription isodose. This index has an ideal value of 1 and plan quality decreases with decreasing index value. The Paddick CI and CIRTOG are inversely related indices which can be defined as $CI_{Paddick} = 0.933/CI_{RTOG}$.

Another alternative CI to the CIRTOG was proposed by Lomax and Scheib [110]. This index is a modification of the stereotactic plan quality criterion initially proposed by the Saint-Anne, Lariboisiere, Tenon (SALT) group for arteriovenous malformations. Lomax and Scheib's modified index, CI_{Lomax} is calculated as $CI_{Lomax} = TV_{PIV}/TV$ where TV_{PIV} is the target volume covered by the prescription isodose and TV is the target volume. This novel index, in effect, shows the proportion of the target volume that receives at minimum the prescription dose. This CI can range from 0 to an optimum value of 1 when the target volume in its entirety receives at least the prescribed dose. This index is the square root of the geometric overlap ratio that is used in the Paddick CI.

The sharpness of the dose fall-off outside the target volume is defined with gradient index (GI) which is calculated by dividing the volume receiving half of the prescribed dose to the volume of prescribed isodose line. Considering the GI, any plan with an excellent CI does not always indicate that it is likewise astounding for the neighboring tissues or OARs, if these structures receive unnecessary excessive doses. Hence, an optimal dose fall-off is likewise essential for minimizing the complication risks notwithstanding to the optimal conformity. In this sense, GI can be thought as an indicator of ideal prescription isodose, so that the steepest conceivable dose fall-off for any given isocenter arrangement is accomplished [107].

Another important index for evaluation of SRS plans is the selectivity index (SI), or just selectivity. CI refers to the fact that the selected isodose conforms to the three-dimensional target volume and the target dose is high. However, selectivity is an equally important aspect of effective SRS and refers to the fact that the integral dose received by the surrounding tissues is low. Plan selectivity is calculated by: $SI = V_{PD}$ n TV/ V_{PD}, where V_{PD} is the total volume receiving prescribed dose and TV is the target volume. An ideal SRS plan should have SI of 1 while any value >1 and <1 refers to overtreatment and undertreatment, respectively (Fig. 7.7).

Recommended parameters and their limits for a typical SRS plan evaluation in regard to the target volume coverage and OAR at risk limits are presented in Tables 7.9 and 7.10.

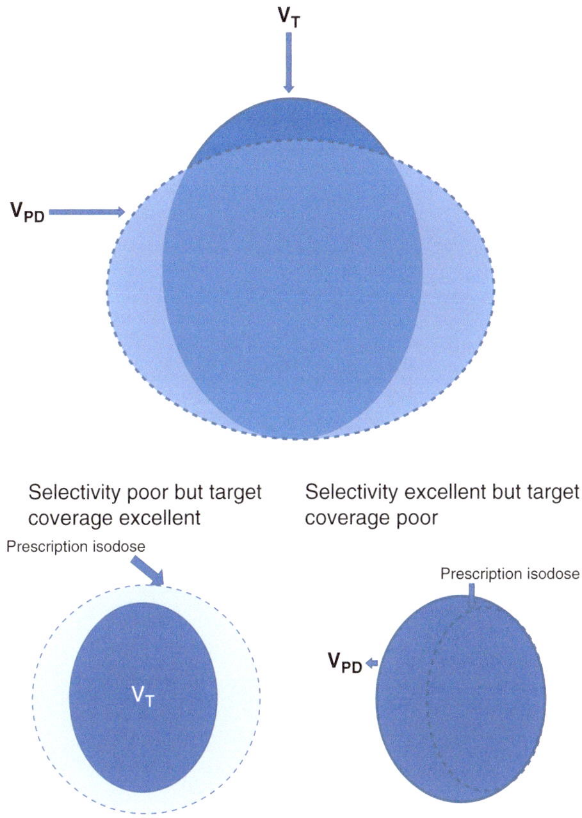

Fig. 7.7 Demonstration of the relationship between target coverage and selectivity: *VT* tumor volume, *VPD* prescription dose volume

Table 7.9 Typical SRS plan assessment specifications

Parameter	No variation	Minor variation (acceptable)	Major deviation (unacceptable)
Target coverage	The 90 % isodose line (90 % of the PD, not TD) completely encompasses target	80 % isodose line covers the target	80 % isodose line does not cover the target
Dose QA (lesion size, PD)	2.0 cm: 20 Gy	–	–
	2.1–3.0 cm: 18 Gy	–	–
	3.1–4.0 cm: 15 Gy	–	–
Dose homogeneity (MD/PD)	≤2	2–2.5	>2.5
Dose conformity (PIV/TV)	1.0–2.0	0.9–1.0 or 2.0–3.5	<0.9 or >3.5

PD prescription dose, *TD* total dose, *QA* quality assurance, *MD* maximum dose, *PIV* volume of prescription isodose line, *TV* target volume

Table 7.10 Dose tolerance limits for SRS and FSRT

Organs	Fractions (n)	Volume (cc)	Volume (%)	Volume limit (Gy)	Max. dose limit (Gy)	Reference
Brainstem	1	1		10	15	[111]
	1	1		18	8	[111]
	1				23	Tradition
	3				31	[111]
	3					[111]
	5					[111]
Chiasma (also for optic nerve)	1	0.2	100	15	15[a]	[112]
	1	0.2		20	13	[113]
	1			20	12	[113]
	1				11	[113]
	1				10[a]	[111]
	3				19.5	[111]
	3				25	[111]
	5					[111]
	5					[111]
	5					[113]
Cochlea	1				12	[111]
	3				20	[111]
	5				27.5	[111]
Brain	5		100	20		[113]
Lens	1				3	[113]
	2				6	[113]
	3				7	[113]
	5				7	[113]

Max maximum, *FSRT* fractionated stereotactic radiotherapy, *SRS* stereotactic radiosurgery
[a]77 % probability of optic neuritis if D_{max} >15 Gy; no risk of optic neuritis if D_{max} <10 Gy

Recommended Treatment Algorithms for SRS

Treatment algorithms for SRS of patients with single and multiple BM are as presented in Figs. 7.8 and 7.9.

Conclusion

Significant advancement has been made over the past three decades for patients with single BM and well-controlled systemic disease. Clear survival advantage has been shown for patients with single BM and favorable prognostic features who underwent neurosurgery or SRS and WBRT versus WBRT alone. On the other hand, for these patients with multiple BM, treatment strategies that prolong survival remain lacking. For this population intracranial disease control, time to

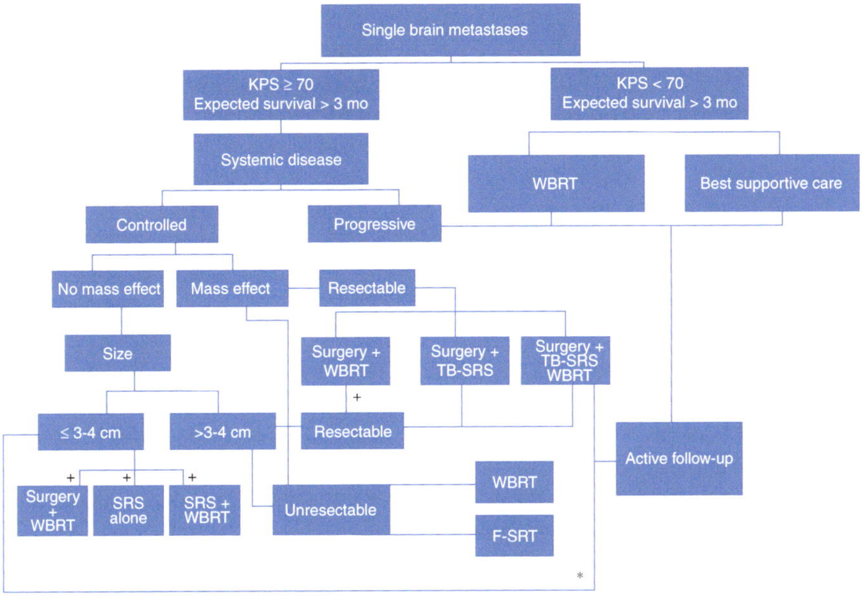

Fig. 7.8 Recommended treatment algorithm for patients with single-brain metastases. *WBRT* whole brain radiation therapy, *TB-SRS* tumor bed stereotactic radiosurgery, (+) level I evidence, (*) level 3 evidence, *FSRT* fractionated radiotherapy

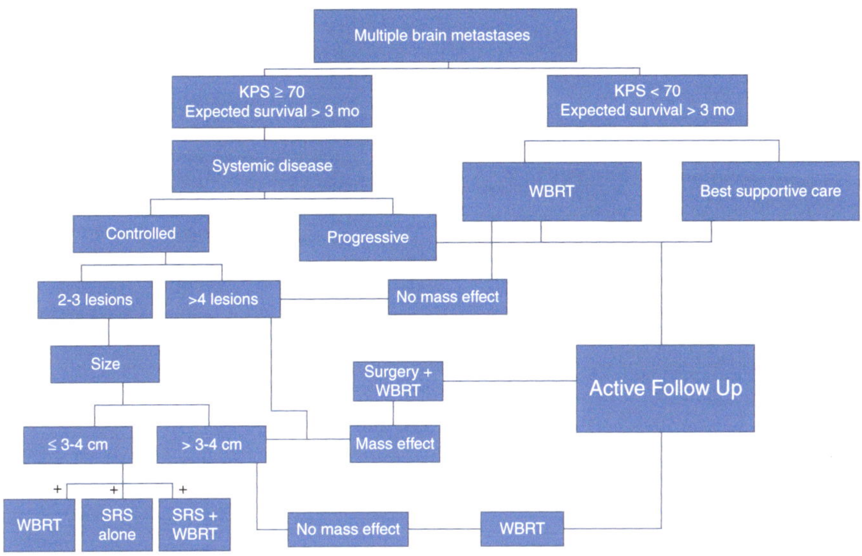

Fig. 7.9 Recommended treatment algorithm for patients with multiple brain metastases. *WBRT* whole brain radiation therapy

neurologic progression, neurologic function, and QOL may be more relevant end points because of the competing risk for death from systemic disease. WBRT remains the standard of care in patients presenting with multiple BM, particularly those with >3 BM. However, addition of SRS may increase the local tumor control rates and may potentially further mitigate tumor-related symptoms.

TB-SRS is a relatively new treatment approach with no randomized data published to date, and only limited prospective data are available. Although the accessible data is encouraging, yet much is still unknown about SRS including the required doses and optimal target volume delineation issues, such as definition of the appropriate margins around the resection cavity. Appropriately designed future TB-SRS studies will most likely provide level 1 proof in clearing some uncertainties and setting the optimal treatment decisions on this particular issue of interest.

Lastly, patients with single or multiple BM will certainly benefit from a multidisciplinary approach focused on the integration of surgical, radiation, and chemotherapeutic options with the goal of preserving neurologic and neurocognitive function and QOL.

References

1. Siegel R, Ward E, Brawley O, Jemal A. Cancer statistics, 2011: the impact of eliminating socioeconomic and racial disparities on premature cancer deaths. CA Cancer J Clin. 2011;61(4):212–36.
2. Liu H, Ma HF, Chen YK. Association between GSTM1 polymorphisms and lung cancer: an updated meta-analysis. Genet Mol Res. 2015;14(1):1385–92.
3. Sorensen JB, Hansen HH, Hansen M, Dombernowsky P. Brain metastases in adenocarcinoma of the lung: frequency, risk groups, and prognosis. J Clin Oncol. 1988;6(9):1474–80.
4. Kocher M, Wittig A, Piroth MD, et al. Stereotactic radiosurgery for treatment of brain metastases. A report of the DEGRO Working Group on Stereotactic Radiotherapy. Strahlenther Onkol. 2014;190(6):521–32.
5. Linskey ME, Andrews DW, Asher AL, et al. The role of stereotactic radiosurgery in the management of patients with newly diagnosed brain metastases: a systematic review and evidence-based clinical practice guideline. J Neurooncol. 2010;96(1):45–68.
6. Eichler AF, Loeffler JS. Multidisciplinary management of brain metastases. Oncologist. 2007;12(7):884–98.
7. Delattre JY, Krol G, Thaler HT, Posner JB. Distribution of brain metastases. Arch Neurol. 1988;45(7):741–4.
8. Chin LS, Regine FW. Principles and practice of stereotactic radiosurgery. New York: Springer; 2008.
9. Berk L. An overview of radiotherapy trials for the treatment of brain metastases. Oncology (Williston Park). 1995;9(11):1205–12; discussion 12–6, 19.
10. Hanahan D, Weinberg RA. Hallmarks of cancer: the next generation. Cell. 2011;144(5):646–74.
11. Langley RR, Fidler IJ. The biology of brain metastasis. Clin Chem. 2013;59(1):180–9.
12. Barsky SH, Siegal GP, Jannotta F, Liotta LA. Loss of basement membrane components by invasive tumors but not by their benign counterparts. Lab Invest. 1983;49(2):140–7.
13. Gavrilovic IT, Posner JB. Brain metastases: epidemiology and pathophysiology. J Neurooncol. 2005;75(1):5–14.

14. Billing PS, Miller DL, Allen MS, Deschamps C, Trastek VF, Pairolero PC. Surgical treatment of primary lung cancer with synchronous brain metastases. J Thorac Cardiovasc Surg. 2001;122(3):548–53.
15. Kocher M, Soffietti R, Abacioglu U, et al. Adjuvant whole-brain radiotherapy versus observation after radiosurgery or surgical resection of one to three cerebral metastases: results of the EORTC 22952-26001 study. J Clin Oncol. 2011;29(2):134–41.
16. DeAngelis LM, Delattre JY, Posner JB. Radiation-induced dementia in patients cured of brain metastases. Neurology. 1989;39(6):789–96.
17. Berghmans T, Paesmans M, Sculier JP. Prognostic factors in stage III non-small cell lung cancer: a review of conventional, metabolic and new biological variables. Ther Adv Med Oncol. 2011;3(3):127–38.
18. Yates JW, Chalmer B, McKegney FP. Evaluation of patients with advanced cancer using the Karnofsky performance status. Cancer. 1980;45(8):2220–4.
19. Sperduto PW, Kased N, Roberge D, et al. Summary report on the graded prognostic assessment: an accurate and facile diagnosis-specific tool to estimate survival for patients with brain metastases. J Clin Oncol. 2012;30(4):419–25.
20. Abrahams JM, Torchia M, Putt M, Kaiser LR, Judy KD. Risk factors affecting survival after brain metastases from non-small cell lung carcinoma: a follow-up study of 70 patients. J Neurosurg. 2001;95(4):595–600.
21. Weltman E, Salvajoli JV, Brandt RA, et al. Radiosurgery for brain metastases: a score index for predicting prognosis. Int J Radiat Oncol Biol Phys. 2000;46(5):1155–61.
22. Venur VA, Ahluwalia MS. Prognostic scores for brain metastasis patients: use in clinical practice and trial design. Chin Clin Oncol. 2015;4(2):18.
23. Komarnicky LT, Phillips TL, Martz K, Asbell S, Isaacson S, Urtasun R. A randomized phase III protocol for the evaluation of misonidazole combined with radiation in the treatment of patients with brain metastases (RTOG-7916). Int J Radiat Oncol Biol Phys. 1991;20(1):53–8.
24. Phillips TL, Scott CB, Leibel SA, Rotman M, Weigensberg IJ. Results of a randomized comparison of radiotherapy and bromodeoxyuridine with radiotherapy alone for brain metastases: report of RTOG trial 89-05. Int J Radiat Oncol Biol Phys. 1995;33(2):339–48.
25. Sause WT, Crowley JJ, Morantz R, et al. Solitary brain metastasis: results of an RTOG/SWOG protocol evaluation surgery + RT versus RT alone. Am J Clin Oncol. 1990;13(5):427–32.
26. Gaspar L, Scott C, Rotman M, et al. Recursive partitioning analysis (RPA) of prognostic factors in three Radiation Therapy Oncology Group (RTOG) brain metastases trials. Int J Radiat Oncol Biol Phys. 1997;37(4):745–51.
27. Park JY, Moon KS, Lee KH, et al. Gamma knife radiosurgery for elderly patients with brain metastases: evaluation of scoring systems that predict survival. BMC Cancer. 2015;15:54.
28. Nieder C, Andratschke N, Grosu AL, Molls M. Recursive partitioning analysis (RPA) class does not predict survival in patients with four or more brain metastases. Strahlenther Onkol. 2003;179(1):16–20.
29. Rades D, Dziggel L, Haatanen T, et al. Scoring systems to estimate intracerebral control and survival rates of patients irradiated for brain metastases. Int J Radiat Oncol Biol Phys. 2011;80(4):1122–7.
30. Lorenzoni J, Devriendt D, Massager N, et al. Radiosurgery for treatment of brain metastases: estimation of patient eligibility using three stratification systems. Int J Radiat Oncol Biol Phys. 2004;60(1):218–24.
31. Nieder C, Geinitz H, Molls M. Validation of the graded prognostic assessment index for surgically treated patients with brain metastases. Anticancer Res. 2008;28(5B):3015–7.
32. Andrews DW, Scott CB, Sperduto PW, et al. Whole brain radiation therapy with or without stereotactic radiosurgery boost for patients with one to three brain metastases: phase III results of the RTOG 9508 randomised trial. Lancet. 2004;363(9422):1665–72.
33. Sperduto PW, Berkey B, Gaspar LE, Mehta M, Curran W. A new prognostic index and comparison to three other indices for patients with brain metastases: an analysis of 1,960 patients in the RTOG database. Int J Radiat Oncol Biol Phys. 2008;70(2):510–4.

34. Antoni D, Noel G. Radiotherapy of brain metastases according to the GPA score (Graded Prognostic Assessment). Cancer Radiother. 2013;17(5–6):424–7.
35. Tabouret E, Metellus P, Goncalves A, et al. Assessment of prognostic scores in brain metastases from breast cancer. Neuro-Oncology. 2014;16(3):421–8.
36. Luo J, Zhu H, Tang Y, et al. Analysis of prognostic factors and comparison of prognostic index scores in patients with brain metastases after whole-brain radiotherapy. Int J Clin Exp Med. 2014;7(12):5217–25.
37. Meyers CA, Weitzner MA, Valentine AD, Levin VA. Methylphenidate therapy improves cognition, mood, and function of brain tumor patients. J Clin Oncol. 1998;16(7):2522–7.
38. Shaw EG, Rosdhal R, D'Agostino Jr RB, et al. Phase II study of donepezil in irradiated brain tumor patients: effect on cognitive function, mood, and quality of life. J Clin Oncol. 2006;24(9):1415–20.
39. Ganz JC. Stereotactic and radiosurgery research in Sweden. Prog Brain Res. 2014; 215:57–66.
40. Thompson BG, Coffey RJ, Flickinger JC, Lunsford LD. Stereotactic radiosurgery of small intracranial tumors: neuropathological correlation in three patients. Surg Neurol. 1990; 33(2):96–104.
41. Brown JM, Carlson DJ, Brenner DJ. The tumor radiobiology of SRS and SBRT: are more than the 5 Rs involved? Int J Radiat Oncol Biol Phys. 2014;88(2):254–62.
42. Patchell RA, Tibbs PA, Walsh JW, et al. A randomized trial of surgery in the treatment of single metastases to the brain. N Engl J Med. 1990;322(8):494–500.
43. Noordijk EM, Vecht CJ, Haaxma-Reiche H, et al. The choice of treatment of single brain metastasis should be based on extracranial tumor activity and age. Int J Radiat Oncol Biol Phys. 1994;29(4):711–7.
44. Muacevic A, Wowra B, Siefert A, Tonn JC, Steiger HJ, Kreth FW. Microsurgery plus whole brain irradiation versus Gamma Knife surgery alone for treatment of single metastases to the brain: a randomized controlled multicentre phase III trial. J Neurooncol. 2008;87(3):299–307.
45. Qin H, Wang C, Jiang Y, Zhang X, Zhang Y, Ruan Z. Patients with single brain metastasis from non-small cell lung cancer equally benefit from stereotactic radiosurgery and surgery: a systematic review. Med Sci Monit. 2015;21:144–52.
46. Vuong DA, Rades D, van Eck AT, Horstmann GA, Busse R. Comparing the cost-effectiveness of two brain metastasis treatment modalities from a payer's perspective: stereotactic radiosurgery versus surgical resection. Clin Neurol Neurosurg. 2013;115(3):276–84.
47. Caruso JP, Moosa S, Fezeu F, Ramesh A, Sheehan JP. A cost comparative study of Gamma Knife radiosurgery versus open surgery for intracranial pathology. J Clin Neurosci. 2015;22(1):184–8.
48. Chang EL, Wefel JS, Hess KR, et al. Neurocognition in patients with brain metastases treated with radiosurgery or radiosurgery plus whole-brain irradiation: a randomised controlled trial. Lancet Oncol. 2009;10(11):1037–44.
49. Meyers CA, Smith JA, Bezjak A, et al. Neurocognitive function and progression in patients with brain metastases treated with whole-brain radiation and motexafin gadolinium: results of a randomized phase III trial. J Clin Oncol. 2004;22(1):157–65.
50. Regine WF, Huhn JL, Patchell RA, et al. Risk of symptomatic brain tumor recurrence and neurologic deficit after radiosurgery alone in patients with newly diagnosed brain metastases: results and implications. Int J Radiat Oncol Biol Phys. 2002;52(2):333–8.
51. Aoyama H, Shirato H, Tago M, et al. Stereotactic radiosurgery plus whole-brain radiation therapy vs stereotactic radiosurgery alone for treatment of brain metastases: a randomized controlled trial. JAMA. 2006;295(21):2483–91.
52. Patchell RA, Regine WF, Loeffler JS, Sawaya R, Andrews DW, Chin LS. Radiosurgery plus whole-brain radiation therapy for brain metastases. JAMA. 2006;296(17):2089–90; author reply 90–1.
53. Wang TJ, Saad S, Qureshi YH, et al. Outcomes of gamma knife radiosurgery, bi-modality & tri-modality treatment regimens for patients with one or multiple brain metastases: the Columbia University Medical Center experience. J Neurooncol. 2015;122(2):399–408.

54. Pinkham MB, Whitfield GA, Brada M. New developments in intracranial stereotactic radiotherapy for metastases. Clin Oncol (R Coll Radiol). 2015;27(5):316–23.
55. Skeie BS, Skeie GO, Enger PO, et al. Gamma knife surgery in brain melanomas: absence of extracranial metastases and tumor volume strongest indicators of prolonged survival. World Neurosurg. 2011;75(5–6):684–91; discussion 598–603.
56. Chen JC, Petrovich Z, O'Day S, et al. Stereotactic radiosurgery in the treatment of metastatic disease to the brain. Neurosurgery. 2000;47(2):268–79; discussion 79–81.
57. Serizawa T, Yamamoto M, Sato Y, et al. Gamma Knife surgery as sole treatment for multiple brain metastases: 2-center retrospective review of 1508 cases meeting the inclusion criteria of the JLGK0901 multi-institutional prospective study. J Neurosurg. 2010;113(Suppl):48–52.
58. Chang WS, Kim HY, Chang JW, Park YG, Chang JH. Analysis of radiosurgical results in patients with brain metastases according to the number of brain lesions: is stereotactic radiosurgery effective for multiple brain metastases? J Neurosurg. 2010;113(Suppl):73–8.
59. Likhacheva A, Pinnix CC, Parikh NR, et al. Predictors of survival in contemporary practice after initial radiosurgery for brain metastases. Int J Radiat Oncol Biol Phys. 2013;85(3):656–61.
60. Schouten LJ, Rutten J, Huveneers HA, Twijnstra A. Incidence of brain metastases in a cohort of patients with carcinoma of the breast, colon, kidney, and lung and melanoma. Cancer. 2002;94(10):2698–705.
61. Vecht CJ, Haaxma-Reiche H, Noordijk EM, et al. Treatment of single brain metastasis: radiotherapy alone or combined with neurosurgery? Ann Neurol. 1993;33(6):583–90.
62. Ebinu JO, Lwu S, Monsalves E, et al. Gamma knife radiosurgery for the treatment of cystic cerebral metastases. Int J Radiat Oncol Biol Phys. 2013;85(3):667–71.
63. Flickinger JC. Radiotherapy and radiosurgical management of brain metastases. Curr Oncol Rep. 2001;3(6):484–9.
64. Kim M, Cheok S, Chung LK, et al. Characteristics and treatments of large cystic brain metastasis: radiosurgery and stereotactic aspiration. Brain Tumor Res Treat. 2015;3(1):1–7.
65. Shaw E, Scott C, Souhami L, et al. Single dose radiosurgical treatment of recurrent previously irradiated primary brain tumors and brain metastases: final report of RTOG protocol 90-05. Int J Radiat Oncol Biol Phys. 2000;47(2):291–8.
66. Murai T, Ogino H, Manabe Y, et al. Fractionated stereotactic radiotherapy using CyberKnife for the treatment of large brain metastases: a dose escalation study. Clin Oncol (R Coll Radiol). 2014;26(3):151–8.
67. O'Neill BP, Iturria NJ, Link MJ, Pollock BE, Ballman KV, O'Fallon JR. A comparison of surgical resection and stereotactic radiosurgery in the treatment of solitary brain metastases. Int J Radiat Oncol Biol Phys. 2003;55(5):1169–76.
68. Amsbaugh MJ, Boling W, Woo S. Tumor bed radiosurgery: an emerging treatment for brain metastases. J Neurooncol. 2015;123(2):197–203.
69. Gans JH, Raper DM, Shah AH, et al. The role of radiosurgery to the tumor bed after resection of brain metastases. Neurosurgery. 2013;72(3):317–25; discussion 25–6.
70. Roberge D, Parney I, Brown PD. Radiosurgery to the postoperative surgical cavity: who needs evidence? Int J Radiat Oncol Biol Phys. 2012;83(2):486–93.
71. Kelly PJ, Lin YB, Yu AY, et al. Stereotactic irradiation of the postoperative resection cavity for brain metastasis: a frameless linear accelerator-based case series and review of the technique. Int J Radiat Oncol Biol Phys. 2012;82(1):95–101.
72. Kim PK, Ellis TL, Stieber VW, et al. Gamma Knife surgery targeting the resection cavity of brain metastasis that has progressed after whole-brain radiotherapy. J Neurosurg. 2006;105(Suppl):75–8.
73. Brennan C, Yang TJ, Hilden P, et al. A phase 2 trial of stereotactic radiosurgery boost after surgical resection for brain metastases. Int J Radiat Oncol Biol Phys. 2014;88(1):130–6.
74. Asher AL, Burri SH, Wiggins WF, et al. A new treatment paradigm: neoadjuvant radiosurgery before surgical resection of brain metastases with analysis of local tumor recurrence. Int J Radiat Oncol Biol Phys. 2014;88(4):899–906.
75. Patchell RA, Tibbs PA, Regine WF, et al. Postoperative radiotherapy in the treatment of single metastases to the brain: a randomized trial. JAMA. 1998;280(17):1485–9.

76. Borgelt B, Gelber R, Kramer S, et al. The palliation of brain metastases: final results of the first two studies by the Radiation Therapy Oncology Group. Int J Radiat Oncol Biol Phys. 1980;6(1):1–9.
77. Zimm S, Wampler GL, Stablein D, Hazra T, Young HF. Intracerebral metastases in solid-tumor patients: natural history and results of treatment. Cancer. 1981;48(2):384–94.
78. Hazuka MB, Kinzie JJ. Brain metastases: results and effects of re-irradiation. Int J Radiat Oncol Biol Phys. 1988;15(2):433–7.
79. Wong WW, Schild SE, Sawyer TE, Shaw EG. Analysis of outcome in patients reirradiated for brain metastases. Int J Radiat Oncol Biol Phys. 1996;34(3):585–90.
80. Kurtz G, Zadeh G, Gingras-Hill G, et al. Salvage radiosurgery for brain metastases: prognostic factors to consider in patient selection. Int J Radiat Oncol Biol Phys. 2014;88(1):137–42.
81. Noel G, Proudhom MA, Valery CA, et al. Radiosurgery for re-irradiation of brain metastasis: results in 54 patients. Radiother Oncol. 2001;60(1):61–7.
82. Alexander 3rd E, Moriarty TM, Davis RB, et al. Stereotactic radiosurgery for the definitive, noninvasive treatment of brain metastases. J Natl Cancer Inst. 1995;87(1):34–40.
83. Weissman DE. Glucocorticoid treatment for brain metastases and epidural spinal cord compression: a review. J Clin Oncol. 1988;6(3):543–51.
84. Valery CA, Cornu P, Noel G, et al. Predictive factors of radiation necrosis after radiosurgery for cerebral metastases. Stereotact Funct Neurosurg. 2003;81(1–4):115–9.
85. Tsao MN, Lloyd N, Wong RK, et al. Whole brain radiotherapy for the treatment of newly diagnosed multiple brain metastases. Cochrane Database Syst Rev. 2012;4:CD003869.
86. Soffietti R, Kocher M, Abacioglu UM, et al. A European Organisation for Research and Treatment of Cancer phase III trial of adjuvant whole-brain radiotherapy versus observation in patients with one to three brain metastases from solid tumors after surgical resection or radiosurgery: quality-of-life results. J Clin Oncol. 2013;31(1):65–72.
87. Slotman BJ, Mauer ME, Bottomley A, et al. Prophylactic cranial irradiation in extensive disease small-cell lung cancer: short-term health-related quality of life and patient reported symptoms: results of an international phase III randomized controlled trial by the EORTC Radiation Oncology and Lung Cancer Groups. J Clin Oncol. 2009;27(1):78–84.
88. Welzel G, Fleckenstein K, Schaefer J, et al. Memory function before and after whole brain radiotherapy in patients with and without brain metastases. Int J Radiat Oncol Biol Phys. 2008;72(5):1311–8.
89. Aoyama H, Tago M, Kato N, et al. Neurocognitive function of patients with brain metastasis who received either whole brain radiotherapy plus stereotactic radiosurgery or radiosurgery alone. Int J Radiat Oncol Biol Phys. 2007;68(5):1388–95.
90. Langley RE, Stephens RJ, Nankivell M, et al. Interim data from the Medical Research Council QUARTZ Trial: does whole brain radiotherapy affect the survival and quality of life of patients with brain metastases from non-small cell lung cancer? Clin Oncol (R Coll Radiol). 2013;25(3):e23–30.
91. Doyle DM, Einhorn LH. Delayed effects of whole brain radiotherapy in germ cell tumor patients with central nervous system metastases. Int J Radiat Oncol Biol Phys. 2008;70(5):1361–4.
92. DiBiase SJ, Chin LS, Ma L. Influence of gamma knife radiosurgery on the quality of life in patients with brain metastases. Am J Clin Oncol. 2002;25(2):131–4.
93. Peschel RE. Notice: recently published book: proton therapy and radiosurgery, H. Breuer, B.J. Smit, springer-verlag; 2000. Int J Cancer. 2000;90(2):112.
94. Wu A, Lindner G, Maitz AH, et al. Physics of gamma knife approach on convergent beams in stereotactic radiosurgery. Int J Radiat Oncol Biol Phys. 1990;18(4):941–9.
95. Gill SS, Thomas DG, Warrington AP, Brada M. Relocatable frame for stereotactic external beam radiotherapy. Int J Radiat Oncol Biol Phys. 1991;20(3):599–603.
96. Fuss M, Salter BJ, Rassiah P, Cheek D, Cavanaugh SX, Herman TS. Repositioning accuracy of a commercially available double-vacuum whole body immobilization system for stereotactic body radiation therapy. Technol Cancer Res Treat. 2004;3(1):59–67.

97. Guckenberger M, Roesch J, Baier K, Sweeney RA, Flentje M. Dosimetric consequences of translational and rotational errors in frame-less image-guided radiosurgery. Radiat Oncol. 2012;7:63.
98. Ramakrishna N, Rosca F, Friesen S, Tezcanli E, Zygmanszki P, Hacker F. A clinical comparison of patient setup and intra-fraction motion using frame-based radiosurgery versus a frameless image-guided radiosurgery system for intracranial lesions. Radiother Oncol. 2010;95(1):109–15.
99. Choi CY, Chang SD, Gibbs IC, et al. Stereotactic radiosurgery of the postoperative resection cavity for brain metastases: prospective evaluation of target margin on tumor control. Int J Radiat Oncol Biol Phys. 2012;84(2):336–42.
100. Wang CC, Floyd SR, Chang CH, et al. Cyberknife hypofractionated stereotactic radiosurgery (HSRS) of resection cavity after excision of large cerebral metastasis: efficacy and safety of an 800 cGy x 3 daily fractions regimen. J Neurooncol. 2012;106(3):601–10.
101. Scoccianti S, Detti B, Gadda D, et al. Organs at risk in the brain and their dose-constraints in adults and in children: a radiation oncologist's guide for delineation in everyday practice. Radiother Oncol. 2015;114(2):230–8.
102. Sadun AA GS, Bose S. Chapter 34: anatomy of the visual sensory system. In: William T, Edward AJ, editors. Duane's ophthalmology, foundations, vol. 1. Philadelphia, USA, Lippincott Williams & Wilkins. 2005.
103. Pacholke HD, Amdur RJ, Schmalfuss IM, Louis D, Mendenhall WM. Contouring the middle and inner ear on radiotherapy planning scans. Am J Clin Oncol. 2005;28(2):143–7.
104. Shehata MK, Young B, Reid B, et al. Stereotactic radiosurgery of 468 brain metastases < or =2 cm: implications for SRS dose and whole brain radiation therapy. Int J Radiat Oncol Biol Phys. 2004;59(1):87–93.
105. Minniti G, Esposito V, Clarke E, et al. Multidose stereotactic radiosurgery (9 Gy x 3) of the postoperative resection cavity for treatment of large brain metastases. Int J Radiat Oncol Biol Phys. 2013;86(4):623–9.
106. Shaw E, Kline R, Gillin M, et al. Radiation Therapy Oncology Group: radiosurgery quality assurance guidelines. Int J Radiat Oncol Biol Phys. 1993;27(5):1231–9.
107. Paddick I, Lippitz B. A simple dose gradient measurement tool to complement the conformity index. J Neurosurg. 2006;105(Suppl):194–201.
108. Feuvret L, Noel G, Mazeron JJ, Bey P. Conformity index: a review. Int J Radiat Oncol Biol Phys. 2006;64(2):333–42.
109. Paddick I. A simple scoring ratio to index the conformity of radiosurgical treatment plans. Technical note. J Neurosurg. 2000;93 Suppl 3:219–22.
110. Lomax NJ, Scheib SG. Quantifying the degree of conformity in radiosurgery treatment planning. Int J Radiat Oncol Biol Phys. 2003;55(5):1409–19.
111. Timmerman RD. An overview of hypofractionation and introduction to this issue of seminars in radiation oncology. Semin Radiat Oncol. 2008;18(4):215–22.
112. Leber KA, Bergloff J, Pendl G. Dose-response tolerance of the visual pathways and cranial nerves of the cavernous sinus to stereotactic radiosurgery. J Neurosurg. 1998;88(1):43–50.
113. Grimm J, LaCouture T, Croce R, Yeo I, Zhu Y, Xue J. Dose tolerance limits and dose volume histogram evaluation for stereotactic body radiotherapy. J Appl Clin Med Phys. 2011; 12(2):3368.

Modern Radiotherapy in Limited and Extensive Stage Small-Cell Lung Cancer

8

Erkan Topkan, Berna Akkus Yildirim, and Ugur Selek

Introduction

Small-cell lung cancer (SCLC), previously called oat-cell carcinoma, accounts for approximately 10–15 % all lung cancers with more than 95 % being associated with tobacco smoking [1]. First recognized in 1926 by Barnard, SCLC is a unique pathological and clinical entity within the range of lung cancers [2]. As later described in detail by Watson and Berg in 1962, SCLC has distinct clinical features, namely, predominance of central location on radiographs, early dissemination tendency, high initial remarkable but temporary chemo- and radiosensitivity, and high propensity for fatal local and/or distant relapses. This first definition still preserves its validity with almost no notable changes since past five decades [3]. Albeit there is no significant difference in outcome by histologic subtype, the World Health Organization classification subdivides SCLC into three cell types: pure or classic, variant cell, and mixed [4].

Typically, SCLC presents in senior patients (>70 years) with a substantial smoking history. The patients usually apply with symptomatic bulky and centrally located masses and accompanying hilar and/or mediastinal enlarged lymph nodes. Albeit numerous local or systemic symptoms may be present at the first admission, the commonest ones are cough (50 %) and weight loss (50 %) trailed by dyspnea (40 %) and generalized weakness (40 %) (Table 8.1). Of note, 15 % of patients present with

E. Topkan, MD (✉) • B.A. Yildirim
Department of Radiation Oncology, Faculty of Medicine, Baskent University, Adana, Turkey
e-mail: docdretopkan@gmail.com;

U. Selek, MD
Department of Radiation Oncology, Faculty of Medicine, Koc University, Istanbul, Turkey

Department of Radiation Oncology, The University of Texas, MD Anderson Cancer Center, Houston, TX, USA
e-mail: uselek@ku.edu.tr; ugurselek@yahoo.com

G. Ozyigit et al. (eds.), *Principles and Practice of Radiotherapy Techniques in Thoracic Malignancies*, DOI 10.1007/978-3-319-28761-4_8

Table 8.1 Symptom frequencies at presentation in SCLC patients

Symptom	Incidence (%)
Cough	50
Weight loss	50
Dyspnea	40
Weakness	40
Chest pain	35
Anorexia	30
Hemoptysis	20
Paraneoplastic syndromes	15
Fever of unknown origin	10
Hoarseness	10

endocrine or neurologic paraneoplastic disorders which may lead to severe morbidity or even fatality, if not intervened timely and appropriately [5]. Disease spread beyond the thorax is diagnosed in up to 75–80 % of cases at initial evaluations, and approximately 20 % of patients present with brain metastases (BM) of which half are symptomatic, while remaining half are detected by radiologic imaging. BM incidence is directly associated with the disease stage, meaning that the risk is higher for patients with extensive stage (ES-SCLC) than the limited stage SCLC (LS-SCLC) that ascends to 69 % at 2-years of diagnosis [6, 7].

Staging

Accurate staging is the initial vital step in the management of SCLC. Although a tumor-lymph node-metastasis (TNM) classification has been proposed for staging, because SCLC rarely presents with sufficiently localized disease that is suitable for surgical resection, this staging system has never gained universal acceptance by the oncologic community and thus is for the most part not utilized. Instead, historic Veteran's Administration Lung Study Group (VALG) staging criteria which simply divides patients into two stages has turned into the preferred staging system in oncology clinics: LS-SCLC and ES-SCLC [8]. LS-SCLC is defined as the disease confined to the ipsilateral hemithorax which can be securely encompassed within a tolerable single radiation port. Involvement of ipsilateral supraclavicular lymph node(s) is also included in LS-SCLC. In contrast, patients with ES-SCLC have disease that is past the ipsilateral hemithorax. In addition to the hematogenous spread, involvement of contralateral supraclavicular lymph node(s) and/or presence of malignant pleural and/or pericardial effusion is also included in ES-SCLC. Unfortunately, only less than one third of SCLC patients present with LS disease, while remaining two thirds have ES disease.

The revised American Joint Committee on Cancer (AJCC) staging system, which was originally implemented the TNM staging for NSCLC, recommended its use for SCLC patients as well in its sixth and seventh editions [9, 10]. Considering the survival outcomes, Vallieres et al. [11] in their recent study on 349 resected

SCLC patients confirmed the utility of TNM-based pathologic staging. However, on the grounds that only 5 % of all SCLC patients present with an operable disease, it seems difficult to adopt TNM-based staging system in routine staging of SCLC patients even in the near future.

Positron emission tomography-computerized tomography (PET-CT) may prove beneficial in detection of CT-occult metastases and/or may alter treatment decisions and/or radiotherapy (RT) port [12]. Therefore, besides the standard staging tools, including the plain chest X-ray, thoracic CT, abdominal CT or ultrasonography, and brain magnetic resonance imaging, the current guidelines of the US National Comprehensive Cancer Network recommend the use of positron emission tomography (PET) or fused PET-CT scanning for the staging of SCLC.

Histologic and Immunohistochemical Markers

Several histologic and immunohistochemical markers have been assessed for their diagnostic, prognostic, and/or predictive roles in SCLC patients, including transcription thyroid factor-1 (TTF-1), cytokeratin 7, chromosome 3 deletions, Leu-7, chromogranin A, synaptophysin, myc amplification, p53 mutations, fragile histidine triad (FHIT), RAS effector homologue (RASSF1), retinoblastoma-1 (RB1), and retinoic acid receptor-beta [13]. Mutations that are often present in NSCLC, such as epidermal growth factor receptor (EGFR) mutations and anaplastic lymphoma kinase (ALK), are rare in SCLC. To our best information, no biomarkers to date have been approved for diagnostic, prognostic, or predictive purposes in SCLC patients.

Prognostic Factors

Regardless of fundamental improvements in imaging and treatment modalities, prognosis of patients with SCLC is still unsatisfactorily poor with median survival ranges of only 15–20 months for LS-SCLC and 8–13 months for ES-SCLC [5]. Moreover, underlining the futility of the condition, 5-year survivors are accounted for to be only in the respective ranges of 10–13 % and 1–2 % [14, 15]. Various variables have been allotted to convey prognostic significance for patients with SCLC; however, the most essential tumor-related variable is the VALG stage (LS- versus ES-SCLC). In LS-SCLC, early stage disease that corresponds to TNM stage 1 carries the best prognosis particularly without raised serum lactate dehydrogenase levels [14, 16]. Like other tumor locales, pretreatment weight loss and poor performance status are significant indicators of unfavorable outcomes [17]. Likewise, men fare poorer than women [5]. In ES-SCLC, the number of organ sites and site of involvement are also strongly associated with prognosis [18]. Compared to other sites, involvement of the bone marrow, liver, or central nervous system signifies unfavorable disease course. SCLC is frequently associated with paraneoplastic syndromes either via antibody-mediated tissue destruction or via ectopic hormone production

Table 8.2 Factors associated with better prognosis in SCLC patients

Good performance status
Limited stage disease
Female sex
Normal serum lactate dehydrogenase
Combination chemotherapy
Early chemoradiotherapy
Prophylactic cranial irradiation
Absence of weight loss
Few sites of metastatic disease
Absence of pleural effusion
Absence of brain metastases
Absence of liver metastases
Age <40 years
Normal serum sodium concentration
Normal liver function tests
Presence of antibody-mediated paraneoplastic syndromes
Lower pretreatment SUVmax value
Low whole-body metabolic tumor volume

[5]. Albeit debated by some, unlike antibody-mediated paraneoplastic syndromes, ectopic hormone production is generally accepted as a predictor of poor outcome. Better prognosis in patients with antibody-mediated paraneoplastic syndromes may be related with presence of a fully competent immune system, indicating the need for exploration of immunotherapy adjunct to standard treatment approaches in this patients group. In summary, as depicted in Table 8.2, although many other factors have been proposed to be useful in stratification of patients with different prognosis, the established factors include: good performance status, limited stage disease, female sex, normal serum lactate dehydrogenase, use of combination chemotherapy, early chemoradiotherapy (CRT), prophylactic cranial irradiation (PCI), absence of weight loss, and few metastatic sites.

Treatment of LS-SCLC

Surgery

Unless diagnosed quite early, which constitutes only less than 5 % of all SCLC patients, surgery currently has little role in the standard management of SCLC. More than four decades ago, The British Medical Research Council study clearly demonstrated the superiority of thoracic radiotherapy (TRT) over surgery by expanding median OS from 6.5 months with surgery to 9.9 months with TRT [19, 20]. Since that time, TRT has become the standard treatment for patients with LS-SCLC.

Radical surgery appears to be predominantly beneficial in LS-SCLC patients with TNM stage I disease [21, 22]. Even such patients should undergo a through radiological and mediastinal staging procedure and assessed for satisfactory pulmonary residual capacity after surgery in order to select appropriate candidates. Currently, surgery is recommended for only medically fit stage I SCLC patients with peripherally located lesions and no hilar/mediastinal nodal involvement. However, adjuvant combination chemotherapy is still strongly recommended for this group of patients. Postoperative CRT should be considered for patients treated with non-anatomic surgery or positive margins or incidentally detected hilar/mediastinal nodal involvement.

Chemotherapy

Although the detailed systemic management of SCLC is beyond the scope of this chapter, the advancements in chemotherapy will shortly be outlined in the following paragraphs. In 1970s, chemotherapy trials of LS-NSCLC demonstrated that the survival was improved from few weeks without to several months with chemotherapy. Several studies conducted past four decades have shown the clear superiority of the combination chemotherapy regimens over single-agent regimens. Response rates of 70–85 %, with complete response of 20–30 %, are encouraging, but virtually almost every patient relapses [5]. Outcomes of randomized controlled trials (RCTs) and meta-analysis in search of the most active regimen indicated the superiority of etoposide plus cisplatin (EP) combination over the other investigated combinations [23–27]. Thusly, the EP combination has turn into the standard chemotherapy combination in United States and Europe since 1980s. In spite of the fact that the cisplatin is the backbone of chemotherapy, carboplatin may be substituted for cisplatin in senior patients or in those with renal insufficiency without an apparent efficacy loss [28]. Combinations constituting a variety of newer agents, like irinotecan, have been tested for enhancing the available outcomes in LS-SCLC. Nevertheless, these agents could not prove to be more active than the older ones. Irinotecan, which was the most promising of them, has been tested in three randomized phase 3 trials [29–31]. The first trial by Noda et al. showed the superiority of cisplatin plus irinotecan (IP) over the standard EP combination in a Japanese Clinical Oncology Group (JCOG) trial [29]. However, two subsequent trials launched in United States could not confirm these results [30, 31]. In both trials response and survival rates in investigational IP arms were found to be equivalent to standard EP. The potential benefit of adding a third agent to standard EP has also been extensively investigated. Higher response rates at a cost of significantly increased toxicity were achieved, with no notable improvement in median survival duration over EP alone [32–34]. In view of these results, four to six cycles o EP combination have been acknowledged to be the present current standard first-line chemotherapy regimen of these patients, and further treatment with either maintenance therapy or four cycles of topotecan following standard EP regimen has not been proved to improve outcomes [35, 36].

Intensification of cytotoxic regimens by either increasing the individual dose size or decreasing dose intervals are promising strategies for improving initial complete response (CR) rates and improving OS durations. In this manner, safe delivery of dose-intensified chemotherapy became possible by utilization of hematopoietic progenitors. The safety and efficacy of intensified chemotherapy with hematopoietic progenitors (ICHP) have been addressed in a single meta-analysis of 5 studies including a total of 641 patients. Unfortunately, although the ICHP receiving patients had higher-grade 3–4 hematologic toxicity (OR:3.71 for hemoglobin; $p<0.001$ and OR:4.9 for platelet; $p<0.001$), no enhancement in either overall response rates (OR:1.29; $p=0.206$) or overall survival (OS) durations (HR:0.94; $p=0.432$) was achieved [37]. Therefore, based on the results of this unique meta-analysis, currently the use of ICHP is not recommended in SCLC patients.

Drug-dose intensification may likewise be conceivable by prophylactic use of granulocyte- (G-CSF) or granulocyte-macrophage colony-stimulating factors (GM-CSF). However, two individual meta-analyses with respective 3 ($n=391$) and 12 RCTs ($n=2{,}107$) failed to demonstrate any notable survival enhancement with either G-CSF or GM-CSF [38, 39], overall suggesting no role for the routine prophylactic use of these agents in the current management of SCLC patients.

Another suggested strategy to improve outcomes of SCLC patients is the use of maintenance or consolidation chemotherapy. Since the results of individual studies are controversial, two meta-analyses have been performed to address its role in this group of patients. In the first meta-analysis by Bozcuk et al. [40], maintenance chemotherapy was shown to improve 1- and 2-year OS from 30 % to 39 % (OR:0.67; $p=0.001$) and from 10 % to 14 % (OR:0.67; $p=0.001$) and 1- (OR:0.49) and 2-year (OR:0.64) progression-free survival (PFS), respectively. However, the authors reported that this survival advantage was at expense of increased toxicity rates. In the second meta-analysis by Rossi et al. [41], in an effort to produce a thorough picture of efficacy related to different pharmacological strategies, the authors evaluated all the investigated maintenance therapy approaches to date. A total of 3,688 LS- and ES-SCLC patients enrolled on 21 trials were included: 11 chemotherapy, 6 interferons, and 4 other biological agents, respectively. Although statistically different effects among the four types of therapy were detected for OS ($p=0.04$) but not for PFS ($p>0.05$ for each), overall, no notable advantage for OS (HR:0.93; $p=0.05$) or PFS (HR:0.98; $p=0.63$) was shown for maintenance or consolidation therapy. Mortality was significantly reduced in chemotherapy (HR:0.89; $p=0.02$) and interferon-alpha studies (HR$=$0.78; $p=0.02$). Considering the increased toxicity rates and associated patient compliance problems, the positive results in OS reported particularly by maintenance chemotherapy and interferon-alpha ought to be interpreted with caution. However, despite the fact that the maintenance treatment cannot be considered for routine use in SCLC patients, such information may demonstrate valuable by proposing value to proceed on exploration of the most potent and safe maintenance or consolidation strategies, if exist.

Thoracic Radiotherapy (TRT)

TRT was the pillar of the oncologic management of LS-SCLC patients before the implementation of chemotherapy in the 1970s [42]. At first, the enthusiasm for TRT was diminished because of aftereffects of chemotherapy success in these patients. Nevertheless, on the grounds that the locoregional relapse rates were unacceptably high with chemotherapy alone, the enthusiasm on TRT was renewed, and the concurrent chemoradiotherapy (C-CRT) became the standard care of SCLC patients, from there on.

Regarding the TRT, current investigations are mainly focused on the relative timing of TRT and chemotherapy, total dose and fractionation, and treatment volumes. These issues will be discussed in detail in the following sections of this chapter. Prophylactic cranial irradiation (PCI) is another essential advancement in management of SCLC with a well-established role in both LS- and ES-SCLC patients which will be discussed in Chap. 10.

Early Versus Delayed Thoracic Radiotherapy

The role of combination of TRT and chemotherapy in LS-SCLC patients is well supported by two meta-analyses [43, 44]. The meta-analysis reported by Pignon et al. [39] reviewed 2,140 patients from 13 trials and demonstrated a 5.4 % improvement in 3-year OS rate with CRT than chemotherapy alone (14.3 % vs. 8.9 %). In the other meta-analysis, Warde and Payne [44] consolidated data from 11 randomized trials with or without CRT and found that the receipt of CRT prompted to better 2-year intrathoracic tumor control rates than did chemotherapy alone (34.1 % vs 16.5 %). The 2-year OS rates were likewise 5.4 % higher in the patients treated with CRT ($P<0.05$). Thusly, the CRT approach has been settled as the standard of care for ES-SCLC patients.

Based on organization timing, TRT and chemotherapy combination is defined as concurrent or sequential. In the C-CRT the TRT and chemotherapy are utilized simultaneously, while in sequential approach, chemotherapy is given either before the initiation of TRT or after the fulfillment of TRT or both. While some of the introductory studies indicated promising results for alternating TRT and chemotherapy, this type of combined approach is mostly surrendered today.

Considering the optimal timing of TRT and chemotherapy, several large studies have shown that the C-CRT produces better disease control than sequential regimes [45–47]. In largest of these studies including 308 patients, Murray et al. [45] treated patients with cyclophosphamide, doxorubicin, and vincristine combination, alternating with EP, and beginning TRT either on week 3 or on week 15. Patients who achieved a complete response also received PCI. Patients who received TRT early during chemotherapy had significantly better median PFS ($p=0.036$), OS ($p=0.008$) and freedom from brain metastases ($p=0.006$) times. Likewise, in the phase 3 trial by the Japanese Clinical Oncology Group (JCOG 9104), Takada et al. [46] compared C-CRT with sequential chemotherapy and TRT in 228 LS-SCLC patients.

Although the clinically apparent differences remained only as a trend approaching statistical significance ($P = 0.097$), patients on C-CRT arm demonstrated superior median (24 vs. 18 months), 2- (54.4 vs 35.1 %), 3- (29.8 vs 20.2 %), and 5-year (23.7 vs. 18.3 %) OS rates than did those on sequential treatment arm. These results were also later confirmed by De Ruysscher et al. [47]. Although it was a retrospective analysis, in the most recent study, Scotti et al. [48] reported the 10-year outcomes of 124 LS-SCLC patients treated with various strategies. In this study, 53 (42.8 %) and 71 patients (57.2 %) received mainly EP-based C-CRT or sequential treatment, respectively. PCI was utilized only in patients with histologically proven complete response to primary treatment. At a mean follow-up of 2.2 years, the authors found that the 10-year OS was significantly longer in who underwent early or late TRT than the sequentially treated counterparts with respective OS rates of 10.0 %, 12.9 %, and 5.6 % ($p = 0.007$).

Although results of available studies, in general, support the early utilization of TRT during the chemotherapy course of LS-SCLC patients, conflicting outcomes have also been reported. Therefore, the impact of timing of TRT relative to chemotherapy has also been addressed by various meta-analyses. The first meta-analysis by Fried et al. assessed the RCTs published after 1985 [49]. In this meta-analysis, TRT was considered early when it was begun before 9 weeks and before the third cycle of chemotherapy. For all studies, OS at 2 years was significantly superior in the early than the late TRT patients (HR = 1.17; $P = 0.03$), with a similar trend at 3 years. In a subset analysis of hyperfractionated TRT, studies revealed superior OS with early TRT at 2 (HR:1.44; $p = 0.001$) and 3 years (HR:1.39; $p = 0.04$) than late TRT. Interestingly, in subset analysis with only the studies using once-daily fractionation, this significant OS advantage favoring early over late TRT disappeared. In summary, the absolute benefit of early vs. late TRT was 5 % for all patients, 10 % for patients who had received cisplatin-based chemotherapy, and 17 % for patients who had received cisplatin-based chemotherapy and twice-daily TRT.

In the meta-analysis by Huncharek and McGarry, data of 8 RCTs enrolling over 1,500 LS-SCLC patients were analyzed and demonstrated that early integration of TRT with systemic chemotherapy was associated with 34–216 % longer OS times, depending on the endpoint of interest [50]. Pooling the 2- and 3-year survival data indicated 60 % and 49 % respective better OS rates with early than late TRT.

In another meta-analysis, De Ruysscher and colleagues analyzed RCTs combining TRT and platinum-based chemotherapy and concluded that the most important predictor of 5-year survival was the interim between the initiations of any treatment and the end of RT (SER). The authors reported that shorter SERs (<30 days) were associated with the highest 5-year OS rates, namely, >20 % [47]. A subsequent meta-analysis, Pijls-Johannesma and colleagues evaluated the impact of timing of TRT by comparing early versus late TRT, by defining early TRT as within 30 days of chemotherapy onset. In presence of platinum-based chemotherapy, the 2- and 5-year survival rates were favoring early TRT, and this difference was significant only if the TRT was administered in a treatment period of less than 30 days. In this study, patient compliance was found to be of paramount importance, indicating the importance of patient selection in clinical trials [51]. These data are in good concordance with the landmark phase 3 ECOG/RTOG trial (INT-096) reported by Turissi et al. [52], which demonstrated that the shortening of total TRT period from 5 to 3 weeks was associated with an absolute 10 % (16 % versus 26 %) increase in 5-year survival rate.

Results of the available studies and meta-analyses suggest a strong interaction between TRT and systemic chemotherapy. Moreover, it has been hypothesized that the accelerated tumor cell repopulation is triggered by the first dose of any active cytotoxic chemotherapy [47] which mandates to kill the last tumor cell before the end of TRT in order to not miss the highest chance for locoregional control [13]. Hence, long-term survival decreases with increased intervals between the initiation of any oncologic treatment and the completion of TRT. In this respect, the novel parameter SER, which takes into account accelerated proliferation of tumor cells during both TRT and chemotherapy, may facilitate a more rational design of combined-modality treatment in rapidly proliferating SCLC.

Dose and Fractionation

As aforementioned in previous sections, TRT was the mainstay of treatment for LS-SCLC before the introduction of chemotherapy in the 1970s [13, 42]. However, despite the great interest in chemotherapy, subsequent studies demonstrated that chemotherapy alone resulted in from 75 % to 90 % intrathoracic failures, which is far beyond acceptable limits [53]. With an end goal to lessening this rates, TRT was added to chemotherapy in a concurrent manner, which decreased the failure rates to as low as 30–60 % [54]. Later, the clinical impressions of such a reduction in intrathoracic failures have been broadly surveyed by two meta-analyses [44, 55]. In the first, Warde and Payne [44] analyzed 1,911 patients enrolled on 11 randomized studies and reported a significantly longer OS favoring the TRT and chemotherapy combination over chemotherapy alone, with an absolute 5.4 % OS benefit at 2-year ($p<0.001$). In the other meta-analysis, Pignon et al. [55] incorporated 13 trials comprising of 2,103 LS-SCLC patients. Combination of TRT and chemotherapy again brought an absolute 5.4 % survival advantage at 3 years compared to chemotherapy alone ($p=0.001$). Based on the results of these two meta-analyses, combination of TRT and chemotherapy turned into the built up standard of consideration in LS-SCLC, at least for those who are fit enough to tolerate the therapy.

Information on the optimum TRT dose and fractionation schedules basically come from retrospective and phase 2 prospective studies. The results of nonrandomized studies indicated a notable increment in local control rates by escalating the TRT dose just from 35 to 40 Gy, and a further slight increase was accomplished at 50 Gy dose level. Preclinical cell line investigations have suggested that regular SCLC cells have radiation survival curves with little shoulders indicating that accelerated fractionation schemes would, in this way, be beneficial [13]. As depicted in Table 8.3, in 1999, two different cooperative groups randomized patients to once-a-day versus twice-a-day TRT with concurrent chemotherapy [52, 56]. In the study of the North Central Cancer Treatment Group (NCCTG) reported by Bonner et al., there was no significant distinction in survival outcomes between the hyperfractionated and conventional TRT arms [56]. However, this study has been criticized

Table 8.3 Outcomes of benchmark NCCTG [56] and ECOG/RTOG [52] randomized trials of limited stage small-cell lung cancer comparing daily versus twice-daily TRT

	NCCTG		p-value	ECOG/RTOG (INT 0096)		p-value
Study arms	Ctx + TRT	Ctx + TRT (b.i.d)		Ctx + RT	Ctx + TRT (b.i.d)	
Patients (N)	176	182		133	130	
Total Ctx cycles (N)	4	4		6	6	
Concurrent Ctx cycles (N)	2	2		2	2	
Median OS (months)	18.6	20.3	0.04	21	21	0.49
2-year OS (%)	42	44		47	45	
3-year OS (%)	–	–		34	29	
5-year OS (%)	16	26		–	–	
≥Grade 3 pneumonitis (%)	4	5	0.97	4.5	6.2	>0.05
≥Grade 3 esophagitis (%)	16	32	<0.001	5.3	12.3	0.05

Ctx chemotherapy, *ECOG* Eastern Cooperative Oncology Group, *N* number, *NCCTG* North Central Cancer Treatment Group, *OS* overall survival, *RTOG* Radiation Therapy Oncology Group, *TRT* thoracic radiotherapy

because of using split-course TRT schedule which is currently an established factor to increase the chance for accelerated repopulation and, therefore, influence treatment outcomes unfavorably. In the benchmark INT-0096 study by Turissi et al. [52], authors reported the long-term outcomes of 358 LS-SCLC patients enrolled onto the cooperative group study of Eastern Cooperative Oncology Group/Radiation Therapy Oncology Group (ECOG/RTOG). Results of this study exhibited that twice-daily 45 Gy (1.5 Gy b.i.d) and concurrent CRT was significantly superior over conventionally fractionated TRT scheme [52]. Based on the results of this latter study, the current standard of care for medically fit LS-SCLC became the 45 Gy (1.5 Gy b.i.d) TRT and concurrent EP. Nonetheless, because of the higher frequency of dose-limiting ≥grade 3 esophagitis in twice-daily TRT scheme, 54 Gy (1.8 Gy per fraction) in 30 days and concurrent EP are also commonly practiced treatment schemes.

The finding that local tumor control rates remain less than optimal at 40–70 % suggested that increasing the radiation dose, either by escalation, hyperfractionation, or a combination of the two, may enhance outcomes. Consequently, several studies assessed the efficacy of higher-dose radiation for LS-SCLC [57–59]. In this respect, Carcinoma and Leukemia Group B (CALGB) conducted two phase 2 trials to research the potential advantage of a higher dosage of 70 Gy given in 35 fractions within 7 weeks [57, 58]. In the first study, median OS time, 2-year OS, and ≥grade 3 esophagitis rates were 22 months, 48 %, and 21 %, respectively [57], while respective rates were 20 months, 35 %, and 30 % in the second study [58]. The maximal tolerated dose (MTD) was reported to be 70 Gy administered in 35 fractions within 7 weeks in a phase 1 study conducted by Choi et al. [59].

In a phase 1 RTOG 97-12 dose escalation study, 36 Gy was delivered in 20 fractions within 4 weeks, followed by a boost of twice-daily RT (1.8 Gy/fraction) to the predetermined total dose levels of 50.4, 54.0, 57.6, 61.2, or 64.8 Gy, respectively [60]. The MTD was determined as the dose that produced grades 3–4 esophagitis and pneumonitis in more than 50 % of patients. The MTD with this approach was 61.2 Gy within 5 weeks. Fifty-four (87 %) of the 62 evaluable patients achieved a complete (68 %) or partial (19 %) tumor response. The 18-month survival was 25 % for patients receiving 50.4 Gy and 82 % for those receiving 61.2 Gy. In a subsequent phase 2 study, RTOG 0239, patients with LS-SCLC and good performance status were given TRT to 61.2 Gy over 5 weeks (daily 1.8-Gy fractions on days 1–22, then twice-daily 1.8-Gy fractions on days 23–33). Cisplatin (60 mg/m^2) was given on day 1 and etoposide (120 mg/m^2) on days 1–3 and days 22–24, followed by two cycles of EP alone [61]. Of eligible 71 patients, 13 (18 %) experienced severe acute esophagitis, and 2 (3 %) of treatment-related deaths were reported. Complete and partial response rates were 41 % and 39 %, respectively. Median and 2-year OS 2-year local control rates were 73 % and 19 months and 36.6, respectively. This treatment strategy is now one of three arms of the ongoing randomized phase 3 trial: RTOG-0538/CALGB 30610 protocol. Based on the promising outcomes of these studies, two ongoing randomized phase 3 trials were conducted to compare standard Turissi protocol (INT-096) with escalated doses of conventionally fractionated TRT. These two landmark trials, namely, intergroup study RTOG-0538/CALGB 30610 and CONVERT (Concurrent Once-daily versus Twice-daily Radiotherapy) will address the answers for the question whether the higher doses conveyed by once-daily scheme in 7 weeks could compensate for the longer interval between the initiation of treatment and the end of TRT in the expense of increased risk for accelerated tumor cell repopulation (Table 8.4).

In summary, until the emergence of better results from ongoing progressing phase 3 RCTs, current evidence recommends the early administration of 45 Gy (1.5 Gy, b.i.d) for medically fit LS-SCLC patients.

Table 8.4 Ongoing landmark trials of chemoradiotherapy for limited stage small-cell lung carcinoma

Trial	Chemotherapy	Standard TRT arm	Experimental TRT arm	Primary endpoint	Expected enrollment
CALGB 30610/ RTOG 0538	4 cycles EP	45 Gy/30 fx, 3 week, b..i.d, starting at first or second course	A: 70 Gy/35 fx, 7 week, once-daily B: 61.2 Gy/34 fx, 5 week, BID, starting at first course	Overall survival	712
CONVERT	4 cycles EP	45 Gy/30 fx, 3 week, b..i.d, starting at second course	66 Gy/33 fx, 6.6 week, once-daily, starting at second course	Overall survival	532

CALGB Carcinoma and Leukemia Group B, *CONVERT* Concurrent Once-daily versus Twice-daily Radiotherapy, *EP* etoposide-cisplatin, *RTOG* Radiation Therapy Oncology Group, *TRT* thoracic radiotherapy

Extensive Stage SCLC

Approximately 70 % of all SCLC patients have disease either spread beyond the thoracic borders or confined to thorax but too large to be encompassed with a tolerable radiation port, namely, ES-SCLC. For quite a long time, combination chemotherapy has been considered to be the standard treatment option for these patients, and TRT has traditionally been reserved for patients who required local palliation. However, prognosis of ES-SCLC patients treated exclusively with chemotherapy remained poor, and almost no striking change has been noted in late decades. An analysis reported by Govindan et al. in 2006 exhibited that the 2-year OS rate was only 5 %, and the median PFS and OS were only in the ranges of 4–6 and 7–11 months, respectively [62]. To overcome poor prognosis with chemotherapy alone, various chemotherapy intensification approaches were investigated; however sadly, neither maintenance chemotherapy beyond initial four to six cycles [35, 63, 64] nor higher chemotherapy dosages [65, 66] proved gainful in this disease setting.

Intrathoracic disease control is a major oncologic challenge to overcome in a significant proportion of ES-SCLC patients, because although almost 90 % of all SCLC patients respond to initial chemotherapy, ≥70 % of them eventually experience intrathoracic recurrences which is almost inevitably fatal. As an excellent example, in the Slotman's benchmark PCI trial 75 % of all study eligible patients had persisting thoracic disease following initial chemotherapy, and roughly 90 % experienced thoracic disease progression within the first year [67]. However, despite this fact, assumedly because of its systemic nature and of inevitable rapid extrathoracic progressions, TRT for such patients did not gain interest for long times. Mainly because of this reason the role of consolidative TRT has been limitedly addressed. In the first commendable trial, Jeremic et al. [68] randomized patients with ES-SCLC to consolidation TRT versus observation arms after three cycles of systemic chemotherapy who responded completely at extrathoracic sites and at least partially at thorax. In experimental arm, accelerated hyperfractionated TRT of 54 Gy (1.5 Gy b.i.d) was given concurrent with EP. The median, 3- and 5-year OS in the TRT, and the chemotherapy-only arms were 17 versus 11 months ($p=0.041$), 22 % and 9 %, and 9.1 % versus 3.7 %, respectively. In a recent retrospective review of 215 patients with ES-SCLC, 19 patients received consolidative TRT [69]. In this favorable subset of patients with one or two metastatic sites, locoregional failure was reported in 26 % at 1 year and 39 % at 2 years. Similarly, Zhu et al. in another retrospective study including 119 patients did a multivariate analysis and reported an improved median OS for patients receiving TRT [70]. These data is supported by the prospective nonrandomized phase 2 study of 32 ES-SCLC patients treated with four cycles of platinum-based chemotherapy and subsequent consolidative 40 Gy TRT (15 daily fractions). Treatment was well tolerated with report of only 15.6 % symptomatic chest recurrences [71].

Efficacy of consolidation TRT has been confirmed by Ou et al. [72] who retrospectively analyzed the data from the Cancer Surveillance programs of Orange, San

Diego, and Imperial countries in southern California. SCLC patients diagnosed between 1991 and 2005 who had complete follow-up data were included in the study. ES-SCLC was defined according to surveillance, epidemiology, and end results summary staging. Of 3,428 such patients, TRT was given to 1,204 (35.1 %) cases. A number of clinicopathological characteristics were analyzed upon their influence on the results. The 1-year, 2-year, and median OS of ES-SCLC patients who received TRT were 27.8, 9.3 %, and 8 months and were significantly better than those who did not receive TRT (16.2, 3.8 %, and 4 months, respectively; $p<0.0001$). Furthermore, multivariate analysis of potential prognosticators confirmed the independent positive influence of TRT on patient outcomes (HR: 0721; $p<0.001$).

In the recently reported phase 3 randomized controlled trial, Chest Radiotherapy in Extensive Disease Small-Cell Lung Cancer Trial (CREST), 498 ES-SCLC patients from 42 hospitals who responded to primary chemotherapy were randomly assigned to receive either TRT of 30 Gy in 3 Gy daily fractions or no TRT [73]. Irrespective of TRT status, all patients underwent PCI. The primary endpoint was OS at 1 year. At median 24 months of follow-up, although a strong trend favored TRT arm over no TRT regarding 1-year OS (33 % vs. 28 %, HR:0·84; $p=0.066$), this difference remained marginally insignificant. However, in a secondary analysis, 2-year OS of 13 % in TRT arm was significantly superior than the 3 % ($p=0.004$) in no-TRT arm. Thoracic disease progression was less likely in the TRT than in the no-TRT group (HR:0·73; $p=0.001$). Additionally, 6 months, PFS was significantly better in the TRT arm (24 % vs. 7 %; $p=0.001$). Based on the results of this study, the authors recommended the addition of TRT to PCI for all ES-SCLC patients who enjoy any objective response after primary chemotherapy.

Although TRT and PCI may reduce thoracic and in-brain failures, many patients present with additional disease progression outside these sites. Therefore, rationally the addition of RT to extrathoracic disease sites might also merit investigation. Such an approach is currently investigated by the phase 2 RTOG 0937 protocol (ClinicalTrials.gov number NCT01055197). In this study, PCI and TRT are combined with TRT to up to four extrathoracic involved sites. The chosen 45 Gy b.i.d or 40 Gy in ten fractions is biologically more effective than the 30 Gy (ten daily fractions) utilized in CREST trial. Results of this interesting study which may potentially redefine the standards of ES-SCLC management are eagerly awaited.

Radiotherapy Techniques

Radiation therapy of SCLC is a complex procedure likewise its non-small-cell counterpart. Regardless of the technique, the main objective of sophisticated RT practice is to deliver the prescribed therapeutic dose to the target (TV) volume in a precise and accurate manner and simultaneously minimize dose to surrounding normal tissues and organs at risk (OARs) in order to increase the therapeutic ratio. As expected, this vital and multistep objective became achievable by the aid of rapid and significant advances in anatomic and metabolic definition of local and regional tumor burden and neighboring critical structures and the technology of RT planning (RTP) and delivery including the verification methods over the past 30 years. During this time period, the RT technology improved step by step from two-dimensional RT (2D-RT) to three-dimensional conformal RT (3D-CRT) and lastly to intensity-modulated radiation therapy (IMRT) together with daily image guidance and four-dimensional (4D) image-based motion management (4D-IGRT). Additionally, the old but highly conformal techniques such as proton therapy and carbon-ion therapy regained interest in the last decade because of technologic advances in hadron therapy planning and delivery methods.

Although some priorities may vary based on the patient's anatomic variations, tumor location, and the available RTP technique, it is imperative to consider several common issues for in order to ensure a safe and effective TRT plan. These are:

- Appropriate patient positioning and target volume imaging
- Accurate image registration
- Accurate target volume delineation
- Proximity of dose-limiting normal structures like ipsi- and contralateral lung, spinal cord, esophagus, heart, brachial plexus, and liver
- Anatomic slope of the chest surface
- Inhomogeneities resulting from the presence of nonuniform tissues on the way of radiation
- Frequent need for irregular field dose calculations
- Respiratory motion of the targeted tumor and normal tissues such as the ipsi- and contralateral lung, esophagus, heart, and liver, depending on the location of the primary tumor and involved lymphatic region(s).
- Appropriate energy selection if IMRT is not used
- Appropriate treatment machine and accessories selection with the capability to serve for intended treatment, such as IMRT and IGRT

The ultimate goal of an optimal TRT plan is to deliver the prescribed dose homogenously to the planning target volume (PTV), such as not cooler than 95 % and not hotter than 107 % (in case of a typical 3D-CRT), and keep the dose to uninvolved normal tissues as minimum as possible respecting their tissue architecture (serial versus parallel) and their radiation tolerance limits. In this setting, with the aid of imaging with anatomic computerized tomography (CT), functional 18-F-fluorodeoxyglucose positron emission tomography (PET), preferably fusion of both (PET-CT), and the use of 3D-CRT, and novel IMRT or 4D-IGRT, it is easier than before to achieve these goals. Additionally, the dose-volume histograms (DVH) created for each patient make it possible to anticipate the potential early and late toxicity risks based on the organ of interest measures and, therefore, modify the treatment plans as necessitated.

3D-Conformal Radiotherapy (3D-CRT)/

RTP is simply the process of arrangement of beams to irradiate a defined TV to the prescribed dose. Accordingly the unique aim is to adequately encompass a predetermined TV with appropriately designed radiation beams. Considering the 2D-RT, this definition is satisfactory as the unique aim is the coverage of empirically determined (by experience) TV by the prescribed dose with little or no respect to the neighboring tissues in absence of image-based TV delineation. Such a treatment plan may theoretically cover the TV adequately with the prescribed dose but is usually handicapped by various factors such as: [1] TV may be larger than the original one and may carry excessive risk of unnecessary but potentially debilitating acute or late toxicity [2], and TV may be larger than the determined one and may carry risk of undercoverage of the real TV and therefore decreased chance for cure or palliation [3], because usually opposing fields or bony landmark-based box/diamond fields are used and large fields receive high doses unnecessarily which increases the risk of radiation-induced second cancers as the possibility for emergence of stochastic effects of radiation increases with doses in the therapeutic range, even not toxic in clinical terms. Because of these disadvantages and improvements in accurate TV and OAR definitions with the implementation of computerized image-based RTP and resultant patient-specific 3D calculations in 1980s the 2D-RT has almost been abandoned in lung cancers. Therefore, since then the 3D-CRT became the minimum standard of care in this patients group.

Treatment planning of LA-NSCLC is complicated by the number of dose-limiting OARs such as the spinal cord, uninvolved lung(s), esophagus, heart, large vessels, and brachial plexus. In this respect, 3D-CRT proves beneficial in reducing the volumes of unavoidably irradiated normal tissues on the way of radiation beams via designing field shapes with the guidance of beam's eye view (BEV) and use of multiple noncoplanar beam arrangements [74]. Moreover, 3D-CRT RTP allows volumetric evaluation of the dose distributions throughout the tumor, OARs, and even the entire patient by use of dose-volume histograms (DVH) and therefore facilitates the chance for achieving intended optimal plan by appropriate rearrangements of the beam angles and weights whenever necessitated.

The vital steps of a typical 3D-CRT of LA-NSCLC are as follows.

Immobilization

For an optimal 3D-CRT plan, the imaging data set should be obtained with the patient set in the simulation and treatment position, if not contraindicated for medical reasons. During the imaging procedure, the patient should lay on a support table in the position that mimics the treatment setup after being immobilized with commercially available custom devices such as commonly used foam cradles. In an effort to prevent passage of radiation beams through the arms and likewise not to restrict the liberty of beam angle selection, the arms should optimally be positioned above their head with the use of available accessory devices, like T-bars (Fig. 8.1).

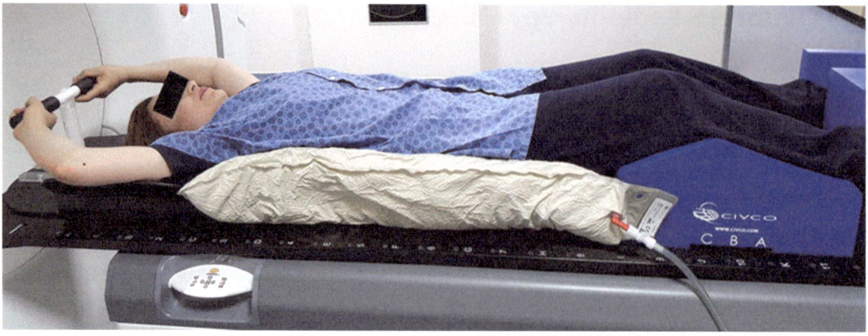

Fig. 8.1 Patient immobilization and positioning during imaging procedure with the use of alpha cradle and T-bar accessories

Target Volume Definition

In order to promote the use of universal terminology and systematic TV definitions through the whole radiation oncology community, the International Commission on Radiation Units and Measurements (ICRU) has published nomenclature and guidelines in 1993 and 1999. For TV delineation procedure, three interconnected volumes have been defined: in case of lung cancers, (a) gross tumor volume (GTV) represents for the visible extent of tumor mass on imaging studies, including any involved nodes; (b) clinical target volume (CTV) is defined as the volume constructed by addition of a margin around the GTV to account for invisible but potentially involved microscopic or subclinical tumor extensions at the periphery of primary tumor or regional nodes; and (c) planning target volume (PTV) is the expansion around the CTV that accounts for the uncertainties of the geographic position of the CTV between fractions, intrafraction tumor motion, organ movements, and setup uncertainties. Although the GTV and CTV are constructed for biologic considerations and therefore represents for biologic volumes, PTV is constructed for nonbiologic but mostly mechanical considerations such as physiologic organ motions and setup problems.

GTV Delineation

The parenchymal and the hilar/mediastinal extent of SCLC should be delineated using pulmonary and mediastinal window, respectively (Figs. 8.2 and 8.3). The best concordance between the CT image and the actual dimensions of the parenchymal tumor has been established at the window width 1,600 and level −600. For lymph nodes and centrally located parenchymal lesions, it is useful to use mediastinal window setting with recommended window width of 400 and level of 20 (Fig. 8.2) [75]. Of note, as calibration of CT may differ between centers, "in-house" measurements of appropriate window settings are strongly recommended for each department. The contrast-enhanced CT may be useful in tumors localized in the hilar region for the purpose of distinguishing of vessels in this area. The bronchoscopy findings should be considered for central locations of tumor with endobronchial component, because

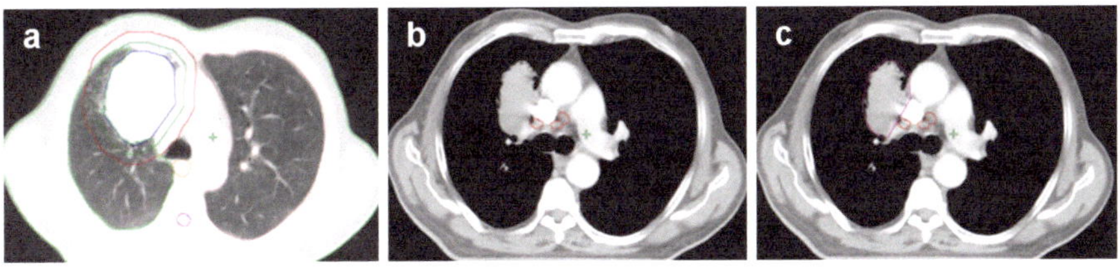

Fig. 8.2 Gross tumor volume (GTV) contouring; (**a**) parenchymal GTV contoured by setting the window width 1,600 and level −600; (**b**) regional nodal GTV contoured by setting the window width 400 and level of 20; (**c**) Total GTV = Parenchymal GTV + Nodal GTV

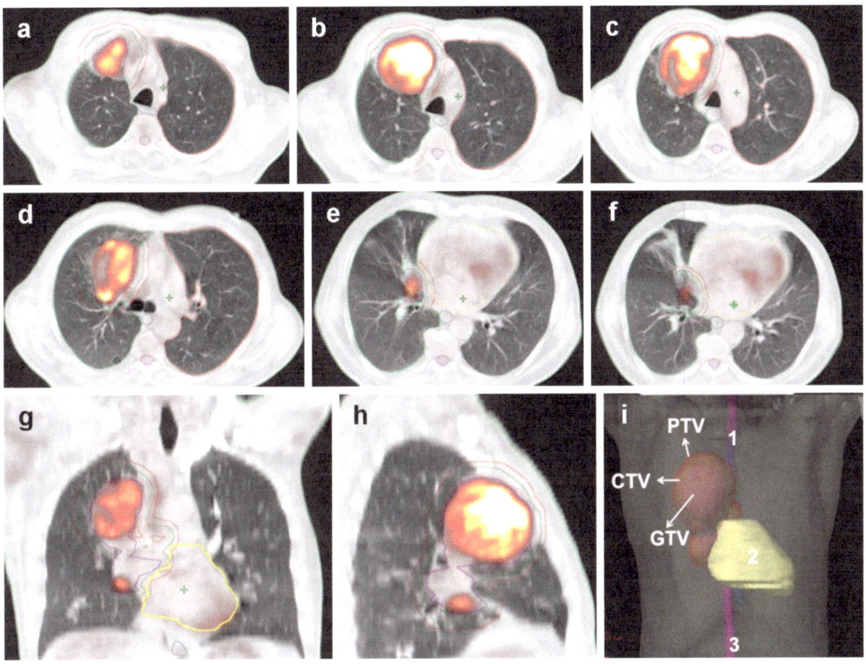

Fig. 8.3 (**a–i**) Target volume and organs at risk contouring: *GTV* gross tumor volume; *CTV* clinical target volume, *PTV* planning target volume; *1* esophagus; *2* heart; *3* spinal cord

even high-resolution CT does not visualize this component and the estimated sensitivity and specificity of FDG-PET are 73 % and 85 %, respectively [76]. If RTP is based on the CT only data, then the usual policy would be to consider all hilar and mediastinal lymph nodes with a diameter at short axis of higher than 10 mm as tumor positive and include in the GTV as the risk is >15 % for tumor cell positivity. Although various algorithms are recommended to define involved primary and nodal GTVs with coregistered PET-CT (e.g., SUV_{max} >2.5), RTOG-11-06 protocol recommends the use of the PET intensity of a 1 cc volume contoured in the aortic arch for NSCLC which is also applicable to SCLC. According to this protocol definition, any primary or nodal disease on PET with an intensity ≥1.5 times the mean of the aortic arch intensity should be included in the GTV.

CTV Delineation

CTV margin represents the effort to cover microscopic disease spread in absence of imaging studies capable of detecting it (Fig. 8.3). Therefore, CTV margins are created mainly on the basis of the correlation of imaging with pathologic data. The CTV has SCLC been investigated relatively in a rarer fashion than the CTV of NSCLC. As it is common also for NSCLC, there are three distinct types of CTV margins for SCLC, which are sources of separate problems. These are: (a) margin for pulmonary primary, (b) margin for endobronchial spread, and (c) margin for extracapsular extension in mediastinal and/or hilar lymph nodes. In absence of SCLC specific data, to be at the safe site, we recommend to define the CTV margins of SCLC patients alike with their adenocarcinoma (AC) counterparts.

Giraud et al. [77] investigated the extent of microscopic disease spread of NSCLC within the pulmonary parenchyma by correlating the pathologic findings with preoperative CT images. For AC histology, the authors reported that a margin of 8 mm around pulmonary GTV was needed to encompass 95 % of microscopic disease. Furthermore, the authors reported that the empirical 5 mm margin was unsatisfactory to adequately cover AC histology in about 20 % cases. Another seminal work evaluating the margins for adequate coverage of microscopic spread in 35 AC patients demonstrated that 9 mm was required for covering 90 % of cases if appropriate pulmonary window was used for GTV definition [78]. Based on our institutional experience, for CTV creation, we recommend 8 mm margins at all directions around the pulmonary GTV.

Microscopic tumor spread along the bronchi may be mucosal, submucosal, intraparietal, or mix type. The endobronchial tumor spread has been extensively addressed in surgical and brachytherapy series, but interestingly, although data of central tumors demonstrated that the proximal microscopic tumor extension is commonly detected with a mean dimension of about 10 mm [79], yet there is no clear recommendation for this issue in the external beam RT literature. Surgical specimen studies suggest 15–20 mm as the appropriate and safe proximal margin from the visible tumor on the bronchial level [80]. Therefore, in the absence of exclusive SCLC RT data, it is reasonable to recommend 15–20 mm safety margin along the bronchotracheal tract for CTV creation in tumors extending to or residing within the bronchial tract.

For both SCLC and NSCLC, the extent of CTV margin around involved lymph nodes has been limitedly studied compared to the margin around the primary parenchymal tumor mass, and the data mainly comes from NSCLC studies. Although Yuan et al. [81] determined the adequate margin at 3 mm for lymph nodes of size up to 20 mm, the authors also reported that the extracapsular microscopic extension might reach 12 mm in lymph nodes between 21 and 30 mm, with no specific comment on lymph nodes >30 mm. In the absence of evidence-based recommendations, different measures are taken to overcome this problem such as inclusion of the whole lymph node station that contains the involved lymph node(s) in the CTV [82]. However, this approach is questionable in the era of "omission of elective irradiation of uninvolved lymph nodes." Therefore, the current common practice is to expand the involved lymph nodes with a margin similar to the primary parenchymal tumor that is 8 mm for AC and SCLC histologies, respectively.

Of note, it is clear that the expansions around the primary tumor and involved lymph nodes should not necessarily be applied uniformly along all axes and should always be individualized respecting their locations and the neighboring OARs. As rule of thumb, the CTV of the primary tumor should not extend into the mediastinum in the absence of radiographic proof of invasion. Likewise, in absence of evidence of CT and/or MRI confirmed invasion, CTV expansions of involved lymph nodes should not extend into the lungs, major airways, chest wall, esophagus, heart, or vertebral bodies.

PTV Delineation

PTV is the margin around the CTV that accounts for the interfraction setup inaccuracies and intrafraction physiologic organ motion (Fig. 8.3). Setup uncertainties should be determined on the institutional premise as it may vary widely depending on the technique being used and expertise of the team on NSCLC treatment. However, if immobilized appropriately by use of commercially available Vac-Loc bag and T-bar and if weekly port film is used, then an empirical 7 mm along the all axes of the CTV will usually be satisfactory to overcome setup errors in more than 95 % cases. This margin may securely be reduced to 5 mm or even to as low as 3 mm if daily kV image or on board image check with utilization of cone beam CT or CT-on-rails, respectively. Additionally, as the tumor motion due to physiologic movements of the lung may cause significant alterations in exact location of the tumor during the irradiation procedure, considerations for compensatory margins may be commanded. The magnitude of the tumor motion may vary significantly relying upon its location and size, which mandates the addition of "tumor movement margin" to the CTV expansion and setup uncertainties [83]. For determination of adequate margins, division of each lung into four quadrants may serve beneficial. A 6 mm margin may be satisfactory for upper lobe lesions regardless of the tumor size and middle lobe lesions <50 mm. A tumor movement margin of 13 mm may be adequate in most cases with tumors <50 mm in size and located in the middle two quadrants of the involved lung or lowest quadrant tumors of 50–80 mm. For lowest quadrant tumors, <50 mm an 18 mm margin will usually be adequate to compensate tumor movement problems. Although most tumors move superior/inferior direction impacting the need for specific care at this direction, yet the best solution to overcome movement problems is its individualized measurement at all dimensions and determination of appropriate margins for each case with the use of specific imaging tools such as regular X-ray fluoroscopy.

Internal Target Volume (ITV) Delineation

An internal margin (IM) must be added to the CTV to adjust for physiological varieties in size, shape, and position of the CTV during treatment in connection to a predetermined reference point and the related coordinate system. The commonly asymmetric IM around the CTV compensates for movements and variations in site, size, and shape of the tissues which contain or are neighboring to the CTV, coming about because of respiration and heart beats in on account of lung cancers. To address this issue, the ICRU-62 Report proposed the notion of ITV which is the volume encompassing the CTV by taking into account the fact that the CTV varies in position, shape, and size. The ITV is defined by the individually measured IM, as described above, and is referred to the patient coordinate system.

The importance of tumor movement and need for ITV has been investigated by various authors. In one of the notable studies, Liu et al. [83] analyzed the 3D-respiration-induced tumor motion and related ITV in 166 tumors from 152 lung cancer patients. All patients underwent 4D-CT during normal breathing TRT. The expiratory phase of 4D-CT images was used as the reference set to GTVs. The GTV on other respiratory phases and resulting ITVs were determined using rigid-body registration of 4D-CT images. Analysis demonstrated that the proportions of tumors that moved >5 mm along the superior-inferior (SI), lateral, and anterior-posterior (AP) axes during normal breathing were 39.2 %, 1.8 %, and 5.4 %, respectively. The magnitude of motion was less than 13.4 mm, 4 mm, and 5.9 mm along the SI, lateral, and AP directions for 95 % of the tumors. The principal component of tumor motion was in the SI direction, with only 10.8 % of tumors moving >10 mm. The tumor movement was discovered to be connected with diaphragm motion, the SI tumor location in the lung, size of the GTV, and disease T stage. On the grounds of these outcomes, the authors concluded that the tumor movement was principally determined by diaphragm motion and the motion of lung tumors was unlikely to surpass 10 mm during quiet normal breathing except for small lesions located in the lower half of the lung.

It is presently conceivable to image patients as they breathe in real time and to evaluate organ motion utilizing 4D-CT with the advent of multislice detectors and faster image reconstruction methods. Although 4D-CT-based ITV methodology may serve helpful in any patients with lung cancer, contingent upon the accessibility of essential supplies, assisted breath-hold or respiratory gating or tumor tracking techniques might likewise be utilized as alternative options to minimize tumor movements during TRT.

Delineation of OAR Volumes

The major critical organs include the lungs, heart, esophagus, spinal cord, and brachial plexus (Fig. 8.3). Contouring of the lungs, spinal cord, esophagus, heart and pericardium, and brachial plexus should be performed by utilizing based the published atlas on OAR that is available on the RTOG website, http://www.rtog.org/CoreLab/ContouringAtlases.aspx. The following recommendations should be considered during OAR contouring:

Lungs: Both lungs should be contoured using pulmonary windows. The right and left lungs can be contoured separately, but they should be considered as one structure for lung dosimetry. All inflated and collapsed, fibrotic, and emphysematic lungs should be contoured; small vessels extending beyond the hilar regions should be included; however, hilars and trachea/main bronchus should not be included in this structure. Total lung volume should be calculated for metric measurements with the formula below:

$$\text{Total lung volume} = (\text{Right lung volume} + \text{Left Lung Volume}) - \text{GTV}$$

Heart: The heart will be contoured along with the pericardial sac. The superior aspect (or base) will begin at the level of the inferior aspect of the pulmonary artery passing the midline and extend inferiorly to the apex of the heart.

Esophagus: The esophagus should be contoured from the beginning at the level just below the cricoid to its entrance to the stomach at GE junction. The esophagus will be contoured using mediastinal window/level on CT to correspond to the mucosal, submucosal, and all muscular layers out to the fatty adventitia.

Spinal cord: The spinal cord will be contoured based on the bony limits of the spinal canal. The spinal cord should be contoured starting at the level just below cricoid (base of skull for apex tumors) and continuing on every CT slice to the bottom of L2. Neural foramens should not be included.

Brachial plexus: This is only required for patients with tumors of upper lobes. Only the ipsilateral brachial plexus is required. This will include the spinal nerves exiting the neuroforamens from top of C5 to top of T2. In contrast to prior RTOG lung studies of contouring the major trunks of the brachial plexus with inclusion of subclavian and axillary vessels, this trial requests contouring the nerves according to the CT anatomy on every other CT slice. The structure should extend at least 3 cm above the PTV.

Pericardium: The structure of pericardium includes pericardial fatty tissue, part of great vessels, normal recesses, pericardial effusion (if applicable), and heart chambers. Pericardium starts at one slice above the top of aortic arch and ends at the last slice of heart apex at diaphragm. Pericardium includes the heart.

TRT Portal Size Without Elective Nodal Irradiation in SCLC

There is extensive debate on the size of the TRT portals of SCLC (Figs. 8.4 and 8.5). Traditionally, the primary tumor, the mediastinum, the hilar, and the supraclavicular regions were included in the treatment volume with generous margins regardless of their clinical and/or radiologic evidence for tumor involvement. This so-called elective nodal irradiation (ENI) approach assumes that all the regional lymph nodes, regardless of the possibility that clinically uninvolved, ought to be irradiated keeping in mind the end goal to treat any potential microscopic spreading. This conventional large volumes were usually irradiated with opposing anterior-posterior and posterior-anterior fields, followed by a boost to the primary tumor and apparently involved nodes by utilizing oblique fields sparing the spinal cord. Albeit such large-field arrangements may ensure the irradiation of target volumes, they are likewise associated with increased acute and late toxicity rates and unplanned treatment delays, which might contrarily affect both quality of life measures and local/regional control rates and associated survival outcomes.

In NSCLC, ENI of hilar and/or mediastinal lymphatic regions has gradually been replaced by treatment limited to nodes recognized by CT or FDG-PET as being involved. However, for SCLC, evidence is too limited to either affirm or negate this

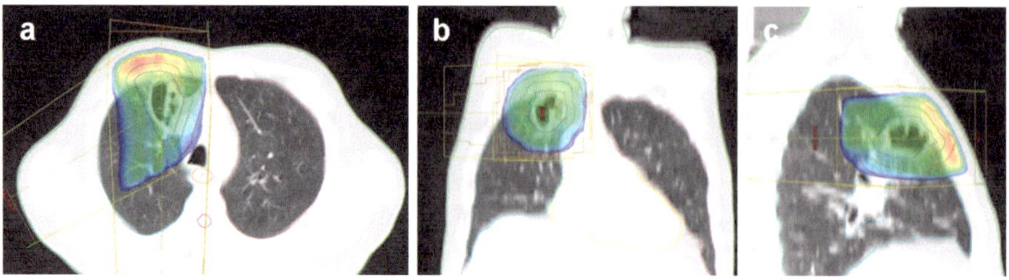

Fig. 8.4 Typical 3D-conformal radiation therapy plans for post-induction chemotherapy target volumes: (**a**) axial; (**b**) coronal; (**c**) sagittal view

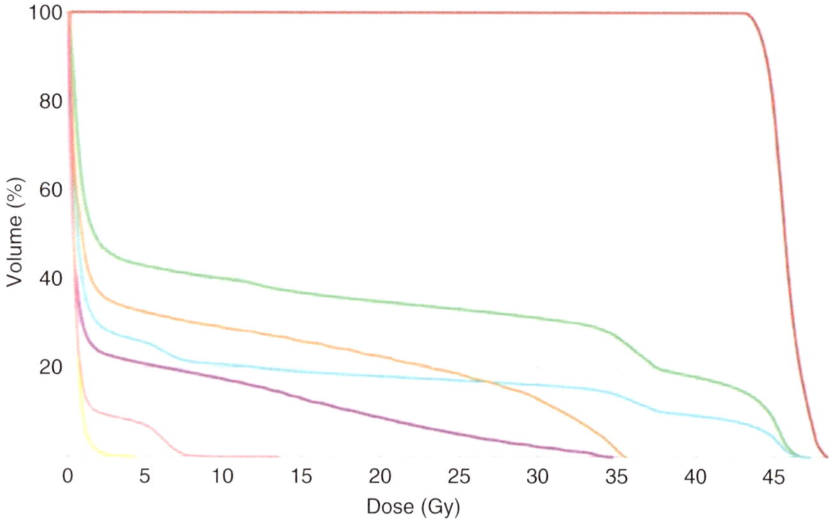

Structure	Min. dose (Gy)	Max. dose (Gy)	Mean dose (Gy)
PTV 45	42.82	48.44	45.71
Total Lung	0.03	47.29	8.24
Right Lung	0.04	47.29	15.09
Left Lung	0.03	13.65	0.92
Esophagus	0.14	35.70	8.46
Heart	0.10	4.53	0.50
Spinal Cord	0.04	34.77	4.25

Fig. 8.5 Dose-volume histogram and related evaluation metrics table for a typical 3D-conformal radiation therapy plan created for post-induction chemotherapy target volumes

approach. In a prospective study by De Ruysscher et al. [84], authors limited the RT fields to only CT-positive mediastinal lymph nodes in a cohort of 27 patients with LS-SCLC with a reported isolated regional recurrence rate of 11 %, which was higher than similar studies using elective mediastinal irradiation. However, no authoritative conclusions can be drawn from this study because of small sample size. In a larger phase 2 study including 60 LS-SCLC patients, van Loon et al. [85] irradiated only the involved lymph nodes based on FDG-PET and reported an isolated nodal failure rate of 3 %. In a more recent study by Shirvani et al. [86] from University of Texas M.D. Anderson Cancer Center, 60 patients with LS-SCLC were treated with IMRT technique, and ENI was intentionally omitted from the PTV (median dose: 45 Gy in 30 fractions; range, 40.5 Gy in 27 fractions to 63.8 Gy in 35 fractions). Eighteen patients (30 %) underwent induction chemotherapy, and 58 patients (97 %) underwent concurrent chemotherapy, usually with a platinum agent and topoisomerase inhibitor. In this study there was only 1 (1.7 %) isolated elective nodal failure. Based on these outcomes, acknowledging the requirement for additional confirmation in bigger study accomplices, accessible data suggest that the omission of ENI in SCLC may be appropriate with lower toxicity rates with no negative effect on either regional failure rates or survival results.

Considering the designation of TRT volumes further benefit can be gained by the use of PET imaging data as the TRT volume defined by CT may alter following PET imaging. Kamel et al. assessed this prospectively in 24 patients with SCLC using PET or PET-CT and found that in 5/15 (33 %) patients with LS disease, the irradiated volume changed due to CT-occult nodal disease in 4 patients and to a CT-occult ipsilateral lung metastasis in another patient, respectively [87]. Likewise, Bradley et al. reported that in 7/24 (29 %) patients with LS-SCLC, the planned TRT volume changed due to CT-occult additional nodal disease ($n=6$) or to a CT-occult ipsilateral lung metastasis in patient, respectively [88]. These findings are in line with the excellent literature review published by Thomson et al. [89] in which the addition of PET to conventional imaging ($n=12$ studies) was reported to result in stage migrations in a median of 13 % of patients, 9 % (range: 0–33 %) upstaged from LS to ES, and 4 % (range: 0–17 %) downstaged from ES to LS disease. Additionally, in a retrospective planning study, van Loon et al. [90] compared CT and PET-CT-based conformal RTP in 21 patients with LS-SCLC and reported that GTV was altered in 24 % cases and PET-CT-defined GTV was smaller in 3/21 cases and larger in 2/21 cases. On the basis of this planning study, 60 patients with LS-SCLC from the same institution were treated with C-CRT ($n=55$) or sequential chemotherapy followed by TRT ($n=5$) with irradiation of primary tumor and involved mediastinal lymph nodes defined by pretreatment PET-CT imaging [85]. Mediastinal staging differed between CT and PET-CT imaging in 30 % of patients. At median 18.5 months of follow-up 65 % of patients developed recurrence. In 2/60 (3 %) patients, this was an isolated regional lymph node failure outside the CTV, in the absence of in-field failure. Therefore, accurate definition of involved sites and accurate designation of TRT portals may potentially enhance the treatment outcomes even with smaller TRT ports.

In the most recent study on subject, Han et al. [91] published the outcomes of an interesting retrospective analysis from Seoul National University College of Medicine. The authors aimed to assess the usefulness of involved-field irradiation and the impact of PET-CT-based staging on treatment outcomes in LS-SCLC patients. Eighty SCLC patients who received definitive chemoradiotherapy were included of whom 50 (62.5 %) were treated with involved-field TRT, while the other 30 (37.5 %) with larger TRT portal which covered the uninvolved mediastinal and/or supraclavicular lymph nodes electively. At a median follow-up of 27 months, no significant differences were observed in 3-year OS (44.6 vs. 54.1 %; $p=0.22$) and 3-year PFS (24.4 vs. 42.8 %; $p=0.13$) between the two groups, respectively. For patients who did not undergo PET-CT scans, 3-year OS (29.3 vs. 56.3 %; $p=0.02$) and 3-year PFS (11.0 vs. 50.0 %, $p=0.04$) were significantly longer in the elective nodal irradiation group. Crude incidences of isolated nodal failure were 6.0 % in the involved-field irradiation group and 0 % in the elective nodal irradiation group, respectively. All isolated nodal failures were reported in group of patients who had not undergone PET-CT scans in their initial workups. This study has specific significance by demonstrating the importance of PET-CT-based staging in SCLC patients in regard to the way that all elective recurrences detected in the involved-field group were fit in to those patients group who did not undergo PET-CT staging.

In summary, available studies suggest that ENI can be omitted, as failures seem to occur within the treated volume, and that encompassing only the residual tumor volume after induction chemotherapy may be sufficient. However, it should be underlined that most patients treated in these old studies had no CT scan-based RTP and PET-CT staging. At our institution we recommend the omission of ENI for all SCLC patients undergoing PET-CT staging prior to initiation of TRT.

TRT Portal Size After Induction Chemotherapy

The definition of TRT portal size in SCLC patients at first treated with induction chemotherapy (ICT), namely, whether to cover pre- versus post-chemotherapy volumes, is another ongoing issue of conflict (Figs. 8.6 and 8.7). Although some authors advocate generous portals encompassing the pre-chemotherapy volumes, others argue that only limited portals encompassing the post-chemotherapy primary tumor and high-risk nodal areas with adequate margins, such as 1-cm, are satisfactorily enough. This latter argument is principally based on the anticipation of the hypothetical possibility of effective chemotherapy to cope with subclinical or microscopic disease which eliminates the requirement for large portals. This approach has the extra potential for diminished treatment-related toxicity, especially in patients undergoing C-CRT. The unique randomized trial that addressed this issue is the one conducted by the South West Oncology Group (SWOG). In this study, patients achieving a partial response or a stable disease after chemotherapy were randomized to pre- versus post-chemotherapy-reduced volume TRT arms. Results of this landmark trial did not demonstrate any superiority for pre-chemotherapy volume irradiation arm over post-chemotherapy irradiation partner in terms of neither local/regional control (32 % for pre- vs. 28 % for post-chemotherapy volumes; $p>0.05$) nor survival rates [92]. In a consequent retrospective analysis of 67 SCLC patients, Liengswangwong and colleagues, with about 30 % local recurrence rates in both groups and no isolated thoracic failure located outside the TRT field, were unable to demonstrate an advantage in favor of pre-chemotherapy large-field TRT [93].

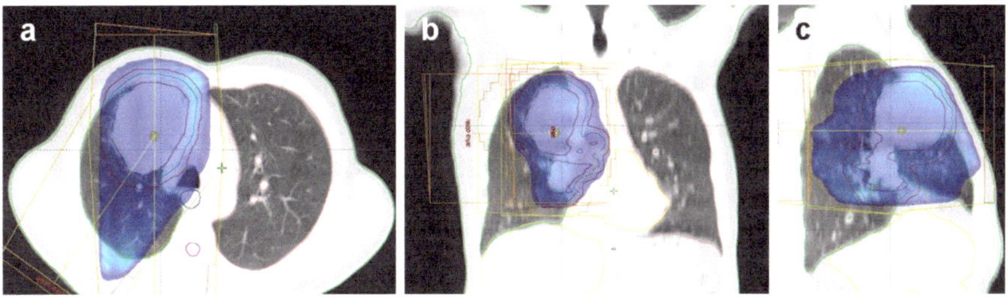

Fig. 8.6 Typical 3D-conformal radiation therapy plans for pre-chemotherapy target volumes: (**a**) axial; (**b**) coronal; (**c**) sagittal view

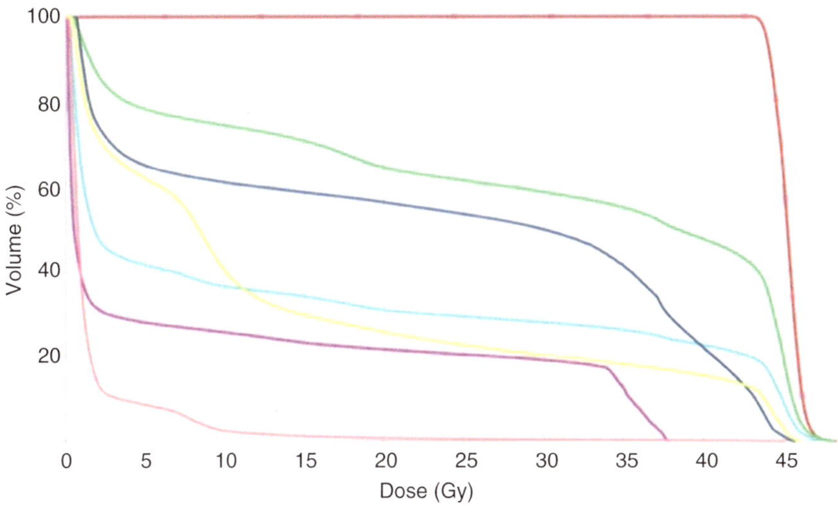

Structure	Min. dose (Gy)	Max. dose (Gy)	Mean dose (Gy)
PTV 45	42.73	48.44	45.28
Total Lung	0.13	48.29	14.57
Right Lung	0.34	48.29	28.86
Left Lung	0.13	45.33	1.74
Esophagus	0.60	45.91	22.66
Heart	0.37	46.25	14.10
Spinal Cord	0.06	37.87	8.55

Fig. 8.7 Dose-volume histogram and related evaluation metrics table for a typical 3D-conformal radiation therapy plan created for pre-chemotherapy target volumes

Although further RCTs addressing the volume of TRT in SCLC patients treated initially with ICT strategies may prove beneficial, yet based on a single RCT and a number of non-RCTs, current evidence suggests that irradiation of post-chemotherapy volumes with adequate margin may provide satisfactory locoregional control rates with a potential for reductions in treatment-related toxicity rates.

Management of Poor Performance Status and Elderly SCLC Patients

The C-CRT, specifically EP chemotherapy with early concurrent twice-daily TRT, is now regarded as the standard treatment for LS-SCLC. However, many clinical trials of potential new treatments for LS-SCLC have excluded elderly patients for various reasons, such as the presence of concomitant chronic illness, a decline in organ function that may interfere with drug clearance, and possible decreased bone marrow tolerance to myelosuppressive agents [94]. Therefore, the optimal management of medically fit, but elderly (>70 years) LS-SCLC patients remained debated in the absence RCTs specifically addressing this issue.

In a small cohort analysis of 25 elderly LS-SCLC patients who had been treated with EP chemotherapy with early concurrent twice-daily TRT were reviewed retrospectively in terms of tolerability and clinical outcomes endpoints [95]. Only 12 (48 %) individuals could receive EP chemotherapy with early concurrent twice-daily TRT. The main toxicities of this treatment regimen were hematologic, with neutropenia of grade 4 being observed in all patients and febrile neutropenia of grade 3 in eight patients during the first cycle of chemoradiotherapy. No treatment-related deaths were observed. The median PFS and OS times were 14.2 months and 24.1 months, respectively. Although the survival outcomes were satisfactory, the protocol was found excessively toxic regarding the 100 % grade 4 myelosuppression rate. In contrast, a recent phase 3 trial specifically designed for elderly or poor-risk patients with ES-SCLC found that split doses of cisplatin plus etoposide (cisplatin at 25 mg/m^2 and etoposide at 80 mg/m^2 on days 1–3) could be safely administered and were effective [96]. Therefore, although further evidence is warranted to determine the optimal treatment of medically fit elderly patients, in absence of conclusive evidence, we suggest treating such patients similar with their younger counterparts by paying great attention on treatment-related toxicities and their timely management.

Treatment of LS-SCLC patients with poor performance status is another debated issue. Initially, single-agent chemotherapy, particularly etoposide, was proposed to provide a more tolerable treatment option for such patients [97]. However, contrasting with this proposal, investigations comparing combination chemotherapy regimens with single-agent oral etoposide demonstrated that patients treated with combination regimens enjoyed significantly longer survival times with no additional toxicities [98, 99]. Accordingly, combination chemotherapy remains the current standard treatment option in this setting. Chemotherapy dose reduction and substitution of carboplatin for cisplatin should be considered if standard dose etoposide and cisplatin is not tolerated.

The issue of radical C-CRT is debated in patients with poor performance status. In a recent study by Manapov et al. [100], the outcomes of a total of 125 patients with initial poor performance score (ECOG 2–3) who successfully completed C-CRT were retrospectively reviewed. Patients received TRT of 54 Gy (1.5 Gy b.i.d) or 45 Gy (1.5 Gy b.i.d) in an ENI fashion either concurrent with chemotherapy or sequentially after chemotherapy. Median PFS and OS were reported to be 11.6 and 14.9 months, which encourages the use of C-CRT in carefully selected SCLC patients with poor performance status at the time of presentation. Therefore, we believe that the palliative chemotherapy and/or RT should be reserved for patients only who are judged to be not suitable for such aggressive procedures or with evident symptomatic evident metastasis.

Plan Evaluation

Although various escalated doses up to 70 Gy have been tested with relatively increased locoregional control rates, all are associated with increased rates of severe toxicities and small but significant increase in mortality rates. Therefore, until the emergence of further evidence supporting usage of a different schedule, the 45 Gy b.i.d (1.5 Gy per fraction) utilized in Turissi protocol (INT0096) is the currently recommended treatment dose schedule which has repeatedly been confirmed to be effective and relatively safer [52].

In patients treated with 3D-CRT, basically the prescribed dose should encompass the defined PTV with isodose lines not "cooler" than 95 % and not "hotter" than 107 % with respecting the OAR limits depicted in Table 8.5. Intensity-modulated radiotherapy is a novel sophisticated radiotherapy option for treatment SCLC patients, which may serve beneficial by reducing the OAR doses and by permitting use of escalated doses. If IMRT is utilized (Figs. 8.8 and 8.9), then the plan should be evaluated utilizing the data provided in Tables 8.5 and 8.6.

Although with the classic 45 Gy b.i.d (1.5 Gy per fraction), most OAR limits are usually not surpassed, typical dose limitations of OARs are presented in Table 8.5 for use in patients treated with higher TRT doses.

Table 8.5 Typical IMRT plan assessment specifications

PTV	No variation	Minor variation
PTV_{45}	95 % of any PTV_{45} is at or above 45 Gy	95 % of PTV_{45} is at or above 45 Gy
	99 % of PTV_{45} is at or above 41.9 Gy	97 % of PTV_{45} is at or above 41.9 Gy
	No more than 20 % of PTV_{66} is at or above 49.5 Gy	No more than 40 % of PTV_{66} is at or above 49.5 Gy
	No more than 5 % of PTV_{66} is at or above 52 Gy	No more than 20 % of PTV_{66} is at or above 52 Gy
	Mean dose ≤47.3 Gy	Mean dose -49.1 Gy

IMRT intensity-modulated radiotherapy, *PTV* planning target volume, *PD* prescription dose

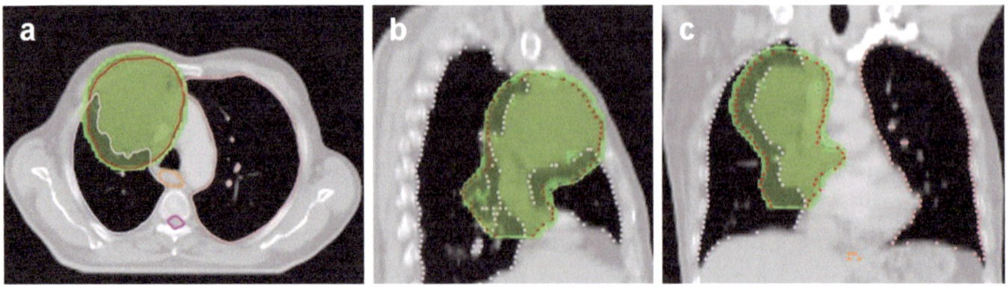

Fig. 8.8 Typical 7-field intensity-modulated radiation therapy plans: (**a**) axial; (**b**) coronal; (**c**) sagittal view; and related dose-volume histogram

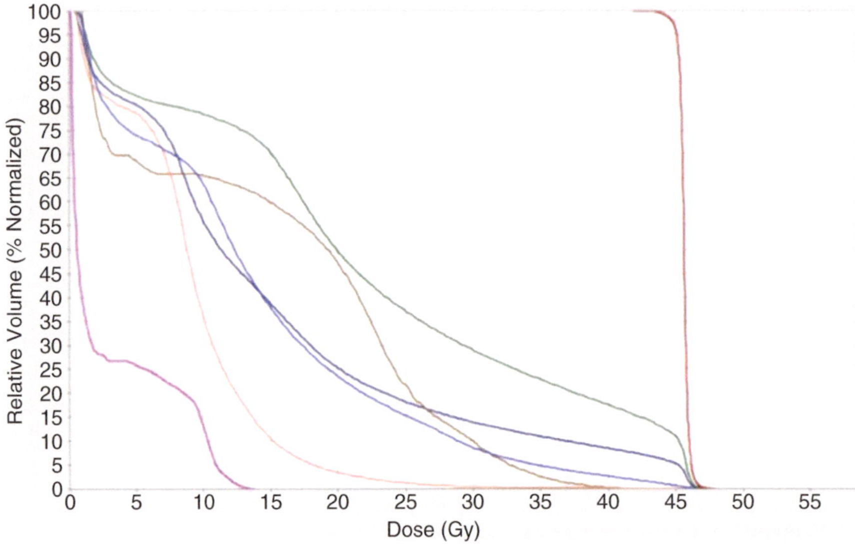

Structure	Min. dose (Gy)	Max. dose (Gy)	Mean dose (Gy)
PTV 45	41.81	47.90	45.62
Total Lung	0.39	47.52	11.39
Right Lung	0.52	47.52	19.93
Left Lung	0.4	46.2	8.9
Esophagus	0.97	42.10	19.37
Heart	0.71	46.43	12.39
Spinal Cord	0.11	13.80	8.79

Fig. 8.9 Dose-volume histogram and related evaluation metrics table for a typical 7-field intensity-modulated radiation therapy plan

Table 8.6 Recommended critical organ dose limits for concurrent chemoradiotherapy

Critical organ	Description	Metric	Per protocol	Variation acceptable	Variation unacceptable
Lungs	Lungs minus GTV	Max dose (0.03 cc)	≤110 % PD	>110 % but ≤113 % PD	>113 % PD
		Mean dose	≤20 Gy	>20 Gy but ≤21 Gy	>21 Gy
		Vol >10 Gy	≤45 %	>45 Gy but ≤50 Gy	>50 Gy
		Vol >20 Gy	≤35 %	>35 % but ≤36 %	>36 %
		Vol >5 Gy	≤65 %	>65 % but ≤75 %	>75 %
Heart	Heart/ pericardium	Max dose (0.03 cc)	≤70 Gy	>70 Gy but ≤75 Gy	>75 %
		Mean dose	≤30 Gy	>30 Gy but ≤31 Gy	>31 Gy
		Vol >30 Gy	≤50 %	>50 % but ≤55 %	>55 %
		Vol >40 Gy	≤35 %	>35 % but ≤40 %	>40 %
Esophagus	Esophagus	Max dose (0.03 cc)	≤74 Gy	>74 Gy but ≤76 Gy	>76 Gy
		Mean dose	≤34 Gy	>34 Gy but ≤35 Gy	>35 Gy
		Vol >70 Gy	≤20 %	>20 % but ≤25 %	>25 %
		Vol >50 Gy	≤40 %	>40 % but ≤45 %	>50 %
Spinal canal	Spinal cord	Max dose (0.03 cc)	≤50 Gy	>50 Gy but ≤52 Gy	>52 Gy
Brachial plexus	Brachial plexus	Max dose (0.03 cc)	≤63 Gy	>63 Gy but ≤65 Gy	>65 Gy
Midline structures	Non-PTV	Max hotspot (1 cc)	≤105 % PD	>105 % but ≤110 % PD	>110 % PD

Max maximum, *GTV* gross tumor volume, *PD* prescription dose

Prophylactic Cranial Irradiation

The PCI in LS- and ES-SCLC is discussed in detail in Chap. 9. In summary, strong evidence coming from RCTs and or meta-analyses which demonstrated prolongation of OS times with addition of PCI to C-CRT in LS-SCLC and ES-SCLC patients who have experienced any degree of favorable response to primary therapy set the PCI as the standard of care for all medically fit SCLC patients irrespective of their initial disease stage [67, 101].

Recommended Treatment Algorithm for SCLC

A summarized algorithm that is utilized in our institution for management of LS- and ES-SCLC patients is as depicted in Fig. 8.10.

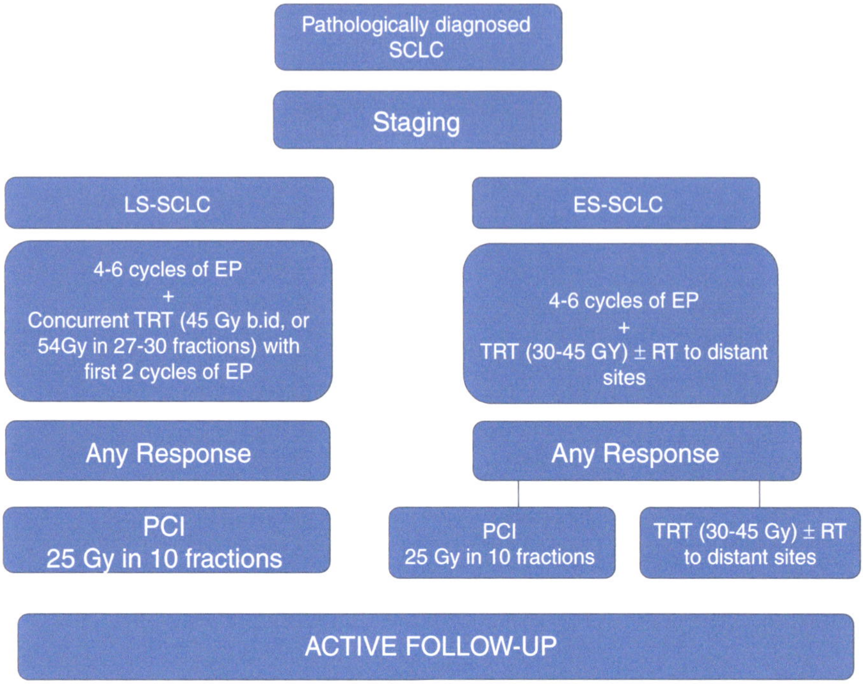

Fig. 8.10 Our institutional treatment algorithm for SCLC patients; *C-CRT* concurrent chemoradiotherapy *ICT* induction chemotherapy, *SCLC* small-cell lung cancer

Conclusion

A summarized algorithm that is utilized in our institution for management of LS- and ES-SCLC patients is as depicted in Fig. 10. In absence of further advancements beyond EP combination chemotherapy, the most progress in the outcome of SCLC in the past decades has come from an improved integration of TRT and PCI in either of LS- and ES-SCLC. Based on the multiple RCTs and/or meta-analyses, the optimal treatment of LS-SCLC appears to be C-CRT (45 Gy b.i.d TRT + concurrent EP combination) followed by PCI (25 Gy in 10 fractions), while EP combination chemotherapy followed by TRT and PCI in patients with any objective response is the current recommendation for ES-SCLC patients. Of note, to achieve the best results, the TRT and chemotherapy should be integrated as soon as possible (preferably at first course of chemotherapy), and the overall interval between the start of chemotherapy and the completion of TRT should be kept as short as possible, namely, <30 days.

References

1. Rosenzweig KE, Chen CP, Yom SS, Krug LM. Tumors of the lung, pleura, and mediastinum. In: Hoppe RT, Phillips TL, Roach III M, editors. Leibel and Phillips textbook of radiation oncology. Philadelphia: Saunders; 2010. p. 737–71. ISBN 978-1-4160-5897-7.
2. Barnard W. The nature of the 'oat-celled sarcoma' of the mediastinum. J Pathol. 1926;29:241–4.
3. Watson WL, Berg JW. Oat cell lung cancer. Cancer. 1962;15:759–68.
4. Brambilla E, Travis WD, Colby TV, Corrin B, Shimosato Y. The new World Health Organization classification of lung tumours. Eur Respir J. 2001;18(6):1059–68.
5. Lally BE, Urbanic JJ, Blackstock AW, Miller AA, Perry MC. Small cell lung cancer: have we made any progress over the last 25 years? Oncologist. 2007;12(9):1096–104.
6. van Oosterhout AG, van de Pol M, ten Velde GP, Twijnstra A. Neurologic disorders in 203 consecutive patients with small cell lung cancer. Results of a longitudinal study. Cancer. 1996;77(8):1434–41.
7. Yang GY, Matthews RH. Prophylactic cranial irradiation in small-cell lung cancer. Oncologist. 2000;5(4):293–8.
8. Zelen M. Keynote address on biostatistics and data retrieval. Cancer Chemother Rep. 1973;4(2):31–42.
9. Greene FL, Page DL, Fleeming ID, et al. AJCC cancer staging manual. 6th ed. New York: Springer; 2002. ISBN 0387952713.
10. Edge SB, Byrd DR, Compton CC, Fritz AG, Greene FL, Trotti A. AJCC cancer staging manual. 7th ed. New York: Springer; 2010. ISBN 0387884408.
11. Vallières E, Shepherd FA, Crowley J, et al. The IASLC Lung Cancer Staging Project: proposals regarding the relevance of TNM in the pathologic staging of small cell lung cancer in the forthcoming (seventh) edition of the TNM classification for lung cancer. J Thorac Oncol. 2009;4(9):1049–59.
12. Fischer BM, Mortensen J, Langer SW, et al. A prospective study of PET/CT in initial staging of small-cell lung cancer: comparison with CT, bone scintigraphy and bone marrow analysis. Ann Oncol. 2007;18(2):338–45.
13. van Meerbeeck JP, Fennell DA, De Ruysscher DK. Small-cell lung cancer. Lancet. 2011;378(9804):1741–55.
14. Lassen U, Osterlind K, Hansen M, et al. Long-term survival in small-cell lung cancer: post-treatment characteristics in patients surviving 5 to 18+ years – an analysis of 1,714 consecutive patients. J Clin Oncol. 1995;13(5):1215–20.
15. Tai P, Tonita J, Yu E, Skarsgard D. Twenty-year follow-up study of long-term survival of limited-stage small-cell lung cancer and overview of prognostic and treatment factors. Int J Radiat Oncol Biol Phys. 2003;56(3):626–33.
16. Byhardt RW, Hartz A, Libnoch JA, Hansen R, Cox JD. Prognostic influence of TNM staging and LDH levels in small cell carcinoma of the lung (SCCL). Int J Radiat Oncol Biol Phys. 1986;12(5):771–7.
17. Paesmans M, Sculier JP, Lecomte J, et al. Prognostic factors for patients with small cell lung carcinoma: analysis of a series of 763 patients included in 4 consecutive prospective trials with a minimum follow-up of 5 years. Cancer. 2000;89(3):523–33.
18. Albain KS, Crowley JJ, Livingston RB. Long-term survival and toxicity in small cell lung cancer. Expanded Southwest Oncology Group experience. Chest. 1991;99(6):1425–32.
19. Fox W, Scadding JG. Medical Research Council comparative trial of surgery and radiotherapy for primary treatment of small-celled or oat-celled carcinoma of bronchus. Ten-year follow-up. Lancet. 1973;2:63–5.

20. Miller AB, Fox W, Tall R. Five-year follow-up of the Medical Research Council comparative trial of surgery and radiotherapy for the primary treatment of small-celled or oat-celled carcinoma of the bronchus. Lancet. 1969;2:501–5.
21. Schreiber D, Rineer J, Weedon J, et al. Survival outcomes with the use of surgery in limited-stage small cell lung cancer: should its role be re-evaluated? Cancer. 2010;116(5):1350–7.
22. Lim E, Belcher E, Yap YK, Nicholson AG, Goldstraw P. The role of surgery in the treatment of limited disease small cell lung cancer: time to reevaluate. J Thorac Oncol. 2008;3(11):1267–71.
23. Fukuoka M, Furuse K, Saijo N, et al. Randomized trial of cyclophosphamide, doxorubicin, and vincristine versus cisplatin and etoposide versus alternation of these regimens in small-cell lung cancer. J Natl Cancer Inst. 1991;83(12):855–61.
24. Amarasena IU, Walters JA, Wood-Baker R, Fong K. Platinum versus non-platinum chemotherapy regimens for small cell lung cancer. Cochrane Database Syst Rev. 2008;4, CD006849.
25. Roth BJ, Johnson DH, Einhorn LH, Randolph JA, Goodlow JL, Broun GO, et al. Randomized study of cyclophosphamide, doxorubicin, and vincristine versus etoposide and cisplatin versus alternation of these two regimens in extensive small-cell lung cancer: a phase III trial of the Southeastern Cancer Study Group. J Clin Oncol. 1992;10(2):282–91.
26. Sundstrom S, Bremnes RM, Kaasa S, et al. Cisplatin and etoposide regimen is superior to cyclophosphamide, epirubicin, and vincristine regimen in small-cell lung cancer: results from a randomized phase III trial with 5 years' follow-up. J Clin Oncol. 2002;20(24):4665–72.
27. Sgambato A, Casaluce F, Maione P. Medical treatment of small cell lung cancer: state of the art and new development. Expert Opin Pharmacother. 2013;14(15):2019–31.
28. Okamoto H, Watanabe K, Kunikane H, et al. Randomized phase III trial of carboplatin(C) plus etoposide (E) vs. split doses of cisplatin (P) plus etoposide (E) in elderly or poorrisk patients with extensive disease small cell lung cancer (ED-SCLC): JCOG9702. J Clin Oncol. 2005;23(Suppl.16):Abstract 7010.
29. Noda K, Nishiwaki Y, Kawahara M, et al. Irinotecan plus cisplatin compared with etoposide plus cisplatin for extensive small-cell lung cancer. N Engl J Med. 2002;346(2):85–91.
30. Lara PN, Natale R, Crowley J, et al. Phase III trial of irinotecan/cisplatin compared with etoposide/cisplatin in extensive-stage small cell lung cancer: clinical and pharmacogenomic results from SWOG S0124. J Clin Oncol. 2009;27(15):2530–5.
31. Hanna N, Bunn PA, Langer C, et al. Randomized phase III trial comparing irinotecan/cisplatin with etoposide/cisplatin in patients with previously untreated extensive-stage disease small-cell lung cancer. J Clin Oncol. 2006;24(13):2038–43.
32. Loehrer PJ, Ansari R, Gonin R, et al. Cisplatin plus etoposide with and without ifosfamide in extensive small-cell lung cancer: a Hoosier Oncology Group study. J Clin Oncol. 1995;13(10):2594–9.
33. Mavroudis D, Papadakis E, Veslemes M, et al. A multicenter randomized clinical trial comparing paclitaxel-cisplatin-etoposide versus cisplatin-etoposide as first-line treatment in patients with small-cell lung cancer. Ann Oncol. 2001;12(4):463–70.
34. Niell HB, Herndon JE, Miller AA, et al. Randomized phase III intergroup trial of etoposide and cisplatin with or without paclitaxel and granulocyte colony-stimulating factor in patients with extensive-stage small-cell lung cancer: Cancer and Leukemia Group B Trial 9732. J Clin Oncol. 2005;23(16):3752–9.
35. Schiller JH, Adak S, Cella D, DeVore RF, Johnson DH. Topotecan versus observation after cisplatin plus etoposide in extensive-stage small-cell lung cancer: E7593 – a phase III trial of the Eastern Cooperative Oncology Group. J Clin Oncol. 2001;19(8):2114–22.
36. Sculier JP, Berghmans T, Castaigne C, et al. Maintenance chemotherapy for small cell lung cancer: a critical review of the literature. Lung Cancer. 1998;19(2):141–51.
37. Jiang J, Shi HZ, Deng JM, et al. Efficacy of intensified chemotherapy with hematopoietic progenitors in small-cell lung cancer: a meta-analysis of the published literature. Lung Cancer. 2009;65(2):214–8.

38. Messori A, Trippoli S, Tendi E. G-CSF for the prophylaxis of neutropenic fever in patients with small cell lung cancer receiving myelosuppressive antineoplastic chemotherapy: meta-analysis and pharmacoeconomic evaluation. J Clin Pharm Ther. 1996;21(2):57–63.
39. Berghmans T, Paesmans M, Lafitte JJ, et al. Role of granulocyte and granulocyte-macrophage colony-stimulating factors in the treatment of small-cell lung cancer: a systematic review of the literature with methodological assessment and meta-analysis. Lung Cancer. 2002;37(2):115–23.
40. Bozcuk H, Artac M, Ozdogan M, Savas B. Does maintenance/consolidation chemotherapy have a role in the management of small cell lung cancer (SCLC)? A meta-analysis of the published controlled trials. Cancer. 2005;104(12):2650–7.
41. Rossi A, Garassino MC, Cinquini M, et al. Maintenance or consolidation therapy in small-cell lung cancer: a systematic review and meta-analysis. Lung Cancer. 2010;70(2):119–28.
42. Slotman BJ, Senan S. Radiotherapy in small-cell lung cancer: lessons learned and future directions. Int J Radiat Oncol Biol Phys. 2011;79(4):998–1003.
43. Pignon JP, Arriagada R. Role of thoracic radiotherapy in limited stage small-cell lung cancer: quantitative review based on the literature versus meta-analysis based on individual data. J Clin Oncol. 1992;10:1819–20.
44. Warde P, Payne D. Does thoracic irradiation improve survival and local control in limited-stage small-cell carcinoma of the lung? A meta-analysis. J Clin Oncol. 1992;10:890–5.
45. Murray N, Coy P, Pater JL, et al. Importance of timing for thoracic irradiation in the combined modality treatment of limited-stage small-cell lung cancer. The National Cancer Institute of Canada Clinical Trials Group. J Clin Oncol. 1993;11:336–44.
46. Takada M, Fukuoka M, Kawahara M, et al. Phase III study of concurrent versus sequential thoracic radiotherapy in combination with cisplatin and etoposide for limited-stage small-cell lung cancer: results of the Japan Clinical Oncology Group Study 9104. J Clin Oncol. 2002;20:3054–60.
47. De Ruysscher D, Pijls-Johannesma M, Bentzen SM, et al. Time between the first day of chemotherapy and the last day of chest radiation is the most important predictor of survival in limited-disease small-cell lung cancer. J Clin Oncol. 2006;24:1057–63.
48. Scotti V, Meattini I, Franzese C, et al. Radiotherapy timing in the treatment of limited-stage small cell lung cancer: the impact of thoracic and brain irradiation on survival. Tumori. 2014;100(3):289–95.
49. Fried DB, Morris DE, Poole C, et al. Systematic review evaluating the timing of thoracic radiation therapy in combined modality therapy for limited-stage small-cell lung cancer. J Clin Oncol. 2004;22:4837–45.
50. Huncharek M, McGarry R. A meta-analysis of the timing of chest irradiation in the combined modality treatment of limited-stage small cell lung cancer. Oncologist. 2004;9(6):665–72.
51. Pijls-Johannesma M, De Ruysscher D, Vansteenkiste J, et al. Timing of chest radiotherapy in patients with limited stage small cell lung cancer: a systematic review and meta-analysis of randomised controlled trials. Cancer Treat Rev. 2007;33(5):461–73.
52. Turrisi AT, Kim K, Blum R, et al. Twice-daily compared with once-daily thoracic radiotherapy in limited small-cell lung cancer treated concurrently with cisplatin and etoposide. N Engl J Med. 1999;340(4):265–71.
53. Faivre-Finn C, Lorigan P, West C, Thatcher N. Thoracic radiation therapy for limited-stage small-cell lung cancer: unanswered questions. Clin Lung Cancer. 2005;7(1):23–9.
54. Topkan E, Parlak C. Radiation therapy in management of small-cell lung cancer. In: Elvisegran EM, editor. Lung diseases – selected state of the art reviews. ISBN: 978-953-51-0180-2, InTech. 2012. doi:10.5772/26433.
55. Pignon JP, Arriagada R, Ihde DC, et al. A meta-analysis of thoracic radiotherapy for small-cell lung cancer. N Engl J Med. 1992;327(23):1618–24.
56. Bonner JA, Sloan JA, Shanahan TG, et al. Phase III comparison of twice-daily split-course irradiation versus once daily irradiation for patients with limited stage small-cell lung carcinoma. J Clin Oncol. 1999;17(9):2681–91.

57. Bogart JA, Herndon 2nd JE, Lyss AP, et al. 70 Gy thoracic radiotherapy is feasible concurrent with chemotherapy for limited-stage small-cell lung cancer: analysis of Cancer and Leukemia Group B study 39808. Int J Radiat Oncol Biol Phys. 2004;59:460–8.
58. Miller AA, Wang XF, Bogart JA, et al. Phase II trial of paclitaxel-topotecan-etoposide followed by consolidation chemoradiotherapy for limited-stage small cell lung cancer: CALGB 30002. J Thorac Oncol. 2007;2(7):645–51.
59. Choi NC, Herndon 2nd JE, Rosenman J, et al. Phase I study to determine the maximum-tolerated dose of radiation in standard Daily and hyperfractionated-accelerated twice-daily radiation schedules with concurrent chemotherapy for limited-stage small-cell lung cancer. J Clin Oncol. 1998;16:3528–36.
60. Komaki R, Swann RS, Ettinger DS, et al. Phase I study of thoracic radiation dose escalation with concurrent chemotherapy for patients with limited small-cell lung cancer: report of Radiation Therapy Oncology Group (RTOG) protocol 97–12. Int J Radiat Oncol Biol Phys. 2005;62:342–50.
61. Komaki R, Paulus R, Ettinger DS, et al. Phase II study of accelerated high-dose radiation therapy with concurrent chemotherapy for patients with limited small-cell lung cancer: RTOG 0239. Int J Radiat Oncol Biol Phys. 2012;83(4):e531–6.
62. Govindan R, Page N, Morgensztern D, et al. Changing epidemiology of small-cell lung cancer in the United States over the last 30 years: analysis of the surveillance, epidemiologic, and end results database. J Clin Oncol. 2006;24(28):4539–44.
63. Splinter TAW. Chemotherapy of small cell lung cancer (SCLC): duration of treatment. Lung Cancer. 1989;5:186–96.
64. Bunn Jr PA, Cohen MH, Ihde DC, et al. Advances in small cell bronchogenic carcinoma: a commentary. Cancer Treat Rep. 1977;61:333–42.
65. Ihde DC, Mulshine JL, Kramer BS, et al. Prospective randomized comparison of high-dose and standard-dose etoposide and cisplatin chemotherapy in patients with extensive-stage small cell lung cancer. J Clin Oncol. 1994;12:2022–34.
66. Leyvraz S, Pampallona S, Martinelli G, et al. Solid tumors working party of the European group for blood and marrow transplantation. A threefold dose intensity treatment with ifosfamide, carboplatin, and etoposide for patients with small cell lung cancer: a randomized trial. J Natl Cancer Inst. 2008;100:533–41.
67. Slotman B, Faivre-Finn C, Kramer G, et al. Prophylactic cranial irradiation in extensive small-cell lung cancer. N Engl J Med. 2007;357(7):664–72.
68. Jeremic B, Shibamoto Y, Nikolic N, et al. The role of radiation therapy in the combined modality treatment of patients with extensive disease small-cell lung cancer (ED SCLC): a randomized study. J Clin Oncol. 1999;17:2092–9.
69. Giuliani ME, Atallah S, Sun A, et al. Clinical outcomes of extensive stage small cell lung carcinoma patients treated with consolidative thoracic radiotherapy. Clin Lung Cancer. 2011;12(6):375–9.
70. Zhu H, Zhou Z, Wang Y, et al. Thoracic radiation therapy improves the overall survival of patients with extensive-stage small cell lung cancer with distant metastasis. Cancer. 2011;117(23):5423–31.
71. Yee D, Butts C, Reiman A, et al. Clinical trial of post-chemotherapy consolidation thoracic radiotherapy for extensive-stage small cell lung cancer. Radiother Oncol. 2012;102(2):234–8.
72. Ou SH, Ziogas A, Zell JA. Prognostic factors for survival in extensive stage small cell lung cancer (ED-SCLC): the importance of smoking history, socioeconomic and marital statuses, and ethnicity. J Thorac Oncol. 2009;4(1):37–43.
73. Slotman BJ, van Tinteren H, Praag JO, et al. Use of thoracic radiotherapy for extensive stage small-cell lung cancer: a phase 3 randomised controlled trial. Lancet. 2015;385(9962):36–42.
74. McShan DL, Fraass BA, Lichter AS. Full integration of the beam's eye view concept into computerized treatment planning. Int J Radiat Oncol Biol Phys. 1990;18(6):1485–94.
75. Spoelstra FO, Senan S, Le Péchoux C, et al. Variations in target volume definition for post-operative radiotherapy in stage III non-small-cell lung cancer: analysis of an international contouring study. Int J Radiat Oncol Biol Phys. 2010;76(4):1106–13.

76. Pasic A, Brokx HA, Comans EF, et al. Detection and staging of preinvasive lesions and occult lung cancer in the central airways with 18F-fluorodeoxyglucose positron emission tomography: a pilot study. Clin Cancer Res. 2005;11(17):6186–9.
77. Giraud P, Antoine M, Larrouy A, et al. Evaluation of microscopic tumor extension in non-small-cell lung cancer for three-dimensional conformal radiotherapy planning. Int J Radiat Oncol Biol Phys. 2000;48:1015–24.
78. Grills IS, Fitch DL, Goldstein NS, et al. Clinicopathologic analysis of microscopic extension in lung adenocarcinoma: defining clinical target volume for radiotherapy. Int J Radiat Oncol Biol Phys. 2007;69:334–41.
79. Kara M, Dizbay Sak S, Orhan D, Kavukcu S. Proximal bronchial extension with special reference to tumor localization in non-small cell lung cancer. Eur J Cardiothorac Surg. 2001;20:350–5.
80. Kara M, Dizbay Sak S, Orhan D, Yavuzer S. Changing patterns of lung cancer; (3/4 in.) 1.9 cm; still a safe length for bronchial resection margin? Lung Cancer. 2000;30:161–8.
81. Yuan S, Meng X, Yu J, et al. Determining optimal clinical target volume margins on the basis of microscopic extracapsular extension of metastatic nodes in patients with non-small-cell lung cancer. Int J Radiat Oncol Biol Phys. 2007;67:727–34.
82. Kepka L, Tatro D, Moran JM, et al. Designing targets for elective nodal irradiation in lung cancer radiotherapy: a planning study. Int J Radiat Oncol Biol Phys. 2009;73:1397–403.
83. Liu HH, Balter P, Tutt T, et al. Assessing respiration induced tumor motion and internal target volume using four-dimensional computed tomography for radiotherapy of lung cancer. Int J Radiat Oncol Biol Phys. 2007;68:531–40.
84. De Ruysscher D, Bremer RH, Koppe F, et al. Omission of elective node irradiation on basis of CT-scans in patients with limited disease small cell lung cancer: a phase II trial. Radiother Oncol. 2006;80(3):307–12.
85. van Loon J, De Ruysscher D, Wanders R, et al. Selective nodal irradiation on basis of (18) FDG-PET scans in limited-disease small-cell lung cancer: a prospective study. Int J Radiat Oncol Biol Phys. 2010;77(2):329–36.
86. Shirvani SM, Komaki R, Heymach JV, Fossella FV, Chang JY. Positron emission tomography/computed tomography-guided intensity-modulated radiotherapy for limited-stage small-cell lung cancer. Int J Radiat Oncol Biol Phys. 2012;82(1):91–7.
87. Kamel EM, Zwahlen D, Wyss MT, et al. Whole-body (18)F-FDG PET improves the management of patients with small cell lung cancer. J Nucl Med. 2003;44:1911–7.
88. Bradley JD, Dehdashti F, Mintun MA, et al. Positron emission tomography in limited-stage small-cell lung cancer: a prospective study. J Clin Oncol. 2004;22:3248–54.
89. Thomson D, Hulse P, Lorigan P, Faivre-Finn C. The role of positron emission tomography in management of small cell lung cancer. Lung Cancer. 2011;73(2):121–6.
90. van Loon J, Offermann C, Bosmans G, et al. 18FDG-PET based radiation planning of mediastinal lymph nodes in limited disease small cell lung cancer changes radiotherapy fields: a planning study. Radiother Oncol. 2008;87:49–54.
91. Han TJ, Kim HJ, Wu HG, et al. Comparison of treatment outcomes between involved-field and elective nodal irradiation in limited-stage small cell lung cancer. Jpn J Clin Oncol. 2012;42(10):948–54.
92. Kies MS, Mira JG, Crowley JJ, et al. Multimodal therapy for limited small-cell lung cancer: a randomized study of induction combination chemotherapy with or without thoracic radiation in complete responders; and with wide-field versus reduced-field radiation in partial responders: a Southwest Oncology Group Study. J Clin Oncol. 1987;5(4):592–600.
93. Liengswangwong V, Bonner JA, Shaw EG, et al. Limited-stage small-cell lung cancer: patterns of intrathoracic recurrence and the implications for thoracic radiotherapy. J Clin Oncol. 1994;12(3):496–502.
94. Talarico L, Chen G, Pazdur R. Enrollment of elderly patients in clinical trials for cancer drug registration: a 7-year experience by the US Food and Drug Administration. J Clin Oncol. 2004;22:4626–31.
95. Okamoto K, Okamoto I, Takezawa K, et al. Cisplatin and etoposide chemotherapy combined with early concurrent twice-daily thoracic radiotherapy for limited-disease small cell lung cancer in elderly patients. Jpn J Clin Oncol. 2010;40(1):54–9.

96. Okamoto H, Watanabe K, Kunikane H, et al. Randomised phase III trial of carboplatin plus etoposide vs split doses of cisplatin plus etoposide in elderly or poor-risk patients with extensive disease small-cell lung cancer: JCOG 9702. Br J Cancer. 2007;97:162–9.
97. Bork E, Ersbøll J, Dombernowsky P, et al. Teniposide and etoposide in previously untreated small-cell lung cancer: a randomized study. J Clin Oncol. 1991;9(9):1627–31.
98. Souhami RL, Spiro SG, Rudd RM, et al. Five-day oral etoposide treatment for advanced small-cell lung cancer: randomized comparison with intravenous chemotherapy. J Natl Cancer Inst. 1997;89(8):577–80.
99. Girling DJ. Comparison of oral etoposide and standard intravenous multidrug chemotherapy for small-cell lung cancer: a stopped multicentre randomised trial. Medical Research Council Lung Cancer Working Party. Lancet. 1996;348(9027):563–6.
100. Manapov F, Klöcking S, Niyazi M, et al. Chemoradiotherapy duration correlates with overall survival in limited disease SCLC patients with poor initial performance status who successfully completed multimodality treatment. Strahlenther Onkol. 2012;188(1):29–34.
101. Auperin A, Arriagada R, Pignon JP, et al. Prophylactic cranial irradiation for patients with small-cell lung cancer in complete remission. Prophylactic Cranial Irradiation Overview Collaborative Group. N Engl J Med. 1999;341:476–84.

Prophylactic Cranial Irradiation in Small- and Non-small-Cell Lung Carcinoma

9

Erkan Topkan and Ugur Selek

PCI in Small-Cell Lung Carcinoma

At initial presentation, approximately 10–14 % of small-cell lung carcinoma (SCLC) patients manifest with radiologically evident brain metastases (BM), and BM incidence is straightforwardly associated with the disease stage [1, 2]. Therefore, patients with extensive-stage SCLC (ES-SCLC) at presentation are more likely than those with limited-stage SCLC (LS-SCLC) to develop BM at 2 years (47 % versus 69 %), and in 20–30 % of those patients, the brain is the only apparent site of relapse [3, 4]. In postmortem examinations, the BM incidence rates are reported to be even far beyond these rates [5].

For patients, the impact of BM on quality of life is essentially more regrettable than the impact of disappointment at other metastatic destinations. Such patients are often obliged to spend significant time hospitalized and endure loss of autonomy which psychosocially affects the patients and their care providers in an adverse manner [6]. Combining this evidence with the limited efficacy of palliative cranial irradiation and/or chemotherapy in clinically settled BM and an overall survival (OS) expectation of only 4–6 months, such data strongly emphasizes the need for earlier interventions targeting the microscopic BM in such patients [7, 8].

Regarding its counteractive actions on BM emergence, the potential beneficial effects of prophylactic cranial irradiation (PCI) in patients with LS-SCLC have been addressed with several randomized trials. Assumably, in patients with controlled extracranial disease, PCI may eradicate the intracranial microscopic tumor cell

E. Topkan, MD (✉)
Department of Radiation Oncology, Baskent University, Adana, Turkey
e-mail: docdretopkan@gmail.com

U. Selek, MD
Department of Radiation Oncology, Faculty of Medicine, Koc University, Istanbul, Turkey

Department of Radiation Oncology, The University of Texas, MD Anderson Cancer Center, Houston, TX, USA

G. Ozyigit et al. (eds.), *Principles and Practice of Radiotherapy Techniques in Thoracic Malignancies*, DOI 10.1007/978-3-319-28761-4_9

deposits with relatively lower and safe radiation doses and, in this way, may potentially lengthen the survival times. Supporting this logical assumption, although neither could reach statistical noteworthiness, the outcomes of two randomized controlled trials (RCT) from France (PCI85) and United Kingdom (UK02) exhibited a trend for better survival with PCI [9, 10]. But unfortunately up till now, no individual RCT has decisively demonstrated a survival advantage for PCI in the LS-SCLC setting, which may be related with their inadequacy in procurement of sufficient statistical power to discriminate moderate differences in survival.

With an end goal to overcome the statistical problems related with the relatively small population sizes and to direct a meta-analysis of trials utilizing PCI and to make proposals for clinical practice, the PCI Overview Collaborative Group was established. The benchmark meta-analysis from this group reported by Auperin et al. in 1999 included individual data from patients enrolled on seven prospective randomized PCI trials [11]. Trials qualified in the meta-analysis were restricted to those, in which patients had been treated with systemic chemotherapy with/without thoracic radiotherapy (TRT) to a complete clinical response and no known BM. PCI doses were for the most part between 24 and 40 Gy given in 2–3 Gy daily fractions. Outcomes of this meta-analysis, for the first time, demonstrated a statistically meaningful survival advantage favoring PCI over non-PCI arms. The relative risk for death in the treated patients, as compared to controls, was 0.84 ($p=0.01$), which corresponds to an absolute 5.4 % higher rate of survival at 3 years (20.7 % versus 15.3 %) which was further preserved over time. As a percent gain over control, this speaks to a 35 % expansion in the extent of surviving patients. There was likewise an absolute 8.8 % increase in disease-free survival at 3 years (22.1 % vs. 13.3 %; $p<0.0001$). PCI was furthermore connected with a 25.3 % absolute decrease in the cumulative incidence of BM at 3 years (33.3 % vs. 58.6 %; $p<0.0001$) [11]. Following publication of this landmark meta-analysis, PCI turned into the standard of consideration in patients with LS-SCLC demonstrating complete response following systemic chemotherapy and TRT. Consequences of this thorough meta-analysis which changed the treatment standards of LS-SCLC have later been affirmed by the audit of information from Surveillance Epidemiology and End Results (SEER) database reported by Patel et al. [12]. Of 7,995 LS-SCLC patients included, 670 received PCI. Better overall and cause-specific survival were observed in patients treated with PCI, and corresponding 2- and 5-year survival rates were 23 % and 11 % without PCI and 42.5 % and 19 % with PCI.

Despite the fact that the useful impacts of PCI on prevention of BM occurrence and on augmentation of overall and disease-free survival have been well established in LS-SCLC, this issue had remained to be answered in ES-SCLC until the publication of the results of the EORTC trial by Slotman et al. [13]. In this benchmark study, patients with ES-SCLC who had a response to chemotherapy were randomized to PCI versus observation arms. The cumulative risk of symptomatic BM and rate of OS at 1 year were 14.6 % vs. 40.4 % ($p<0.001$) and 27.1 % vs. 13.3 % ($p=0.003$), both favoring the PCI arm excluding those experiencing disease progression during the chemotherapy PCI turned into the standard of consideration for ES-SCLC patients after the publication of this RCT, likewise the LS-SCLC.

Table 9.1 Characteristics of the trials included in the meta-analysis by Zhang et al. [14] and Viani et al. [4]

Author	Year	Patients (N)	Total dose (dose per fraction, Gy)	Disease stage
Zhang et al. [14]	2014	1,601	8–36 (1.8–8)	Limited/extensive
Gregor et al. [10]	1997	314	8–36 (1–18)	Limited/extensive
Laplanche et al.	1998	211	24 (3)	Limited/extensive
Cao et al.	2005	51	25.2–30.6 (1.8–1.9)	Limited
Slotman et al. [13]	2007	286	20–30 (5–12)	Extensive
Schild et al.	2012	739	25–30 (2–2.5)	Limited/extensive
Viani et al.	2014	1,983	8–40 (1.8–8)	Limited/extensive
Aisner et al.	1982	29	30 (3)	Limited/extensive
Arriagada et al. [9]	1995	300	24 (3)	Limited/extensive
Beiler et al.	1979	54	24 (3)	Limited/extensive
Cao et al.	2005	51	25.2–30.6 (1.8–1.9)	Limited
Kristjansen et al.	1993	55	24 (3)	Limited/extensive
Eagan et al.	1981	30	36 (1.8)	Limited
Gregor et al. [10]	1997	314	8–36 (1–18)	Limited/extensive
Hansen et al.	1980	109	40 (2)	Limited
Jackson et al.	1977	29	30 (3)	Limited/extensive
Laplanche et al.	1998	211	24 (3)	Limited/extensive
Maurer et al.	1980	153	30 (3)	Limited/extensive
Niiranen et al.	1989	51	40 (2)	Limited
Ohonoshi et al.	1993	46	40 (2)	Limited/extensive
Seydel et al.	1985	217	30 (3)	Limited
Slotman et al.	2007	286	20–30 (5–12)	Extensive
Wagner et al.	1996	32	24 (3)	Limited/extensive

The results of the landmark study by Slotman et al. [13], which represents the first randomized trial to demonstrate survival advantage with PCI, were recently confirmed by two large meta-analyses [4, 14]. In the first meta-analysis by Zhang et al. [14], 1,601 LS- and ES-SCLC patients enrolled on five randomized controlled trials between 1997 and 2012 were identified to compare BM incidence and OS between PCI and non-PCI arms (Table 9.1). In two trials reporting the 1-year incidence of BM, PCI was reported to reduce the BM incidence in 1 year with a pooled relative risk of 0.45 ($p<0.00001$). The 1-year OS rate was noted in four trials which demonstrated a significant OS benefit favoring the PCI over the non-PCI group with a pooled relative risk of 0.87 ($p=0.01$). The 3- and 5-year OS rates were reported in respective three and four trials, which cumulatively revealed a significant OS advantage in the PCI group with pooled relative risks of 0.87 ($p<0.00001$) and 0.92 ($p<0.00001$), respectively.

In the second meta-analysis by Viani et al. [4], 16 randomized clinical trials, collectively involving 1,983 patients, were analyzed. Of those patients, 1,021 received PCI, while 962 did not. Overall, compared to non-PCI group, the PCI utilization revealed 4.4 % absolute reduction in rates of mortality (OR = 0.73; $p = 0.01$), especially among the patients enjoying a complete response after chemotherapy (OR = 0.68; $p = 0.02$) and in those submitted to PCI after that treatment (OR = 0.68; $p = 0.03$). This survival advantage was further found to be independent of the disease stage: LS-SCLC (OR = 0.73; $p = 0.03$) and ES-SCLC (OR = 0.48; $p = 0.02$).

Although the aforementioned strong data supports the standard use of PCI in patients with any SCLC enjoying at least disease stabilization following the intended locoregional and/or systemic treatment, an existing vital worry about the utilization of PCI is the requirement for determination of a built non-harmful yet compelling fractionation scheme and total dose. Accessible information has demonstrated that lower dosages of PCI may be less effective in avoiding CNS failures [10, 11]. As of late, Le Pechoux et al. [15] published the results of benchmark international PCI trial assessing the radiation dose for PCI in LS-SCLC. The study randomized 720 patients with LS-SCLC from 157 centers to one of two PCI arms: Arm 1 included patients receiving standard-dose PCI to 25 Gy in 2.5 Gy per fraction, and Arm 2 included patients receiving higher-dose PCI to 36 Gy in 2 Gy once-daily or 1.5 Gy twice-daily fractions. No significant difference of BM incidence was reported between two study arms, yet there was a significantly higher rate of cancer-related mortality in the higher-dose arm as a consequence of unexplained finding of more deaths from extracranial disease progression [15]. Based on the results of this study, 25 Gy delivered at 2.5 Gy per fraction per day remains the standard of care for PCI in LS-SCLC patients.

PCI for Geriatric SCLC Patients

Lung cancer is mainly a disease of elderly patients with a median age of 67 years. Unfortunately, in spite of the proven survival benefit, many eligible senior patients with SCLC do not receive PCI mainly due physicians and to a lesser degree to patients concerns on an increased risk of radiation-induced neurotoxicity. As a result, in most PCI trials, patients with advanced age were excluded from protocols and, therefore, did not receive this potentially life-prolonging treatment option.

In clinical practice, although the dilemma of whether to administer PCI in older individuals remains controversial, available literature supports its use in elderly patients just similar to their younger counterparts [12, 16]. In the aforementioned SEER analysis [12], multiple age groups were analyzed (age <60, 60–66, 67–72, and ≥73) and PCI was reported to be beneficial in all age groups. The 5-year OS for the 67–72- and ≥73-year cohorts were 16 % vs. 10 % ($p = 0.0005$) and 10 % vs. 5 % ($p < 0.0001$), both favoring the PCI group. In the second analysis of patients with LS-SCLC >70 years (median age, 75 years), PCI was demonstrated to strongly associate with improved survival rates (33 % vs. 23 %; $p = 0.028$). Additionally, PCI was reported to be an independent predictor of longer OS (HR = 0.72; $p = 0.032$) in those patients >75 years of age [16].

In the recently published pooled analysis of North Central Cancer Treatment Group experience [17], the outcomes of 155 patients with ≥70 years of age and LS-SCLC or ES-SCLC who participated in four phase II or III trials were retrospectively analyzed according to their PCI status. Of those, 91 patients received PCI (30 Gy/15 or 25 Gy/10 fractions), while 64 patients did not, and served as controls. Survival analysis included the patients with any objective response (stable disease or better) to prescribed primary locoregional and/or systemic therapy. Results of this analysis proved that compared to non-PCI, the survival outcomes were significantly better in PCI group, namely, median OS (12.0 vs. 7.6 months; $p=0.001$) and 3-year OS (13.2 % vs. 3.1 %; $p=0.001$). The only factor that remained significant for longer survival was stage (LS-SCLC vs. ES-SCLC; $p=0.0072$) on multivariate analysis of the entire cohort, while same analysis limited to ES-SCLC demonstrated the PCI utilization as the sole predictor to associate with longer survival times (HR=0.47; $p=0.03$).

In summary, enlightened with the strong evidence which supports the use of PCI as a life-prolonging treatment option for both LS-SCLC and ES-SCLC, we believe that chronologic age should not solely be considered as a contraindication for PCI. Therefore, alike with their younger counterparts, we recommend the use of PCI for all medically fit elderly SCLC patients who have experienced any degree of favorable response to primary therapy irrespective of their initial disease stage.

PCI in Locally Advanced Non-small-Cell Lung Carcinoma

Non-small-cell lung carcinoma (NSCLC), with its particular histologies, namely, adenocarcinoma (AC), squamous cell carcinoma (SCC), and large cell carcinoma (LCC), accounts for more than 85 % of all lung cancers. Based on the outcomes of two phase III randomized studies, the current standard treatment approach for the locally advanced NSCLC (LA-NSCLC) is definitive concurrent chemoradiotherapy (C-CRT), while surgery and stereotactic radiosurgery are appropriate treatment options for early stage disease [18, 19]. Although aggressive C-CRT has been shown to result in particular superb results with ≥50 % locoregional control rates and approximately 2-year median survival times in LA-NSCLC [18–22], yet starkly contrasting with the tumor control and survival advantages gained, this approach has proved no noteworthy viability in lessening of overall brain failure (21–54 %) or brain as the first site of relapse (15–30 %) rates [23, 24], stressing the prerequisite for earlier interventions targeting the microscopic BM.

Patients at Higher Risk of BM Development

Disease stage (IIIA/B vs. I–II) is the strongest factor predicting the incidence of BM development at some point during the course of treatment where the risk is <10 % for stage I–II and >50 % for stage III patients, respectively. In stage IIIA/B NSCLC patients who have the highest risk for brain first and overall brain failures after aggressive combination therapies, several factors associate with an increased risk of BM including the histology (non-SCC vs. SCC), gender (female vs. male), age at presentation (<60 years vs. older), nodal status (N2-3 vs. N0-1), performance score

(Zubrod <70 vs. ≥70), lymph node bulk (bulky vs. non-bulky), duration of survival (longer vs. short), lactate dehydrogenase (LDH) levels (high vs. normal), chemotherapy regimen (taxane–platinum vs. other platinum-based combinations), and usage of targeted therapies [23, 25–35]. Age <60 or 70 years was shown to be associated with an increased risk of BM in various studies [30, 33, 35]. In the subgroup analysis of the study by Keith et al. [36], female gender and elevated LDH levels were found to be the factors to relate with a higher risk of BM. Primary tumor stage of T4 was associated with increased risk of BM in a multivariate analysis of 305 patients with localized NSCLC [35], and the N2 status was found to be predictive of BM by Jacobs et al. [37] and Tang et al. [38]. In the study by Jacobs et al. [38], the risk of BM was significantly higher in the presence of hilar (N1) and ipsilateral mediastinal (N2) lymph nodes than in the N0 patients. Similarly, in the Italian multivariate analysis, there was a trend toward a higher risk of BM in the presence of bulky (6.2 cm) mediastinal lymph nodes [30]. Although the Italian study failed to report a relationship between tumor histology and BM development [30], in view of the results of the other studies demonstrating higher BM rates in AC than SCC, with its reported BM incidence range of 24–35.7 % [23, 37, 38], the AC histology has gained general acceptance for being associated with higher BM development than SCC [25, 26, 28, 39–41].

In a recent retrospective report by Ji et al., risk factors for BM in LA-NSCLC patients treated with definitive chest irradiation have been investigated [42]. Stage III 346 patients treated between 2008 and 2010 were included with a median follow-up of 48.3 months for the surviving patients. Seventy-four (21.4 %) patients were reported to experience BM with a median time from the treatment to BM diagnosis of 9 months and respective BM incidence rates of 15 % and 28.1 % at 1- and 3-year time points. In univariate analysis, female sex, age 60 years, non-SCC, T3-4, N3, >3 areas of lymph node metastasis, and high LDH and serum levels of tumor markers (CEA, NSE, CA125) before treatment were found as significant associates of BM ($p<0.05$). In multivariate analysis, age <60 years ($p=0.004$; HR=0.491), non-SCC histology ($p=0.0001$; HR=3.726), NSE >18 ng/mL ($p\leq0.008$; HR=1.968), and CA125 ≥35 U/mL ($p=0.002$, HR=2.129) were found as the independent risk factors for BM. Stratification of patients according to these factors revealed that patients with no or lesser risk factors had significantly reduced BM rates at 3 years, 7.3 % for 0, 18.9 % for 1, 35.8 % for 2, and 70.3 % for 3–4 risk factors, respectively ($p<0.001$).

Rationale of PCI in NSCLC

Platinum-based combination chemotherapy, which enhanced survival rates by reducing the locoregional and distant failures, is the current standard systemic regime for LA-NSCLC patients [25, 43, 44]; in any case, chemotherapy seems to have little or no effect on brain failure rates [25]. The lack of further significant improvements in survival may relate with the increased incidence of isolated BM and the absence of cure promising therapies for this almost exclusively fatal disease state [26, 28, 29, 31, 45]. It is critical to point out that preoperative induction chemotherapy has been exhibited to decrease the risk of visceral metastases in many series but could not attain the same impact on BM and, in certain cases, was even suggested to associate with isolated raised BM rates, such as in the series of Andre et al. [26]. In this report compared to upfront surgery, preoperative induction chemotherapy was associated with doubled rates of isolated BM (22 % vs. 11 %) and (39 % vs. 20 %) in that of Robnett et al. [28]. Because micrometastasis in brain parenchyma was not successfully treated with induction chemotherapy, PCI was suggested as a possible solution. Stuschke et al. [46] introduced PCI to eradicate potential disease in a phase II trial on trimodality treatment of locally advanced NSCLC, achieving a reduced incidence of BM as the first site of relapse and a reduced rate of overall brain relapse. The recent series of the Adjuvant Navelbine International Trialist Association (ANITA) investing adjuvant chemotherapy underscored that adjuvant chemotherapies seem to be ineffective in preventing BM, even in operable NSCLC [47] which was followed by a similar conclusion of the International Adjuvant Lung Cancer Trial Collaborative Group [48]. ANITA trial demonstrated that distant metastases were more frequent in patients receiving postoperative radiotherapy (PORT) for both the observation and the chemotherapy groups; this seemed to be more pronounced for patients with pN2 disease in the observation group [47]. Furthermore, although PORT reduced the local relapse rate in both groups, more patients receiving PORT presented with BM (16.4 % vs. 9.5 %), which might probably be related to increased referral to PORT in cases of more advanced disease.

The failure of available chemotherapeutic agents to prevent brain failures may be associated with their poor ability to cross the blood–brain barrier (BBB) and relative poor response rates at this sanctuary site. Cisplatin has been proven to cross the BBB, but the response rate in BM from primary NSCLC was shown to be only 15–30 % in patients treated with cisplatin-based combination regimens [49]. Although the temozolomide may achieve high concentrations in the central nervous system, its activity in BM of NSCLC is only less than 10 % [50]. Topotecan appears to be a promising agent in this setting [51]. The BBB permeability modulation is currently under research which may potentially alter the response to present chemotherapeutics in a positive manner with the hope of increase of PCI effectiveness when concurrently administered [52].

The failure of chemotherapy to reduce the BM incidence provides a rationale for the possible use of PCI in stage III NSCLC patients. Furthermore, the emergence of almost half of all BM at posttreatment 4 and more than 80 % at 12 months supports the need for urgent preventive interventions, such as PCI, against BM in such patients. For example, in a recent retrospective review of the Southwest Oncology Group (SWOG) database reported by Gaspar et al. [31], of 422 patients with stage IIIA/IIIB NSCLC who were treated with concurrent cisplatin–etoposide and thoracic RT (TRT), 268 (64 %) experienced disease progression; 54 (20 %) of these affected the brain only and 17 (6.5 %) the brain and other sites simultaneously. In these 71 patients, time from treatment to disease progression in the brain was reported as follows: during treatment, 16 relapses (22.5 %); 0–16 weeks after treatment, 17 relapses (24 %); 16 weeks to 6 months after treatment, 10 relapses (14 %); 6–12 months after treatment, 16 relapses (22.5 %); and more than 12 months after treatment, 12 relapses (17 %). Thus, it seems that 46.5 % and 83 % of all brain relapses develop within 16 weeks and 12 months after the completion of treatment, respectively.

Efficacy of PCI in High-Risk NSCLC Patients

Several nonrandomized and randomized studies have addressed the efficacy of PCI in delaying or reducing the incidence of BM in high-risk NSCLC patients.

Nonrandomized Studies

As summarized in Table 9.2, several nonrandomized multimodality studies have suggested a potential beneficial role for PCI in patients with LA-NSCLC [24, 26, 46, 53, 54]. In one of the most notable studies by Stuschke et al. [46], 75 LA-NSCLC patients were treated with trimodality therapy consisting of induction chemotherapy, preoperative CRT, and surgery. PCI of 30 Gy (2 Gy/day) was introduced after the first half of the study because of a high incidence of BM and reduced the rate of BM as the first site of relapse from 30 % to 8 % at 4 years ($p=0.005$) and the rate of overall brain relapse from 54 % to 13 % ($p=0.0004$).

In a recently reported SEER database analysis by Park et al. [55], a total of 17,852 NSCLC patients were included, among whom 326 (1.8 %) received PCI. The authors reported that patients <60 years of age and those with AC were significantly

Table 9.2 Outcomes of nonrandomized trials on prophylactic cranial irradiation of locally advanced non-small-cell lung carcinoma

Reference	Patients (N)	Histology	Primary tx	PCI dose (Gy)	BM PCI- (%)	BM PCI+ (%)	P-value
Strauss et al. [24]	54	Non-SCC	Trimodality	30 (2 Gy/fx)	12	0	0.32
Albain et al. [22]	126	Any NSCLC	Trimodality	36 (2 Gy/fx)	16	8	0.36
Skarin et al. [54]	41	Any NSCLC	Trimodality	NS	27	14	–
Stuschke et al. [46]	75	Any NSCLC	Trimodality	30 (2 Gy/fx)	54	13	0.0004
Rusch et al. [53]	75	NS	Ctx + RT	36 (2 Gy/fx) 30 (2 Gy/fx)	–	0	–
Topkan et al. [57]	134	AC + SCC	ICT + C-CRT	30 (2 Gy/fx)	–	13.8	0.03
			C-CRT	30 (2 Gy/fx)	–	3.9	

AC adenocarcinoma, *BM* brain metastasis, *C-CRT* concurrent chemoradiotherapy, *Ctx* chemotherapy, *fx* fraction, *ICT* induction chemotherapy, *NS* not specified, *NSCLC* non-small-cell lung carcinoma, *PCI* prophylactic cranial irradiation, *RT* radiotherapy, *SCC* squamous cell carcinoma, *tx* treatment more likely to receive PCI. Median OS for the entire population was 8 months with no statistically significant survival difference between PCI and non-PCI patients (9 vs. 8 months; HR, 1.04; $p=0.646$). Similar results were found in all subgroup analyses of high-risk patients for BM, including the age <60 years (10 months vs. 11 months; $p=0.124$), AC histology (9 vs. 8 months; $p=0.304$), and those with stage IIIB (8 months vs. 6 months; $p=0.075$) patients. However, the results of this analysis should be interpreted with great caution, because the reported median OS of only 8 months for the whole study population is almost only one-third of those achieved with modern C-CRT. Although it was not given in the original manuscript, this may potentially be related with inclusion of patients with poor performance status and with significant weight loss who are the strong candidates for poorest prognosis after any oncological intervention.

In another systemic review and meta-analysis of 12 trials (6 randomized and 6 nonrandomized) published by Xie et al. [56] with a total of 1,718 NSCLC patients, PCI was noted to significantly reduce BM incidence (HR, 0.30; $p<0.00001$). However, interestingly in the same analysis, the use of PCI in NSCLC patients was reported to be associated with worse OS than non-PCI patients (OR, 1.19; $p=0.004$).

In an interesting recent study from Turkey, Topkan et al. [57] analyzed the outcomes of 134 stage IIIB NSCLC patients. All patients were Group 1 according to the recursive partitioning analysis grouping system and were treated with PCI (30 Gy at 2 Gy/fx) following one of two CRT regimes. Patients in Regime 1 ($n=58$) and 2 ($n=76$) received three cycles of induction chemotherapy followed by C-CRT or immediate definitive C-CRT, respectively. At a median follow-up of 27.6 months, 65 patients were alive. Median OS, progression-free survival, and brain metastasis-free survival (BMFS) times for the whole study cohort were 23.4, 15.4, and 23.0 months, respectively. Median survival time and the 3-year survival rate for regimes 1 and 2 were 19.3 vs. 26.1 months ($p=0.001$) and 14.4 % vs. 34.4 % ($p<0.001$), respectively. Median time from the initiation of primary treatment to PCI was 123.2 (range, 97–161) and 63.4 (range, 55–74) days for regimes 1 and 2, respectively ($p<0.001$). Overall, 11 (8.2 %) patients developed brain metastasis (BM) during the follow-up period: 8 (13.8 %) in regime 1 and 3 (3.9 %) in regime 2 ($p=0.03$). Median BMFS for regimes 1 and 2 were 17.4 versus 26.0 months, respectively ($p<0.001$). The results of this study suggested that immediate C-CRT rather than induction-first regime was associated with lower BM incidence and longer survival rates in stage IIIB NSCLC patients treated with PCI. This study is important by addressing the timing of PCI in LA-NSCLC patients and by indicating maximum benefit of PCI with its earlier use without delay caused by induction strategies, which is quite similar with the well-established superiority of immediate definitive C-CRT over induction-first protocols for thoracic primaries.

In general, the use of PCI reduced the rates of BM compared with non-PCI groups. In any case, albeit such nonrandomized data might be utilized as a base for larger randomized trials, results ought to be interpreted with caution because of potential biasing impacts; for instance, it is quite surprising to observe a 0 % BM rate in one of the treatment groups, as reported by Strauss et al. [24], or a

Table 9.3 Outcomes of randomized controlled trials on prophylactic cranial irradiation of locally advanced non-small-cell lung carcinoma

Reference	Patients (N)	Histology	Primary tx	PCI dose (Gy)	BM PCI- (%)	BM PCI+ (%)	P-value
Unsawasdi et al.	97	Any NSCLC	Trimodality	30 (3 Gy/fx)	27	4	0.002
			Ctx + RT				
Cox et al.	281	Any NSCLC	RT	20 (2 Gy/fx)	13	6	0.038
Mira et al.	111	Any NSCLC	Ctx + RT	30 (2 Gy/fx)	11	0	0.0001
				37.5 (2.5 Gy/fx)			
Russell et al.	187	Non-SCC	RT	30 (3 Gy/fx)	19	9	0.06
Pöttgen et al.	112	Any NSCLC (all stage IIIA)	Ctx + RT	30 (2 Gy/fx)	34.7 (FSF)	7.8 (FSF)	0.02
					27.2	9.1	0.04
Gore et al.	340	AC + SCC	Any combination	30 (2 Gy/fx)	18.0	7.7	0.004
Li [63]	156	Any NSCLC (all stage IIIA)	Sx + Ctx	30 (3 Gy/fx)	49.9 (5 years)	20.3 (5 years)	<0.001

AC adenocarcinoma, *BM* brain metastasis, *C-CRT* concurrent chemoradiotherapy, *Ctx* chemotherapy, *FSF* first site of failure, *fx* fraction, *ICT* induction chemotherapy, *NS* not specified, *NSCLC* non-small-cell lung carcinoma, *PCI* prophylactic cranial irradiation, *RT* radiotherapy, *SCC* squamous cell carcinoma, *Sx* surgery, *tx* treatment

large difference in one relatively small study, such as that reported by Stuschke et al. [46].

Randomized Studies

Outcomes of reported randomized trials of PCI in patients with LA-NSCLC are as summarized in Table 9.3 [27, 58–63]. The first study conducted by the Veterans Administration Lung Group (VALG) also included small-cell lung carcinoma (SCLC) patients [60], and patients were randomized to receive PCI (20 Gy in ten fractions) or no PCI and to receive one of two regimens of TRT. In the NSCLC group, PCI decreased the incidence of BM from 13 % to 6 % ($p = 0.038$) in all NSCLC and from 29 % to 0 % in adenocarcinomas ($p = 0.04$).

In a series of 97 LA-NSCLC patients, Umsawasdi et al. [59] administered combined CRT and randomized patients to PCI (30 Gy in ten fractions) or non-PCI arms. PCI increased the BMFS and significantly reduced the incidence of BM from 27 % to 4 % ($p = 0.002$). In a SWOG randomized study, Mira et al. [61] randomized 232 localized NSCLC patients to compare TRT with TRT plus chemotherapy, with or without PCI arms. Patients in the PCI arm received 30 or 37.5 Gy (2 Gy or 2.5 Gy in 15 fractions, respectively). PCI significantly reduced the brain relapse rate from 11 % to 0 % ($p = 0.001$).

Russell et al. [58] in a RTOG prospective randomized study randomized 187 NSCLC patients into groups receiving TRT alone or TRT plus PCI (30 Gy in ten fractions). This study included patients with inoperable or unresectable T1-4 N1-3M0 and resected T1-3 N2-3M0 non-epidermoid NSCLC. Manifestation of symptomatic BM was delayed in the PCI group, but the overall incidence of BM was not significantly decreased. Subgroup analysis revealed that in a small subgroup of patients with prior complete surgical resection, PCI reduced the incidence of BM from 25 % to 0 % ($p=0.06$). However, the results of this study should be considered with caution for the following reasons: first, the study population was highly heterogeneous regarding the T and N stage; second, systemic therapy was not used and locoregional therapy was ineffective compared with current standards; third, the median survival in this study was only 8 months due to ineffective therapy and relatively poor prognostic factors which may have prevented these patients from living long enough to develop BM; and finally, the ineffectiveness of locoregional therapy and lack of systemic therapy might have resulted in an increased incidence of locoregional and distant failures that served as sources of secondary seeding of the brain after delivery of PCI.

In the German multicenter randomized trial, Pöttgen et al. [27] enrolled 112 operable stage IIIA NSCLC patients to receive either primary resection followed by adjuvant TRT or preoperative chemotherapy followed by C-CRT and definitive surgery. Patients in the second group were also scheduled to receive PCI (30 Gy in 15 fractions). At the 5-year follow-up, PCI significantly reduced the incidence of BM as the first site of failure from 34.7 % to 7.8 % ($p=0.02$) and the overall brain relapse rate from 27.2 % to 9.1 % ($p=0.04$).

In general, the promising results of these randomized studies suggest a beneficial role for PCI in prevention of BM in NSCLC patients, especially those treated with multimodality aggressive treatment protocols. However, the vital question of whether the reduction in the rate of BM is associated with improved OS rates has not been answered yet. The RTOG-0214 phase III trial was built to address this question in stage IIIA/B NSCLC patients [62]. This study did not only investigate the effect of PCI on survival rates but also intended to focus on determining the impact of PCI on the incidence of BM, quality of life (QOL), and neurocognitive functions in more than 1,058 patients. However, the trial was closed earlier because of poor accrual with only 356 patients included, of which 340 were eligible for analysis. The survival times with and without PCI arms, namely, 1-year OS (75.6 % vs.76.9 %; $p=0.86$) and DFS (56.4 % vs. 51.2 %; $p=0.11$), were not different. The 1-year rates of BM were significantly different favoring the PCI arm over the non-PCI (7.7 % vs. 18.0 %; $p=0.004$). Patients in the observation arm were 2.52 times more likely to develop BM than those in the PCI arm (unadjusted OR=2.52). Therefore, the authors concluded the PCI in patients with stage III NSCLC without disease progression after therapy reduced the rates of BM but did not improve OS or DFS. Nevertheless, considering the fact that eligible 340 patients accounted only for 32 % of the targeted accrual, results of this benchmark study should be interpreted with caution and should not be perceived as decisive as it lacks the intended statistical power to demonstrate potentially present modest survival advantage with PCI.

The most recent randomized study of PCI in LA-NSCLC was reported by Li et al. [63]. The authors compared PCI against observation in resected stage IIIA NSCLC patients ($n=156$) and high risk of BM after adjuvant chemotherapy. Similar with the RTOG 0214, this study was also terminated earlier due to slow accrual. Patients in the PCI ($n=81$) arm received 30 Gy in ten fractions. The primary end point was DFS. The secondary end points included the incidence of BM, OS, toxicity, and QOL measures. The patients in the PCI group had significantly longer median DFS compared with the observation group (28.5 vs. 21.2 months; HR=0.67; $p=0.037$). The median 31.2 months of OS in the PCI arm was numerically superior than the 27.4 months in the observation arm but could not reach statistical significance (HR=0.81; $p=0.31$), respectively. PCI was associated with an actuarial 5-year decrease in the risk of BM (20.3 % vs. 49.9 %; HR=0.28; $p<0.001$).

Treatment Techniques

Standard PCI Technique and Doses

Several techniques can be utilized to irradiate whole brain content for the purpose of PCI. Regardless of the teletherapy machine and energy in use, patients are typically first fixed by the use of commercially available thermoplastic head masks to avoid unintentional motion and related target coverage or critical organ overdosage problems (Fig. 9.1). If tomographic check on-treatment opportunities are not available below, suggested steps should be followed, while simulation step may be avoided if such opportunities are readily available:

- Each patient must undergo simulation procedure prior to the start of PCI for accurate definition of the target borders and to avoid critical structures.
- Patients should lay supine with radiopaque markers placed at the lateral orbital canthi to assist in blocking the lenses from the therapy portal (Fig. 9.2a).
- The clinical target volume (CTV) must include the entire intracranial contents (Fig. 9.2b).

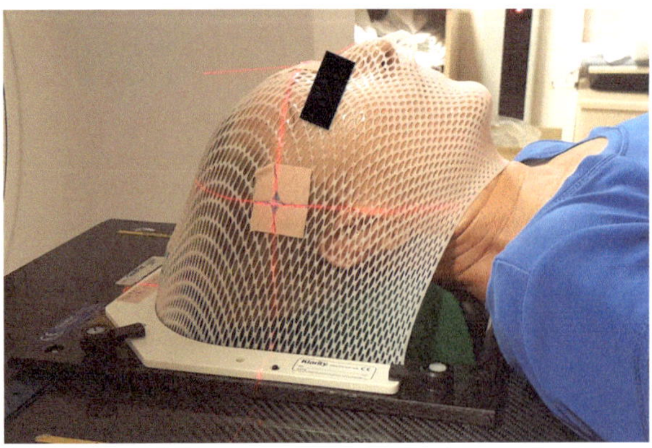

Fig. 9.1 Patient immobilization and positioning during imaging procedure with the use of commercially available head mask

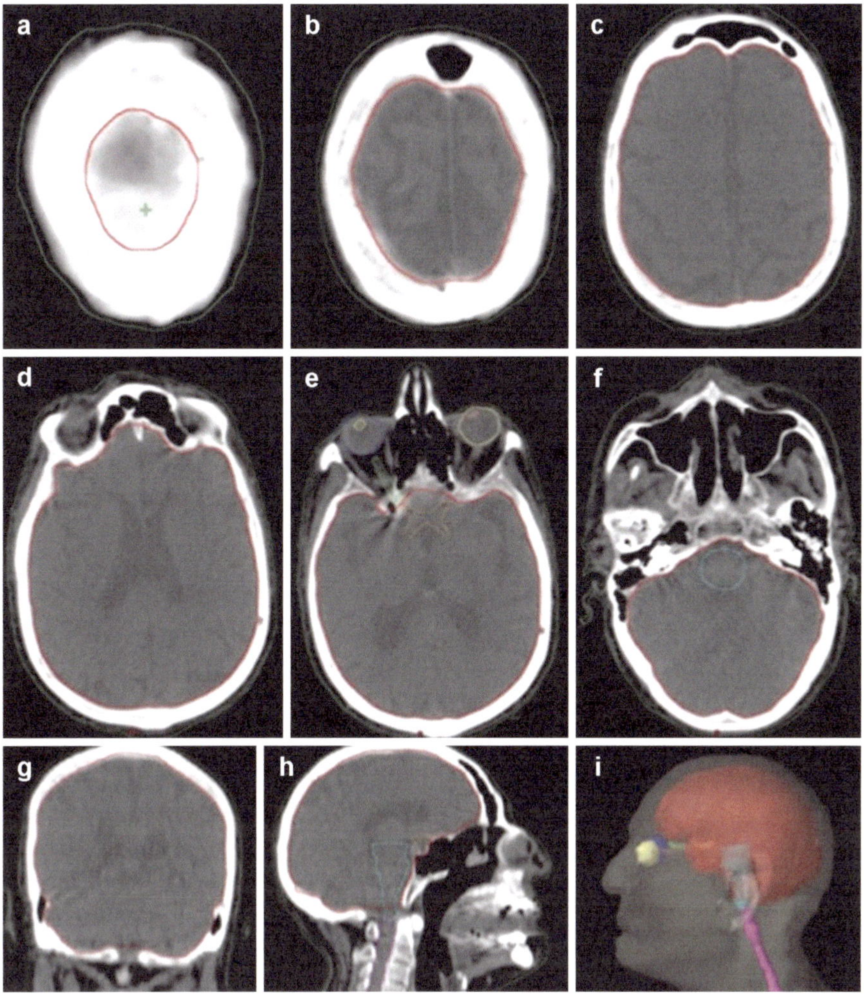

Fig. 9.2 (**a–i**) Contouring of target volumes and organs at risk and target volume shaping for a standard prophylactic cranial irradiation procedure: *CTV* clinical target volume, *PTV* planning target volume

- At least 1 cm margin at all directions around the bony skull, namely, superiorly, inferiorly, anteriorly, and posteriorly, should be given to delineate planning target volume (PTV) which is the target to receive the whole prescribed dose. The inferior border at the cervical vertebral bodies should be at the C1–C2 interspace (Fig. 9.2c).
- A small lead block or multileaf collimator is carefully placed to shield globes while still allowing adequate coverage of the anterior–inferior extents of the cranial contents (Fig. 9.2d).
- In contrast with tumors with high risk of cerebrospinal fluid seeding such as leukemias, lymphomas, and primitive neuroectodermal tumors, the significance

of involving the cribriform plate in the PTV is questionable, but the traditional approach recommends its adequate coverage inferiorly (Fig. 9.2e).

- Individually shaped ports with tailor-made lead blocks or multileaf collimators must be utilized to assist in defining the irradiation target volume (Fig. 9.2f).
- To avoid both the over- and underdosage of the particular parts of the intracranial contents, appropriate energy should have carefully been selected. A 6 MV photon energy will usually be satisfactory to overcome such problems in most cases.
- Wedge blocks must be used to achieve a homogenous dose distribution where necessitated. For this purpose, field-in-field (FIF) technique may also be utilized separately or in conjunction with wedge blocks.
- The PTV should be covered by no less than 95 % and no more than 107 % of the prescribed dose, and the dose to lens and globe should be kept as low as possible (Figs. 9.3 and 9.4).
- Either of 30 Gy in 2 Gy (15 days) or 25 Gy in 2.5 Gy (10 days) may be chosen for PCI of LS-SCLC, ES-SCLC, and LA-NSCLC patients. However, higher doses beyond these should be avoided because of the related increased risk of neurotoxicity in the absence of further reductions in BM emergence rates and even handicapped survival outcomes.

Novel Cranial Irradiation Techniques to Avoid Neurocognitive and Scalp Toxicity

Hippocampal Avoidance PCI

Long-term serious and permanent toxic effects of cranial irradiation, including cognitive deterioration and cerebellar dysfunction, have been described [64]. As many as 11 % of long-term (112 months) BM survivors treated with whole brain RT (WBRT) were suggested to develop dementia, especially with the use of higher-dose/fraction regimens [65]. Hippocampal dysfunction seems to be an important component of cognitive disturbances which are the hallmark of diffuse encephalopathy syndrome. Supporting this suggestion, recent studies have demonstrated that the functions of learning, memory, and spatial information processing are influenced by irradiation of the hippocampus. Abayomi [66] noted emergence of progressive severe deficits in hippocampal-dependent functions after WBRT. The mechanisms of chronic radiation damage involve the changes in exquisitely radiosensitive stem cells residing within the subgranular zone of the hippocampus. Changes in the microenvironment induced by radiation injury in combination with metabolic derangements, glial reactions, and inflammatory response force the remaining neuronal progenitor cells to adopt glial rather than neuronal fates. Irradiation of this area causes depletion of cells necessary for neurogenesis, especially for the memory domains [67]. Therefore, rationally, avoidance of the hippocampus during WBRT has been hypothesized to potentially delay and/or reduce the incidence and severity of neurocognitive deficits in survivors by selectively sparing the stem cells responsible for post-WBRT neurogenesis.

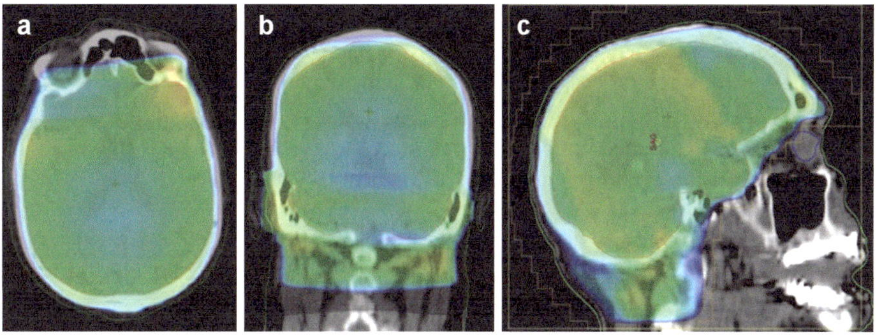

Fig. 9.3 Typical 3D conformal radiation therapy plan: (**a**) axial, (**b**) coronal, (**c**) sagittal view

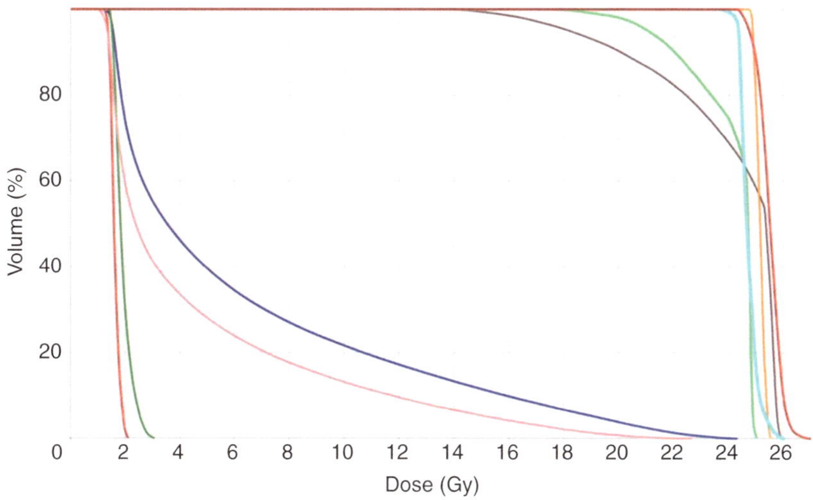

Structure	Min. dose (Gy)	Max. dose (Gy)	Mean dose (Gy)
CTV = Brain	23.76	28.09	25.50
Right Lens	1.36	3.11	1.89
Left Lens	1.22	2.13	1.60
Right Optic Nerve	16.79	25.08	24.05
Left Optic Nerve	13.00	25.95	24.01
Right Eye	1.13	24.32	6.20
Left Eye	0.95	22.67	4.56
Optic Chiasm	24.70	25.59	25.14
Brainstem	23.52	26.10	24.71

Fig. 9.4 Dose–volume histogram and related evaluation metrics table for a typical 3D conformal radiation therapy plan

Combination of advancements in preclinical and clinical evidence impacting the neurocognitive importance of hippocampi, the accurate anatomic definition and therefore delineation of hippocampi by the use of modern imaging techniques, and irradiation technology lead to rapid conduction of hippocampal avoidance studies in PCI or metastatic brain tumors. In the first study by Gutierrez et al. [68], the feasibility of composite tomotherapy to achieve homogenous whole brain dose distribution equivalent to conventional WBRT with conformal hippocampal avoidance was demonstrated, which was followed by others [69–73]. In one of the earliest studies, Gondi et al. demonstrated that the mean doses to the hippocampus could be reduced by 81–87 % to doses of 0.49–0.73 Gy with preserved target volume coverage and homogeneity by utilizing IMRT technique for PCI [69].

Comparison of the outcomes of two recently reported landmark WBRT studies may prove beneficial regarding the impact of hippocampal avoidance on neurocognitive functions and QOL measures [71, 74]. In the phase III RTOG 0214 study (discussed in detail in this chapter) where hippocampal sparing was not intended, the investigators focused on the impact of PCI on neurocognitive function (NCF) and QOL measures [74]. NCF was assessed with mini-mental status examination (MMSE), activities of daily living scale (ADLS), and Hopkins Verbal Learning Test (HVLT). QOL was assessed with the European Organisation for Research and Treatment of Cancer (EORTC) core tool (QOL Questionnaire-QLQC30) and brain module (QLQBN20). Although a trend for greater decline in patient-reported cognitive functioning with PCI was noted, no statistically significant differences were detected between the PCI and non-PCI arms at 1 year in any component of the EORTC-QLQC30 or QLQBN20 ($p>0.05$). Additionally, there were no significant differences in MMSE ($p=0.60$) or ADLS ($p=0.88$). Nevertheless, for HVLT, there was greater decline in immediate recall ($p=0.03$) and delayed recall ($p=0.008$) in the PCI arm at 1-year follow-up.

The RTOG 0933, reported by Gondi et al., was a single-arm phase II study of hippocampal avoidance WBRT for brain metastases with prespecified comparison with a historical control of patients treated with WBRT without hippocampal avoidance [71]. Eligible adult patients with established BM received hippocampal avoidance WBRT to 30 Gy in ten fractions. Standardized NCF and QOL assessments were performed at baseline and 2, 4, and 6 months. The primary end point was the Hopkins Verbal Learning Test–Revised Delayed Recall (HVLT-R DR) at 4 months. Of 113 patients accrued, 42 were analyzable at 4 months. Mean relative decline in HVLT-R DR from baseline to 4 months was 7.0 % which was significantly lower than the historical control of 30 % ($p<0.001$). No decline in QOL scores and grade 4–5 toxicities was reported in this study with a median OS of 6.8 months. Considering the only 4.5 % progression report in the hippocampal region with relatively excellent NCF preservation, compared to the historic controls and indirectly to RTOG 0214 patients, these outcomes strongly support the relatively safer use of HA-WBRT in the PCI or TCI settings.

Considering the fact that the contouring of hippocampus is problematic because of its difficult to demonstrate curved shape on 2D projections, we strongly recommend to use available atlases for accurate delineation of hippocampi, such as "Hippocampal Contouring: A Contouring Atlas for RTOG 0933" which can be accessed online via https://www.rtog.org/CoreLab/ContouringAtlases/HippocampalSparing.aspx and the

"A Radiation Oncologist's Guide to Contouring the Hippocampus" published by Chera et al. [75]. Typical contouring of hippocampi, related treatment plan with hippocampal avoidance PCI, and dose–volume histogram are as presented in Figs. 9.5, 9.6, and 9.7, respectively. In summary, to achieve the best plan, hippocampal avoidance regions must be generated by three-dimensionally expanding the hippocampal contours by 5 mm with ≤2-mm deviation per protocol, and the maximum dose to hippocampi must be kept ≤16 Gy with D100 % ≤9 Gy (Table 9.4).

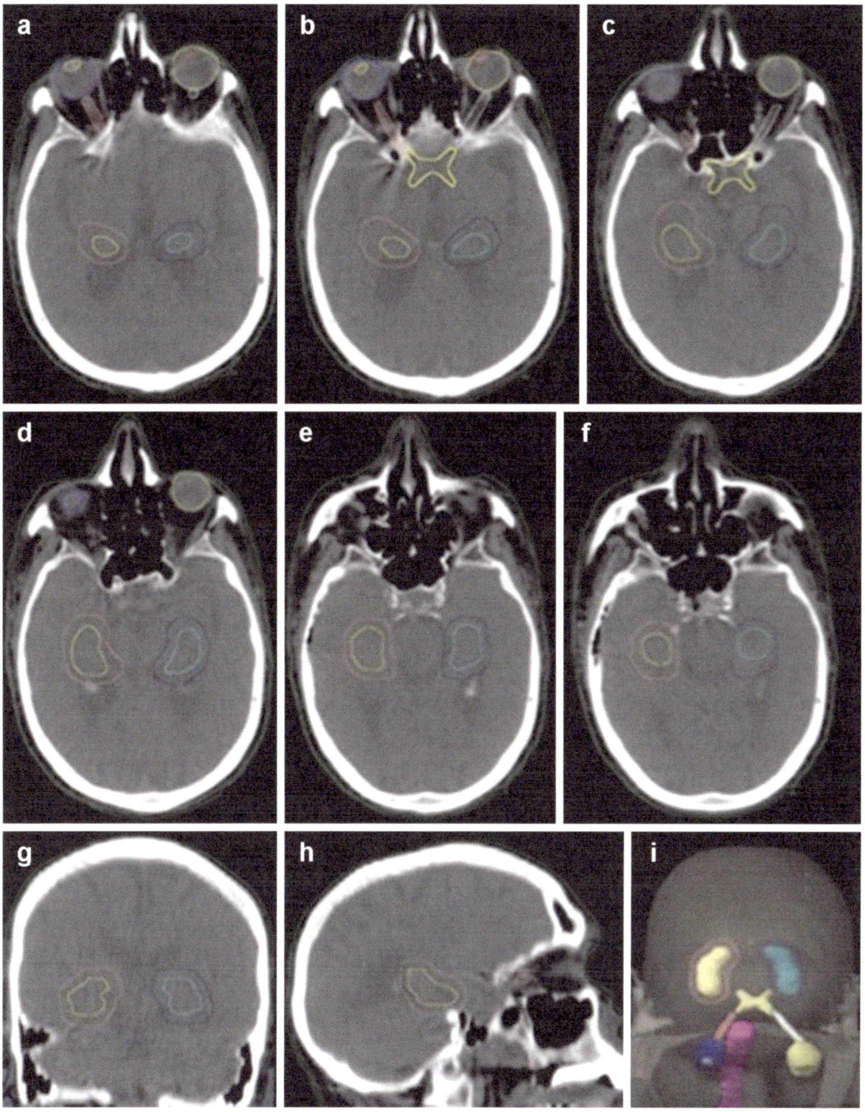

Fig. 9.5 (**a–i**) Contouring of hippocampi and its three-dimensional view

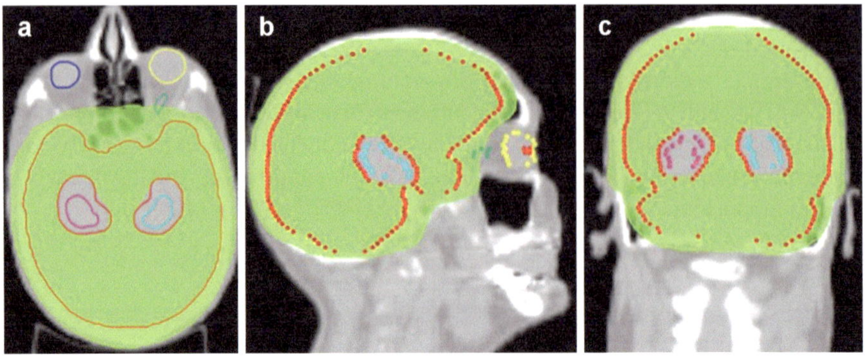

Fig. 9.6 Typical tomotherapy plan for hippocampal avoidance prophylactic cranial irradiation: (**a**) axial, (**b**) coronal, and (**c**) sagittal view

Scalp-Sparing PCI

Novel irradiation techniques may also better spare the scalp without any detriment on tumor control or prophylactic actions of therapeutic WBRT or PCI, respectively. Such a maneuver may prevent permanent hair loss, which significantly decreases QOL of both female and male cancer patients. Roberge et al. demonstrated the possibility to reduce scalp doses with IMRT. The authors validated their scalp-sparing WBRT plans with thermoluminescent dosimetry and showed that the median dose to the scalp can be reduced by nearly 40 % without affecting target volume doses [76]. These results were later confirmed by Kao et al. [77]. The author reported that, compared to conventional WBRT, IMRT WBRT reduced the mean scalp dose from 26.2 to 16.4 Gy ($p<0.001$). Using Olsen hair loss score criteria, 4 of 15 (26.7 %) assessable patients preserved at least 50 % of hair coverage at 1–3 months after treatment, while 6 (40 %) patients preserved between 25 % and 50 % hair coverage. These results suggest that although scalp-sparing WBRT may not effectively prevent transient alopecia in most of the treated patients, it may be of benefit for those with a priori risk factors for increased alopecia, such as previous or concomitant chemotherapy.

For scalp-sparing PCI, the CTV must be defined and delineated as the contents of the cranium bordered by the internal table of the skull. The hair-bearing skin volume should be defined as a 5-mm outer rind of soft tissue within the confines of the marked hairline and contoured accordingly [76]. Alternatively, as demonstrated in Fig. 9.8, the scalp contour can be defined as the skin + 3-mm depth from the level of the canthi to the vertex [77]. For a typical PCI plan, the eyes and lens must be contoured as critical structures. PTV should be created by adding a 2-mm generous margin around the CTV at all directions (Fig. 9.8). For an acceptable scalp-sparing PCI plan, the dose to the scalp must be kept <18 Gy, while the maximum eye and lens doses must be limited at 7 Gy and 5 Gy, respectively (Figs. 9.9 and 9.10).

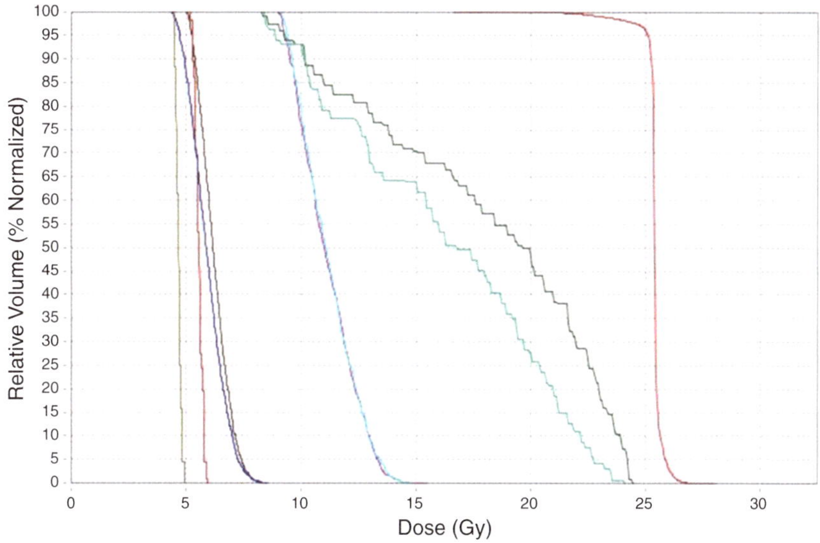

Structure	Min. dose (Gy)	Max. dose (Gy)	Mean dose (Gy)
CTV = Brain	22.8	27.98	25.41
Right Lens	4.37	4.94	4.65
Left Lens	5.14	5.91	5.51
Right Optic Nerve	8.30	24.43	19.71
Left Optic Nerve	8.42	24.11	16.59
Right Eye	4.37	8.55	5.86
Left Eye	4.97	8.38	6.16
Right Hippocampus	9.01	15.45	11.04
Left Hippocampus	9.10	14.72	11.11

Fig. 9.7 Dose–volume histogram and related evaluation metrics table for a typical tomotherapy plan for hippocampal avoidance prophylactic cranial irradiation

Table 9.4 Hippocampal avoidance PCI plan compliance criteria

Protocol compliance	Hippocampal contouring	Hippocampal dose	PTV
Best protocol fit	≤2-mm deviation	D100 % ≤9 Gy	D2 % ≤31 Gy
		Maximum dose ≤16 Gy	D98 % ≥21 Gy
Variation acceptable	2–7-mm deviation	D100 %: 9–10 Gy	D2 % >31 but ≤33 Gy
		Maximum dose 16–17 Gy	D98 % <21 Gy
Deviation unacceptable	>7-mm deviation	D100 % >10 Gy	V_{25} <90 %
		Maximum dose >17 Gy	D2 % >33 Gy

DX% dose received by the X% volume, *V25* volume receiving 25 Gy, *PCI* prophylactic cranial irradiation, *PTV* planning target volume

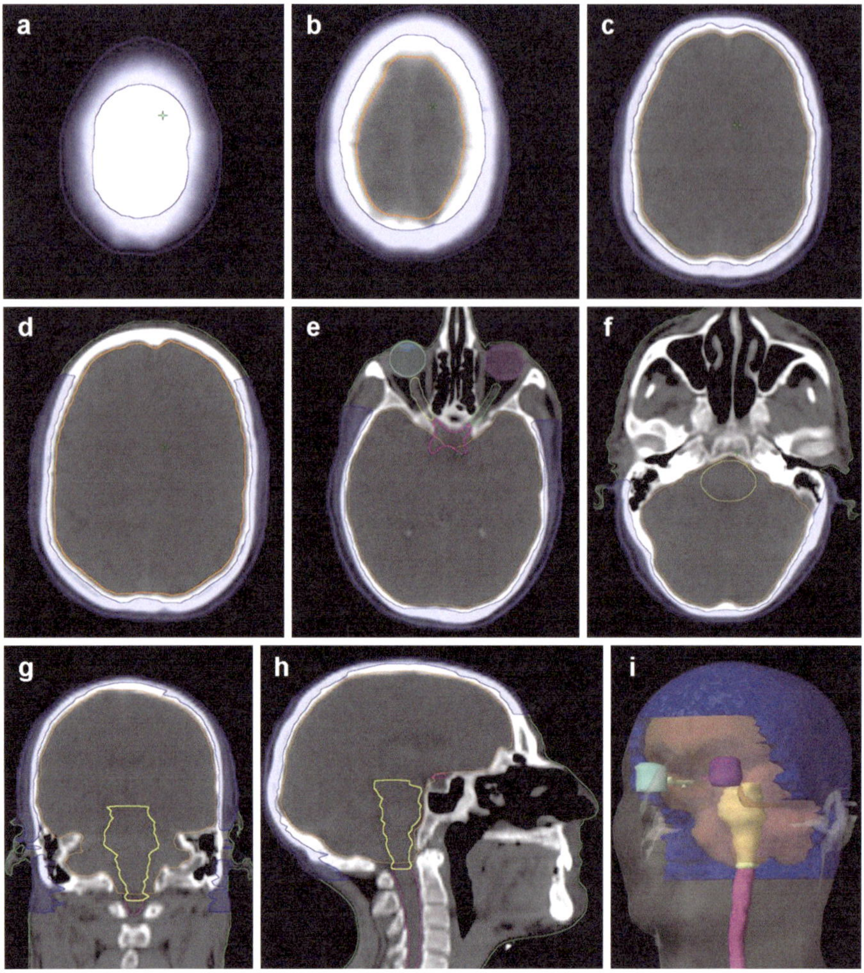

Fig. 9.8 (**a**–**i**) Contouring scalp and other organs at risk for a typical scalp-sparing prophylactic cranial irradiation procedure

Key Points on PCI-Related Toxicity Assessment

The incidence of PCI-related toxicities is likely dependent on certain risk factors already present before onset of PCI, including the patient's age, preceding or concomitant chemotherapy, and other putative risk factors that are to date not exactly defined such as smoking, diabetes mellitus, radiation hypersensitivity syndromes, hypothalamo–hypophyseal abnormalities, and/or atherosclerosis. Because many of the classical PCI toxicity data are derived from SCLC patients those primarily treated with chemotherapy which is followed by PCI, caution is advised when diagnosing PCI toxicity. The influence of chemotherapy on cognitive functions of many cancer patients remained underestimated for a long time [78]. The phenomenon has been termed "chemo-fog" or "chemo brain" to reflect

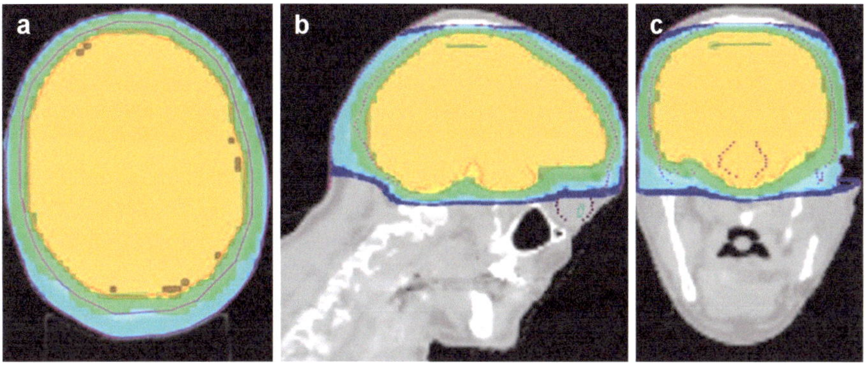

Fig. 9.9 Typical tomotherapy plan for scalp-sparing prophylactic cranial irradiation: (**a**) axial, (**b**) coronal, and (**c**) sagittal view

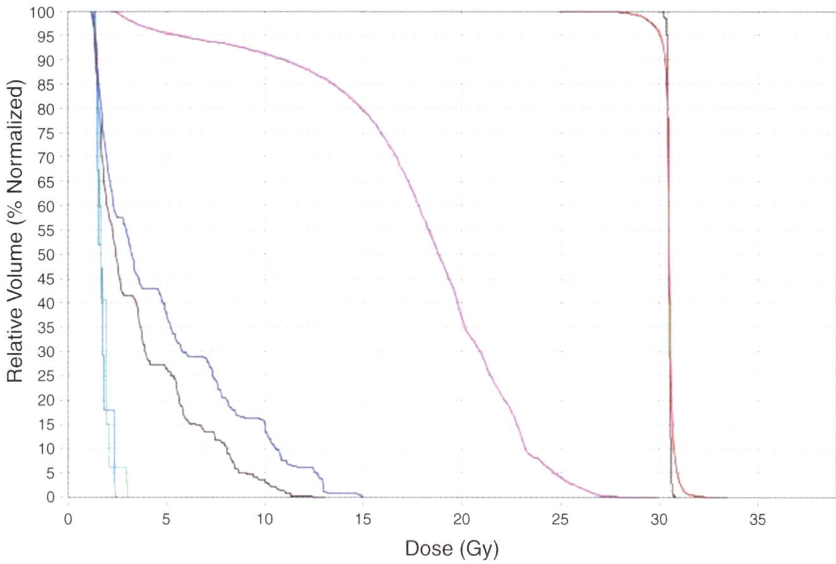

Structure	Min. dose (Gy)	Max. dose (Gy)	Mean dose (Gy)
CTV = Brain	23.40	28.33	25.51
Right Lens	1.03	1.68	1.26
Left Lens	1.09	2.34	1.29
Scalp	1.77	25.05	15.69
Right Eye	0.93	6.49	1.74
Left Eye	0.97	8.93	2.43
Optic Chiasm	25.38	25.57	25.47
Brainstem	25.10	26.16	25.48

Fig. 9.10 Dose–volume histogram and related evaluation metrics table for a typical tomotherapy plan for scalp-sparing prophylactic cranial irradiation

the fact that the symptoms of the cognitive dysfunction are usually mild to moderate and generally not global, i.e., specific domains of cognition are affected, such as attention, concentration, speed of information processing, verbal and visual memory, multitasking, and ability to organize information [78–81]. However, these deficits undoubtedly have negative impacts on the patients' QOL [82]. Therefore, as the side effects evoked by cranial irradiation are largely similar, it is not surprising that the effects were rather attributed to the radiation than to chemotherapy. However, already more than a decade ago, it has been noted that patients receiving standard-dose adjuvant chemotherapy for breast cancer exhibit decreased cognitive memory and language functions as compared to matched control groups [83]. This data is of paramount importance for radiation oncologists considering the fact that almost all toxicities following therapeutic WBRT or PCI are almost invariably attributed to cranial irradiation by the other oncologic disciplines.

In a key notifying prospective study by Komaki et al., SCLC patients who finished combination chemotherapy and TRT were asked to perform neuropsychological tests just before inception and completion of PCI [84]. The authors noticed that roughly half of patients had neurocognitive shortages before PCI and observed a somewhat noteworthy decay in executive function and language after 1 year which turned inconsequential in later assessments. This study underlines the importance of implementation of neurocognitive function tests prior to WBRT in order to reflect the actual impact of therapeutic WBRT or PCI following treatment. To further underline the fact, it is important to remind that currently chemotherapy alone is accepted to induce white matter changes particularly in the frontal, parietal, and occipital lobes, which is consistent with the notion of chemotherapy-related axonal degeneration and demyelination. Additionally, it has been confirmed that chemotherapy-related intellectual shortfalls endure for over 10 years, which can overlay most (if not all) PCI-incited toxicities.

Conclusion

PCI should be recommended for all medically fit LS- and ES-SCLC patients with any objective response to primary therapy, including the disease stabilization, in order to reduce BM incidence rates and to prolong OS times. Although it is difficult to conclude in a solid manner regarding the available data which suggests significant reductions in BM incidence rates with PCI but with no established survival benefit, it appears that there is insufficient evidence to support routine use of PCI in LA-NSCLC patients. However, considering the fact that results of retrospective analyses and necropsies have revealed that roughly 50 % of non-SCC patients will experience BM, it appears mandatory to identify the subgroup of patients with higher BM risk who may potentially benefit from PCI. On the way to find a subgroup, it is important to mention that tumor size and lymph node status are the key determinants for assessing the risk of BM in NSCLC. In this regard, a recent analysis by Ding et al. revealed that nearly 60 % of patients with NSCLC stage IIIA-N2 developed BM within 5 years if more than 30 % of all excised lymph nodes were involved, which decreased to 30 % if less than 30 % were affected [85]. Therefore, studies involving high-risk patients are needed in order to reliably comment on the issue of PCI in LA-NSCLC patients.

References

1. Hardy J, Smith I, Cherryman G, et al. The value of computed tomographic (CT) scan surveillance in the detection and management of brain metastases in patients with small cell lung cancer. Br J Cancer. 1990;62:684–6.
2. Yang GY, Matthews RH. Prophylactic cranial irradiation in small-cell lung cancer. Oncologist. 2000;5(4):293–8.
3. van Oosterhout AG, van de Pol M, ten Velde GP, Twijnstra A. Neurologic disorders in 203 consecutive patients with small cell lung cancer. Results of a longitudinal study. Cancer. 1996;77:1434–41.
4. Viani GA, Boin AC, Ikeda VY, et al. Thirty years of prophylactic cranial irradiation in patients with small cell lung cancer: a meta-analysis of randomized clinical trials. J Bras Pneumol. 2012;38(3):372–81.
5. Hirsch FR, Paulson OB, Hansen HH, et al. Intracranial metastases in small cell carcinoma of the lung. Cancer. 1982;50:2433–7.
6. Felletti R, Souhami RL, Spiro SG, et al. Social consequences of brain or liver relapse in small cell carcinoma of the bronchus. Radiother Oncol. 1985;4(4):335–9.
7. Carmichael J, Crane JM, Bunn PA, Glatstein E, Ihde DC. Results of therapeutic cranial irradiation in small cell lung cancer. Int J Radiat Oncol Biol Phys. 1988;14(3):455–9.
8. Postmus PE, Haaxma-Reiche H, Sleijfer DT, et al. High dose etoposide for brain metastases of small cell lung cancer. A phase II study. The EORTC Lung Cancer Cooperative Group. Br J Cancer. 1989;59(2):254–6.
9. Arriagada R, Le Chevalier T, Borie F, et al. Prophylactic cranial irradiation for patients with small-cell lung cancer in complete remission. J Natl Cancer Inst. 1995;87:183–90.
10. Gregor A, Cull A, Stephens RJ, et al. Prophylactic cranial irradiation is indicated following complete response to induction therapy in small cell lung cancer: results of a multicentre randomised trial. United Kingdom Coordinating Committee for Cancer Research (UKCCCR) and the European Organization for Research and Treatment of Cancer (EORTC). Eur J Cancer. 1997;33:1752–8.
11. Auperin A, Arriagada R, Pignon JP, et al. Prophylactic cranial irradiation for patients with small-cell lung cancer in complete remission. Prophylactic Cranial Irradiation Overview Collaborative Group. N Engl J Med. 1999;341:476–84.
12. Patel S, Macdonald OK, Suntharalingam M. Evaluation of the use of prophylactic cranial irradiation in small cell lung cancer. Cancer. 2009;115(4):842–50.
13. Slotman B, Faivre-Finn C, Kramer G, et al. Prophylactic cranial irradiation in extensive small-cell lung cancer. N Engl J Med. 2007;357(7):664–72.
14. Zhang W, Jiang W, Luan L, et al. Prophylactic cranial irradiation for patients with small-cell lung cancer: a systematic review of the literature with meta-analysis. BMC Cancer. 2014;14:793.
15. Le Péchoux C, Dunant A, Senan S, et al. Standard-dose versus higher-dose prophylactic cranial irradiation (PCI) in patients with limited-stage small-cell lung cancer in complete remission after chemotherapy and thoracic radiotherapy (PCI 99-01, EORTC 22003-08004, RTOG 0212, and IFCT 99-01): a randomised clinical trial. Lancet Oncol. 2009;10(5):467–74.
16. Eaton BR, Kim S, Marcus DM, et al. Effect of prophylactic cranial irradiation on survival in elderly patients with limited-stage small cell lung cancer. Cancer. 2013;119(21):3753–60.
17. Rule WG, Foster NR, Meyers JP, et al. Prophylactic cranial irradiation in elderly patients with small cell lung cancer: findings from a North Central Cancer Treatment Group pooled analysis. J Geriatr Oncol. 2015;6(2):119–26.

18. Furuse K, Fukuoka M, Kawahara M, et al. Phase III study of concurrent versus sequential thoracic radiotherapy in combination with mitomycin, vindesine, and cisplatin in unresectable stage III non-small-cell lung cancer. J Clin Oncol. 1999;17:2692–9.
19. Curran Jr WJ, Paulus R, Langer CJ, et al. Sequential vs. concurrent chemoradiation for stage III non-small cell lung cancer: randomized phase III trial RTOG 9410. J Natl Cancer Inst. 2011;103(19):1452–60.
20. Choi NC, Carey RW, Daly W, et al. Potential impact on survival of improved tumor downstaging and resection rate by preoperative twice-daily radiation and concurrent chemotherapy in stage IIIA non-small cell lung cancer. J Clin Oncol. 1997;15:712–22.
21. Eberhardt W, Wilke H, Stuschke M, et al. Preoperative chemotherapy followed by concurrent chemoradiation therapy based on hyperfractionated accelerated radiation therapy and definitive surgery in locally advanced non-small-cell lung cancer: mature results of a phase II trial. J Clin Oncol. 1998;16:622–34.
22. Albain KS, Rusch VW, Crowley JJ, et al. Concurrent cisplatin/etoposide plus chest radiotherapy followed by surgery for stages IIIA (N2) and IIIB non-small-cell lung cancer: mature results of Southwest Oncology Group phase II study 8805. J Clin Oncol. 1995;13:1880–92.
23. Komaki R, Scott CB, Byhardt R, et al. Failure patterns by prognostic group determined by recursive partitioning analysis (RPA) of 1547 patients on four Radiation Therapy Oncology Group (RTOG) studies in inoperable non-small-cell lung cancer. Int J Radiat Oncol Biol Phys. 1998;42:263–7.
24. Strauss GM, Herndon JE, Sherman DD, et al. Neoadjuvant chemotherapy and radiotherapy followed by surgery in stage IIIA non-small cell carcinoma of the lung: report of a Cancer and Leukemia Group B phase II study. J Clin Oncol. 1992;10:1237–44.
25. Cox JD, Scott CB, Byhardt RW, et al. Addition of chemotherapy to radiation therapy alters failure patterns by cell type within non-small cell carcinoma of lung (NSCCL): analysis of Radiation Therapy Oncology Group (RTOG) trials. Int J Radiat Oncol Biol Phys. 1999;43:505–9.
26. Andre F, Grunenwald D, Pujol JL, et al. Patterns of relapse of N2 non-small-cell lung carcinoma patients treated with preoperative chemotherapy: should prophylactic cranial irradiation be reconsidered? Cancer. 2001;91:2394–400.
27. Pöttgen C, Eberhardt W, Grannass A, et al. Prophylactic cranial irradiation in operable stage IIIA non-small-cell lung cancer treated with neoadjuvant chemoradiotherapy: results from a German multicenter trial. J Clin Oncol. 2007;25:4987–92.
28. Robnett TJ, Machtay M, Stevenson JP, Algazy KM, Hahn SM. Factors affecting the risk of brain metastases after definitive chemoradiation for locally advanced non-small-cell lung carcinoma. J Clin Oncol. 2001;19:1344–9.
29. Law A, Karp DD, Dipetrillo T, Daly BT. Emergence of increased cerebral metastasis after high-dose preoperative radiotherapy with chemotherapy in patients with locally advanced non-small cell lung carcinoma. Cancer. 2001;92:160–4.
30. Ceresoli GL, Reni M, Chiesa G, et al. Brain metastases in locally advanced non-small cell lung carcinoma after multimodality treatment: risk factors analysis. Cancer. 2002;95:605–12.
31. Gaspar LE, Chansky K, Albain KS, et al. Time from treatment to subsequent diagnosis of brain metastasis in stage III non-small-cell lung cancer. A retrospective review by the Southwest Oncology Group. J Clin Oncol. 2005;23:2955–61.
32. Mamon HJ, Yeap BY, Janne PA, et al. High risk of brain metastases in surgically staged IIIA non-small-cell lung cancer patients treated with surgery, chemotherapy, and radiation. J Clin Oncol. 2005;23:1530–7.
33. Schouten LJ, Rutten J, Huveneers HA, Twinjstra A. Incidence of brain metastases in a cohort of patients with carcinoma of the breast, colon, kidney, and lung and melanoma. Cancer. 2002;94:2698–705.
34. Carolan H, Sun AY, Bezjak A, et al. Does the incidence and outcome of brain metastases in locally advanced non-small cell lung cancer justify prophylactic cranial irradiation or early detection? Lung Cancer. 2005;49:109–15.

35. Bajard A, Westeel V, Dubiez A, et al. Multivariate analysis of factors predictive of brain metastases in localised non-small cell lung carcinoma. Lung Cancer. 2004;45:317–23.
36. Keith B, Vincent M, Stitt L, et al. Subsets more likely to benefit from surgery or prophylactic cranial irradiation after chemoradiation for localized non-small cell lung cancer. Am J Clin Oncol. 2002;25:583–7.
37. Jacobs RH, Awan A, Bitran JD, et al. Prophylactic cranial irradiation in adenocarcinoma of the lung: a possible role. Cancer. 1987;59:2016–9.
38. Tang SG, Lin FJ, Leung VM. Impact of cranial irradiation in adenocarcinoma of the lung. J Formos Med Assoc. 1993;92:413–9.
39. Milleron B, Guigay J, Rugeri L, et al. Le bilan d'extension des adenocarcinomes bronchiques doit-il differer de celui des autres cancers bronchiques non a petites cellulies? Rev Pneumol Clin. 1992;48:159–62.
40. Salbeck R, Grau HC, Artmann H. Cerebral tumor staging in patients with bronchial carcinoma by computed tomography. Cancer. 1990;66:2007–11.
41. Salvatierra A, Bahamonde C, Llamas J, Cruz F, Lopez-Pujol J. Extrathoracic staging of bronchogenic carcinoma. Chest. 1990;97:1052–8.
42. Ji Z, Bi N, Wang J, et al. Risk factors for brain metastases in locally advanced non-small cell lung cancer with definitive chest radiation. Int J Radiat Oncol Biol Phys. 2014;89(2):330–7.
43. Arriagada R, Le Chevalier T, Quiox E, et al. ASTRO plenary. Effect of chemotherapy on locally advanced non-small cell lung carcinoma: a randomized study on 353 patients. GETCB (Groupe d'Etude et Traitement des Cancers Bronchiques), FNCLCC (Féderation Nationale des Centres de Lutte contre le Cancer) and the CEBI trialists. Int J Radiat Oncol Biol Phys. 1991;20:1183–90.
44. Non Small Cell Lung Cancer Collaborative Group: Chemotherapy in non-small cell lung cancer: a meta-analysis using updated individual patient data from 52 randomised clinical trials. BMJ. 1995;311:899–909.
45. Kumar P, Herndon II J, Langer M, et al. Patterns of disease failure after trimodality therapy of non small cell lung carcinoma pathologic stage IIIa (N2). Analysis of Cancer and Leukemia Group B Protocol 8935. Cancer. 1996;77:2393–9.
46. Stuschke M, Eberhardt W, Pottgen C, et al. Prophylactic cranial irradiation in locally advanced non-small-cell lung cancer after multimodality treatment: long-term follow-up and investigations of late neuropsychologic effects. J Clin Oncol. 1999;17:2700–9.
47. Douillard JY, Rosell R, De Lena M, et al. Impact of postoperative radiation therapy on survival in patients with complete resection and stage I, II, or IIIA non-small-cell lung cancer treated with adjuvant chemotherapy: the Adjuvant Navelbine International Trialist Association (ANITA) randomized trial. Int J Radiat Oncol Biol Phys. 2008;72:695–701.
48. The International Lung Cancer Trial Collaborative Group. Cisplatin-based adjuvant chemotherapy in patients with completely resected non-small-cell lung cancer. N Engl J Med. 2004;350:351–60.
49. Postmus PE, Smit EF. Chemotherapy for brain metastases of lung cancer. A review. Ann Oncol. 1999;10:753–9.
50. Abrey LE, Olson JD, Raizer JJ, et al. A phase II trial of temozolamide for patients with recurrent or progressive brain metastases. J Neurooncol. 2001;53:259–65.
51. Schutte W, Manegold C, Von Pawl JV, et al. Topotecan: a new treatment option in the therapy of brain metastases of lung cancer. Front Radiat Ther Oncol. 1999;33:354–63.
52. Griffin BR, Livingston RB, Stewart GR, et al. Prophylactic cranial irradiation for limited non-small cell lung cancer. Cancer. 1988;62:36–9.
53. Rusch VW, Griffin BR, Liv Rusch VW, Griffin BR, Livingston RB. The role of prophylactic cranial irradiation in regionally advanced non-small cell lung cancer. A Southwest Oncology Group Study. J Thorac Cardiovasc Surg. 1989;98:535–9.
54. Skarin A, Jochelson M, Sheldon T, et al. Neoadjuvant chemotherapy in marginally resectable stage III M0 non-small cell lung cancer: long-term follow-up in 41 patients. J Surg Oncol. 1989;40:266–74.

55. Park HS, Decker RH, Wilson LD, Yu JB. Prophylactic cranial irradiation for patients with locally advanced non-small-cell lung cancer at high risk for brain metastases. Clin Lung Cancer. 2015;16(4):292–7.
56. Xie SS, Li M, Zhou CC, Song XL, Wang CH. Prophylactic cranial irradiation may impose a detrimental effect on overall survival of patients with nonsmall cell lung cancer: a systematic review and meta-analysis. PLoS One. 2014;9(7):e103431.
57. Topkan E, Parlak C, Kotek A, et al. Impact of prophylactic cranial irradiation timing on brain relapse rates in patients with stage IIIB non-small-cell lung carcinoma treated with two different chemoradiotherapy regimens. Int J Radiat Oncol Biol Phys. 2012;83(4):1264–71.
58. Russell AH, Pajak TE, Selim HM, et al. Prophylactic cranial irradiation for lung cancer patients at high risk for development of cerebral metastasis: results of a prospective randomized trial conducted by the Radiation Therapy Oncology Group. Int J Radiat Oncol Biol Phys. 1991;21:637–43.
59. Umsawasdi T, Valdivieso M, Chen TT, et al. Role of elective brain irradiation during combined chemoradiotherapy for limited disease non-small cell lung cancer. J Neurooncol. 1984;2:253–9.
60. Cox JD, Stanley K, Petrovich Z, Paig C, Yesner R. Cranial irradiation in cancer of the lung of all cell types. JAMA. 1981;245:469–72.
61. Mira JG, Miller TP, Crowley JJ. Chest irradiation vs. chest irradiation plus chemotherapy with or without cranial prophylactic brain radiotherapy in localized non small cell lung cancer. A South West Oncology Group randomized study. Int J Radiat Oncol Biol Phys. 1990;19:145.
62. Gore EM, Bae K, Wong SJ, et al. Phase III comparison of prophylactic cranial irradiation versus observation in patients with locally advanced non-small-cell lung cancer: primary analysis of radiation therapy oncology group study RTOG 0214. J Clin Oncol. 2011;29(3):272–8.
63. Li N, Zeng ZF, Wang SY, et al. Randomized phase III trial of prophylactic cranial irradiation versus observation in patients with fully resected stage IIIA-N2 nonsmall-cell lung cancer and high risk of cerebral metastases after adjuvant chemotherapy. Ann Oncol. 2015;26(3):504–9.
64. Roman DD, Sperduto PW. Neuropsychological effects of cranial radiation: current knowledge and future directions. Int J Radiat Oncol Biol Phys. 1995;31:983–98.
65. De Angelis LM, Delattre JY, Posner JB. Radiation-induced dementia in patients cured of brain metastases. Neurology. 1989;39:789–96.
66. Abayomi OK. Pathogenesis of irradiation induced cognitive dysfunction. Acta Oncol. 1996;35:659–63.
67. Monje ML, Mizumatsu S, Fike JR. Irradiation induces neural precursor-cell dysfunction. Nat Med. 2002;8:955–62.
68. Gutierrez AN, Westerly DC, Tome WA, et al. Whole brain radiotherapy with hippocampal avoidance and simultaneously integrated brain metastases boost: a planning study. Int J Radiat Oncol Biol Phys. 2007;69:589–97.
69. Gondi V, Tolakanahalli R, Mehta MP, et al. Hippocampal-sparing whole-brain radiotherapy: a "how-to" technique using helical tomotherapy and linear accelerator-based intensity-modulated radiotherapy. Int J Radiat Oncol Biol Phys. 2010;78(4):1244–52.
70. Suh JH. Hippocampal-avoidance whole-brain radiation therapy: a new standard for patients with brain metastases? J Clin Oncol. 2014;32(34):3789–91.
71. Gondi V, Pugh SL, Tome WA, et al. Preservation of memory with conformal avoidance of the hippocampal neural stem-cell compartment during whole-brain radiotherapy for brain metastases (RTOG 0933): a phase II multi-institutional trial. J Clin Oncol. 2014; 32(34):3810–6.
72. Oehlke O, Wucherpfennig D, Fels F, et al. Whole brain irradiation with hippocampal sparing and dose escalation on multiple brain metastases: local tumour control and survival. Strahlenther Onkol. 2015;191(6):461–9.
73. Kundapur V, Ellchuk T, Ahmed S, Gondi V. Risk of hippocampal metastases in small cell lung cancer patients at presentation and after cranial irradiation: a safety profile study for

hippocampal sparing during prophylactic or therapeutic cranial irradiation. Int J Radiat Oncol Biol Phys. 2015;91(4):781–6.
74. Sun A, Bae K, Gore EM, et al. Phase III trial of prophylactic cranial irradiation compared with observation in patients with locally advanced non-small-cell lung cancer: neurocognitive and quality-of-life analysis. J Clin Oncol. 2011;29(3):279–86.
75. Chera BS, Amdur RJ, Patel P, Mendenhall WM. A radiation oncologist's guide to contouring the hippocampus. Am J Clin Oncol. 2009;32(1):20–2.
76. Roberge D, Parker W, Niazi TM, Olivares M. Treating the contents and not the container: dosimetric study of hair-sparing whole brain intensity modulated radiation therapy. Technol Cancer Res Treat. 2005;4(5):567–70.
77. Kao J, Darakchiev B, Conboy L, et al. Tumor directed, scalp sparing intensity modulated whole brain radiotherapy for brain metastases. Technol Cancer Res Treat. 2015;14(5): 547–55.
78. Vardy J, Tannock I. Cognitive function after chemotherapy in adults with solid tumours. Crit Rev Oncol Hematol. 2007;63(3):183–202.
79. van Dam FS, Schagen SB, Muller MJ, et al. Impairment of cognitive function in women receiving adjuvant treatment for high-risk breast cancer: high-dose versus standard-dose chemotherapy. J Natl Cancer Inst. 1998;90(3):210–8.
80. Schagen SB, van Dam FS, Muller MJ, et al. Cognitive deficits after postoperative adjuvant chemotherapy for breast carcinoma. Cancer. 1999;85(3):640–50.
81. Brezden CB, Phillips KA, Abdolell M, Bunston T, Tannock IF. Cognitive function in breast cancer patients receiving adjuvant chemotherapy. J Clin Oncol. 2000;18(14):2695–701.
82. Ganz PA, Desmond KA, Leedham B, et al. Quality of life in long-term, disease-free survivors of breast cancer: a follow-up study. J Natl Cancer Inst. 2002;94(1):39–49.
83. Wefel JS, Lenzi R, Theriault RL, Davis RN, Meyers CA. The cognitive sequelae of standard-dose adjuvant chemotherapy in women with breast carcinoma: results of a prospective, randomized, longitudinal trial. Cancer. 2004;100(11):2292–9.
84. Komaki R, Meyers CA, Shin DM, et al. Evaluation of cognitive function in patients with limited small cell lung cancer prior to and shortly following prophylactic cranial irradiation. Int J Radiat Oncol Biol Phys. 1995;33(1):179–82.
85. Ding X, Dai H, Hui Z, et al. Risk factors of brain metastases in completely resected pathological stage IIIA-N2 non-small cell lung cancer. Radiat Oncol. 2012;7:119.

Systemic Therapy for Lung Cancer

10

Nil Molinas Mandel

Non-small Cell Lung Cancer (NSCLC)

Early Stage Non-small Cell Lung Cancer

Adjuvant Therapy for Resected NSCLC

Lung cancer is one of the leading causes of cancer-related mortality in industrialized countries. In appropriate patients, surgery is the primary treatment modality for early stage (stage IA–IIB) NSCLC. However, only 20–25 % of patients with NSCLC are candidates for surgery at initial presentation. Stereotactic radiotherapy, if especially the lesion(s) is (are) small, is a treatment option to those patients who have contraindications (e.g., medical comorbidities) for a curative surgery. Unfortunately, more than half of the patients treated with local therapies recur within the first two years, either as a local relapse or systemic metastases. Five-year survival for stage I, II, and IIIA diseases is 60–70 %, 40–50 %, and 15–30 %, respectively (Table 10.1). Meaning that even more than one-third of patients with stage I disease are lost within 5 years due to systemic recurrence [1–4]. Despite the improvements of survival with therapies directed for a relapsed disease, in most cases, eradication of relapsed NSCLC is impossible. Therefore an adjuvant systemic chemotherapy is recommended to curatively resected NSCLC patients with certain characteristics hoping to eradicate the microscopic metastases present initially.

Chemotherapy, so-called adjuvant, has become the standard of care after curative resection of early stage breast or colon cancers. This treatment has a goal to prolong the disease free as well as the overall survival of the patients. The absolute benefit

N. Molinas Mandel, MD
Department of Medical Oncology, American Hospital, Istanbul, Turkey

Department of Medical Oncology, Koc University Hospital,
Davutpasa Caddesi, No: 4, Topkapi, Istanbul 34010, Turkey
e-mail: nmmandel@gmail.com

G. Ozyigit et al. (eds.), *Principles and Practice of Radiotherapy Techniques in Thoracic Malignancies*, DOI 10.1007/978-3-319-28761-4_10

Table 10.1 Five-year survival of NSCLC according to pathological stage

Pathological stage	Five-year survival (%)
IA	73
IB	58
IIA	46
IIB	36
IIIA	24
IIIB	9

of adjuvant chemotherapy is 5 % within 10 years, which seems a small but a statistically significant effect. Adjuvant chemotherapy strategy is also applicable for colon, gastric, and ovarian cancers.

The first meta-analysis regarding the effect of adjuvant chemotherapy in lung cancer was published in 1995, which examined the data of 52 randomized clinical trials [5]. In this meta-analysis, eight randomized trials that assessed the effect of cisplatin-based combination therapies showed a 5 % increase in survival and 13 % reduction in mortality which was not statistically significant ($p=0.08$). Adjuvant platinum-based therapy resulted a 6 % decrease in mortality when compared with adjuvant radiotherapy only ($p=0.46$). No benefit was shown when alkylating agents are used as adjuvant therapy. Although the benefit of adjuvant platinum-based therapies were not statistically significant, experts who believe otherwise try to explain this with the use of old generation drugs, small patient populations, staging errors, and heterogeneity of surgical techniques in these trials.

Since 2004, three key randomized clinical trials have been published showing the efficacy of cisplatin-based combination therapy in resected lung cancer: the IALT (International Adjuvant Lung Cancer Trial), ANITA (Adjuvant Navelbine International Trialist Association), and NCIC-CTG JBR 10 studies [6–8]. While the JBR 10 study included only stage I and II patients, the ANITA and IALT studies included stage IIIA patients, also. In these last two studies, adjuvant therapy especially had a beneficial effect in those patients who had N2 disease detected at surgery.

In the ANITA trial (Adjuvant Navelbine International Trialist Association), 367 patients were treated with adjuvant vinorelbine plus cisplatin and 431 patients were followed without adjuvant therapy [8]. Percentages of stage IB, II, and IIIA patients were, 24 %, 26 %, and 39 %, respectively. N2 positivity rate was 29 % in stage IIIA patients. Frequency of neutropenia and febrile neutropenia were 92 % and 9 %, respectively, and 2 % toxic deaths were reported due to adjuvant chemotherapy. After a median follow-up of 76 months, overall survival rates were 65.7 versus 43.7 months in chemo and no chemo arms, respectively. Despite the presence of treatment-related side effects and toxic deaths, adjuvant chemotherapy with cisplatin and vinorelbine decreased the risk of death (hazard ratio 0.80) and increased the five-year survival rates by 8.6 %.

The CALGB 9633 (Cancer and Leukemia Group B) trial was also designed to address the efficacy of adjuvant treatment in resected lung cancer [9]. Three hundred and forty four patients randomized either to postsurgical four cycles of paclitaxel plus carboplatin or follow-up. After median 74 months of follow-up, preliminary results showed no difference in overall survival between the study arms. But subgroup analyses depicted that adjuvant chemo was statistically beneficial in tumors ≥4 cm. According to the results, there was no place for adjuvant chemo in stage IA patients ($p = 0.43$). The efficacy of adjuvant treatment in stage IB lung cancer is debatable; neither the LACE meta-analyses nor most of other studies recommend adjuvant chemo for this stage of disease [10]. According to the newer staging classification, tumors ≥4 cm are reclassified as stage IIB, which benefits from adjuvant therapy [11].

Postoperative adjuvant chemotherapy is recommended for curatively resected stage II and III NSCLC. The beneficial effects of cisplatin-based combination chemo were showed in ANITA, IALT, and NCIC-CTG JBR 10 studies [6–8]. Despite the fact that JBR 10 study included only stage IB and II patients, the ratio of N2 patients was 29 % and 25 % in ANITA and IALT studies, respectively. Adjuvant chemo was shown to be efficacious (HR 0.89) in these trials ($p = 0.005$). Since staging was done with computerized tomography in older trials, this might have had an effect on results in general [12].

A retrospective study done by researchers from Birmingham Alabama University addressed the staging and incidental N2 positivity [13]. This trial included 148 patients who were staged with the same modalities and were N2 negative. All patients were staged with integrated positron emission tomography (PET) and computerized tomography (CT) and undergone wide mediastinal dissection plus R0 resection. Ninety-three percent of patients with incidental N2 disease received adjuvant chemotherapy, whereas 13 % received both chemo and radiotherapy. Two- and five-year survivals were 58 % and 35 %, respectively, and five-year median survivals were 40 % in single N2 node-positive and 25 % in multiple N2 node-positive patients ($p = 0.028$). The number of metastatic lymph nodes was found to be an independent prognostic factor for overall survival ($p = 0.032$).

Although research had been undertaken to find predictive biomarkers of adjuvant chemotherapy efficacy, no single biomarker could be defined so far. Studies that assessed the importance of K-RAS, p53, and p27 mutations were futile [14]. The level of ERCC1 (a DNA repair gene) expression was questioned as a predictive biomarker [15]. A high level of ERCC1 expression was linked with poor survival rates, whereas patients whose tumors showed low ERCC1 expression and treated with cisplatin experienced longer survival.

When we look into details of the randomized trials, some patients benefit from adjuvant therapies while surgery might achieve a cure for the others. Unfortunately, no further conclusive results could be generated from the ERCC1 studies, which might enable us to define the right patient population for the adjuvant chemo. With adding vinorelbine to cisplatin in ANITA and JBR 10 studies, paclitaxel in CALGB 9633, and vinorelbine, vinblastine, vindesine, or etoposide in IALT study, adjuvant chemo resulted to a 5 % increase in 5 years survival [6–9].

Class-III beta-tubulin (TUBB3) expression was also studied as a predictive biomarker of antitubulin drugs in lung cancer [16]. Studies conducted in advanced NSCLC showed overexpression of TUBB3 decreased the efficacy of treatments and therefore had detrimental effects on overall survival.

Table 10.2 Adjuvant chemotherapy studies in resected NSCLC

Study	n (number of patients)	Hazard ratio (95 % CI)
BMJ meta [5]	1,394	0.70 (0.52–0.92)
IALT [6]	1,867	0.62 (0.41–0.95)
ANITA [7]	1,840	0.79 (0.66–0.95)
NCIC-CTG JBR 10 [8]	482	0.74 (0.61–0.88)
CALGB 9633 [9]	330	0.62 (0.41–0.95)
ALPI [18]	1,209	0.80 (0.60–1.07)
E3590 [19, 20]	488	0.79 (0.66–0.95)
UFT meta [21]	2,003	0.74 (0.61–0.88)

Postoperative adjuvant chemotherapy provided 12 % and 15 % benefit in disease-free survival (DFS) and overall survival (OS) of patients in JBR 10 study. The treatment regimen was cisplatin plus vinorelbine in this trial. Tumor tissues of 265 patients out of 482 were analyzed for TUBB3 expression. Patients with high TUBB3 expression had lower DFS and OS rates but also benefited more from the adjuvant chemotherapy.

Some other studies revealed that overexpression of TUBB3 caused taxane and vinorelbine resistance and therefore resulted in worse prognosis. Researchers from the LACE-Bio group analyzed tumor tissues of 1,149 patients from ANITA, CALGB 9633, IALT, and JBR 10 studies in terms of TUBB3 expression with immunohistochemistry [17]. The importance of low and high TUBB3 expression was questioned for DFS and OS. Findings suggest that high TUBB3 expression was prognostic but did not have a predictive value for paclitaxel or vinorelbine efficacy.

Besides the cisplatin studies, a meta-analysis of six adjuvant chemo studies with UFT (tegafur/uracil) from Japan was reported [21]. In these trials, 1–2-year adjuvant postoperative UFT 400–600 mg/day was compared with surgery only and UFT showed superior survival rates. Over 2,000 patients randomized in these trials and HR was 0.74 with UFT ($p=0.001$). Since European and North American experts needed confirmatory studies, currently fluoropyrimidines are not in use for adjuvant treatment in resected NSCLC. The results of the adjuvant studies are summarized in Table 10.2. Adjuvant treatment with platinum-pemetrexed combination gives positive results in nonsquamous subtype of NSCLC [22].

Recently, researchers have been trying to develop a molecular risk-scoring model to define the best population that will benefit from the adjuvant chemotherapy [22, 23]. Tang et al. conducted a prospective randomized trial in resected lung adenocarcinoma in this manner. The predictive value of a 12 gene set for chemotherapy was assessed in 442 patients with resected stage I–III NSCLC. According to the JBR 10 study results, high-risk patients were treated with chemo and an increase in survival was reported ($p=0.017$). On the other side, the group which was expected to not benefit from chemo, no survival advantage was noted (p=0.70). Hazard ratios were 0.36 and 0.80, respectively.

In conclusion, there is no well-defined predictive biomarker to show the efficacy of adjuvant chemotherapy. For patients with curatively resected stage IB disease, tumors ≥4 cm, and stage II and III NSCLC, adjuvant chemotherapy with a platinum combination is recommended [24, 25].

Targeted therapies showed success in certain subgroups of advanced NSCLC. Especially studies with tyrosine kinase inhibitors (TKI) for epidermal growth factor receptor (EGFR) and anaplastic lymphoma kinase (ALK) caused dramatic benefits [26, 27]. Despite these, there is no role for targeted therapies in the adjuvant or locally advanced setting unless this practice is in a clinical trial [28].

Neoadjuvant Chemotherapy

Neoadjuvant chemotherapy is a preoperative treatment model for preoperative patients or stage III patients. Stage III disease is approximately one-third of all lung cancers and is a highly heterogeneous disease. For stage IIIA, chemotherapy alone is the chosen way of treatment; however for some selected cases, chemoradiotherapy is performed. The main purpose is to decrease the size of the tumor, so the patient would have a safer and restricted surgery. The prognosis of lung cancer is not satisfactory even after a good surgery; therefore, many clinical trials have been performed regarding adjuvant and neoadjuvant treatments. Taking precautions toward systemic micrometastatic disease, seeing the biology as well as the response to treatment of the tumor, and the fact that drugs are tolerated better during the preoperative stage are a few measures where neoadjuvant treatment is superior to adjuvant treatment. The situation where it is contrary is that staging is only clinical rather than pathological; the chance of surgery may be missed when there is no response to neoadjuvant treatment and the possible increase of morbidity and mortality of surgery after the treatment.

With the seventh classification made by IASLC, the TNM system of local progressive disease is redefined. According to the new version; T4 N0-1 M0 and T3 N1 M0 diseases are considered as stage IIIA. When defined as T4 tumor, it states that the tumor has invaded the mediastina, heart and major vessels, trachea, recurrent nerve, esophagus, or vertebra or the tumor is present on the same side of the lung however at different lobes. T4 N2-3 M0 tumors are now defined as stage IIIB [29].

The first neoadjuvant chemotherapy trials, randomized with surgery, were started during the 1990s and were done solely with chemotherapy, without any radiotherapy. Of these trials, the one conducted by Roth et al. consisted of 60 patients who either had surgery or preoperative cisplatin, etoposide, and cyclophosphamide neoadjuvant chemotherapy and then surgery [30]. The patients, who had a positive response, continued three more cycles of chemotherapy after the surgery. The median survival for patients who only had surgery was 11 months, while the median survival for patients who had neoadjuvant treatment was found to be 64 months ($p<0.008$). This trial was highly criticized due to the low number of patients. It is notable that with the follow-ups, it was seen that the median survival for only surgery patients was 14 months, while it was down to 21 months for patients who had neoadjuvant treatment ($p=0.056$) [31].

There are many trials where the benefits of postoperative and preoperative treatments in lung cancer are researched. Most of these studies looked into the effectiveness of postoperative chemotherapy, while others questioned the preoperative treatment. The meta-analysis conducted by Lim et al. evaluated 32 randomized studies including more than 10,000 cases. Of these, 22 were postoperative and 10 were preoperative chemotherapy cases. After the evaluation of all these cases, it is stated that whether it is preoperative or postoperative, the overall survival and disease-free survival increase [32]. The decrease of risks for postoperative and preoperative chemotherapy is 0.80 ($p<0.001$) and 0.81 ($p=0.024$), respectively.

The study conducted by Scagliotti and friends looks into surgery alone and preoperative chemotherapy. Stage IB–IIIA cases were randomized into surgery branches after either surgery alone or after three cycles of cisplatin and gemcitabine-combined therapy. Preoperative chemotherapy proved to be superior at both progression-free survival and overall survival, and this effect is higher specifically at stages IIB/IIIA [33]. While the study was proceeding, there were publications stating the superiority of adjuvant treatment; therefore, the continuation of the only surgery arm of the study was found to be ethically inappropriate and it was discontinued.

Neoadjuvant or Adjuvant Taxol/Carbo Hope (NATCH) study is a study where 624 non-small cell lung cancer patients at stages IA/IIIA are treated randomly [34]. There are three arms to this randomized study: patients either had just surgery or preoperative- or postoperative chemotherapy (paclitaxel/carboplatin). This study shows no significant superiority between induction chemotherapy and adjuvant treatment for early stage lung cancer. Patients who received induction chemotherapy had a slight increase at overall survival, which was found to be statistically insignificant, compared to those who had surgery alone (HR 0.88; 95 % CI, 0.69–1.12; $P=0.31$).

Recently published French intergroup study investigates the timing of chemotherapy [35]. In this study, 528 patients were randomized to receiving preoperative or perioperative chemotherapy. The patients were administered either cisplatin and gemcitabine or paclitaxel and carboplatin for a total of four cycles. The preoperative group received the entire treatment prior to surgery, while the perioperative group received two cycles before the surgery and two cycles after the surgery. There were no differences in the efficacy of the treatments. Even though there were different toxicities, the timing difference of the treatment had no effect on the overall survival. Moreover, the response rate did not change whether the patient received two or four cycles of treatment. The increase of surgical morbidity was not reported for preoperative chemotherapy group.

In the light of these results, whether the chemotherapy was administered as adjuvant or neoadjuvant showed no difference in overall survival for early stage non-small cell lung cancer. Chemotherapy, if given as neoadjuvant, is tolerated well, and the dose intensity of the planned treatment is close to 100 %. While planning an adjuvant treatment, it is of most importance to consider the comorbidities and choose the patient accordingly. It is the same for the elderly; age is not a contraindication for chemotherapy. For platinum, doublet combinations must be preferred. For adjuvant treatment, cisplatin dose should be at least 300 mg/m^2. Neoadjuvant chemotherapy is an appropriate choice in order to decrease the tumor volume [36].

Advanced Stage Non-Small Cell Lung Cancer

Lung cancer is the most frequent cause of cancer-related mortality in the world. Lung adenocarcinoma is the most diagnosed histological subtype of non-small cell lung cancer (NSCLC) accounting almost 85 % of all lung cancers, followed by squamous cell carcinoma. For stage I, II, and III non-small cell lung cancer, the aim of therapy is to cure the cancer. The curative intent treatment requires usually surgery, chemotherapy, radiation therapy, and sometimes combination of different treatment modalities. But metastatic-advanced lung cancers are not curable by surgery or radiotherapy. Disseminated NSCLC patients are treated with systemic chemotherapy, targeted therapies, or biologic therapy. The goal of treatment for metastatic lung cancer is to prolong survival and improve quality of life and symptom control while minimizing the side effects related with the treatment. All stage IV lung cancer patients should have early palliative supportive care to prolong survival and to improve the well-being.

For oligometastatic disease (solitary adrenal gland or cranial metastasis), metastasectomy or definitive radiotherapy with stereotactic body radiation therapy (SBRT) may be the options. Systemic chemotherapy or biologic therapy and/or surgical resection of metastatic lesion are also used for patients who have recurrent disease following prior definitive treatment.

During the past 20 years, remarkable progress has been made in the treatment of the non-small cell lung cancer. Advances in the use of chemotherapy, targeted agents, and immunotherapies have offered to the new options of multiple therapies to control symptoms and prolong survival in patients with advanced NSCLC. Treatment selection and sequencing of modalities of therapies and the specific approach to different patients groups will be reviewed here.

Initial Systemic Treatment for Advanced NSCLC

Until 1995, there was no consensus regarding the benefit of systemic chemotherapy for advanced stage NSCLC. The standard of care was to give supportive care to those patients. Platinum-containing regimens showed better but modest improvements in survival. According to a large meta-analysis in 1995, conducted by Non-small Cell Lung Cancer Collaborative Group, chemotherapy plus best supportive care showed 10 % increase in one-year survival rate. Response rates were 30 % for first-line and 10 % for second-line treatments. Platinum-containing regimens are better than nonplatinum combination regimens [5].

Meta-analyses have shown higher response rates for cisplatin combinations compared to those including carboplatin. In the subgroup of nonsquamous tumors, the overall survival was higher for cisplatin. However, carboplatin can be tolerated better when compared to cisplatin, making it a better option for palliative care, even though it has a hematologic toxicity risk. The cisplatin-based combinations can cause nausea and vomiting, neurotoxicity, ototoxicity, and nephrotoxicity.

Although the response rate is higher with three drug regimens, there is no difference in overall survival when compared to doublets regimens.

The combination of platinum compounds with either etoposide or second-generation cytotoxic drugs (docetaxel, gemcitabine, vinorelbine, and paclitaxel) is considered as the standard treatment. For nonsquamous NSCLC treatment, pemetrexed is another option. It is an antimetabolite, antifolate, and anticancer drug. It can either be used as a first-line or a second-line treatment or maintenance therapy. It is solely used in patients who have nonsquamous cell subtype of NSCLC [37].

Maintenance Therapy

The cytotoxic chemotherapy is administered in order to stabilize the tumor or reduce it in metastatic NSCLC. However due to its cumulative toxicity or increase in drug resistance, the administration is limited to four to six cycles. Maintenance therapy can delay the progression of the tumor while prolonging the survival and increasing the quality of life.

The maintenance therapy done with gemcitabine and docetaxel showed an increase in toxicity; however, no survival benefits were seen [37]. The results of a phase III, double-blind study showed that there is a significant increase of progression-free survival (PFS) if the maintenance chemotherapy is with pemetrexed. Pemetrexed showed significantly prolonged OS (13.4 vs 10.6 months $P=0.012$), better PFS ($P<0.00001$), and response ($P<0.001$). Such improvements were seen mostly in patients with nonsquamous subtype NSCLC (PFS HR = 0.47 and OS HR = 0.70). The effect of treatment by histology interaction for OS was significant ($P=0.038$) [38].

"Sequential Tarceva in Unresectable NSCLC (SATURN; BO18192) study", another phase III, placebo-controlled trial, showed that using erlotinib as maintenance therapy following a first-line platinum-doublet chemotherapy can prolong progression-free survival when compared to placebo. There was a small difference in the erlotinib group; PFS was longer in this group of patients. PFS was 12·3 weeks for those in the erlotinib group versus 11·1 weeks for patients in the placebo group (HR 0·71, 95 % CI 0·62–0·82; $p<0·0001$). OS was significantly prolonged with erlotinib maintenance in the stable disease group only (HR = 0.72; $P=0.0019$) median OS 11.9 versus 9.6 months, respectively [39].

Second-Line Treatment

The second-line therapies for NSCLC contain docetaxel, erlotinib, and pemetrexed. When compared to best supportive care, docetaxel had improved overall survival. When compared to placebo, erlotinib had improved overall survival [40, 41]. Pemetrexed had no difference from docetaxel in an efficacy standpoint, and it approved in nonsquamous NSCLC. The objective response rates however are less than 10 %, median progression-free survival is less than 4 months, and the median overall survival is 7–9 months [37]. The addition of a cytotoxic or targeted agent in a previously treated patient showed no improvement in overall survival [42].

Targeted Therapies

The cell subtype and genetic mutations as well as the patients' functional status play a critical role in making a treatment decision.

The most common histological subtype of NSCLC is adenocarcinoma, followed by squamous cell carcinoma. The Cancer Genome Atlas (TCGA), the International Cancer Genome Consortium (ICGC), and some other groups have identified many novel driver mutations and potentially targetable genes [43].

Driver mutations, which are the genetic changes in lung cancer patients, have been identified in some subsets of NSCLC. Such genetic alterations are of great importance for targeted therapies. Patients with advanced NSCLC should be advised to have their tumor assessed for certain driver mutations epidermal growth factor receptor (EGFR), anaplastic lymphoma kinase (ALK), oncogene, and ROS1. The presence of such mutations changes the treatment plan completely [44]. The American Society of Clinical Oncology (ASCO) Guidelines recommend analysis of either the primary tumor or of the metastatic lesions for all patients whose tumor contains adenocarcinoma components (pure lung adenocarcinoma or mixed adenocarcinoma-containing component) before deciding the treatment protocol [45].

EGFR mutation points toward the activity of tyrosine kinase inhibitors (TKI). Patients with advanced EGFR-mutated NSCLC show higher response rates of 56–74 % and a median progression-free survival of 10–14 months when treated with EGFR TKIs such as gefitinib, erlotinib, and afatinib [46, 47].

Although the response rates are higher when compared to doublet platinum-containing regimens, the progressive disease can reoccur in 1–2 years. The development of an additional EGFR mutation (EGFR T790M) is the source of such outcome [48]. This second mutation decreases the ability of ATP-competitive reversible EGFR TKIs to bind to the tyrosine kinase domain of EGFR [47]. In a trial with advanced or metastatic NSCLC patients with positive EGFR mutations, gefitinib or carboplatin and paclitaxel was administered. It showed that when compared to standard chemotherapy, gefitinib improved progression-free survival, while having an acceptable toxicity [49].

The phase III EURTAC trial was a first-line treatment with advanced EGFR-mutation-positive NSCLC. Patients with EGFR-mutated nonsquamous cell NSCLC (with exon 19 deletion or L858R mutation in exon 21) were randomized for erlotinib 150 mg/day or standard first-line chemotherapy with platinum-containing doublets. The median PFS was 9·7 months in the erlotinib group and 5·2 months in the standard platinum-containing chemotherapy group. There was 63 % risk reduction with first-line erlotinib ($p < 0{\cdot}0001$) [50].

First-line treatment with a TKI (erlotinib, gefitinib, or afatinib) is the preferred treatment for patients with tumors bearing an activating (sensitizing) EGFR mutation. If the EGFR tyrosine kinase inhibitor treatments fail, there are limited options left such as cytotoxic chemotherapy or supportive care. A newly developed TKI, AZD9291, is shown to be highly active in patients with lung cancer who have positive EGFR T790M mutation. This molecule is effective if the treatment failed with prior TKI treatment [44, 51].

In adenocarcinomas, testing for ALK fusion gene mutations is a standard of care. Such oncogenic drivers are mostly present in younger patients, never smokers, and adenocarcinoma subtypes. Crizotinib is an ALK TKI, targeting the activity of ALK [27, 51].

Antiangiogenic Therapies

Inhibition of angiogenesis is one of the main targets of cancer treatment. The regulation of angiogenesis in normal and cancer patients is related with vascular endothelial growth factor (VEGF). In most of the tumors, including NSCLC, VEGF expression is increased, and it is related with tumor growth and progression. High levels of VEGF are related with increased risks of recurrence, metastasis, and death. A humanized variant of VEGF antibody bevacizumab showed clinical activity in cancer and increases survival when combined to standard chemotherapy in metastatic lung cancer. When added to platinum-based chemotherapy regimen, bevacizumab not only increases the response rates, but also prolongs PFS and OS [52].

OS was significantly longer in patients receiving bevacizumab and carboplatin-paclitaxel than in those receiving chemotherapy alone (median OS, 12.3 versus 10.3 months; $p = 0.013$). With the increase of response rates, the side effects become more common in bevacizumab-receiving patients. When bevacizumab is added to the regimen, side effects such as hypertension, proteinuria, bleeding, neutropenia, febrile neutropenia, thrombocytopenia, hyponatremia, rash, and headache were more obvious and frequent.

There are two meta-analyses showing the improvement of RR, PFS, and OS once the bevacizumab is added to a platinum-containing doublet regimen for nonsquamous NSCLC [52]. Due to the increased risk of bleeding, the addition of bevacizumab is not recommended for squamous subtype [53].

Ramucirumab, another angiogenesis inhibitor, is a human IgG1 monoclonal antibody. The main target of this antibody is the extracellular domain of VEGFR-2 and thus inhibits the formation, proliferation, and migration of new blood vessels [54].

The randomized trial REVEL applied docetaxel plus placebo or docetaxel plus ramucirumab as second line of treatment to patients who progressed after platinum-based chemotherapy. Ramucirumab plus docetaxel group had higher survival with stage IV NSCLC. Both nonsquamous and squamous subgroups had the same response rate. Since there are no driver mutations in patients with squamous tumor histology, ramucirumab plus docetaxel combination became an option [55].

Immunotherapy for Non-small Cell Lung Cancer Progressing After Platinum-Based Chemotherapy

The standard of care for patients with advanced NSCLC without a driver mutation is platinum-based chemotherapy. If the progression continues during or after the platinum-based chemotherapy, immunotherapy becomes an option. For that, anti-PD-1 antibodies (nivolumab) of anti-PDL-1 antibodies (pembrolizumab) can be recommended [56, 57].

For advanced or metastatic squamous cell lung cancer patients, a phase III trial (CheckMate-017) pointed out that nivolumab is superior to docetaxel, median overall survival is 12.2 months and 9.4 months, objective response rates were 19 % vs 12 %, and the duration of response were 17.2 months vs 5.8 months, respectively [57]. Nivolumab proves to be more effective in PDL-1 positive patients, presenting as a new therapeutic possibility for those who are resistant to platinum treatments [57].

CheckMate-057 trial, another phase III trial, compared nivolumab and docetaxel in second-line treatment for nonsquamous NSCLC, showing that nivolumab reduces the risk of death by 27 % vs docetaxel. For those who have higher levels of PD-L1 expression, the risk of death reduction rate was about 60 % [58, 59].

Increased PD-L1 expression (more than 50 % of all tumor cells) improves the efficacy of pembrolizumab and increases the overall survival rate [60].

Systemic Treatment for Small Cell Lung Cancer (SCLC)

Limited Disease

15–20 % of primary lung carcinomas present as small cell lung cancers (SCLC). Rapid doubling time, early metastatic presentation, and sensitivity to chemotherapy and radiotherapy are some of the characteristics of SCLC. Development of drug resistance is highly common and frequent [61].

The standard approach for the treatment of SCLC is platinum-based chemotherapy. For a certain group of patients who are unable to tolerate platinum-containing regimens, nonplatinum regimens can be offered. However, even if the patient appears to tolerate platinum-based chemotherapy, due to its high toxicity risk, a maximum number of four to six cycles of first-line treatment are recommended [62].

Even though there are many randomized studies and researches, there is no consensus among the caregivers regarding a standard approach. The studies varied from the most effective treatment strategy to best agents or treatment duration, etc. However, these trials mostly showed contrasting results. Cisplatin and irinotecan combination did not show superiority to standard cisplatin and etoposide combination [63].

According to two meta-analyses, the thoracic radiotherapy should be initiated as early as possible, either at the beginning with the first or second cycle of platinum-based chemotherapy regimen [64, 65]. For localized disease, even though there is higher toxicity, thoracic radiotherapy, if given early and in combination with chemotherapy, improves long-term results [66].

Extensive Disease

According to the received results of meta-analyses, platinum-based chemotherapy should be the standard of care in the treatment of SCLC. Cisplatin and carboplatin have shown similar efficacy, and the choice of the platinum compound for the treatment of patients with extensive stage SCLC should consider the expected toxicity profile, organ function, performance status, and comorbidities [66, 67].

The palliative treatment of stage IV SCLC shows high response rates (60–70 %); however, because of the rapid and frequent relapses and limited activity of second-line treatment, the overall survival (OS) remains poor. Three-drug regimens and increased dose intensity showed no improvement in OS. Moreover, such cases are mostly associated with high toxicity in this group of patient population [68]. These regimens are not recommended as first-line treatment.

Prophylactic cranial irradiation after induction treatment is standard of care for patients who have limited disease or patients who show good partial response and have extensive disease [68]. Maintenance treatment, intensified chemotherapy, or the usage of growth factors showed no significant efficacy [69].

Second-Line Treatment

If the relapse occurs 3–6 months after the treatment is completed, the patient may benefit from reintroduction of the first-line regimen. If the relapse occurs prior to 3 months, topotecan or CAV (cyclophosphamide-doxorubicin-vincristine) can be used. However, the clinical benefit of such regimen for patients relapsed after first-line treatment is very limited. And if the relapse occurs within 6 weeks after completing the first-line treatment, chemotherapy is not recommended [70].

References

1. Gibbons D, Pisters K, Johnson F, Eapen GA. Non small cell lung cancer. In: Kantarjian HM, Wolff R, Koller CA, editors. The MD Anderson manual of medical oncology. 2nd ed. New York: McGraw-Hill Companies; 2011. p. 35.
2. Detterbeck FC, Boffa DJ, Tanoue LT. The new lung cancer staging system. Chest. 2009;136(1):260–71.
3. Boffa DJ, Detterbeck F, Smith EJ, Rami-Porta R, Crowley J, Zelterman D, et al. Should the 7th edition of the lung cancer stage classification system change treatment algorithms in non-small cell lung cancer? J Thorac Oncol. 2010;5(11):4.
4. Blum RH. Adjuvant chemotherapy for lung cancer – a new standard of care. N Engl J Med. 2004;350(4):404–5.
5. Chemotherapy in non-small cell lung cancer: a meta-analysis using updated data on individual patients from 52 randomised clinical trials. Non-small Cell Lung Cancer Collaborative Group. BMJ. 1995;311(7010):899–909.
6. Arriagada R, et al. Cisplatin-based adjuvant chemotherapy in patients with completely resected non-small-cell lung cancer. N Engl J Med. 2004;350(4):351–60.

7. Douillard JY, et al. Adjuvant vinorelbine plus cisplatin versus observation in patients with completely resected stage IB–IIIA non-small-cell lung cancer (Adjuvant Navelbine International Trialist Association [ANITA]): a randomised controlled trial. Lancet Oncol. 2006;7(9):719–27.
8. Winton T, et al. Vinorelbine plus cisplatin vs. observation in resected non-small-cell lung cancer. N Engl J Med. 2005;352(25):2589–97.
9. Strauss GM, et al. Adjuvant paclitaxel plus carboplatin compared with observation in stage IB non-small-cell lung cancer: CALGB 9633 with the Cancer and Leukemia Group B, Radiation Therapy Oncology Group, and North Central Cancer Treatment Group Study Groups. J Clin Oncol. 2008;26(31):5043–51.
10. Pignon JP, et al. Lung adjuvant cisplatin evaluation: a pooled analysis by the LACE Collaborative Group. J Clin Oncol. 2008;26(21):3552–9.
11. Douillard JY, et al. Adjuvant cisplatin and vinorelbine for completely resected non-small cell lung cancer: subgroup analysis of the Lung Adjuvant Cisplatin Evaluation. J Thorac Oncol. 2010;5(2):220–8.
12. Cerfolio RJ, Bryant AS. Survival of patients with unsuspected N2 (stage IIIA) nonsmall-cell lung cancer. Ann Thorac Surg. 2008;86(2):362–6; discussion 366–7.
13. Besse B, Le Chevalier T. Adjuvant chemotherapy for non-small-cell lung cancer: a fading effect? J Clin Oncol. 2008;26(31):5014–7.
14. Schiller JH, et al. Lack of prognostic significance of p53 and K-ras mutations in primary resected non-small-cell lung cancer on E4592: a Laboratory Ancillary Study on an Eastern Cooperative Oncology Group Prospective Randomized Trial of Postoperative Adjuvant Therapy. J Clin Oncol. 2001;19(2):448–57.
15. Olaussen KA, et al. DNA repair by ERCC1 in non-small-cell lung cancer and cisplatin-based adjuvant chemotherapy. N Engl J Med. 2006;355(10):983–91.
16. Seve P, et al. Class III beta-tubulin expression and benefit from adjuvant cisplatin/vinorelbine chemotherapy in operable non-small cell lung cancer: analysis of NCIC JBR.10. Clin Cancer Res. 2007;13(3):994–9.
17. Reiman T, et al. Cross-validation study of class III beta-tubulin as a predictive marker for benefit from adjuvant chemotherapy in resected non-small-cell lung cancer: analysis of four randomized trials. Ann Oncol. 2012;23(1):86–93.
18. Scagliotti GV. The ALPI trial: the Italian/European experience with adjuvant chemotherapy in resectable non-small lung cancer. Clin Cancer Res. 2005;11(13):5011s–6.
19. Keller SM, AS, Wagner H, et al. Prospective randomized trial of postoperative adjuvant therapy in patients with completely resected stages II and IIIa non-small cell lung cancer: an Intergroup Trial (E3590). Chicago: ASCO meeting abst; 1999. p. 1793.
20. Wagner Jr H. Postoperative adjuvant therapy for patients with resected non-small cell lung cancer: still controversial after all these years. Chest. 2000;117(4 Suppl 1):110s–8.
21. Hamada C, et al. Meta-analysis of postoperative adjuvant chemotherapy with tegafur-uracil in non-small-cell lung cancer. J Clin Oncol. 2005;23(22):4999–5006.
22. Leong D, Rai R, Nguyen B, Lee A, Yip D. Advances in adjuvant systemic therapy for non-small-cell lung cancer. World J Clin Oncol. 2014;5(4):633.
23. Zuccato JA, Ellis PM. Improving referral of patients for consideration of adjuvant chemotherapy after surgical resection of lung cancer. Curr Oncol. 2012;19(6):e422–7.
24. Tang H, et al. A 12-gene set predicts survival benefits from adjuvant chemotherapy in non-small cell lung cancer patients. Clin Cancer Res. 2013;19(6):1577–86.
25. Booth CM, et al. Time to adjuvant chemotherapy and survival in non-small cell lung cancer: a population-based study. Cancer. 2013;119(6):1243–50.
26. Mok TS, et al. Gefitinib or carboplatin-paclitaxel in pulmonary adenocarcinoma. N Engl J Med. 2009;361(10):947–57.
27. Shaw AT, et al. Crizotinib versus chemotherapy in advanced ALK-positive lung cancer. N Engl J Med. 2013;368(25):2385–94.
28. Martinez P, et al. Molecular targeted therapy for early-stage non-small-cell lung cancer: will it increase the cure rate? Lung Cancer. 2014;84(2):97–100.

29. Baik CS, VrE, Martins GR. The role of chemotherapy in the management of stage IIIA non-small cell lung cancer. in American Society of Clinical Oncology. Chicago; 2013, http://tr.scribd.com/doc/283509665/2015-Asco-Edbook#scribd.
30. Goldstraw P, et al. The IASLC Lung Cancer Staging Project: proposals for the revision of the TNM stage groupings in the forthcoming (seventh) edition of the TNM Classification of malignant tumours. J Thorac Oncol. 2007;2(8):706–14.
31. Roth JA, et al. A randomized trial comparing perioperative chemotherapy and surgery with surgery alone in resectable stage IIIA non-small-cell lung cancer. J Natl Cancer Inst. 1994;86(9):673–80.
32. Roth JA, et al. Long-term follow-up of patients enrolled in a randomized trial comparing perioperative chemotherapy and surgery with surgery alone in resectable stage IIIA non-small-cell lung cancer. Lung Cancer. 1998;21(1):1–6.
33. Lim E, et al. Preoperative versus postoperative chemotherapy in patients with resectable non-small cell lung cancer: systematic review and indirect comparison meta-analysis of randomized trials. J Thorac Oncol. 2009;4(11):1380–8.
34. Scagliotti GV, et al. Randomized phase III study of surgery alone or surgery plus preoperative cisplatin and gemcitabine in stages IB to IIIA non-small-cell lung cancer. J Clin Oncol. 2012;30(2):172–8.
35. Felip E, et al. Preoperative chemotherapy plus surgery versus surgery plus adjuvant chemotherapy versus surgery alone in early-stage non-small-cell lung cancer. J Clin Oncol. 2010;28(19):3138–45.
36. Westeel V, et al. A randomised trial comparing preoperative to perioperative chemotherapy in early-stage non-small-cell lung cancer (IFCT 0002 trial). Eur J Cancer. 2013;49(12): 2654–64.
37. Vansteenkiste J, De Ruysscher D, Eberhardt EWE, Lim E, Senan S, Felip E, Peters S, on behalf of the ESMO Guidelines Working Group. Early and locally advanced non-small-cell lung cancer (NSCLC): ESMO clinical practice guidelines for diagnosis, treatment and follow-up. Ann Oncol. 2013;24(Supplement 6):9.
38. Ciuleanu T, et al. Maintenance pemetrexed plus best supportive care versus placebo plus best supportive care for non-small-cell lung cancer: a randomised, double-blind, phase 3 study. Lancet. 2009;374(9699):1432–40.
39. Gentzler RD, Patel JD. Maintenance treatment after induction therapy in non-small cell lung cancer: latest evidence and clinical implications. Ther Adv Med Oncol. 2014;6(1):4–15.
40. Coudert B, et al. Survival benefit with erlotinib maintenance therapy in patients with advanced non-small-cell lung cancer (NSCLC) according to response to first-line chemotherapy. Ann Oncol. 2012;23(2):388–94.
41. Cohen MH, et al. Approval summary: erlotinib maintenance therapy of advanced/metastatic non-small cell lung cancer (NSCLC). Oncologist. 2010;15(12):1344–51.
42. Stinchcombe TE, Socinski MA. Maintenance therapy in advanced non-small cell lung cancer: current status and future implications. J Thorac Oncol. 2011;6(1):174–82.
43. Comprehensive genomic characterization of squamous cell lung cancers. Nature. 2012. 489(7417):519–25.
44. Aisner DL, Marshall CB. Molecular pathology of non-small cell lung cancer: a practical guide. Am J Clin Pathol. 2012;138(3):332–46.
45. Leighl NB, et al. Molecular testing for selection of patients with lung cancer for epidermal growth factor receptor and anaplastic lymphoma kinase tyrosine kinase inhibitors: American Society of Clinical Oncology endorsement of the College of American Pathologists/International Association for the study of lung cancer/association for molecular pathology guideline. J Clin Oncol. 2014;32(32):3673–9.
46. Janne PA RS, Yang JC-H, Ahn M-J, Kim D-W, Kim S-W, Planchard D, Ohe Y, Felip E, Watkins C, Cantarini M, Ghiorghiu S, Ranson M. Clinical activity of the mutant-selective EGFR inhibitor AZD9291 in patients (pts) with EGFR inhibitor-resistant non-small cell lung cancer (NSCLC) [abstract]. J Clin Oncol. 2014;32:5s.
47. Janne PA, et al. AZD9291 in EGFR inhibitor-resistant non-small-cell lung cancer. N Engl J Med. 2015;372(18):1689–99.

48. Nguyen K-SH, Kobayashi S, Costa DB. Acquired resistance to epidermal growth factor receptor tyrosine kinase inhibitors in non-small-cell lung cancers dependent on the epidermal growth factor receptor pathway. Clin Lung Cancer. 2009;10(4):281–9.
49. Maemondo M, et al. Gefitinib or chemotherapy for non-small-cell lung cancer with mutated EGFR. N Engl J Med. 2010;362(25):2380–8.
50. Rosell R, et al. Erlotinib versus standard chemotherapy as first-line treatment for European patients with advanced EGFR mutation-positive non-small-cell lung cancer (EURTAC): a multicentre, open-label, randomised phase 3 trial. Lancet Oncol. 2012;13(3):239–46.
51. Ou SH, et al. Clinical benefit of continuing ALK inhibition with crizotinib beyond initial disease progression in patients with advanced ALK-positive NSCLC. Ann Oncol. 2014;25(2): 415–22.
52. Sandler A, et al. Paclitaxel-carboplatin alone or with bevacizumab for non-small-cell lung cancer. N Engl J Med. 2006;355(24):2542–50.
53. Lima AB, Macedo LT, Sasse AD. Addition of bevacizumab to chemotherapy in advanced non-small cell lung cancer: a systematic review and meta-analysis. PLoS One. 2011;6(8):e22681.
54. Soria JC, et al. Systematic review and meta-analysis of randomised, phase II/III trials adding bevacizumab to platinum-based chemotherapy as first-line treatment in patients with advanced non-small-cell lung cancer. Ann Oncol. 2013;24(1):20–30.
55. Garon EB, et al. Ramucirumab plus docetaxel versus placebo plus docetaxel for second-line treatment of stage IV non-small-cell lung cancer after disease progression on platinum-based therapy (REVEL): a multicentre, double-blind, randomised phase 3 trial. Lancet. 2014;384(9944):665–73.
56. Spigel DR, Reckamp KL, Rizvi NA, Poddubskaya E, West HJ, Eberhardt WEE, … Brahmer, JR. A phase III study (CheckMate 017) of nivolumab (NIVO; anti-programmed death-1 [PD-1]) vs docetaxel (DOC) in previously treated advanced or metastatic squamous (SQ) cell non-small cell lung cancer (NSCLC). In: ASCO Annual Meeting Proceeding (vol. 33, no. 15_ suppl, Chicago; p. 8009). 2015.
57. Rizvi NA, et al. Activity and safety of nivolumab, an anti-PD-1 immune checkpoint inhibitor, for patients with advanced, refractory squamous non-small-cell lung cancer (CheckMate 063): a phase 2, single-arm trial. Lancet Oncol. 2015;16(3):257–65.
58. Brahmer J, et al. Nivolumab versus docetaxel in advanced squamous-cell non-small-cell lung cancer. N Engl J Med. 2015;373(2):123–35.
59. Luis Paz-Ares, LH, Borghaei H, Spigel DR, Steins M, Ready N, Chow LQM, Vokes EE, Felip E, Holgado E, Barlesi F, Kohlhaeufl M, Rodriguez O, Burgio MA, Fayette J, Gettinger SN, Harbison C, Dorange C, Finckenstein FG, Brahmer JR.. Phase III, randomized trial (CheckMate 057) of nivolumab (NIVO) versus docetaxel (DOC) in advanced non-squamous cell (non-SQ) non-small cell lung cancer (NSCLC) in ASCO Annual Meeting 2015. J Clin Oncol. 2015 (suppl; abstr LBA109).
60. Garon EB, et al. Pembrolizumab for the treatment of non-small-cell lung cancer. N Engl J Med. 2015;372(21):2018–28.
61. Planchard D, Le Pechoux C. Small cell lung cancer: new clinical recommendations and current status of biomarker assessment. Eur J Cancer. 2011;47 Suppl 3:S272–83.
62. Thatcher N, Faivre-Finn C, Lorigan P. Management of small-cell lung cancer. Ann Oncol. 2005;16 suppl 2:235–9.
63. Ohe Y, Ohashi Y, Kubota K, Tamura T, Nakagawa K, Negoro S, … Fukuoka M. Randomized phase III study of cisplatin plus irinotecan versus carboplatin plus paclitaxel, cisplatin plus gemcitabine, and cisplatin plus vinorelbine for advanced non-small-cell lung cancer: Four-Arm Cooperative Study in Japan. Ann Oncol. 2007;18(2):317–23.
64. Fruh M, et al. Small-cell lung cancer (SCLC): ESMO clinical practice guidelines for diagnosis, treatment and follow-up. Ann Oncol. 2013;24 Suppl 6:vi99–105.
65. Murray N, et al. Importance of timing for thoracic irradiation in the combined modality treatment of limited-stage small-cell lung cancer. The National Cancer Institute of Canada Clinical Trials Group. J Clin Oncol. 1993;11(2):336–44.
66. Pignon JP, et al. A meta-analysis of thoracic radiotherapy for small-cell lung cancer. N Engl J Med. 1992;327(23):1618–24.

67. Rossi A, et al. Carboplatin- or cisplatin-based chemotherapy in first-line treatment of small-cell lung cancer: the COCIS meta-analysis of individual patient data. J Clin Oncol. 2012;30(14):1692–8.
68. Rossi A, Martelli O, Di Maio M. Treatment of patients with small-cell lung cancer: from meta-analyses to clinical practice. Cancer Treat Rev. 2013;39(5):498–506.
69. Hanna N, et al. Randomized phase III trial comparing irinotecan/cisplatin with etoposide/cisplatin in patients with previously untreated extensive-stage disease small-cell lung cancer. J Clin Oncol. 2006;24(13):2038–43.
70. Schiller JH. Current standards of care in small-cell and non-small-cell lung cancer. Oncology. 2001;61 Suppl 1:3–13.

11 Surgical Staging and Advanced Surgical Techniques in Early Stage Non-small Cell Lung Cancers

Sukru Dilege, Serhan Tanju, and Suat Erus

Case Presentation

Case 1

A 70-year-old female patient, who did not have any symptoms, was admitted to the hospital for routine health checkup. She had no significant past medical history other than a 40 pack-year history of smoking. Systematic physical examination was normal. Chest X-ray revealed a suspected opacity in the left upper zone. Thoracic computerized tomography showed peripheral solitary pulmonary nodule in the left lung upper lobe. FDG PET/CT demonstrated high FDG uptake in the left upper lobe nodule with maximal standard uptake value (SUVmax) 7,4 (Fig. 11.1). There was no FDG uptake in the other systems. Cranial MRI did not reveal any metastatic lesion. The patient was clinically staged as cT1aN0M0. Minimally invasive surgery was recommended to patient for diagnosis and treatment.

Robot-assisted thoracic surgical left upper lobe wedge resection was performed. Intraoperative frozen-section analysis of the nodule confirmed the diagnosis of adenocarcinoma; thus, robot-assisted thoracic surgical left upper lobectomy with mediastinal lymph dissection was performed. Postoperative period was uneventful. She was discharged on postoperative day 3. Pathologic stage was T1aN0M0.

S. Dilege, MD (✉) • S. Tanju, MD • S. Erus
Department of Thoracic Surgery, Koc University Hospital,
Davutpasa Caddesi, No: 4, Topkapi, Istanbul 34010, Turkey
e-mail: sdilege@gmail.com; stanju@ku.edu.tr; serus@kuh.ku.edu.tr

G. Ozyigit et al. (eds.), *Principles and Practice of Radiotherapy Techniques in Thoracic Malignancies*, DOI 10.1007/978-3-319-28761-4_11

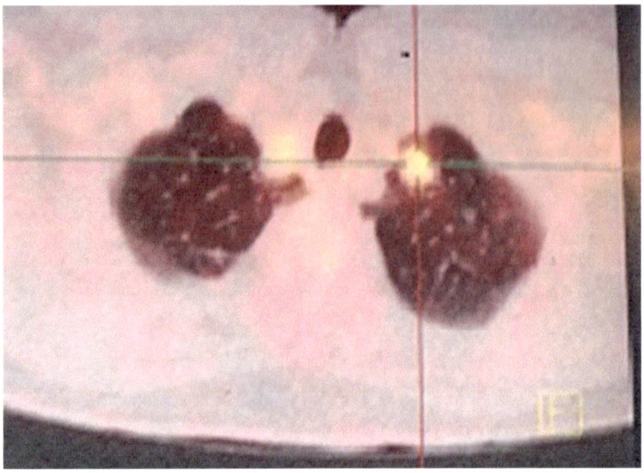

Fig. 11.1 FDG PET/CT revealed high FDG uptake in the *left* upper lobe nodule

Case 2

A 54-year-old female patient presented with solitary pulmonary nodule in the right lung lower lobe. FDG PET/CT revealed right lower lobe nodule with high FDG uptake (SUV max:4,5). The patient was clinically staged as cT1bN0M0. Video-assisted thoracoscopic surgery (VATS) was performed for diagnosis and treatment. Wedge resection of the nodule was analyzed with frozen section, and the diagnosis was confirmed as non-small cell lung carcinoma. VATS lower lobectomy and mediastinal lymph node dissection (Figs. 11.2a, b and 11.3a, b) was performed. The patient was discharged on postoperative day 3. Pathologic stage was T1bN0M0.

Evidence-Based Surgical Approaches

Lung resection with mediastinal lymph node dissection or systematic sampling is widely accepted as gold therapeutic standard for patients with early stage non-small cell lung cancer. Although there is a growing trend toward a minimally invasive surgical approach in early stage, thoracoscopic lung resection is performed only in 23–30 % of patients undergoing surgical treatment for lung cancer [1, 2], so vast majority of patients with operable lung cancer still have open surgery. However, many studies and reviews published over the past decade demonstrated the feasibility and benefits of minimally invasive surgical techniques including VATS and robot-assisted thoracoscopic surgery (RATS) in lung cancer.

A propensity-matched analysis of outcome of VATS versus open lobectomy for primary non-small cell lung cancer from the European Society of Thoracic Surgeon's database published in this year included two matched groups of 2,721 patients among 28,771 cases. The study confirmed that VATS lobectomy was associated with a significantly lower morbidity than open lobectomy (29.1 % vs 31.7 %, $p=0.0357$), and length of stay was shorter by a mean of 2 days for patients who had VATS lobectomy (mean: 7.8 days vs 9.8 days, $P=0.0003$). Mortality at hospital

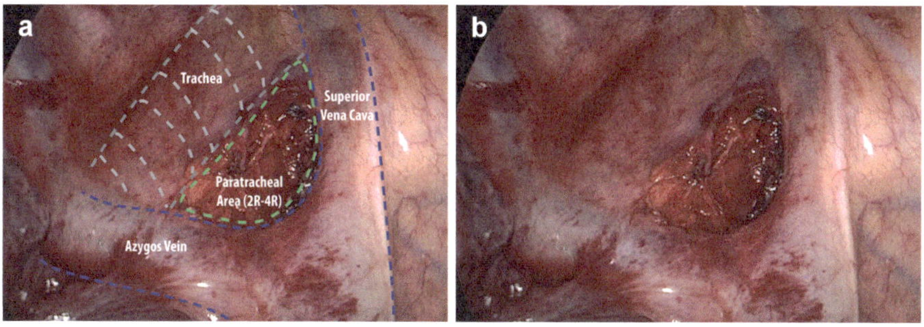

Fig. 11.2 (**a**, **b**) Intraoperative view of right paratracheal lymph node dissection

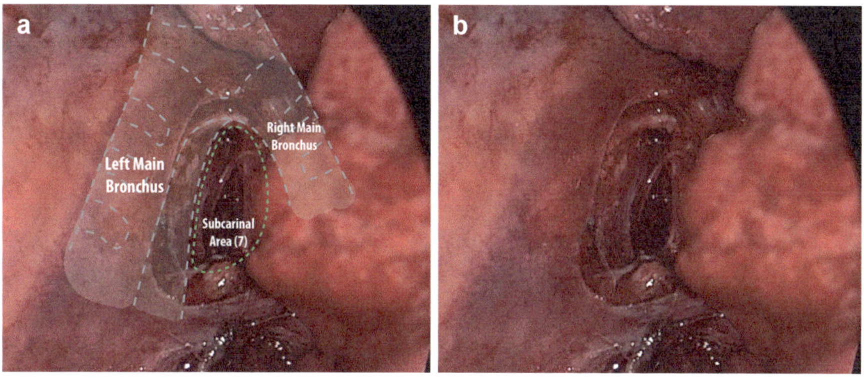

Fig. 11.3 (**a**, **b**) Intraoperative view of subcarinal lymph node dissection

discharge was significantly lower in the VATS lobectomy group (27 patients (1.0 %) vs 50 patients (1.9 %), $P=0.002$). VATS lobectomy group had also favorable results with significantly less complications (32.8 vs 38.5 %, $P<0.0001$), reduced mortality at hospital discharge by one-third (1.9 vs 2.9 %, $P=0.0011$), and shorter length of stay by a median of 1 day (median: 7 days vs 8 days, $P<0.0001$) in patients older than 70 years [1].

Numerous studies (Table 11.1) showed the benefits of VATS; however, there is lack of randomized studies. In 1995, Kirby et al. [3] randomized 61 stage I lung cancer patients into either VATS (n:30) or muscle-sparing thoracotomy (MST, n:31) for lung resection. In VATS group, operative time (175 ± 93 min vs 161 ± 61 min), average duration of chest tube drainage (6.5 ± 4.8 days vs 4 .6 ± 3.3 days), and average duration of hospital stay (8.3 ± 5.7 days vs 7.1 ± 5.5 days) are less than MST group; however, there were no significant differences ($p>0.05$). Postoperative complication rate was found to be significantly high in MST group (n:6 vs n:16, $p<0.05$) especially in terms of prolonged air leak.

Sugi et al. [4] randomized 100 consecutive patients with early stage lung cancer into VATS group (n:48) and conventional lobectomy by thoracotomy (n:52) in 2000. There were no significant differences in terms of tumor size (22.6 ± 1.2 mm vs

Table 11.1 Comparison studies between VATS and thoracotomy

Author	Patients (VATS vs T) (N)	OT (min) (VATS vs T)	DT (days) (VATS vs T)	LHS (days) (VATS vs T)	Complication (%) (VATS vs T)	Survival (VATS vs T)	Design
Whitson et al. [7]	3,114 vs 3,256	–	4.2 vs 5.7 ($p=0.025$)	8.3 vs 13.3 ($p=0.016$)	16.4 vs 31.2 ($p=0.018$)	80.1 vs 65.6 (5-year)	Rev
Yim et al. [5]	18 vs 18	78 ± 36 vs 82 ± 27 ($p>0.05$)	3.2 ± 2.8 vs 4.1 ± 3.5 ($p>0.05$)	4.1 ± 3.6 vs 5.3 ± 4.8 ($p>0.05$)	5.5 vs 5.5 ($p>0.05$)	–	P
Muraoka et al. [8]	43 vs 42	288 ± 66 vs 293 ± 83 ($P=0.56$)	3.0 ± 2.1 vs 3.9 vs 2.9 ($P=0.016$)	–	25.6 vs 47.6 ($p=0.011$)	–	R
Park et al. [9]	136 vs 136	–	–	8.8 ± 6.5 vs. 6.3 ± 3.3 $p<0.05$	12.5 vs 16.1 $p=0.65$	85.3 vs 81.8 $p=0.43$	R
Flores et al. [10]	398 vs 343	220 vs 224	–	5 vs 7 $P<0.0001$	24 vs 30 $p=0.05$	79 vs 75 (5-year) ($p=0.08$)	R
Cajipe et al. [11]	46 vs 45	268 vs 229 $p=0.17$	3 vs 4 $p<0.001$	7 vs 10 $p=0.02$	30 vs 58 $P=0.01$	–	R
Stephens et al. [12]	307 vs 307	173 ± 57 vs 159 ± 56 $p=0.0001$	2 ± 4 vs 3 ± 19 $p=0.0001$	4 ± 8 vs 6 ± 8 $p=0.0001$	19 vs 37 $p=0.0001$	78 vs 73 (5-year) $p=0.071$	R
Paul et al. [13]	1,281 vs 1,281	173 vs 143 $p<0.0001$	3 vs 4 $p<0.0001$	4 vs 6 $p<0.0001$	26.23 vs 34.66 $p<0.0001$	–	R
Farjah et al. [14]	721 vs 12,237	–	–	4 vs 8 $p<0.001$	–	48 vs 44 $p=0.02$	R
Scott et al. [15]	66 vs 686	117.5 vs 171.5 $p<0.001$	–	5 vs 7 $p<0.001$	27.3 vs 47.8 $p=0.05$	–	R

T Thoracotomy, *OT* operation time, *DT* drainage time, *LHS* length of hospital stay, *Rev* review, *P* prospective, *R* retrospective

20.2 ± 1.8 mm, $p = 0.30$), tumor histology, and the number of dissected lymph nodes (hilar – 8.4 ± 1.0 vs 8.2 ± 1.5, $p = 0.88$; mediastinal – 13.4 ± 1.7 vs 13.0 ± 2.5, $p = 0.88$) between the open group and the VATS group. Seven patients (13 %) from the open group developed distant recurrences, whereas three patients (6 %) developed local or regional recurrences. In the VATS group, two patients (4 %) developed distant recurrences, and three patients (6 %) developed locoregional recurrences. There were no significant differences in the incidence of the recurrences between the two groups. The overall survival rates 3 and 5 years after surgery were 93 % and 85 % in the open group and 90 % and 90 % in the VATS group, respectively. There were no significant differences in the survival rates between the two groups ($p = 0.91$).

The other prospective study published by Yim APC [5] in 2000 demonstrated that VATS lobectomy is associated with reduced postoperative release of both proinflammatory and antiinflammatory cytokines compared with the open lobectomy. In 2014, Erus et al. [6] also showed that postoperative C-reactive protein levels were significantly lower for the VATS group compared with axillary thoracotomy for lung resection in patients with lung cancer. These findings were similar with the study by Yim et al.

RATS has become increasingly popular all over the world since the development of robotic surgical system (RSS) (Fig. 11.4a–c) more than 10 years ago. RSS has several advantageous when compared with conventional endoscopic surgical systems used in VATS. During the last 10 years, robotic systems are still developing that provide the thoracic surgeon with 7° of freedom of the instrumentation which allow to replicate the human wrist without tremor. This greater instrument maneuverability cannot be achieved with VATS procedure. RSS also provides three-dimensional view of the surgical site. As the RSS is a high-tech surgical tool, it is crucial to have dedicated team include experienced thoracic surgeons and nurses as well.

In 2002, preliminary results of RATS were published by Melfi FMA et al. [16]. Following these results, analysis of robotic lung resections were done in many studies (Table 11.2). Meyer et al. [17] in 2012, reported on robotic lobectomy performed in 185 consecutive patients. The mean operative time was 211 ± 60 min within the range 102–454 min. The rate of conversion to thoracotomy was 1.6 % due to bleeding from proximal pulmonary artery. Complications were seen in 31 patients (16.8 %). Mortality rate was 1.6 %. Two patients died of respiratory insufficiency and one patient died of cardiac arrest. Duration of hospital stay ranged from 2 to 21 days with a median of 4 days. In this study, authors concluded that operative time, mortality, and surgeon comfort were found to be key parameters for the learning curve of robotic lobectomy. The overall learning curve was 18 ± 3 cases.

Dylewski et al. [18] presented 200 consecutive patients who had robotic lung resection in between 2006 and 2010. Three patient required conversion to open procedure (1.5 %). Median operative time, median operating room time, and median docking time were 90 min (30–279), 175 min (82–370), and 12 min [6–20], respectively. The complication rate of this cohort was 26 % with 60-day mortality of 1.5 %. Median length of stay was 3 days (1–44). This study showed that robotic lung resection is technically feasible and able to be done with low morbidity and mortality.

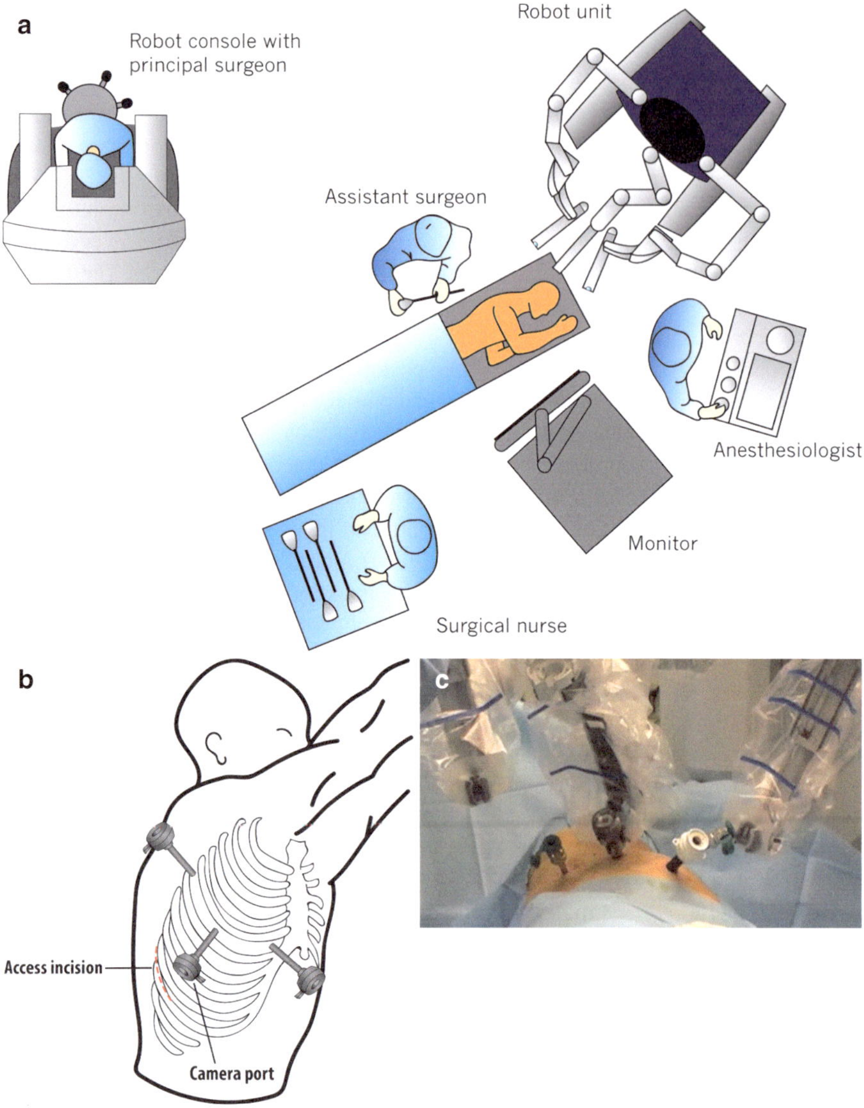

Fig. 11.4 (**a–c**) RSS setup and positions of ports for right-sided resections

Comparative studies between robotic approach and conventional thoracoscopic procedures or open techniques have been published in recent years. Cerfolio et al. [23], in 2011, presented a propensity matched analysis of 106 patients who underwent completely portal robotic lobectomy with 317 patients who had rib- and nerve-sparing thoracotomy for lobectomy. This study showed that there was no statistically difference in median number of mediastinal and hilar lymph nodes removed. In the robotic group, there were less blood loss (35 mL vs 90 mL; $P=0.03$), shorter chest

Table 11.2 Outcome of robotic lung resection

Author	Year	Patients (n)	Lob./seg. (n)	OT (min)	Conversion rate (%)	LHS (days)	Complication rate (%)	Mortality rate (%)
Nasir et al. [19]	2014	394	282/71	107	10 %	2	27	0.25
Park et al. [20]	2012	325	325	206	8 %	5	25	0.3
Toker et al. [21]	2015	100	54/46	104	4 %	5	24	2
Veronesi et al. [22]	2010	54	54/–	–	13 %	4.5	20	0

Lob lobectomy, *seg* segmentectomy, *OT* operation time, *LHS* length of hospital stay

tube duration (1.5 vs 3.0 days; $P<0.001$), and shorter hospital stay (2 days vs 4 days). In 2014, Lee et al. [24] reported the results of a total of 69 (35 robotic-34 VATS) patients who underwent minimally invasive lobectomy. When comparing two minimally invasive technique, there was no difference in the median operative time for lower lobectomies (140 vs 123 min); however, operative time for upper lobectomies in robotic group was significantly longer (172 vs 134 min, $p=0.001$).

The other most important concern about robotic lung resections is long-term oncologic outcome in patients with primary lung cancer. One of the largest experiences about long-term outcome after robotic lobectomy was published in 2012 by Park et al. [20]. In this retrospective multi-institutional review, a total of 325 consecutive patients who had robotic lobectomy for non-small cell lung cancer were analyzed. Overall morbidity rate was 25.2 %, and major complication rate was 3.7 % (12/325) with 5 days of median length of stay. In this cohort, pathologic stage distribution was 54 % (176) IA, 22 % (72) IB, 13 % (41) IIA, 5 % [15] IIB, and 6 % [21] IIIA. Median follow-up was 27 months. Overall 5-year survival was 80 %. According to the pathologic stages IA, IB, and II, 5-year survival was 91 %, 88 %, and 49 %, respectively. The authors of this study concluded that lobectomy with robotic approach is a feasible and oncologically sound surgical treatment option for non-small cell lung cancer.

Surgical Staging

Adequate surgical mediastinal and hilar lymph node (Figs. 11.2 and 11.3) assessment is crucial to obtain accurate stage in patient who had surgical treatment for non-small cell lung cancer (Fig. 11.5). Mediastinoscopy (Fig. 11.6) is one of the conventional surgical staging method used for obtaining mediastinal lymph node biopsies mainly include 2R, 2L, 4R, 4L, and 7. For the assessment of sub- and para-aortic nodes (number 5 and 6), extended mediastinoscopy is a surgical method of choice (Fig. 11.7). There are also two extensive techniques, video-assisted mediastinoscopic lymphadenectomy (VAMLA) – transcervical extended mediastinal lymphadenectomy (TEMLA) also referred as "supermediastinoscopies" [25]

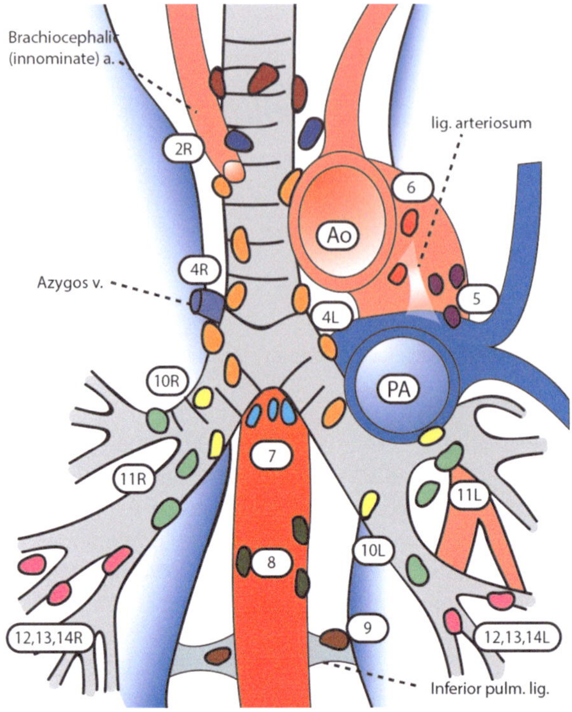

Fig. 11.5 Mediastinal-hilar lymph node map

(Fig. 11.8). Hürtgen developed VAMLA and published initial results in 2002 [26]. This technique is defined as the complete dissection of the whole fatty and lymphatic tissue of both paratracheal and the subcarinal area with bimanually dissection through advance mediastinoscope with spreadable blades. In this prospective study, 46 patients underwent VAMLA for non-small cell lung carcinoma. The mean total number of lymph nodes resected using VAMLA was 20.7 (SD 11.1, minimum 5, maximum 60). In one patient, a left-sided recurrent nerve palsy occurred.

Kim et al. [27] presented 649 consecutive patients who underwent VATS pulmonary resection for lung cancer in 2015. Among the group, 225 patients had VAMLA combined with VATS, and the other group (n:424) underwent VATS pulmonary resection only. There was significantly shorter operative time (116.8 ± 39.8 vs 159.8 ± 44.0 min; $P<0.001$), and more extensive lymph node dissection (total number of removed lymph nodes, 29.7 ± 10.8 vs 23.0 ± 8.6; $P<0.001$) in patients underwent VATS + VAMLA when compared with VATS group. Also, the patients in the VATS + VAMLA group tended to have higher rates of being upstaged with mediastinal involvement (8.0 vs 5.7 %; $P=0.31$).

Perioperative accurate staging is another critical aspect of treatment in non-small cell lung carcinoma. It is still under debate which of the resection guideline has to be followed for better survival. Guidelines from the American College of Surgeons Oncology Group (ACOSOG), the National Comprehensive Cancer Network (NCCN), and the International Association for the Study of Lung Cancer

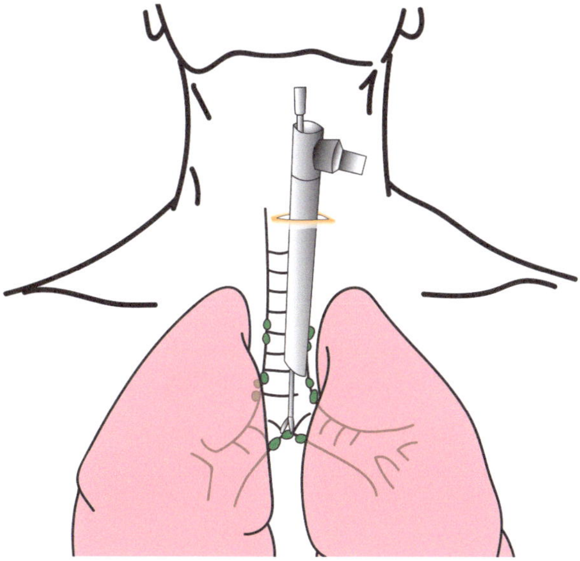

Fig. 11.6 Insertion of mediastinoscope through cervical incision

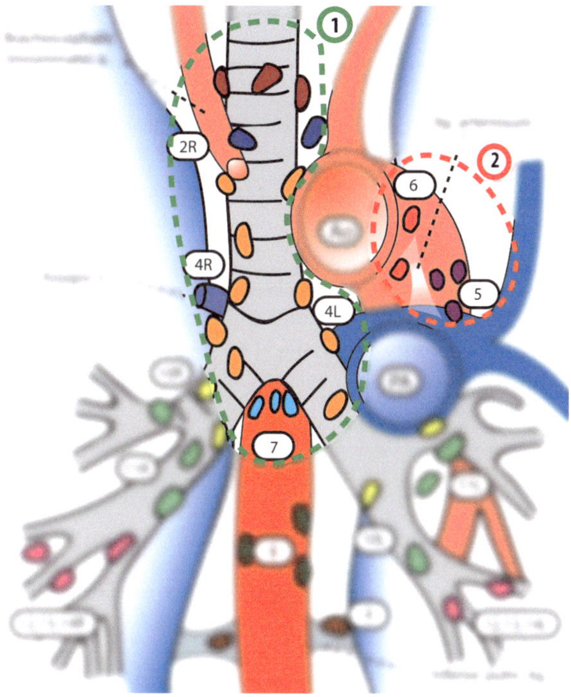

Fig. 11.7 Lymph node stations that can be reached with conventional mediastinoscopy (*1*) and extended mediastinoscopy (*2*)

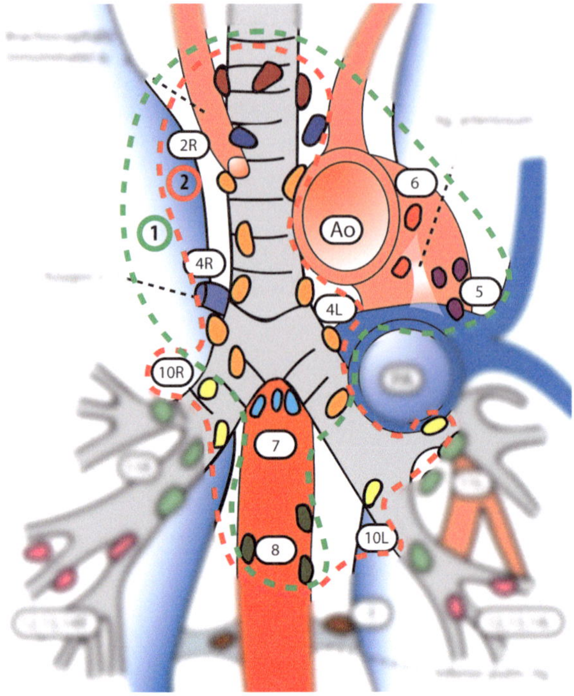

Fig. 11.8 Lymph node stations that can be reached with TEMLA (*1*) and VAMLA (*2*)

(IASLC) vary depending on the degree of lymph node sampling and resection [28–30].

Yue et al. [31], in 2014, reported on 2,711 patients who underwent surgical resection for non-small cell lung carcinoma. Univariate analysis and log-rank test showed that surgical resection following the guidelines proposed by the IASLC, NCCN, and ACOSOG trials was associated with higher cumulative overall survival rates (OS). Multivariate analysis revealed that there was a significant improvement in OS only when IASLC resection guidelines (complete resection) were followed ($p = 0.032$).

References

1. Falcoz PE, Puyraveau M, Thomas PA, Decaluwe H, Hürtgen M, Petersen RH, Hansen H, Brunelli A, ESTS Database Committee and ESTS Minimally Invasive Interest Group. Video-assisted thoracoscopic surgery versus open lobectomy for primary non-small-cell lung cancer: a propensity-matched analysis of outcome from the European Society of Thoracic Surgeon database. Eur J Cardiothorac Surg. 2016;49:602–9.
2. Boffa DJ, Allen MS, Grab JD, et al. Data from the Society of Thoracic Surgeons General Thoracic Surgery database: the surgical management of primary lung tumors. J Thorac Cardiovasc Surg. 2008;135:247–54.
3. Kirby TJ, Mack MJ, Landreneau RJ, Rice TW. Lobectomy. Video-assisted thoracic surgery versus muscle-sparing thoracotomy. A randomized trial. J Thorac Cardiovasc Surg. 1995;109:997–1001.

4. Sugi K, Kaneda Y, Esato K. Video-assisted thoracoscopic lobectomy achieves a satisfactory long-term prognosis in patients with clinical stage IA lung cancer. World J Surg. 2000;24:27–30.
5. Yim AP, Wan S, Lee TW, et al. VATS lobectomy reduces cytokine responses compared with conventional surgery. Ann Thorac Surg. 2000;70:243–7.
6. Erus S, Tanju S, Kapdagli M, Ozkan B, Dilege S, Toker A. The comparison of complication, pain, quality of life, and performance after lung resections with thoracoscopy and axillary thoracotomy. Eur J Cardiothorac Surg. 2014;46:619–09.
7. Whitson BA, Groth SS, Duval SJ, Swanson SJ, Maddaus MA. Surgery for early stage non-small cell lung cancer: a systematic review of the video-assisted thoracoscopic surgery versus thoracotomy approaches to lobectomy. Ann Thorac Surg. 2008;86:2008–16.
8. Muraoka M, Oka T, Akamine S, et al. Video-assisted thoracic surgery lobectomy reduces the morbidity after surgery for stage I non-small cell lung cancer. Jpn J Thorac Cardiovasc Surg. 2006;54:49–55.
9. Park JS, Kim K, Choi MS, et al. Video-assisted thoracic surgery lobectomy for pathologic stage non-small cell lung cancer: a comparative study with thoracotomy lobectomy. Kor J Thorac Cardiovasc Surg. 2011;44:32–8.
10. Flores RM, Park BJ, Dycoco J, et al. Lobectomy by video-assisted thoracic surgery (VATS) versus thoracotomy for lung cancer. J Thorac Cardiovasc Surg. 2009;138:11–8.
11. Cajipe MD, Chu D, Bakaeen FG, Casal RF, LeMarie SA, Coselli JS, Cornwell LD. Video-assisted thoracoscopic lobectomy is associated with better perioperative outcomes than open lobectomy in a veteran population. Am J Surg. 2012;204:607–12.
12. Stephens N, Rice D, Correa A, Hofstetter W, Mehran R, Roth J, Walsh G, Vaporciyan A, Swisher S. Thoracoscopic lobectomy is associated with improved short-term and equivalent oncological outcomes compared with open lobectomy for clinical stage I non-small-cell lung cancer: a propensity match analysis of 963 cases. Eur J Cardiothorac Surg. 2014;46:607–13.
13. Paul S, Altorki NK, Sheng S, Lee PC, Harpole DH, Onaitis MW, Stiles BM, Port JL, D'Amico TA. Thoracoscopic lobectomy associated with lower morbidity than open lobectomy: a propensity matched analysis from the STS database. J Thorac Cardiovasc Surg. 2010;139:366–78.
14. Farjah F, Wood DE, Mulligan MS, Krishnadasan B, Heagerty PJ, Symons RG, et al. Safety and efficacy of video-assisted versus conventional lung resection for lung cancer. J Thorac Cardiovasc Surg. 2009;137:1415–21.
15. Scott WJ, Allen MS, Darling G, Meyers B, Decker PA, Putnam JB et al. Video-assisted thoracic surgery versus open lobectomy for lung cancer: a secondary analysis of data from the American College of Surgeons Oncology Group Z0030 randomized clinical trial. J Thorac Cardiovasc Surg. 2010;139:976–81; discussion 981–3.
16. Melfi FMA, Menconi GF, Mariani AM, Angeletti CA. Early experience with robotic technology for thoracoscopic surgery. Eur J Cardiothorac Surg. 2002;21:864–8.
17. Meyer M, Gharagozloo F, Tempesta P, Margolis M, Strother E, Christenson D. The learning curve of robotic lobectomy. Int J Med Robot. 2012;8:448–52.
18. Dylewski MR, Ohaeto AC, ARNP, Pereira JF. Pulmonary resection using a total endoscopic robotic video-assisted approach. Semin Thorac Surg. 2011;23:36–42.
19. Nasir BS, Bryant AS, Minnich DJ, Wei B, Cerfolio RJ. Performing robotic obectomy and segmentectomy: cost, profitability and outcomes. Ann Thorac Surg. 2014;98:203–9.
20. Park BJ, Melfi F, Mussi A, Maisonneuve P, Spaggiari L, Da Silva RKC, Veronesi G. Robotic lobectomy for non-small cell lung cancer (NSCLC). Long-term oncologic results. J Thorac Cardiovasc Surg. 2012;143:383–9.
21. Toker A, Ozyurtkan MO, Kaba E, Ayalp K, Demirhan O, Uyumaz E. Robotic anatomic lung resections: the initial experience and description of learning in 102 cases. Surg Endosc. 2016;30:676–83.
22. Veronesi G, Galetta D, Maisonneuve P, Melfi F, Schmid RA, Borri A, Vannucci F, Spaggiari L. Four-arm robotic lobectomy for the treatment of early-stage lung cancer. J Thorac Cardiovasc Surg. 2010;140:19–25.

23. Cerfolio RJ, Byrant AS, Skylizard L, Minnich DJ. Initial consecutive experience of completely portal robotic pulmonary resection with 4 arms. J Thorac Cardiovasc Surg. 2011;142:740–6.
24. Lee BE, Korst RJ, Kletsman E, Rutledge JR. Transitioning from video-assisted thoracic surgical lobectomy to robotics for lung cancer: are there outcomes advantages? J Thorac Surg. 2014;147:724–9.
25. Rami-Porta R. Supermediastinoscopies: a step forward in lung cancer staging. J Thorac Oncol. 2007;4:355–6.
26. Hürtgen M, Friedel G, Toomes H, Fritz P. Radical video-assisted mediastinoscopic lymphadenectomy (VAMLA)-technique and first results. Eur J Cardiothorac Surg. 2002;21:348–51.
27. Kim HJ, Kim YH, Choi SH, Kim HR, Kim DK, Park SI. Video-assisted mediastinoscopic lymphadenectomy combined with minimally invasive pulmonary resection for left-sided lung cancer: feasibility and clinical impacts on surgical outcomes. Eur J Cardiothorac Surg. 2016;49:308–13.
28. Darling GE, Allen MS, Decker PA, Ballman K, Malthaner RA, Inculet RI, Jones DR, McKenna RJ, Landreneau RJ, Putnam Jr JB. Number of lymph nodes harvested from a mediastinal lymphadenectomy: results of the randomized, prospective American College of Surgeons Oncology Group Z0030 trial. Chest. 2011;139:1124–9.
29. NCCN Clinical Practice Guidelines in Oncology. Non-small cell lung cancer (v.2.2013). 2013. http://www.nccn.org/professionals/physician_gls/pdf/nscl.pdf. Accessed 2 July 2013.
30. Rami-Porta R, Wittekind C, Goldstraw P. International Association for the Study of Lung Cancer (IASLC) Staging Committee: complete resection in lung cancer surgery: proposed definition. Lung Cancer. 2005;49:25–33.
31. Yue D, Gong L, You J, Su Y, Zhang Z, Zhang Z, Gu F, Wang M, Wang C. Survival analysis of patients with non-small cell lung cancer who underwent surgical resection following 4 lung cancer resection guidelines. BMC Cancer. 2014;14:422.

Translational Research and Immunotherapy in Lung Cancer

12

Jonathan E. Schoenhals, Eric D. Brooks, Maria A. Cortez, Steven N. Seyedin, Sharareh Niknam, Xiaohong Wang, Alexandra P. Cadena, Xuan Shirley Li, Daniel R. Gomez, Zhongxing Liao, and James W. Welsh

Overview: Targeted Therapy for Lung Cancer

Lung cancer is a disease process often initiated by carcinogens from tobacco smoke. Chronic exposure to carcinogens over time is thought to prompt genetic changes in DNA that facilitate progression from a precancerous state to cancer formation and spread. Although tobacco smoke is by far the most common cause of lung cancer, lung cancer can also arise in individuals who have never smoked, and these cancers often involve aberrant driving mutations in the epidermal growth factor receptor (EGFR) [12].

J.E. Schoenhals • M.A. Cortez • S. Niknam • D.R. Gomez • Z. Liao, MD
J.W. Welsh, MD (✉)
Division of Radiation Oncology, The University of Texas MD Anderson Cancer Center, 1515 Holcombe Blvd, B24595, Unit 97, Houston, TX, USA
e-mail: jwelsh@mdanderson.org

E.D. Brooks
Department of Medicine, Memorial Sloan Kettering Cancer Center, 1275 York Avenue, New York, NY 10065, USA

S.N. Seyedin
Department of Radiation Oncology, University of Iowa Hospitals and Clinics, LL PFPW 200 Hawkins Dr, Iowa City, IA 52242, USA

X. Wang
Institute for Applied Cancer Science, The University of Texas MD Anderson Cancer Center, 1901 East Road, Houston, TX, USA

A.P. Cadena
Yale University,
New Haven, CT 06520, USA

X.S. Li
Biomedical Informatics at Molecular Match Inc., TMC X+ 220 2450 Holcombe Blvd, Houston TX 77021, USA

G. Ozyigit et al. (eds.), *Principles and Practice of Radiotherapy Techniques in Thoracic Malignancies*, DOI 10.1007/978-3-319-28761-4_12

EGFR is a transmembrane kinase receptor that becomes activated through interaction with its ligands EGF or transforming growth factor-alpha (TGFα). Activation of EGFR leads to downstream signaling via the PI3K/mTOR pathways, which in turn leads to transcription of genes that result in proliferation and malignant transformation. EGFR mutations are implicated in about 30 % of epithelial cancers and in about 15 % of non-small cell lung cancer (NSCLC). Information on drivers of carcinogenesis has prompted the development of targeted therapeutics such as small molecules or antibodies intended to target or halt signaling in these aberrant pathways. Erlotinib (Tarceva) has been approved by the US FDA for the treatment of NSCLC in three specific conditions: for patients with NSCLC, regardless of mutation status, that has been previously treated [189]; as maintenance therapy for patients with nonprogressing disease that had previously been treated with platinum-based chemotherapy [24]; and as upfront therapy for patients whose tumors have either an *EGFR* exon 19 deletion or an exon 21 L858R-activating mutation [84]. Mutations associated with the development of resistance to EGFR-targeted therapy have been studied extensively, and the overwhelming majority seem to be a T790M gatekeeper mutation in *EGFR*. Fortunately second- and third-generation EGFR-targeted therapies have been developed such as afatinib that seem to be effective against some of these resistance mutations [90].

The benefits of blocking kinase signaling pathways such as EGFR can also be enhanced by the use of other antitumor agents, particularly radiation. EGFR blockade has been shown to be an effective radiation sensitizer in several types of cancer, including that of the head and neck and lung (see "Clinical Relevance" below).

Another important driver of malignant transformation in lung cancer is ALK translocation. ALK is a kinase gene that is activated in about 3–5 % of lung cancers through fusion of *EML4* and *ALK*. This translocation is most common in lung adenocarcinoma and seems to be mutually exclusive of other mutations such as *EGFR* and *KRAS*. Crizotinib, a small-molecule ALK inhibitor that also targets ROS-1 and c-Met, was approved for second-line treatment of ALK-positive NSCLC based on results from a phase III trial demonstrating a 7.7-month benefit in progression-free survival from crizotinib versus a 3-month benefit from chemotherapy alone [154]. Although the response rate to crizotinib was high at 65 %, no difference in survival was seen between treatment groups. As is true of other kinase-targeted therapies, resistance to crizotinib often develops after 12–18 months of treatment, and second-generation ALK inhibitors are being tested in clinical trials for crizotinib-refractory disease.

Mutations in *KRAS* are present in about 15–30 % of patients with lung cancer and confer a poor prognosis. Historically few therapeutic strategies have been effective against *KRAS*-mutated lung cancer, but two new classes of therapeutic targets are showing some promise: cyclin-dependent kinase (CDK)-4 or CDK-6 inhibitors and MEK inhibitors. CDKs have key roles in regulating cell cycle progression. Acquisition of *KRAS* mutations leads to constitutive activation of the RAS-RAF-MEK-ERK pathway, leading to increased expression of CDK-4 and cyclin D1 [4]. The rationale is that CDK-4/CDK-6 inhibitors could produce a synthetic lethal interaction between *KRAS* oncogenes and CDK-4 [138]. Another way to exploit dependence on mitogen-activated protein kinase (MAPK) signaling would be to directly block the downstream substrate MEK. Small-molecule inhibitors of MEK (such as trametinib) are showing some clinical activity against *KRAS*-mutated tumors. As is true for other genes, mutation-specific variants can have significantly different responses to pathway inhibition [71]. Cancer with *KRAS* mutation G12C seems to respond better to MEK inhibitors and is biologically unique among variants [75].

More recently, tumor characterization has expanded beyond histologic analysis of tumor tissues for mutations in single pathways. Genomic profiling analysis, for example, can test hundreds of genes and millions of variants of potential functional significance. Given the difficulty of sorting through millions of potential variants, while keeping up with advances in treatment options for patients with multiple mutations, several services have arisen to offer patients and their oncologists the opportunity to match an individual's cancer with relevant therapeutic options. One such service, FoundationOne (www.foundationone.com), is a website sponsored by Foundation Medicine to help patients and their physicians identify the molecular growth drivers of the patient's cancer by analyzing large genomic panels. Other services make use of artificial intelligence decision support systems to help physicians make sense of the massive amounts of data needed to efficiently match patients to appropriate therapeutic options; MolecularMatch is another such tool, providing free access to databases of clinical trials and a service to match patients with appropriate trials.

Another advance that can greatly facilitate analysis of mutations as well as identify biomarkers to aid in diagnosis and choice of treatment is the ability to analyze circulating tumor DNA (ctDNA) in blood or urine samples. Although these panels were initially limited in terms of the numbers of mutations that could be analyzed, they are rapidly expanding to offer in-depth analyses that more closely match the characteristics of the tumor tissue itself. Although the sensitivity and specificity of many of these analyses have yet to be established, these so-called liquid tumor biopsies offer many advantages over the more invasive option of sampling lung tumor tissues, as described further in the paragraphs that follow.

Alternatives to Tumor Sampling: "Liquid Tumor Biopsies"

Sampling of bodily fluids for genetic testing has several advantages over solid tissue biopsies. Blood and urine are easier to access, abundant, conducive to serial sampling over time, and likely to contain metastatic clones from heterogeneous solid tumors [115]. Isolation and analysis of normal leukocytes also allows genetic profiles of tumors to be compared directly with normal genetic profiles, which enables filtering of patient-specific germline mutations [79]. Blood-based diagnostic tests targeting 68 genes are currently offered by Guardant Health in their Guardant360 test and by Personal Genome Diagnostics (PGDx) PlasmaSelect [7, 96]. PGDx also offers LungSelect, which is more sensitive (<0.2 %) but is limited to nine genes.

Another alternative to tumor sampling has been the characterization of circulating tumor cells (CTCs), an area of active research over the past decade. Unfortunately the rarity of CTCs has limited the broader application of this approach [19]. Several currently available diagnostic tests are based on isolating ctDNA, with analyses based on exomes and even platelets now in development [82]. In the United States, certification by the Clinical Laboratory Improvement Amendments is sufficient for laboratory-derived tests to be offered commercially, which has led to a crowded field of technologies and vendors. Before ctDNA isolation, blood cells and other components that may contribute to degradation or contamination of the ctDNA must be removed. The ctDNA can then be purified, amplified, and sequenced [150]. High-throughput methods of dilution or physically separating individual DNA molecules through beads (BEAMing) before amplification have significantly reduced signal-to-noise and error rates. At this time, technologies differ mainly in whether the amplification step is based on polymerase chain reaction (PCR) techniques (e.g., amplification refractory mutation system [ARMS], digital PCR) or integrated with the sequencing (e.g., CAPP-Seq Roche and TAm-Seq) [57, 123].

These advances have accelerated the development and adoption of blood- or urine-based diagnostic tests for monitoring mutations indicative of resistance to tyrosine kinase inhibitors like EGFR T790M or ALK L1196M [124, 134]. Concordance between the initial biopsy findings and ctDNA is an area of ongoing research because of tumor heterogeneity, but most studies have suggested that liquid biopsies may be more sensitive [141, 165]. Because liquid biopsies are designed to detect metastatic subclones, definitive concordance studies may need to be single-cell comparisons.

With regard to immunotherapy, liquid biopsies could be used to monitor treatment efficacy or disease progression by deep sequencing of the T-cell receptor (TCR) repertoire at the CDR3 locus [148]. For example, preliminary studies indicate that CTLA4 inhibition increases TCR diversity, whereas PD1 blockade stimulates TCR post-antigen engagement [31, 128].

Biomarkers of Toxicity: Single Nucleotide Polymorphisms and Radiation Pneumonitis

NSCLC is the most common type of lung cancer and is often diagnosed at advanced stages. The current standard of care for locally advanced NSCLC, for those who can tolerate it, is concurrent chemoradiation therapy. However, only 15–20 % of patients are rendered cancer-free by this treatment, in part because radiation doses must be limited to avoid causing radiation pneumonitis (RP), a severe, sometimes fatal inflammatory reaction of normal lung tissue. Because the radiation dose distribution to normal (undiseased) lung tissue in NSCLC treatment is known to affect the risk of RP, currently the risk of RP is minimized by keeping the mean dose to normal lung (MLD) and the normal lung volume exposed to at least 20 Gy (V_{20}) below certain limits [109]. Unfortunately, achieving these dosimetric limits forces reductions in the radiation dose to the tumor, eroding the probability of cure.

Individuals differ in their intrinsic sensitivity to radiation [11]; clinically, only a subset of patients with NSCLC treated with similar radiation dose distributions experience severe RP. Genetic variations in cellular signaling pathways may affect radiosensitivity and thereby risk of toxicity [39, 200]. The Genetic Predictors of Adverse Radiotherapy Effects (Gene-PARE) project reported positive associations between radiosensitivity and functional polymorphisms in genes involved in inflammation (e.g., *TGFβ1*) and in DNA double-strand break and base-excision repair (e.g., *XRCC1*, *XRCC3*) [71]. In clinical practice, standardized radiation doses are necessarily determined by the most sensitive patients because of the need to avoid lethal or disabling toxicity and because no way has yet been found to identify, before treatment, who will be at high risk of toxicity.

Yuan et al. discovered that patients with different genotypes of rs1982073:T869C in *TGFβ1* are at lower risk of RP after radiation therapy for NSCLC [197]. This association was independent of dosimetric factors such as V_{20} and MLD. Patients with the CT or CC genotype in *TGFβ1* rs1982073:T869C had a significantly lower incidence of severe RP than did those with the TT genotype, especially patients who had received an MLD <20 Gy or a V_{20} <30 %; indeed, this single nucleotide polymorphism (SNP) in *TGFβ1* was able to separate patients into different risk groups even after correction for MLD. These authors further found that the tumor necrosis factor-alpha (*TNFα*) 0629:308 G>A AA genotype was associated with severe RP, although the number of patients in that study was small [172]. Among four patients with the AA genotype, three (75 %) experienced severe RP versus 21 of 92 patients (23 %) with the AG/GG genotype. This difference was not accounted for by differences in MLD.

Other investigations have shown that functional polymorphisms of the base-excision repair genes *XRCC1* and *APEX1* and genetic variants of the nonhomologous end joining gene *LIG4* also predict the risk of RP, not only in whites but also in Han Chinese patients [102, 195, 196]. Our group further found that polymorphisms in vascular endothelial growth factor (VEGF) may modulate the risk of RP and that the CC genotype of *HSPB1* rs2868371 was associated with higher risk of severe RP [65, 129]. Subsequent analyses of patients treated with chemoradiation showed that XRCC1 Q399R=WW (versus PP or PW), VEGF4032 CT/TT, and TNF0629=AA all conferred higher risk of severe RP. Another gene, *ATM*, is a master regulator mediating DNA damage detection and repair. Patients carrying the *ATM* rs189037 variant AA genotype were at high risk of developing severe RP, particularly those receiving an MLD of ≥19.0 Gy [193]. Other SNPs associated with RP include oxidative stress genes including *MTHFR* (methylenetetrahydrofolate reductase; rs1801131, rs1801133, AA versus AC/CC) (hazard ratio [HR] for grade ≥2 RP=0.37, 95 % confidence interval [CI] 0.18–0.76, $P=0.006$, corrected $P=0.018$ and HR for grade ≥3 RP=0.21, 95 % CI 0.06–0.70, $P=0.01$, corrected $P=0.03$) [107]. Ethnic differences have also been noted in genotypes within the same gene and risk of RP [184, 193, 198].

Incorporating SNPs into predictive models such as the Lyman model has been shown to improve the model's ability to predict the likelihood of RP [172]. In one study, 16 potentially functional SNPs in genes related to DNA repair, cell cycling, TGF-β, TNF and TNFR, folic acid metabolism, and angiogenesis were genotyped from 143 patients. Five SNPs were selected for inclusion in a multivariate normal tissue complication probability model based on MLD alone. SNPs associated with an increased risk of severe RP were found in *TGFβ*, *VEGF*, *TNFα*, *XRCC1*, and *APEX1*. When smoking status was included in the multivariate model, the SNPs associated with increased risk of RP were found in *TGFβ*, *VEGF*, and *XRCC3*. The SNP that most significantly improved the fit of the Lyman model based on MLD alone was XRCC_NCI. Patients with XRCC_NCI=WW had an increased risk of RP, with a TD_{50} of 21.5 Gy versus 30.6 Gy for patients with the PP or PW genotype ($P=0.013$). Inclusion of the VEGF4039 SNP further improved the model ($P=0.035$), with the CT/TT genotypes conferring increased risk of RP. Patients with both XRCC_NCI=WW and VEGF4039=CT/TT had a TD_{50} of only 16.7 Gy, half that for patients with XRCC_NCI=PP/PW and VEGF4039=CC (33.8 Gy). Further improvement was noted with inclusion of TNF0629=AA as a risk factor ($P=0.048$), but only four patients had this genotype. The SNP previously identified by our group as being associated with increased risk of RP, TGFB073=TT, was marginally significant when included in the model containing XRCC_NCI and VEGF4039 ($P=0.064$) or XRCC_NCI, VEGF4039, and TNF0629 ($P=0.071$) [172]. These findings provide evidence that SNPs can significantly improve the predictive ability of the Lyman MLD model. Even with a small number of SNPs, it was possible to distinguish cohorts with >50 % risk versus <10 % risk of RP when they were exposed to high MLDs [172].

Next, to provide proof of principle, a virtual clinical study was done using the SNPs from the study reported by Tucker et al. [178]. The prescribed radiation dose for each patient was scaled according to normal tissue constraints. The conventional dose-volume constraints for the spinal cord, esophagus, and heart and a personalized iso-complication MLD limit from a mathematical prediction model were used. The difference between the model-determined prescribed dose and the dose originally prescribed for 32 patients was then compared. The original dose-volume values for the spinal cord, esophagus, and heart exceeded the dose-volume limits imposed for the study (before the model-determined MLD limit being applied), because at the time of treatment the clinician chose to exceed the dose-volume constraints in the hopes of better tumor control. This simulation study was performed both with and without patients who had exceeded dose-volume constraints (before the MLD being applied), because including the 32 patients provides a clinically realistic scenario, whereas excluding them helped to isolate the effect of the personalized MLD limit. The original prescribed tumor dose was then scaled (with no change in beam orientation) based on the model-determined MLD limit and other treatment planning parameters. If all dose-volume parameters were below the applied limits, the dose could be escalated; conversely, if one of the parameters exceeded the limits, the dose needed to be lowered. The model predicted that, for most of the patients who developed RP, the prescribed doses needed to be reduced using the model based on SNPs, and the difference in prescribed dose exceeded the clinically significant value of 5 Gy [178].

If these SNP findings can be verified with independent patient groups, the changes to prescribed doses illustrated in this study would be expected to reduce toxicity in some patients and help to push the prescribed dose to the maximum tolerable value. However, independent validation of these findings has been challenging, because of differences in endpoints, patient populations, and toxicity scoring criteria [180, 184]. For this reason, the National Cancer Institute National Human Genome Research Institute Working Group on Replication in Association Studies has published a comprehensive set of guidelines that include important points to consider in reporting (and evaluating) initial genotype-phenotype findings and in designing positive replication studies [35].

In summary, SNPs can be used as genetic markers to screen for known (and unknown) genetic variants in a given region of a specific gene. These preliminary reports of using SNPs as predictive biomarkers for the risk of radiation-induced normal tissue toxicity suggest that this approach has the potential to guide clinical decisions. “Big data” with objective and consistent measurements of endpoints and tightly controlled variables are needed to validate these findings and to prospectively test the models developed in clinical settings.

Biomarkers of Response to Therapy: MicroRNAs

Another emerging method for detecting response to therapy is the detection of microRNAs. In 1993, Victor Ambros [98] and Gary Ruvkun [190] discovered during a study of *C. elegans* development that LIN-14 protein abundance was regulated by a small RNA product encoded by the *lin-4* gene. It was not until 2000, when another small RNA, *let-7*, was identified and found to be conserved in many species [131, 144] that a new layer of complexity in the regulation of gene expression was unveiled. The discovery of the posttranscriptional silencing of target messenger RNAs [55] by these small RNAs was a revolutionary step in the understanding of genetic information control. Further studies provided evidence that these small RNAs are members of a large class of tiny noncoding RNAs of approximately 22 nucleotides known as microRNAs (miRNAs), which regulate most of the genes in the human genome [101]. miRNAs are strongly conserved among vertebrates, invertebrates, and plants [6], and most are transcribed from individual miRNA genes, introns or exons of protein-coding genes, or the polycistronic transcripts that encode miRNAs involved in interconnected molecular pathways [99]. Biogenesis of miRNA involves maturation of miRNA precursors, assembly of the mature miRNA into microprocessor complexes, and regulating the expression of protein-coding genes by degrading or blocking translation of messenger RNA targets [13]. Because a single miRNA can target hundreds of mRNAs and because miRNAs are involved in virtually all biologic processes, aberrant miRNA expression is involved in the initiation of many diseases, including cancer. Genome-wide miRNA expression profiling studies using high-throughput techniques have shown that almost all types of cancer present a specific profile of upregulated and downregulated miRNAs and a global reduction in miRNA expression [106]. Exosomes containing miRNAs have been found not only in blood [160] but in other types of body fluids such as saliva [111]. Exosomes represent a newly discovered mechanism by which donor cells can communicate and influence the gene expression of recipient cells. Growing evidence indicates that *exosomal miRNA packaging occurs nonrandomly based on differential expression of exosomal miRNA compared with that of donor cells* [174]. Indeed, recent studies have demonstrated that nearly 30 % of miRNAs released in vitro and in vivo do not reflect the expression profile found in donor cells, suggesting that specific miRNAs are selected to be intracellularly retained or released by exosomes [81]. The secretion of oncogenic miRNAs by tumor cells is associated with their ability to influence the local and distant environment to facilitate tumor progression, metastasis [133], and tumor immunity [147]. Tumor-secreted miRNA targeting of immune cells and the immune system have been shown in several studies to represent an active pathway for tumor immune evasion.

These findings have led to exploration of the use of miRNAs and exosomes as biomarkers of response to therapy or as a therapeutic approach themselves. Clinical studies suggest that miRNAs can be used to predict sensitivity to radiation therapy and anticancer agents [119]. For example, the loss of heterozygosity in miR-128b, an EGFR regulator, was found to correlate with response to the EGFR inhibitor gefitinib in patients with relapsed NSCLC [186]. Recently, various strategies for restoring miRNA function have yielded the first miRNA replacement therapeutic in the clinical pipeline: MRX34, an intravenously injected liposome-formulated miR-34 mimic with a diameter of ~120 nm, which is now in clinical trials for patients with advanced or metastatic liver cancer. Preclinical studies have shown that tail-vein injection of MRX34 reduced tumor growth and enhanced survival, with a favorable safety profile, in orthotopic mouse models of hepatocellular carcinoma [53, 85, 86, 117]. We showed that therapeutic delivery of MRX34 downregulated tumor PDL1 expression. Moreover, giving MRX34 in combination with radiation increased CD8+ cell numbers "while reducing PD1 expression on these T-cells" and delivery of miR-34a has been shown to reduce the numbers of radiation-induced macrophages and T-regulatory cells (Tregs) (*J Natl Cancer Inst* 2015, PMID 26577528, doi 10.1093/jnci/dv303). Collectively, these findings suggest that combining immunoregulatory miRNAs with immunotherapy could be a powerful therapeutic approach. However, larger prospective clinical trials are needed to validate the previous results, since most published studies had relatively small sample sizes and lack information on long-term outcomes. Further studies are also needed to establish a well-characterized panel of exosomal miRNAs specific to each type of tumor, disease stage (early or advanced), response to treatment, outcomes, and recurrence.

Immunotherapy for Lung Cancer

How Tumors Evade the Immune System

Traditional methods for treating lung cancer are resection, targeted radiation therapy, or chemotherapy. However, recent findings have illuminated the potential power of immunotherapy, which we believe will help to move healthcare toward personalized medicine. Other exciting approaches involve combining radiation therapy with therapies targeted to specific immune pathways used by many lung tumors to escape the patient's immune system, particularly the antitumor T-cells.

Precancerous cells are likely produced on a regular basis; fortunately, most are rapidly detected and destroyed by the host's immune system. This raises the question, why do we get cancer at all? For a cancerous cell to survive and expand, it must gain several unique properties, such as unchecked proliferation and the ability to resist and overcome hypoxia through stimulation of angiogenesis. Tumor cells must also learn how to evade host immunity so that they can proliferate and expand. Moreover, the fact that cancer cells are derived from and share significant overlap with normal cells further complicates the ability of the immune system to identify and destroy malignant cells. Cancer cells develop several unique mechanisms under selective pressure to facilitate immune evasion. One such mechanism is for a tumor cell to modify itself, for example, by overexpressing PDL1, which can blunt to T-cell responses. Tumor cells can also evade immune detection by downregulating the major histocompatibility complex (MHC) receptors required for antigen presentation and by suppressing the penetration of T-cells into the tumor. Cytokines produced by tumors can also profoundly influence the negative regulatory cell populations in the tumor and stroma, which can affect the ratio of M1/M2 myeloid cells and increase the proportions of inhibitory myeloid-derived suppressor cells (MDSCs) and regulatory T-cells (Tregs). Finally, as tumors grow, they tend to develop a hypoxic center, which itself has unique ways of blunting immune responses. The secretion of factors such as VEGF by hypoxic tumors can also contribute to blunting an immune response.

Ironically, many of the kinase-driven signaling pathways mentioned above (e.g., EGFR and ALK) can serve as unique tumor antigens for distinguishing tumor from self, which is needed to mount an effective immune response. Many of these kinase mutations can contribute to immune escape. For example, some tumor cell lines that are resistant to EGFR-targeting drugs like erlotinib have unregulated PD1 expression [37]. Resistance to other kinases such as c-Met has also implicated PD1 in other pathways of resistance. Our laboratory recently discovered a mechanism by which P53 mutations lead to overexpression of PD1 as mediated through loss of microRNA34a (JNCI PMID 26577528).

Targeting PD1/PDL1

One signaling pathway currently under intense investigation is PD1/PDL1. PD1/PDL1 is an immune checkpoint that is normally involved in cell-mediated immunity via T-cells; upregulation of PD1/PDL1 by tumors can create an immunosuppressive environment in which cancer cells can thrive. PD1 (programmed cell death-1) in particular has crucial roles in the immune system; it is found on virtually all types of immune cells, including B cells, NK-cells, T-cells, dendritic cells, and macrophages [169]. The two ligands related to PD1, PDL1 and PDL2, are expressed by different cell types, including tumor cells [169].

Early studies of the PD1/PDL1 pathway focused on treatments for autoimmune diseases such as rheumatoid arthritis. The premise was that the negative signal transmitted by PD1, which ultimately blocks the production of T-cells, could be exploited in conditions in which overproduction of T-cells was detrimental to patients' health. Now this pathway is being exploited in a different way for the treatment of cancer.

Tumors interact with the immune system "and evade its effects" in a variety of ways. Tumor antigens on the surface of tumor cells trigger the recruitment of antigen-presenting cells (APCs), which ultimately prime T-cells to attack the tumor. Unfortunately, tumors can make use of feedback systems, such as the PD1/PDL1 checkpoint, to evade such attacks [116]. Consequently, the abundance of PD1 and PDL1 typically suppresses the production of tumor-infiltrating lymphocytes and generally confers a poor prognosis. In addition to facilitating tumor immune escape, the PD1/PDL1 pathway also participates in the differentiation of Tregs so as to promote their immune-suppressive function [116]. Induction of PD1 expression can also suppress B-cell activation and interleukin-8 (IL-8) production, which in turn blocks NK-cell function. The race to find therapies that specifically target PD1/

PDL1 is intense because PDL1 expression can be activated by various oncogenic signaling pathways (e.g., interferon [IFN], Stat3, MYD88) and thus serves as a gateway for potential immunotherapies [116].

Targeting TGFβ

TGFβ is a member of a cytokine superfamily that includes activins, inhibins, nodals, bone morphogenetic proteins (BMPs), anti-Müllerian hormone or Müllerian-inhibiting factor, and a variety of growth and differentiation factors [130]. A multifunctional polypeptide, TGFβ, regulates a broad variety of processes including immune function, proliferation, differentiation, adhesion, migration, and the epithelial-mesenchymal transition (Fig. 12.1). Each of the four known isotypes (e.g., TGFβ1, TGFβ2, TGFβ3, and TGFβ5) has different functions.

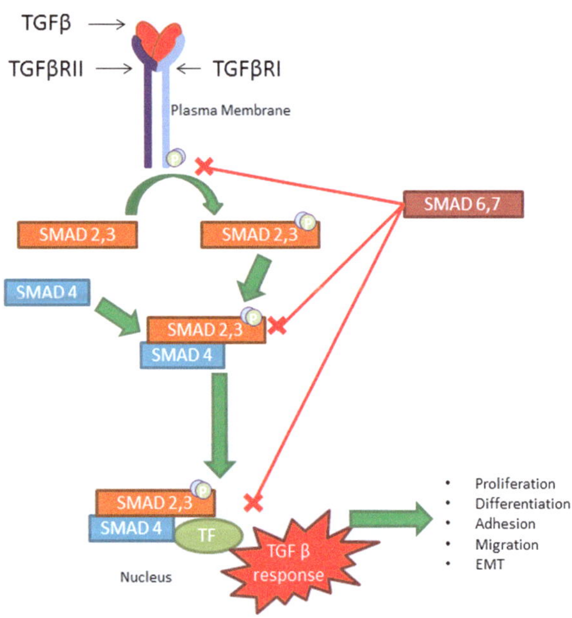

Fig. 12.1 *TGFβ signaling*. As shown to the right, TGFβ signaling begins when TGFβ binds to its receptors TGFβRI or TGFβRII; phosphorylation of TGFβRI regulates SMAD2/SMAD3, which in turn binds to SMAD4, causing the translocation of SMAD2/SMAD3 and other transcription factors from the cytoplasm to the nucleus. Inhibitory SMADs (SMAD6/SMAD7) inhibit SMAD2/SMAD3 and other transcription factors. Regulation of miRNAs also directly affects SMAD2/SMAD3 and regulates posttranscriptional factors for TGFβ response

TGFβ and the Immune System

TGFβ suppresses T-cell proliferation, induces B-cell apoptosis, and hinders B-cell proliferation and IgA secretion. TGFβ further inhibits the function of NK-cells by suppressing NK-cell-mediated production of IFNγ, which is necessary for NK-cell tumor-killing activity through transcriptional effects of SMAD3 on the IFNγ promoter. In general, the immunosuppressive effects of TGFβ result from its weakening the antitumor functions of CD8+ T-cells, CD4+ T-cells, and dendritic cells and can affect immune cell differentiation by blocking key "cytotoxic program" proteins such as perforin, granzymes, and cytotoxins. TGFβ further blocks the development of type I macrophages and neutrophils, but upholds type II macrophages and neutrophils, which have reduced effector functions but produce large amounts of anti-inflammatory molecules such as IL-6, IL-11, and TGFβ [3].

TGFβ, Lung Cancer, and Radiation Therapy

TGFβ has complex dual functions in that it acts as a tumor suppressor in early stages of tumor progression but in later stages is associated with metastatic invasion and immune evasion. As a result, TGFβ controls various critical factors in tumor progression like proliferation, apoptosis, and equilibrium [118]. Although most lung cancer cells secrete TGFβ, malignant transformation often results in loss of its tumor-suppressive effects, which has been linked with tumor development and progression in several types of cancer. In lung cancer, overexpression of TGFβ has been linked with better 5-year survival rates [78]; however, others have found TGFB1 protein levels to be negatively correlated with prognosis in NSCLC [46, 175]. Radiation activates TGFβ via the induction of reactive oxygen species (ROS), which is thought to enhance tumor cell radioresistance. Radiation has been shown to increase serum TGFβ1 levels, and, as noted previously, SNPs in *TGFβ1* have been associated with risk of RP after radiation therapy for NSCLC.

Immunotherapy and the Abscopal Effect

In 1953, RH Mole first reported the occurrence of an unexpected, systemic regression of tumor metastases when localized radiation was given to a primary tumor [114]. Mole termed the "abscopal" effect, derived from the Latin prefix *ab* ("position away from") and the Greek suffix *scopos* ("the target"). During the decades since that time, a few isolated reports of systemic responses to localized radiation have appeared, but only in the past 10 years has this phenomenon begun to be explored in clinical trials. Abscopal effects occurring after radiation therapy are now thought to be mediated by the immune system; because such effects can be greatly enhanced by immunotherapy agents, this offers a powerful new treatment option for a variety of cancers, including NSCLC.

Evading Immune Surveillance

As noted previously, the surveillance functions of the innate and adaptive immune systems normally recognize and eradicate tumor cells that arise from unavoidable and naturally occurring DNA damage throughout an individual's lifetime [25, 26, 191]. However, during neoplastic progression, tumor cells can evade detection and destruction by the adaptive immune system in several ways. One is by down-regulating MHC1 receptors, which make the tumor invisible to antitumor CD8+ lymphocytes [36, 59, 170]. Another is through attracting immunosuppressive MDSCs, tumor-associated macrophages, and Tregs to the tumor microenvironment, which then release factors that conceal the tumor from the immune system and suppress immune function (e.g., IL-6, CSF1, TGF-β, Fig. 12.2) [43, 58, 132, 149, 158, 167]. A third method is for the tumor to express cytotoxic cell death receptors on the tumor cell surface (e.g., PD1/PDL1) that kill antitumor cytotoxic T lymphocytes when they come in contact with the tumor [50, 199]. When these and other evasive tumor changes occur, tumor cells are, under certain circumstances, able to elude the immune system to the point that the tumor advances to significant disease [51, 52, 151].

Radiation and the Immune System

Radiation affects the ability of tumor cells to evade immune destruction by acting as a sort of tumor-specific, in vivo "vaccine" that allows re-recognition of the hidden tumor mass and penetration of immune cells into the tumor cell environment, thereby prompting resurrection of the necessary antitumor response [47]. Radiation also has been found to prompt expression of MHC1 receptors and calreticulin on the tumor cell surface, which make the tumor cells visible to dendritic cells and macrophages that can then consume them and present tumor cell antigens to CD8+ lymphocytes to mount an attack (Fig. 12.2) [125, 145]. Radiation improves the immune system's ability to recognize the tumor by releasing previously hidden tumor-associated antigens (TAAs) and kills tumor cells in a way that releases compounds from within tumor cells that activate the immune system (Fig. 12.2) (e.g., ATP, HMGB1, uric acid, heat shock proteins) and lead to maturation of dendritic cells for T-cell activation [9, 60, 156, 163]. Finally, radiation allows activated immune cells back into the tumor environment by (1) altering the vascular endothelium of tumor blood vessels so as to increase expression of intercellular cellular adhesion molecules and (2) causing the release of chemokines that attract and allow extravasation of immune cells into the tumor bed (Fig. 12.2) [67]. Ultimately, radiation-induced changes in tumors, including release of TAAs and immune-stimulatory signals, cause a local tumor immune response that would not be possible without the radiation. This response and invasion of a locally irradiated tumor site leads to a system-wide antitumor response as TAAs released at the primary site are

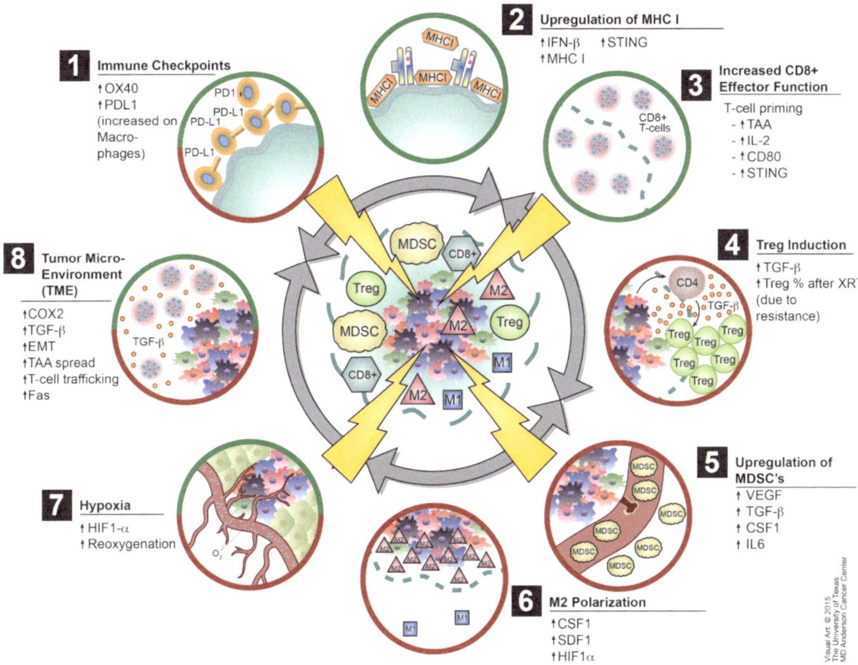

Fig. 12.2 Radiation has multiple effects on the tumor microenvironment. *1* PDL1 increases on tumor-associated macrophages (TAMs), and OX40 expression on various immune cell subsets increases (our unpublished data). *2* MHC I is upregulated via the type I IFN pathway. *3* Lymphocyte priming is increased and there is increased activation at the tumor site. *4* Higher Treg percentages are seen, possibly due to Treg radioresistance. *5* MDSC's are recruited to the tumor site through CSF1 and TGF-β secretion by the tumor. Additionally, IL-6 and TGF-β are important for MDSC survival once at the irradiated site. *6* TAMs are polarized to M2 phenotype after radiation due to CSF1 and SDF1 secretion by the tumor. HIF1a expression also causes this repolarization. *7* HIF1a is upregulated after radiation, even though there is increased oxygenation to the tumor site. *8* Various immunosuppressive factors are increased at and around the tumor site after radiation. This includes COX2 and TGF-β, which can lead to enhanced EMT. However, there is increased tumor-associated antigen spread, T-cell trafficking, and Fas expression

recognized at areas of distant disease. Therefore, immune activation at the locally irradiated site can lead to regression and resolution of distant, nonirradiated masses as well as locally treated tumor masses.

Enhancing the Abscopal Effect by Combining Radiation with Immunotherapy

Despite its effects on unveiling and TAA release, radiation therapy alone is only weakly immunogenic and only rarely produces an abscopal effect. The abscopal effect was originally reported in patients with leukemia or lymphoma after splenic or visceral irradiation [8, 74, 142]. However, during the past few decades, reports of this rare phenomenon have increased, with abscopal effects reported in solid tumors such as melanoma [127, 137], breast cancer [112], adenocarcinoma [143], hepatocellular carcinoma [121, 126], Merkel cell carcinoma [40], renal cell cancer [77], cervical cancer [166], and NSCLC. Reasons for this increased frequency and for the growing interest in reports of abscopal effects lie in part in the advent and wider implementation of novel immunotherapy checkpoint inhibitors in the treatment of solid tumors.

Three Phases of Immune Activation for an Abscopal Effect

Preclinical and clinical studies have shown that inducing a successful abscopal response requires at least three phases of clinical immune activation. First, the release of previously hidden tumor antigens is required for the immune system to initially detect the tumor to be targeted. Environmental changes within the tumor itself are also required so that the antigens that are released can be taken up by APCs and presented to CD8+ effector lymphocytes to stimulate an initial activating response. As discussed above, these initial steps are accomplished through radiation-induced changes to the tumor microenvironment and the release of TAAs (i.e., the "battering ram" and "release" phenomena).

Second, the population of activated CD8+ cytotoxic T-cells directed against the various released TAAs must expand sufficiently to mount a body-wide response to distant areas of disease sharing the same antigenic signature. This is now being accomplished through one or more immune-stimulatory agents administered around the time of radiation (e.g., Toll-like receptor [TLR] agonists, dendritic cell injections, granulocyte-macrophage colony-stimulating factor [GM-CSF], or checkpoint inhibitors). Two of the most commonly reported agents used for this purpose are the checkpoint inhibitors anti-CTLA4 and anti-PD1 antibodies. Briefly, CTLA4, a potent inhibitory receptor on the surface of T-cells that interacts with CD80 on the surface of APCs to prevent co-stimulation or activation, functions to naturally prevent a permanent immune response once immune activation has begun [183]. However, inhibiting CTLA4 leads to fervent activation of the immune system and clinically significant destruction of tumor burden. Theoretically, antibodies to these inhibitory proteins (CTLA4 and PD1/PDL1) would lead to increased immune activation, and their use for patients receiving radiation has led to numerous abscopal responses, as the cytotoxic T lymphocyte populations directed against the TAAs after radiation are expanded via increased activation after administration of these two potent immunostimulatory therapies (i.e., "army expansion").

Third, preserving a pool of cytotoxic T-cells after activation is probably necessary to achieve a sustained, long-term, and successful attack on distant tumor sites that would lead to resolution of disease. Essentially, the argument is that radiation plus a single immunotherapeutic agent is not sufficient because tumor cells continue to express immune-inhibitory signals or adapt to express new ones that can blunt or abort an initiated abscopal response [44, 69, 173]. Thus after the initial delivery of radiation and a single immunotherapy agent, a second agent (e.g., anti-PD1) should be incorporated to sustain the immune response at distant sites so as to complete the abscopal effect (i.e., "keeping troops deployed"). This process is called immune "reinvigoration," and it is only now being studied in relation to the induction and sustainment of an abscopal effect. An important aspect of this third step, however, is that dual checkpoint immunotherapy may be necessary to achieve abscopal response on a grand scale in clinical practice, and to this end numerous phase III studies of radiation plus dual checkpoint therapy are currently underway. Questions also remain as to the optimal timing of radiation with immunotherapy (whether the sequence should be concurrent, preceding, or successive), appropriate radiation fractionation and dose, and the location and number of sites that require irradiation to optimize response. So far, preclinical and case study findings suggest that hypofractionated radiation to visceral lesions may provide the best outcomes [49].

Abscopal Effects in NSCLC

New evidence suggests that NSCLC is more immunogenic than was previously thought, and two case reports have been published describing abscopal effects in NSCLC. The first involved a 78-year-old woman who received stereotactic ablative radiation therapy (SABR) for NSCLC in a right lower-lobe primary and 60 Gy in 30 fractions to a left upper-lobe primary. At 70 days after treatment of the right-lobe lesion, the disease had progressed to involve the bone and adrenal glands. At 12 months, however, testing showed a complete metabolic response (resolution) in all sites of previously abnormal uptake of fluorodeoxyglucose (FDG), a result attributed to a delayed abscopal response to the SABR [159]. The second case was a 64-year-old man with stage IV NSCLC that continued to progress despite initial treatment with six cycles of pemetrexed/carboplatin and subsequent radiation to 59.4 Gy to the lymph nodes, hilum, and mediastinum. The cancer spread to the liver and bones and continued to progress after additional rounds of chemotherapy. At that point, a palliative radiation dose (30 Gy to the most metabolically active liver metastasis) with concurrent immunotherapy (ipilimumab) produced drastic regression of disease burden. The patient was without evidence of disease (per RECIST criteria) at 1 year after the concurrent radiation and immunotherapy [63].

In addition to these two case reports, a recent proof-of-principle study evaluating abscopal effects in solid tumors demonstrated that 4 of 18 patients with NSCLC (22 %) experienced a partial or a complete abscopal response after receiving GM-CSF and concurrent radiation, with a partial abscopal effect defined as a decrease of at least 30 % in the longest diameter of the best-responding lesion [62]. These promising preliminary findings have led to several ongoing trials to evaluate abscopal effects in NSCLC.

Although abscopal effects are rare, interest is growing in determining how to increase their frequency. Clinical studies are currently underway to assess and optimize the use of combined radiation and new-age immunobiologics. The abscopal effect offers the exciting possibility of transforming radiation therapy—once considered strictly local therapy—into an effective systemic treatment.

Radiation Therapy and the Tumor Microenvironment

The advent of immunotherapy has underscored the importance of clarifying the positive and negative effects of radiation and the immune system on the tumor microenvironment. As noted previously, radiation has many positive effects, aside from direct cell killing, on the tumor microenvironment and the immune system: radiation increases antigen presentation, T-cell priming, T-cell activation, and T-cell trafficking (Fig. 12.2). However, radiation can also influence pathways that impair immune responses via recruitment of Tregs, MDSCs, or tumor-associated macrophages; polarization of M2 macrophages; and upregulation of hypoxia-inducible factors (HIFs). Various methods must be considered to target and overcome these problems without interfering with the antitumor immune response.

Regulatory T-Cell Radioresistance

Tregs have been well studied with regard to their role in immune suppression. This subset of CD4+ T-helper cells express the transcription factor Foxp3 and are heavily involved in immune regulation at various sites throughout the body. Although radiation effectively kills tumor cells, it also kills immune cell populations present at the tumor site. The relative radioresistance of Tregs cause higher proportions of Tregs at tumor sites after radiation [22, 80, 93]. However, the numbers of Tregs still decline in response to radiation, even though their relative percentage among the lymphocyte population increases [140]. Some studies have shown increased numbers of circulating Tregs after radiation and that those Tregs are highly immunosuppressive [15, 139, 152]. The magnitude of the effect that these Tregs have at the tumor site after radiation remains unclear; however, two preclinical studies thus far have shown synergy between radiation and Treg depletion" (Bos et al 2013 "Transient regulatory T-cell ablation deters oncogene-driven breast cancer and enhances radiotherapy", and Son et al 2015 "Combination effect of regulatory T-cell depletion and ionizing radiation in mouse models of lung and colon cancer.

Recruitment of MDSCs After Radiation Therapy

MDSCs are immature myeloid cells that are highly immunosuppressive. "Recruitment of MDSCs to the tumor" was recently shown to vary was recently shown to vary depending on fractionation, with the suggestion that stereotactic doses may be better for controlling the influx of MDSCs to the tumor [54]. However, this probably depends on the type of cancer, as another group showed an influx of myeloid cells after 20 Gy in the FaDu xenograft nasopharyngeal cancer model [2]. The mechanism by which this recruitment/influx is thought to occur is through increased levels of colony-stimulating factor 1 (CSF1), which is upregulated after radiation and acts as a chemokine for MDSCs, encouraging them to travel to the tumor site [194].

Recruitment of Tumor-Associated Macrophages and M2 Polarization of Macrophages After Radiation Therapy

Macrophages are an important part of the innate immune system and help to clear cellular debris, respond to extracellular stimuli, and dictate the direction of an immune response. Macrophages are polarized into general types, M1 or M2. M1 macrophages promote anti-tumor immune responses and M2 macrophages promote tumor growth and protection [176]. Like MDSCs, tumor-associated macrophages are recruited to tumor sites after radiation via CSF1 secretion or by HIF-1a-dependent secretion of stromal cell-derived factor 1 (SDF1), which binds to CXCR4 [30]. Both of these mechanisms are involved in migration of macrophages to the tumor site. However, because tumor-associated macrophages are already present at the tumor site and are typically M2 polarized, radiation tends to push even more macrophages toward the M2 phenotype.

Upregulation of Hypoxia-Inducing Factors After Radiation Therapy

HIFs can respond quickly to decreases in oxygen concentration. Under normoxic conditions, they are quickly degraded in proteasomes. However, as oxygen levels drop, these factors are stabilized and relocate to the nucleus, where they become transcriptionally active. HIFs lead to enhanced angiogenesis, proliferation, and invasion of the tumor [83]. Traditionally, larger, hypoxic tumors require higher doses of radiation to produce antitumor effects. Hypoxia confers resistance to radiation because less oxygen is available for the creation of ROS. Also, radiation leads to upregulation of HIF1a by the tumor despite enhanced oxygenation, which can exert pro-tumorigenic effects [113].

As discussed in the previous sections and illustrated graphically in Fig. 12.2, radiation activates the immune system in several ways. By using combination therapies to target negative side effects, we expect to tip the scale in favor of complete tumor rejection and immune memory thereafter, with the ultimate goal of producing complete cures.

Clinical Relevance: Non-Small Cell Lung Cancer

Targeted Therapies

Two general categories of clinical trials were ongoing when this chapter was written: those that are genetically based and those that focus on reactivation of the immune system. Future trials are likely to involve combinations of these two approaches. Given that the local or regional therapeutic options for thoracic tumors have been around for quite some time, many trials now are focusing on resistance to kinase inhibitors and evaluating second- and third-generation kinase inhibitors that may be susceptible to some mechanisms of resistance but may also be less toxic. Interestingly, mechanisms of resistance to kinase pathways such as EGFR may not overlap with mechanisms of resistance to immune checkpoint inhibitors, and as such therapeutic combinations of kinase inhibitors and checkpoint inhibitors are being pursued with great interest.

EGFR Inhibitors

EGFR inhibitors such as gefitinib (Iressa) and erlotinib (Tarceva) were the first personalized therapeutics to be approved for the treatment of lung cancer, and as such they have been the most thoroughly studied. Although initial responses to these agents can be quite dramatic in some patients, most will develop progression because of the development of resistance within a few months and in many cases that resistance arises from a T790M mutation in *EGFR*. Second- or third-generation tyrosine kinase inhibitors are being developed in the hopes of overcoming this resistance. At this time, 28 experimental EGFR therapeutic agents are being evaluated, some of which are AZD-9291 and CO-1686. Clinical trials addressing EGFR resistance include Clovis Oncology's "TIGER" trials, such as TIGER-3 (NCT02322281) and TIGER-2 (NCT02147990). Tiger 3 is a phase III trial comparing rociletinib (CO-1686) monotherapy versus single-agent chemotherapy for patients with mutant-EGFR NSCLC that has not responded to at least one EGFR-directed tyrosine kinase inhibitor. These EGFR-targeting agents are also effective radiation sensitizers for thoracic tumors; indeed, our group did a trial with erlotinib plus whole-brain radiation therapy. This combination was found to enhance tumor control in patients with brain metastases as well as median survival time, especially in patients with mutated *EGFR* [187]. The RTOG 0320 trial took a different approach, combining erlotinib with stereotactic radiosurgery and whole-brain radiation therapy; the findings for this trial were negative, and outcomes were not categorized according to an *EGFR* mutation status [162]. Nevertheless, these findings suggest that radiosensitizers like erlotinib may be best used when high radiation doses cannot be used, as high-dose stereotactic approaches already achieve high rates of local control. These and other trial results suggest that a high proportion of patients with brain metastases from lung cancer have *EGFR* mutations, raising the possibility that *EGFR*-mutated tumors may have a higher proclivity to produce brain metastases. Another important phase II trial exploring the value of combining tyrosine kinase inhibitors with radiation showed that adding erlotinib to chemoradiation for patients with stage III NSCLC extended the median survival time to 36.5 months, a significant improvement over the historical precedent of 17 months set by RTOG 9410 [92]. Finally, although adding erlotinib to radiation for brain or chest lesions has shown a reasonable safety profile with no increases in neurotoxicity or pneumonitis, definitive information on potential benefits from this approach is still lacking.

ALK Translocations

The story for ALK translocations is similar to that for *EGFR*; two therapeutics have been approved by the US FDA for NSCLC, ceritinib and crizotinib. Shortly after these agents were approved, resistance pathways were identified, and the search began for second-generation inhibitors for patients whose disease progressed on ceritinib or crizotinib. Seven experimental agents are currently being tested for resistance to first-generation ALK inhibitors, among which alectinib is the most prominent. A Genentech-sponsored trial (NCT02271139) is evaluating rates of response to alectinib among patients with NSCLC and ALK rearrangement who cannot tolerate or experience progression on prior ALK tyrosine kinase inhibitor therapy. Like the EGFR inhibitors, some evidence is emerging that ALK inhibitors can cause radiosensitization. Preclinical studies have shown that crizotinib can sensitize NSCLC cell lines in vitro and in vivo [164]. Clinically, the NRG trial group is now running a trial (RTOG 1306) in which crizotinib is given to patients with ALK translocations before chemoradiation, with the goal of shrinking the tumor. Because this drug is not being used concurrently with radiation, no evaluation of its potential for radiosensitization is possible in this trial.

KRAS Mutations

Although *KRAS* is one of the most common mutations in lung cancer, until recently few therapeutic options were available. For *KRAS*, it has become clear that the unique variants such as G12C have quite distinct effects, and thus the development of therapeutics will need to account for this specificity [75]. At present, no drugs have been approved for KRAS-mutated lung cancer, but trametinib was recently approved for metastatic melanoma with BRAF mutations and is gaining attention in lung cancer. When this chapter was written, 41 trials were underway for *KRAS*-mutated lung cancer.

Given the challenges of finding and enrolling ever-smaller subsets of patients with specific mutations, many investigators have turned to "basket trials" that include an array of targeted therapies in a single trial, so that patients can get the best therapeutics for them based on their tumor biology. Such trials, like the NCI-Molecular Analysis for Therapy Choice (NCI-MATCH) trial, are important for bringing precision medicine to larger numbers of patients, while simultaneously making it easier for patients to find an appropriate genomically based trial. As noted previously in this chapter, companies like MolecularMatch.com aggregate all of the currently approved target therapies and clinical trials in one place and provide free access to this information so that both patients and physicians can find targeted therapies and trials on the basis of information on genomic variants.

Clinical Studies of Immunotherapy

Clinically, the impact of immunotherapy on thoracic tumors has been both rapid and profound, and thus we expect to see a proliferation of new immunological agents being tested alone and in combination with other therapies such as biologics, chemotherapy, and radiation. Clinical immunotherapy was largely pioneered in melanoma, in which the importance of a tumor being able to evade immune detection to survive and progress is clear. The first FDA-approved checkpoint inhibitor, ipilimumab (anti-CTLA4), was approved for melanoma, which was followed by the first approval of the PD1 inhibitors nivolumab and pembrolizumab. After these approvals for melanoma, attention turned to tumors such as prostate cancer, lymphoma, and lung cancer. Interest in checkpoint inhibitors for lung cancer is considerable because of the prevalence, morbidity, and global impact of lung cancer; however, the importance of checkpoint inhibitors for lung cancer was initially unclear. Although studies undertaken within the past two decades have focused largely on genomics and the personalization of lung cancer treatments through the identification of unique driver mutations such as *EGFR* and/or ALK translocations, we are now seeing a rapid shift to the importance of immunotherapy for thoracic diseases. In fact, the first PD1 inhibitor to be approved for indications other than melanoma was nivolumab for NSCLC. This approval was based on a pivotal phase III trial in which 272 patients with metastatic squamous cell lung cancer that had progressed on chemotherapy were randomly assigned to nivolumab or docetaxel. Nivolumab produced a median survival time of 9.2 months versus 6 months for docetaxel [23]. Nivolumab was also superior in terms of toxicity, with only 7 % of patients experiencing any grade 3 or 4 toxicity compared with 55 % among patients given docetaxel. Studies of nivolumab are also undergoing for patients with adenocarcinoma NSCLC; pembrolizumab was recently approved for this purpose as well, with a companion finding that tumors that expressed PDL1 in more than 50 % of cells were more likely to respond to pembrolizumab [61]. Agents such as these are already being tested for other thoracic tumors such as small cell lung cancer and mesothelioma, both of which have shown signs of responding to checkpoint inhibition. This is a particularly revolutionary finding, because these two histologic tumor types have shown little benefit from personalized genomics during the past decade.

Despite the excitement surrounding immunotherapy for thoracic disease, the current reality remains that most patients do not benefit from checkpoint inhibitors used as monotherapy. As such, attention needs to turn to combination therapies targeting other mechanisms of immune escape and rational combinations of immunotherapy, chemotherapy, radiation therapy, and targeted therapies. During the brief time these agents have been studied in the clinic, much has been revealed about toxicity. Much of the known information about toxicity has come from melanoma trials, where it became apparent that pneumonitis was a toxic effect of checkpoint inhibitors that could be quite serious and, in some cases, even fatal. The risk of pneumonitis is of particular concern as these agents are being tested in patients with thoracic cancer, who often have a history of tobacco smoking and worsening lung function. Although early experience with using PD1 inhibition as monotherapy seemed to be relatively safe, the combination of CTLA4 and PD1 inhibitors has proven to have substantially greater toxicity. As immunotherapy expands, with increasing numbers of combinations of therapies with multiple agents, toxicity will become more apparent and may ultimately prove to be one of the greatest challenges for implementing immunotherapy for thoracic tumors.

Considerable attention is now being focused on expanding the use of immunotherapy for NSCLC at all stages, as outlined briefly in the sections that follow.

Stage I NSCLC

Patients with early-stage disease are typically treated with surgical resection or with SABR, with the latter technique being considerably less invasive but achieving very high rates of local control. A recent randomized trial showed that outcomes after surgery versus SABR were comparable for patients with early-stage disease [34]. Yet despite high rates of local control, these patients remain at risk of regional and distant failure, although one could imagine using SABR in combination with immunotherapy to essentially turn the tumor into an in situ vaccine that could induce T-cell responses that would address distant metastatic disease. This approach is likely to be reasonably safe, given the tight fields used in SABR and the minimal volumes of lung tissue treated.

Another trial that is attempting to quantify T-cell induction in these two techniques is NCT02488850, which is evaluating 40 patients with T1-2aN0M0 NSCLC to study the effect of surgery and SABR on immunostimulatory functions, with the primary endpoint being CD8+ cytotoxic T-cells.

Stage II NSCLC

Stage II NSCLC is typically treated with surgery up front followed by adjuvant chemotherapy, although induction therapy is occasionally used to shrink larger tumors before surgery. This would be an interesting setting for which to consider immunotherapy becuase such patients are at risk of local, regional, and distant failure, all of which could potentially be improved by immunotherapy. Induction therapy with checkpoint inhibitors before surgery could be used to prime the T-cell response before the tumor is removed. This approach could be taken one step further through the use of induction immunotherapy and radiation, with the radiation used not to shrink or downstage a tumor but rather to induce the production of neoantigens. The added risk would need to be considered carefully, because conventional treatment in some cases could be curative, and thus additional treatment that could delay or make surgery more complicated would be challenging to justify. Adjuvant immunotherapy after surgery may be a safer approach; however, because the tumor is removed, the primary source of antigens would not be present and immunotherapy thus may be less effective.

An ongoing phase III trial of adjuvant immunotherapy for completely resected NSCLC, NCT02273375, is a double-blind randomized trial in which MEDI4736 is given after surgical resection by the National Cancer Institute of Canada Clinical Trials Group. This approach may also be attractive for other types of thoracic tumors such as small cell lung cancer, mesothelioma, or esophageal cancer.

Stage III NSCLC

The standard of care for stage III (locally advanced) NSCLC, for patients who can tolerate it, is chemoradiation, which produces a median survival time of about 17 months. Given the high prevalence of both local and distant failure, combination approaches are warranted. The challenge for combining immunotherapy with radiation is that the radiation fields needed to encompass all gross disease are sufficiently large as to greatly increase the risk of RP, which could be enhanced by the potential pneumonitis caused by many checkpoint inhibitors. Thus combining chemoradiation with checkpoint inhibitors (which can further increase pneumonitis) raises considerable concern for safety. As described for treating stage II disease, adjuvant immunotherapy trials may be a safer alternative for getting immunotherapy to patients with stage III NSCLC; this strategy is currently being discussed in US cooperative groups such as the NRG. The same concerns as for stage II disease apply here: because radiation stimulates antigen production, giving a checkpoint inhibitor days to weeks after T-cell priming has already occurred may not be particularly effective.

Another approach, combining anti-PD1 therapy concurrently with chemoradiation, is being tested in a phase I/II clinical trial at The University of Texas MD Anderson Cancer Center. This Genentech-sponsored trial combines the PDL1 inhibitor atezolizumab with chemoradiation for stage III lung cancer to evaluate the safety and efficacy of this combination. It will be interesting to see how the safety profile of this anti-PDL1 agent differs from previously approved PD1 inhibitors. Certainly stage III disease is one of the riskiest stages for combining radiation with immunotherapy because of the often-large tumor burden within the radiation field.

Stage IV NSCLC

Perhaps the greatest amount of interest has been expressed in testing combinations of radiation and immunotherapy for metastatic (stage IV) NSCLC, given the inability of current targeted therapy to provide durable long-term tumor control. This stands in contrast to findings in patients with melanoma, for whom immunotherapy such as ipilimumab has provided durable control for years in some cases. With this realization, we must also question some of our current practices such as frequent use of steroids, which blunt immune responses but nevertheless are often given with chemotherapy, if immunotherapy is to be given as well.

The landscape has changed rapidly for squamous cell NSCLC, for which the FDA-approved nivolumab (Opdivo) in December 2014 [23]. More recently, pembrolizumab (Keytruda) was approved for both squamous and adenocarcinomatous NSCLC, where objective response rates have reached 19.4 %. This was also the first immunotherapeutic agent approved for lung cancer that included a companion diagnostic, in that tumors that express PDL1 in more than 50 % of cells are more likely to respond to pembrolizumab [61].

After FDA approval of nivolumab and pembrolizumab, attention shifted to using one or more of these agents in combination with other forms of therapy, because in about 75 % of cases, stage IV NSCLC does not respond to PD1 inhibition alone. One of the first combination immunotherapy strategies to be extensively tested in such patients is that of blocking both CLTA4 and PD1, a combination that has proven highly effective for melanoma but has been associated with greatly increased toxicity relative to the use of single checkpoint inhibitors. This strategy is being pursued by Bristol-Myers-Squibb, which now has several ongoing trials testing optimal doses and sequences to combine CTLA4 inhibition (ipilimumab) with PD1 inhibition (nivolumab).

Many other combinations are now entering clinical trials, with drugs targeting the CD28 homolog inducible costimulatory molecule (ICOS), OX40, TIM-3, GITR, IDO, and STAT3 being tested alone or in combination with PD1. Combinations of anti-PD1 with targeted therapies are also underway, as are novel immunotherapy approaches such as dendritic cell vaccines, the use of adoptive T-cells, or chimeric antigen receptor (CAR) T-cell therapy (described further under section "Future Directions").

Another aspect to be considered in integrating immunotherapy into future therapeutic strategies is the prevalence of brain metastasis from NSCLC. Traditionally, radiation has been the treatment of choice in such cases because chemoradiation and most biologics cannot penetrate the blood-brain barrier. However, several case reports have shown that aspects of the immunologic response can penetrate from the body into the brain and vice versa; indeed, many immunotherapy trials allow patients with asymptomatic brain metastasis to participate. A clinical challenge today is what to do with a patient on immunotherapy with disease that progressed or spread to the brain: can whole-brain radiation therapy or stereotactic radiosurgery be offered safely while the immunotherapy continues? Or could these agents further worsen mental status or even contribute to radionecrosis? These and other related questions are being addressed in a phase I/II trial at MD Anderson in which patients with NSCLC and brain metastasis will be treated with a combination of whole-brain radiation therapy, stereotactic radiosurgery, anti-PD1, and anti-PD1 plus anti-CTLA4.

Clinical Relevance: Small Cell Lung Cancer

The beneficial effects of checkpoint inhibitors in small cell lung cancer came as a surprise to many. Yet some of the first clinical findings that small cell tumors could respond to checkpoint inhibitors were reported at the 2015 meeting of the American Society of Clinical Oncology [161]. Perhaps in retrospect this should not have been so surprising because the experience with melanoma showed that mutational burden can correlate with response to immunotherapy; these mutations can serve as tumor antigens. Interestingly, small cell lung cancer is one of the most heavily mutated tumors, having mutation rates in some series that are higher than in melanoma.

This work is now being taken one step further in trials involving immunotherapy for both limited-stage and extensive-stage small cell lung cancers. Trials at MD Anderson are evaluating both the safety and efficacy of anti-PD1 therapy in combination with chemoradiation for patients with limited-stage disease; patients with extensive-stage disease receive induction chemotherapy first, followed by concurrent consolidative radiation therapy and anti-PD1 therapy to induce systemic response and enhance progression-free survival.

Clinical Relevance: Mesothelioma

Increasing preclinical evidence has suggested that immune checkpoint blockade can be effective in malignant pleural mesothelioma. In one study involving a subcutaneous murine mesothelioma model, a CTLA4 blocking antibody was given after each cycle of chemotherapy, and the antitumor effect was compared with that in control mice. The anti-CTLA4 monoclonal antibody inhibited growth at an early stage of tumor development, attenuated cell repopulation, and increased CD4+ and CD8+ infiltration and expression of IL-2, IFN-γ, and granzyme B [192]. In another study using a non-immunogenic murine model of mesothelioma, mice that had initially shown tumor resolution after anti-CTLA4, singly or with other agents, were then rechallenged with a mesothelioma cell line; those mice demonstrated protective antitumor immunological memory and expressed memory T-cells [100].

Prior clinical and translational studies have demonstrated important paradigms that can serve as the foundation of future studies. About 20–70 % of tumors express increased PDL1, which is typically associated with worse outcomes [29, 41, 108]. A phase II single-arm clinical study of the CTLA-4 inhibitor tremelimumab was given at 15 mg/kg intravenously every 90 days to 29 patients with chemotherapy-resistant mesothelioma until disease progression or severe toxicity. Two patients in that trial had a durable partial response, with a median progression-free survival time of 6.2 months and a median overall survival time of 10.7 months [27]. The same investigators then studied the efficacy of a different regimen of tremelimumab, 10 mg/kg once every 4 weeks × 6 doses, then every 12 weeks until disease progression, for patients with mesothelioma. At a median follow-up time of 21.3 months, four RECIST partial responses were attributed to immunotherapy, and 52 % of patients experienced disease control. The median interval for disease control was 10.9 months [28]. The toxicity profile in these studies was similar to those observed in studies of other malignancies. For instance, in the initial phase II trial, almost all patients experienced low-grade toxicity (primarily skin reactions or colitis/diarrhea); 4 of 29 patients had a grade ≥3 event (two gastrointestinal, one neurological, two hepatic, and one pancreatic) [27, 28].

Results from the KEYNOTE-028 trial of pembrolizumab for malignant pleural mesothelioma were reported recently in abstract form. In that phase I study, 25 patients with mesothelioma and at least 1 % PDL1 expression in tumors were treated with pembrolizumab, 10 mg/kg every 2 weeks for up to 2 years or until confirmed disease progression or toxicity. Almost 90 % of patients had received at least 1 prior therapy (80 % had platinum and pemetrexed). The overall response rate was 24 %, 52 % of patients had stable disease (disease control rate 76 %), and 64 % of patients remained on treatment at the time of the report. Toxicity was considered acceptable, with the most common side effects being nausea (40 %), fatigue (32 %), and reduced appetite (28 %). Three patients (12 %) had grade ≥3 drug-related toxicity. The authors concluded that pembrolizumab is "generally well tolerated and provides robust antitumor activity in patients with advanced PDL1-positive mesothelioma" [5].

Several phase I and II clinical trials have emerged based on this evidence and via extrapolation from other types of tumor; trials specific to mesothelioma are listed in Table 12.1.

Table 12.1 Upcoming or active mesothelioma-specific trials with immunotherapy

Test agent	Target	Institution	Phase	Clinical trial ID number	Details
Pembrolizumab	PD1	University of Chicago	II	NCT02399371	Examines agent in both unselected patients and those with PDL1 positivity
Pembrolizumab	PD1	MD Anderson Cancer Center	I	TBD	Examines safety and efficacy in patients who cannot undergo pneumonectomy and who will receive radiation
Tremelimumab	CTLA4	Azienda Ospedaliera Universitaria Senese	II	NCT01655888	For patients who have received one prior platinum-based regimen for mesothelioma
Tremelimumab	CTLA4	Azienda Ospedaliera Universitaria Senese	II	NCT01843374	Randomized comparison of tremelimumab versus placebo for unresectable pleural or peritoneal mesothelioma

Future Directions

Chimeric Antigen Receptor T-Cell Therapy

With the importance of the immune system in battling cancer now recognized, novel immunotherapeutic approaches are being investigated involving T-cells with engineered chimeric antigen receptors (CARs). CAR T-cells contain genetically customizable monoclonal antibodies that serve as receptors for various TAAs. Their specificity comes from the single-chain antibody variable fragment (scFv); the resulting antigen receptor activation does not require MHC binding and is advantageous because tumors can decrease MHC-1 expression to evade immune-mediated killing by endogenous T-cells [146]. However, MHC signaling also enhances T-cell activation, and thus costimulatory domains have been added to the intracellular domain of CARs, resulting in second- and third-generation CAR T-cells [87].

One of the first case reports on the effects of CAR T-cells involved a patient with stage I chronic lymphocytic leukemia [136]. Diagnosed in 1996, this patient's leukemia relapsed after several types of chemotherapy, including rituximab and fludarabine. The patient was given CAR T-cells targeting CD19 (an antigen expressed by malignant B cells), which led to resolution of adenopathy within 31 days and a remission that was sustained for 10 months. Since that time, CAR T-cells have been expanded to target TAAs of a variety of solid malignancies, including renal cell carcinoma (CAIX), ovarian (αFR), and some sarcomas (HER2+) [1, 88, 95]. However, only a few patients in those trials have experienced clinical response. Used as adjunct therapy, radiation could increase the clinical efficacy of CAR T-cells by promoting TAA expression by tumors.

The ability of radiation to enhance the expression of various TAAs on tumor cells has been verified in several preclinical studies. c-Met, a receptor tyrosine kinase, is overexpressed in several types of cancer, including colorectal, lung, and glioma [20], with some studies linking worse clinical outcomes with higher c-Met expression levels in NSCLC [110, 120]. In one preclinical study, radiation was found to increase c-Met production in low-expressing NSCLC cell lines [21]. The cell surface receptor mesothelin has been found to be upregulated in mesothelioma, ovarian cancer, and pancreatic cancer. Like c-Met, transfection of epidermoid carcinoma cell lines with mesothelin increased their mesothelin production upon irradiation [70]. These results suggest that radiation can be used to selectively raise TAA expression, which could promote CAR T-cell-mediated tumor destruction. However, several questions remain to be answered, such as whether multiple fractions of low-dose radiation or a single high-dose fraction would promote the optimal amounts of TAA production and CAR T-cell tumor penetration. The sequence and timing of CAR T-cell therapy in relation to radiation to achieve tumor regression also requires further elucidation. Clinical trials in which radiation is combined with CAR T-cell therapy can shed light on these questions.

NK-Cell Therapy

Although CD8+ T-cells are critical for antitumor immunity, NK-cells have recently gained attention as a potential contributor to antitumor immunity as well. Part of the innate immune system, NK-cells are large granular lymphocytes that use cytotoxic mediators to induce destruction of foreign cells, including virus-infected and malignant cells. NK-cells express a variety of cell surface receptors, among them killer immunoglobulin-like receptors (KIRs), which can promote either quiescence or activation of NK-cells when they bind to ligands. This balance of stimulatory and inhibitory signals determines whether or not NK-cells eliminate cells that they encounter [179]. Healthy cells avoid NK-cell-mediated death by expressing MHC-I, which binds to inhibitory KIRs (e.g., KIRS2DL1, KIRS2DL2, or KIRS2DL3) [17]. When MHC-I is not present, NK-cells are activated and promote cell lysis, resulting in a process known as "missing self" recognition. A cancer cell's ability to suppress expression of MHC-I molecules to avoid T-cell-mediated death makes use of NK-cells an appealing option for therapy. Analyses of tumor samples from patients with breast, colorectal, or head and neck cancer showed that NK-cells not only participate in antitumor activity but also communicate with other T-cells to augment tumor cell death [14, 135, 153].

Donor NK-cells can be delivered in one of two common approaches, one involving haploidentical (i.e., MHC matched) hematopoietic stem cell transplantation and the other direct NK-cell infusion. The first approach involves a conditioning regimen of chemoradiation followed by transplantation of donated stem cells. The latter approach entails isolating NK-cells from a donor (or patient), expanding them, and reinfusing them into the patient. In either case, the donated NK-cells do not recognize the MHC-I expressed by tumor cells, resulting in their activation. Clinical trials of NK-cell therapy for solid tumors have produced variable outcomes. One group administered NK-cells that had been expanded in vitro to 16 patients with locally advanced lung cancer that had not responded to first- and second-line chemotherapy; only two patients had a clinical response, and seven had disease progression [76]. Similar trials for patients with other types of cancer such as renal cell carcinoma and melanoma have produced similar results [10, 168].

The effects of radiation on NK-cells are not well known. One study found no difference in the numbers of NK-cells before and after chemoradiation for advanced (T3–T4) rectal cancer [104], possibly because radiation also increases tumor expression of MHC-I [56], which induces NK-cell inactivation. A recent phase II clinical trial investigating the use of targeted NK-cell therapy after chemoradiation for inoperable stage III lung cancer (NCT02118415) could provide further insight. A possible solution may be to block the interaction of MHC-I with KIRs by using the monoclonal antibody IPH2101. One phase I trial found that IPH2101 promoted NK-cell activation ex vivo but did not result in objective clinical response in patients with multiple myeloma [18]. Another phase I trial of IPH2101 for acute myeloid leukemia noted an improvement in overall survival relative to patients with similar disease who did not receive IPH2101 [177]. The question of whether anti-KIR monoclonal antibodies enhance radiation therapy is becoming crucial because those antibodies are being incorporated with other immunotherapies already known to have synergistic effects with radiation [48]. One such trial, a phase I trial combining lirilumab, a second-generation anti-KIR antibody, and nivolumab for advanced solid malignancies, is currently underway (NCT01714739). Further preclinical experiments are needed to clarify the effects of anti-KIR antibodies and radiation on tumor microenvironment.

Tumor Vaccines and Other Immune Agents

Recent years have seen increased interest in the unique roles of radiation in inducing immunogenic tumor cell death, inflammatory responses, and cross-priming of tumor-specific T-cells, with numerous preclinical and clinical studies of various combinations of radiotherapy with different immunomodulatory agents. Successful combinations could achieve robust systemic antitumor responses, which would not only control local disease but also eliminate metastatic disease and provide long-term immune protection against cancer.

Cancer Vaccines

Both preclinical and clinical evidence support the idea that radiation can be a powerful adjunct to active therapeutic cancer vaccines, including vaccines based on dendritic cells (e.g., Sipuleucel-T) [38, 89, 157, 185], whole-tumor cell vaccines (e.g., GVAX) [122], viral vaccines (e.g., a recombinant avipoxvirus expressing CEA and three T-cell costimulatory molecules) [32, 65, 72, 97], peptide or protein vaccines (HLA-A2-restricted glioma antigen peptides) [188], DNA vaccines [33, 171], and live attenuated vaccines based on *Listeria monocytogenes* [68].

In addition to enhancing the therapeutic value of current cancer vaccines, another potential benefit is that radiation may help in the development of new cancer vaccines, which remains a major challenge because little is known as to which tumor antigens are the best to target. One approach to increasing this knowledge is the creation of an antigen discovery platform that combines data from mass spectrometry, genomics, biochemistry, and immunology with the goal of generating valid candidate tumor-associated peptides. One such platform XPRESIDENT (Immatics) was used to create the multipeptide vaccine IMA901, which in phase III trials with immunotherapy for renal cell carcinoma is showing significant clinical benefit [91, 182]. Because radiation can generate mutations and increase the number and diversity of the peptide pool [145], localized radiotherapy presumably would increase the diversity of novel tumor-associated peptides, especially for tumors with little or no immunogenicity.

Immune Agents Targeting the TNF Receptor Superfamily

In addition to CTLA4 and PD1, several TNF receptors, including OX40, 4-1BB, GITR, and CD27, are important in controlling T-cell activation and function. The theory is that binding of these glycoproteins with agonist antibodies conveys activating signals to lymphocytes, which have produced antitumor effects in mouse models. Antibodies targeting OX40, 4-1BB, GITR, and CD27 have recently entered clinical trials. Preclinical studies suggest that the greatest potential of these agents will likely be achieved in combined treatment strategies.

Previous research [94, 103] and our own unpublished data indicate that radiation increases OX40L/OX40 expression on tumor-infiltrating T-cells and peripheral blood cells (Fig. 12.2). Costimulatory signals from OX40 to a conventional T-cell promote division and survival, augmenting the clonal expansion of antigen-specific effector and memory populations [42]. Conversely, stimulating OX40 on Tregs is thought to inactivate Treg function [181]. One anti-OX40 agonist antibody was shown to increase local control and to reduce systemic metastasis after radiation therapy in a preclinical mouse model [64]. Early clinical trial findings suggest that this agent has an acceptable toxicity profile and has prompted regression of at least one metastatic lesion in 12 of 30 patients [45]. Because radiation can increase OX40 expression, future combinations of radiation with anti-OX40 could significantly increase the abscopal effects of radiation in treating advanced disease. Combinations of radiation and antibodies targeting 4-1BB have also shown promising antitumor outcomes in preclinical models [16, 105, 155], warranting future trials to test the ability of these agents to induce abscopal effects.

References

1. Ahmed N, Brawley VS, Hegde M, Robertson C, Ghazi A, Gerken C, Liu E, Dakhova O, Ashoori A, Corder A, Gray T, Wu MF, Liu H, Hicks J, Rainusso N, Dotti G, Mei Z, Grilley B, Gee A, Rooney CM, Brenner MK, Heslop HE, Wels WS, Wang LL, Anderson P, Gottschalk S. Human epidermal growth factor receptor 2 (HER2) -specific chimeric antigen receptor-modified T cells for the immunotherapy of HER2-positive sarcoma. J Clin Oncol: Off J Am Soc Clin Oncol. 2015;33(15):1688–96. doi:10.1200/JCO.2014.58.0225.
2. Ahn GO, Tseng D, Liao CH, Dorie MJ, Czechowicz A, Brown JM. Inhibition of Mac-1 (CD11b/CD18) enhances tumor response to radiation by reducing myeloid cell recruitment. Proc Natl Acad Sci U S A. 2010;107(18):8363–8. doi:10.1073/pnas.0911378107.
3. Akhurst RJ, Hata A. Targeting the TGFbeta signalling pathway in disease. Nat Rev Drug Discov. 2012;11(10):790–811. doi:10.1038/nrd3810.
4. Aktas H, Cai H, Cooper GM. Ras links growth factor signaling to the cell cycle machinery via regulation of cyclin D1 and the Cdk inhibitor p27KIP1. Mol Cell Biol. 1997; 17(7):3850–7.
5. Alley EA, Rhoda Molife L, Santoro A, Beckey K, Yuan S, Cheng JD, Piperdi B, Schellens JHM. Clinical safety and efficacy of pembrolizumab (MK-3475) in patients with malignant pleural mesothelioma: preliminary results from KEYNOTE-028. Proceedings of the American Association of Cancer Research, Philadelphia; 2015.
6. Ambros V. MicroRNA pathways in flies and worms: growth, death, fat, stress, and timing. Cell. 2003;113(6):673–6.
7. Talasaz A, Mortimer S, Sebisanovic D, Siew LM, Zapanta A, Mei G, Schiller B, Eltoukhy H. Use of the GUARDANT360 noninvasive tumor sequencing assay on 300 patients across colorectal, melanoma, lung, breast, and prostate cancers and its clinical utility. 2014 ASCO Annual Meeting. J Clin Oncol. 2014;32(suppl; abstr e22041).
8. Antoniades J, Brady LW, Lightfoot DA. Lymphangiographic demonstration of the abscopal effect in patients with malignant lymphomas. Int J Radiat Oncol Biol Phys. 1977;2(1–2):141–7.
9. Apetoh L, Ghiringhelli F, Tesniere A, Obeid M, Ortiz C, Criollo A, Mignot G, Maiuri MC, Ullrich E, Saulnier P, Yang H, Amigorena S, Ryffel B, Barrat FJ, Saftig P, Levi F, Lidereau R, Nogues C, Mira JP, Chompret A, Joulin V, Clavel-Chapelon F, Bourhis J, Andre F, Delaloge S, Tursz T, Kroemer G, Zitvogel L. Toll-like receptor 4-dependent contribution of the immune system to anticancer chemotherapy and radiotherapy. Nat Med. 2007;13(9): 1050–9. doi:10.1038/nm1622.
10. Arai S, Meagher R, Swearingen M, Myint H, Rich E, Martinson J, Klingemann H. Infusion of the allogeneic cell line NK-92 in patients with advanced renal cell cancer or melanoma: a phase I trial. Cytotherapy. 2008;10(6):625–32. doi:10.1080/14653240802301872.
11. Awwad HK. Normal tissue radiosensitivity: prediction on deterministic or stochastic basis? J Egypt Natl Cancer Inst. 2005;17(4):221–30.
12. Baik CS, Pritchard CC, Eaton KD, Chow LQ. EGFR mutations in squamous cell lung cancer in never-smokers. J Thorac Oncol. 2013;8(1):e6–7. doi:10.1097/JTO.0b013e3182762d49.
13. Bartel DP. MicroRNAs: genomics, biogenesis, mechanism, and function. Cell. 2004;116(2):281–97.
14. Baskic D, Vujanovic L, Arsenijevic N, Whiteside TL, Myers EN, Vujanovic NL. Suppression of natural killer-cell and dendritic-cell apoptotic tumoricidal activity in patients with head and neck cancer. Head Neck. 2013;35(3):388–98. doi:10.1002/hed.22968.
15. Battaglia A, Buzzonetti A, Martinelli E, Fanelli M, Petrillo M, Ferrandina G, Scambia G, Fattorossi A. Selective changes in the immune profile of tumor-draining lymph nodes after different neoadjuvant chemoradiation regimens for locally advanced cervical cancer. Int J Radiat Oncol Biol Phys. 2010;76(5):1546–53. doi:10.1016/j.ijrobp.2009.10.014.

16. Belcaid Z, Phallen JA, Zeng J, See AP, Mathios D, Gottschalk C, Nicholas S, Kellett M, Ruzevick J, Jackson C, Albesiano E, Durham NM, Ye X, Tran PT, Tyler B, Wong JW, Brem H, Pardoll DM, Drake CG, Lim M. Focal radiation therapy combined with 4-1BB activation and CTLA-4 blockade yields long-term survival and a protective antigen-specific memory response in a murine glioma model. PLoS ONE. 2014;9(7), e101764. doi:10.1371/journal.pone.0101764.
17. Benson Jr DM, Caligiuri MA. Killer immunoglobulin-like receptors and tumor immunity. Cancer Immunol Res. 2014;2(2):99–104. doi:10.1158/2326-6066.CIR-13-0219.
18. Benson Jr DM, Hofmeister CC, Padmanabhan S, Suvannasankha A, Jagannath S, Abonour R, Bakan C, Andre P, Efebera Y, Tiollier J, Caligiuri MA, Farag SS. A phase 1 trial of the anti-KIR antibody IPH2101 in patients with relapsed/refractory multiple myeloma. Blood. 2012;120(22):4324–33. doi:10.1182/blood-2012-06-438028.
19. Bettegowda C, Sausen M, Leary RJ, Kinde I, Wang Y, Agrawal N, Bartlett BR, Wang H, Luber B, Alani RM, Antonarakis ES, Azad NS, Bardelli A, Brem H, Cameron JL, Lee CC, Fecher LA, Gallia GL, Gibbs P, Le D, Giuntoli RL, Goggins M, Hogarty MD, Holdhoff M, Hong SM, Jiao Y, Juhl HH, Kim JJ, Siravegna G, Laheru DA, Lauricella C, Lim M, Lipson EJ, Marie SK, Netto GJ, Oliner KS, Olivi A, Olsson L, Riggins GJ, Sartore-Bianchi A, Schmidt K, Shih IM, Oba-Shinjo SM, Siena S, Theodorescu D, Tie J, Harkins TT, Veronese S, Wang TL, Weingart JD, Wolfgang CL, Wood LD, Xing D, Hruban RH, Wu J, Allen PJ, Schmidt CM, Choti MA, Velculescu VE, Kinzler KW, Vogelstein B, Papadopoulos N, Diaz Jr LA. Detection of circulating tumor DNA in early- and late-stage human malignancies. Sci Transl Med. 2014;6(224):224ra224. doi:10.1126/scitranslmed.3007094.
20. Bhardwaj V, Cascone T, Cortez MA, Amini A, Evans J, Komaki RU, Heymach JV, Welsh JW. Modulation of c-Met signaling and cellular sensitivity to radiation: potential implications for therapy. Cancer. 2013;119(10):1768–75. doi:10.1002/cncr.27965.
21. Bhardwaj V, Zhan Y, Cortez MA, Ang KK, Molkentine D, Munshi A, Raju U, Komaki R, Heymach JV, Welsh J. C-Met inhibitor MK-8003 radiosensitizes c-Met-expressing non-small-cell lung cancer cells with radiation-induced c-Met-expression. J Thorac Oncol: Off Publ Int Assoc Stud Lung Cancer. 2012;7(8):1211–7. doi:10.1097/JTO.0b013e318257cc89.
22. Bogdandi EN, Balogh A, Felgyinszki N, Szatmari T, Persa E, Hildebrandt G, Safrany G, Lumniczky K. Effects of low-dose radiation on the immune system of mice after total-body irradiation. Radiat Res. 2010;174(4):480–9. doi:10.1667/RR2160.1.
23. Brahmer J, Reckamp KL, Baas P, Crino L, Eberhardt WE, Poddubskaya E, Antonia S, Pluzanski A, Vokes EE, Holgado E, Waterhouse D, Ready N, Gainor J, Aren Frontera O, Havel L, Steins M, Garassino MC, Aerts JG, Domine M, Paz-Ares L, Reck M, Baudelet C, Harbison CT, Lestini B, Spigel DR. Nivolumab versus docetaxel in advanced squamous-cell non-small-cell lung cancer. N Engl J Med. 2015;373(2):123–35. doi:10.1056/NEJMoa1504627.
24. Brugger W, Triller N, Blasinska-Morawiec M, Curescu S, Sakalauskas R, Manikhas GM, Mazieres J, Whittom R, Ward C, Mayne K, Trunzer K, Cappuzzo F. Prospective molecular marker analyses of EGFR and KRAS from a randomized, placebo-controlled study of erlotinib maintenance therapy in advanced non-small-cell lung cancer. J Clin Oncol. 2011;29(31):4113–20. doi:10.1200/JCO.2010.31.8162.
25. Burnet FM. Immunological surveillance in neoplasia. Transplant Rev. 1971;7:3–25.
26. Burnet M. Cancer; a biological approach. I The processes of control. Br Med J. 1957;1(5022):779–86.
27. Calabro L, Morra A, Fonsatti E, Cutaia O, Amato G, Giannarelli D, Di Giacomo AM, Danielli R, Altomonte M, Mutti L, Maio M. Tremelimumab for patients with chemotherapy-resistant advanced malignant mesothelioma: an open-label, single-arm, phase 2 trial. Lancet Oncol. 2013;14(11):1104–11. doi:10.1016/S1470-2045(13)70381-4.
28. Calabro L, Morra A, Fonsatti E, Cutaia O, Fazio C, Annesi D, Lenoci M, Amato G, Danielli R, Altomonte M, Giannarelli D, Di Giacomo AM, Maio M. Efficacy and safety of an intensified schedule of tremelimumab for chemotherapy-resistant malignant mesothelioma: an

open-label, single-arm, phase 2 study. Lancet Respir Med. 2015;3(4):301–9. doi:10.1016/S2213-2600(15)00092-2.

29. Cedres S, Ponce-Aix S, Zugazagoitia J, Sansano I, Enguita A, Navarro-Mendivil A, Martinez-Marti A, Martinez P, Felip E. Analysis of expression of programmed cell death 1 ligand 1 (PD-L1) in malignant pleural mesothelioma (MPM). PLoS ONE. 2015;10(3), e0121071. doi:10.1371/journal.pone.0121071.
30. Ceradini DJ, Kulkarni AR, Callaghan MJ, Tepper OM, Bastidas N, Kleinman ME, Capla JM, Galiano RD, Levine JP, Gurtner GC. Progenitor cell trafficking is regulated by hypoxic gradients through HIF-1 induction of SDF-1. Nat Med. 2004;10(8):858–64. doi:10.1038/nm1075.
31. Cha E, Klinger M, Hou Y, Cummings C, Ribas A, Faham M, Fong L. Improved survival with T cell clonotype stability after anti-CTLA-4 treatment in cancer patients. Sci Transl Med. 2014;6(238):238ra270. doi:10.1126/scitranslmed.3008211.
32. Chakraborty M, Abrams SI, Coleman CN, Camphausen K, Schlom J, Hodge JW. External beam radiation of tumors alters phenotype of tumor cells to render them susceptible to vaccine-mediated T-cell killing. Cancer Res. 2004;64(12):4328–37. doi:10.1158/0008-5472.CAN-04-0073.
33. Chamoto K, Takeshima T, Wakita D, Ohkuri T, Ashino S, Omatsu T, Shirato H, Kitamura H, Togashi Y, Nishimura T. Combination immunotherapy with radiation and CpG-based tumor vaccination for the eradication of radio- and immuno-resistant lung carcinoma cells. Cancer Sci. 2009;100(5):934–9. doi:10.1111/j.1349-7006.2009.01114.x.
34. Chang JY, Senan S, Paul MA, Mehran RJ, Louie AV, Balter P, Groen HJ, McRae SE, Widder J, Feng L, van den Borne BE, Munsell MF, Hurkmans C, Berry DA, van Werkhoven E, Kresl JJ, Dingemans AM, Dawood O, Haasbeek CJ, Carpenter LS, De Jaeger K, Komaki R, Slotman BJ, Smit EF, Roth JA. Stereotactic ablative radiotherapy versus lobectomy for operable stage I non-small-cell lung cancer: a pooled analysis of two randomised trials. Lancet Oncol. 2015;16(6):630–7. doi:10.1016/s1470-2045(15)70168-3.
35. Chanock SJ, Manolio T, Boehnke M, Boerwinkle E, Hunter DJ, Thomas G, Hirschhorn JN, Abecasis G, Altshuler D, Bailey-Wilson JE, Brooks LD, Cardon LR, Daly M, Donnelly P, Fraumeni Jr JF, Freimer NB, Gerhard DS, Gunter C, Guttmacher AE, Guyer MS, Harris EL, Hoh J, Hoover R, Kong CA, Merikangas KR, Morton CC, Palmer LJ, Phimister EG, Rice JP, Roberts J, Rotimi C, Tucker MA, Vogan KJ, Wacholder S, Wijsman EM, Winn DM, Collins FS. Replicating genotype-phenotype associations. Nature. 2007;447(7145):655–60. doi:10.1038/447655a.
36. Chen L, Ashe S, Brady WA, Hellstrom I, Hellstrom KE, Ledbetter JA, McGowan P, Linsley PS. Costimulation of antitumor immunity by the B7 counterreceptor for the T lymphocyte molecules CD28 and CTLA-4. Cell. 1992;71(7):1093–102.
37. Chen N, Fang W, Zhan J, Hong S, Tang Y, Kang S, Zhang Y, He X, Zhou T, Qin T, Huang Y, Yi X, Zhang L. Upregulation of PD-L1 by EGFR activation mediates the immune escape in EGFR-driven NSCLC: implication for optional immune targeted therapy for NSCLC patients with EGFR mutation. J Thorac Oncol. 2015;10(6):910–23. doi:10.1097/JTO.0000000000000500.
38. Chi KH, Liu SJ, Li CP, Kuo HP, Wang YS, Chao Y, Hsieh SL. Combination of conformal radiotherapy and intratumoral injection of adoptive dendritic cell immunotherapy in refractory hepatoma. J Immunother. 2005;28(2):129–35.
39. Chistiakov DA, Voronova NV, Chistiakov PA. Genetic variations in DNA repair genes, radiosensitivity to cancer and susceptibility to acute tissue reactions in radiotherapy-treated cancer patients. Acta Oncol. 2008;47(5):809–24. doi:10.1080/02841860801885969.
40. Cotter SE, Dunn GP, Collins KM, Sahni D, Zukotynski KA, Hansen JL, O'Farrell DA, Ng AK, Devlin PM, Wang LC. Abscopal effect in a patient with metastatic Merkel cell carcinoma following radiation therapy: potential role of induced antitumor immunity. Arch Dermatol. 2011;147(7):870–2. doi:10.1001/archdermatol.2011.176.
41. Cowan MI, Forde PM, Taube JM, Illei PB. PD-L1 expression in malignant mesothelioma: an immunohistochemical analysis of 33 cases. Lab Invest. 2014;94:276A.

42. Croft M, So T, Duan W, Soroosh P. The significance of OX40 and OX40L to T-cell biology and immune disease. Immunol Rev. 2009;229(1):173–91. doi:10.1111/j.1600-065X.2009.00766.x.
43. Cuenca A, Cheng F, Wang H, Brayer J, Horna P, Gu L, Bien H, Borrello IM, Levitsky HI, Sotomayor EM. Extra-lymphatic solid tumor growth is not immunologically ignored and results in early induction of antigen-specific T-cell anergy: dominant role of cross-tolerance to tumor antigens. Cancer Res. 2003;63(24):9007–15.
44. Curran MA, Montalvo W, Yagita H, Allison JP. PD-1 and CTLA-4 combination blockade expands infiltrating T cells and reduces regulatory T and myeloid cells within B16 melanoma tumors. Proc Natl Acad Sci U S A. 2010;107(9):4275–80. doi:10.1073/pnas.0915174107.
45. Curti BD, Kovacsovics-Bankowski M, Morris N, Walker E, Chisholm L, Floyd K, Walker J, Gonzalez I, Meeuwsen T, Fox BA, Moudgil T, Miller W, Haley D, Coffey T, Fisher B, Delanty-Miller L, Rymarchyk N, Kelly T, Crocenzi T, Bernstein E, Sanborn R, Urba WJ, Weinberg AD. OX40 is a potent immune-stimulating target in late-stage cancer patients. Cancer Res. 2013;73(24):7189–98. doi:10.1158/0008-5472.CAN-12-4174.
46. Dancea HC, Shareef MM, Ahmed MM. Role of radiation-induced TGF-beta signaling in cancer therapy. Mol Cell Pharmacol. 2009;1(1):44–56.
47. Demaria S, Ng B, Devitt ML, Babb JS, Kawashima N, Liebes L, Formenti SC. Ionizing radiation inhibition of distant untreated tumors (abscopal effect) is immune mediated. Int J Radiat Oncol Biol Phys. 2004;58(3):862–70. doi:10.1016/j.ijrobp.2003.09.012.
48. Deng L, Liang H, Burnette B, Beckett M, Darga T, Weichselbaum RR, Fu YX. Irradiation and anti-PD-L1 treatment synergistically promote antitumor immunity in mice. J Clin Invest. 2014;124(2):687–95. doi:10.1172/JCI67313.
49. Dewan MZ, Galloway AE, Kawashima N, Dewyngaert JK, Babb JS, Formenti SC, Demaria S. Fractionated but not single-dose radiotherapy induces an immune-mediated abscopal effect when combined with anti-CTLA-4 antibody. Clin Cancer Res: Off J Am Assoc Cancer Res. 2009;15(17):5379–88. doi:10.1158/1078-0432.CCR-09-0265.
50. Dong H, Strome SE, Salomao DR, Tamura H, Hirano F, Flies DB, Roche PC, Lu J, Zhu G, Tamada K, Lennon VA, Celis E, Chen L. Tumor-associated B7-H1 promotes T-cell apoptosis: a potential mechanism of immune evasion. Nat Med. 2002;8(8):793–800. doi:10.1038/nm730.
51. Dunn GP, Bruce AT, Ikeda H, Old LJ, Schreiber RD. Cancer immunoediting: from immunosurveillance to tumor escape. Nat Immunol. 2002;3(11):991–8. doi:10.1038/ni1102-991.
52. Dunn GP, Old LJ, Schreiber RD. The immunobiology of cancer immunosurveillance and immunoediting. Immunity. 2004;21(2):137–48. doi:10.1016/j.immuni.2004.07.017.
53. Farooqi AA, Fayyaz S, Shatynska-Mytsyk I, Javed Z, Jabeen S, Yaylim I, Gasparri ML, Panici PB. Is miR-34a a well equipped swordsman to conquer temple of molecular oncology? Chem Biol Drug Des. 2015. doi:10.1111/cbdd.12634.
54. Filatenkov A, Baker J, Mueller AM, Kenkel J, Ahn GO, Dutt S, Zhang N, Kohrt H, Jensen K, Dejbakhsh-Jones S, Shizuru JA, Negrin RN, Engleman EG, Strober S. Ablative tumor radiation can change the tumor immune cell microenvironment to induce durable complete remissions. Clin Cancer Res. 2015;21(16):3727–39. doi:10.1158/1078-0432.CCR-14-2824.
55. Fire A, Xu S, Montgomery MK, Kostas SA, Driver SE, Mello CC. Potent and specific genetic interference by double-stranded RNA in Caenorhabditis elegans. Nature. 1998;391(6669): 806–11. doi:10.1038/35888.
56. Formenti SC, Demaria S. Combining radiotherapy and cancer immunotherapy: a paradigm shift. J Natl Cancer Inst. 2013;105(4):256–65. doi:10.1093/jnci/djs629.
57. Forshew T, Murtaza M, Parkinson C, Gale D, Tsui DW, Kaper F, Dawson SJ, Piskorz AM, Jimenez-Linan M, Bentley D, Hadfield J, May AP, Caldas C, Brenton JD, Rosenfeld N. Noninvasive identification and monitoring of cancer mutations by targeted deep sequencing of plasma DNA. Sci Transl Med. 2012;4(136):136ra168. doi:10.1126/scitranslmed.3003726.
58. Gajewski TF, Meng Y, Blank C, Brown I, Kacha A, Kline J, Harlin H. Immune resistance orchestrated by the tumor microenvironment. Immunol Rev. 2006;213:131–45. doi:10.1111/j.1600-065X.2006.00442.x.

59. Garcia-Lora A, Algarra I, Garrido F. MHC class I antigens, immune surveillance, and tumor immune escape. J Cell Physiol. 2003;195(3):346–55. doi:10.1002/jcp.10290.
60. Garg AD, Nowis D, Golab J, Vandenabeele P, Krysko DV, Agostinis P. Immunogenic cell death, DAMPs and anticancer therapeutics: an emerging amalgamation. Biochim Biophys Acta. 2010;1805(1):53–71. doi:10.1016/j.bbcan.2009.08.003.
61. Garon EB, Rizvi NA, Hui R, Leighl N, Balmanoukian AS, Eder JP, Patnaik A, Aggarwal C, Gubens M, Horn L, Carcereny E, Ahn MJ, Felip E, Lee JS, Hellmann MD, Hamid O, Goldman JW, Soria JC, Dolled-Filhart M, Rutledge RZ, Zhang J, Lunceford JK, Rangwala R, Lubiniecki GM, Roach C, Emancipator K, Gandhi L, Investigators K. Pembrolizumab for the treatment of non-small-cell lung cancer. N Engl J Med. 2015;372(21):2018–28. doi:10.1056/NEJMoa1501824.
62. Golden EB, Chhabra A, Chachoua A, Adams S, Donach M, Fenton-Kerimian M, Friedman K, Ponzo F, Babb JS, Goldberg J, Demaria S, Formenti SC. Local radiotherapy and granulocyte-macrophage colony-stimulating factor to generate abscopal responses in patients with metastatic solid tumours: a proof-of-principle trial. Lancet Oncol. 2015;16(7):795–803. doi:10.1016/S1470-2045(15)00054-6.
63. Golden EB, Demaria S, Schiff PB, Chachoua A, Formenti SC. An abscopal response to radiation and ipilimumab in a patient with metastatic non-small cell lung cancer. Cancer Immunol Res. 2013;1(6):365–72. doi:10.1158/2326-6066.CIR-13-0115.
64. Gough MJ, Crittenden MR, Sarff M, Pang P, Seung SK, Vetto JT, Hu HM, Redmond WL, Holland J, Weinberg AD. Adjuvant therapy with agonistic antibodies to CD134 (OX40) increases local control after surgical or radiation therapy of cancer in mice. J Immunother. 2010;33(8):798–809. doi:10.1097/CJI.0b013e3181ee7095.
65. Guan X, Yin M, Wei Q, Zhao H, Liu Z, Wang LE, Yuan X, O'Reilly MS, Komaki R, Liao Z. Genotypes and haplotypes of the VEGF gene and survival in locally advanced non-small cell lung cancer patients treated with chemoradiotherapy. BMC Cancer. 2010;10:431. doi:10.1186/1471-2407-10-431.
66. Gulley JL, Arlen PM, Bastian A, Morin S, Marte J, Beetham P, Tsang KY, Yokokawa J, Hodge JW, Menard C, Camphausen K, Coleman CN, Sullivan F, Steinberg SM, Schlom J, Dahut W. Combining a recombinant cancer vaccine with standard definitive radiotherapy in patients with localized prostate cancer. Clin Cancer Res: Off J Am Assoc Cancer Res. 2005;11(9):3353–62. doi:10.1158/1078-0432.CCR-04-2062.
67. Hallahan D, Kuchibhotla J, Wyble C. Cell adhesion molecules mediate radiation-induced leukocyte adhesion to the vascular endothelium. Cancer Res. 1996;56(22):5150–5.
68. Hannan R, Zhang H, Wallecha A, Singh R, Liu L, Cohen P, Alfieri A, Rothman J, Guha C. Combined immunotherapy with Listeria monocytogenes-based PSA vaccine and radiation therapy leads to a therapeutic response in a murine model of prostate cancer. Cancer Immunol Immunother: CII. 2012;61(12):2227–38. doi:10.1007/s00262-012-1257-x.
69. Harper J, Sainson RC. Regulation of the anti-tumour immune response by cancer-associated fibroblasts. Semin Cancer Biol. 2014;25:69–77. doi:10.1016/j.semcancer.2013.12.005.
70. Hassan R, Williams-Gould J, Steinberg SM, Liewehr DJ, Yokokawa J, Tsang KY, Surawski RJ, Scott T, Camphausen K. Tumor-directed radiation and the immunotoxin SS1P in the treatment of mesothelin-expressing tumor xenografts. Clin Cancer Res: Off J Am Assoc Cancer Res. 2006;12(16):4983–8. doi:10.1158/1078-0432.CCR-06-0441.
71. Helwick C. Targeting KRAS mutations in lung cancer: no longer impossible. ASCO Post. 2014;5(14). http://www.ascopost.com/issues/september-1,-2014/targeting-kras-mutations-in-lung-cancer-no-longer-impossible.aspx.
72. Ho AY, Atencio DP, Peters S, Stock RG, Formenti SC, Cesaretti JA, Green S, Haffty B, Drumea K, Leitzin L, Kuten A, Azria D, Ozsahin M, Overgaard J, Andreassen CN, Trop CS, Park J, Rosenstein BS. Genetic predictors of adverse radiotherapy effects: the Gene-PARE project. Int J Radiat Oncol Biol Phys. 2006;65(3):646–55. doi:10.1016/j.ijrobp.2006.03.006.
73. Hodge JW, Sharp HJ, Gameiro SR. Abscopal regression of antigen disparate tumors by antigen cascade after systemic tumor vaccination in combination with local tumor radiation. Cancer Biother Radiopharm. 2012;27(1):12–22. doi:10.1089/cbr.2012.1202.

74. Horiuhi T, Nomura J, Okuda M, Ichinohasama R. Abscopal effect of small intestinal NK/T--cell lymphoma. Rinsho Ketsueki. 2003;44(9):940–5.
75. Ihle NT, Byers LA, Kim ES, Saintigny P, Lee JJ, Blumenschein GR, Tsao A, Liu S, Larsen JE, Wang J, Diao L, Coombes KR, Chen L, Zhang S, Abdelmelek MF, Tang X, Papadimitrakopoulou V, Minna JD, Lippman SM, Hong WK, Herbst RS, Wistuba II, Heymach JV, Powis G. Effect of KRAS oncogene substitutions on protein behavior: implications for signaling and clinical outcome. J Natl Cancer Inst. 2012;104(3):228–39. doi:10.1093/jnci/djr523.
76. Iliopoulou EG, Kountourakis P, Karamouzis MV, Doufexis D, Ardavanis A, Baxevanis CN, Rigatos G, Papamichail M, Perez SA. A phase I trial of adoptive transfer of allogeneic natural killer cells in patients with advanced non-small cell lung cancer. Cancer Immunol Immunother: CII. 2010;59(12):1781–9. doi:10.1007/s00262-010-0904-3.
77. Ishiyama H, Teh BS, Ren H, Chiang S, Tann A, Blanco AI, Paulino AC, Amato R. Spontaneous regression of thoracic metastases while progression of brain metastases after stereotactic radiosurgery and stereotactic body radiotherapy for metastatic renal cell carcinoma: abscopal effect prevented by the blood-brain barrier? Clin Genitourin Cancer. 2012;10(3):196–8. doi:10.1016/j.clgc.2012.01.004.
78. Jeon HS, Jen J. TGF-beta signaling and the role of inhibitory Smads in non-small cell lung cancer. J Thorac Oncol: Off Publ Int Assoc Stud Lung Cancer. 2010;5(4):417–9. doi:10.1097/JTO.0b013e3181ce3afd.
79. Jones S, Anagnostou V, Lytle K, Parpart-Li S, Nesselbush M, Riley DR, Shukla M, Chesnick B, Kadan M, Papp E, Galens KG, Murphy D, Zhang T, Kann L, Sausen M, Angiuoli SV, Diaz Jr LA, Velculescu VE. Personalized genomic analyses for cancer mutation discovery and interpretation. Sci Transl Med. 2015;7(283):283ra253. doi:10.1126/scitranslmed.aaa7161.
80. Kachikwu EL, Iwamoto KS, Liao YP, DeMarco JJ, Agazaryan N, Economou JS, McBride WH, Schaue D. Radiation enhances regulatory T cell representation. Int J Radiat Oncol Biol Phys. 2011;81(4):1128–35. doi:10.1016/j.ijrobp.2010.09.034.
81. Kahlert C, Kalluri R. Exosomes in tumor microenvironment influence cancer progression and metastasis. J Mol Med. 2013;91(4):431–7. doi:10.1007/s00109-013-1020-6.
82. Karachaliou N, Mayo-de-Las-Casas C, Molina-Vila MA, Rosell R. Real-time liquid biopsies become a reality in cancer treatment. Ann Transl Med. 2015;3(3):36. doi:10.3978/j.issn.2305-5839.2015.01.16.
83. Keith B, Johnson RS, Simon MC. HIF1alpha and HIF2alpha: sibling rivalry in hypoxic tumour growth and progression. Nat Rev Cancer. 2012;12(1):9–22. doi:10.1038/nrc3183.
84. Kelly K, Altorki NK, Eberhardt WE, O'Brien ME, Spigel DR, Crino L, Tsai CM, Kim JH, Cho EK, Hoffman PC, Orlov SV, Serwatowski P, Wang J, Foley MA, Horan JD, Shepherd FA. Adjuvant erlotinib versus placebo in patients with stage IB-IIIA non-small-cell lung cancer (RADIANT): a randomized, double-blind. Phase III trial. J Clin Oncol. 2015. doi:10.1200/JCO.2015.61.8918.
85. Kelnar K, Bader AG. A qRT-PCR method for determining the biodistribution profile of a miR-34a mimic. Methods Mol Biol. 2015;1317:125–33. doi:10.1007/978-1-4939-2727-2_8.
86. Kelnar K, Peltier HJ, Leatherbury N, Stoudemire J, Bader AG. Quantification of therapeutic miRNA mimics in whole blood from nonhuman primates. Anal Chem. 2014;86(3):1534–42. doi:10.1021/ac403044t.
87. Kershaw MH, Westwood JA, Darcy PK. Gene-engineered T cells for cancer therapy. Nat Rev Cancer. 2013;13(8):525–41. doi:10.1038/nrc3565.
88. Kershaw MH, Westwood JA, Parker LL, Wang G, Eshhar Z, Mavroukakis SA, White DE, Wunderlich JR, Canevari S, Rogers-Freezer L, Chen CC, Yang JC, Rosenberg SA, Hwu P. A phase I study on adoptive immunotherapy using gene-modified T cells for ovarian cancer. Clin Cancer Res: Off J Am Assoc Cancer Res. 2006;12(20 Pt 1):6106–15. doi:10.1158/1078-0432.CCR-06-1183.
89. Kim KW, Kim SH, Shin JG, Kim GS, Son YO, Park SW, Kwon BH, Kim DW, Lee CH, Sol MY, Jeong MH, Chung BS, Kang CD. Direct injection of immature dendritic cells into irradiated tumor induces efficient antitumor immunity. Int J Cancer J Int Cancer. 2004;109(5):685–90. doi:10.1002/ijc.20036.

90. Kim Y, Ko J, Cui Z, Abolhoda A, Ahn JS, Ou SH, Ahn MJ, Park K. The EGFR T790M mutation in acquired resistance to an irreversible second-generation EGFR inhibitor. Mol Cancer Ther. 2012;11(3):784–91. doi:10.1158/1535-7163.MCT-11-0750.
91. Kirner A, Mayer-Mokler A, Reinhardt C. IMA901: a multi-peptide cancer vaccine for treatment of renal cell cancer. Hum Vaccines Immunother. 2014;10(11):3179–89. doi:10.4161/21645515.2014.983857.
92. Komaki R, Allen PK, Wei X, Blumenschein GR, Tang X, Lee JJ, Welsh JW, Wistuba II, Liu DD, Hong WK. Adding erlotinib to chemoradiation improves overall survival but not progression-free survival in stage III non-small cell lung cancer. Int J Radiat Oncol Biol Phys. 2015;92(2):317–24. doi:10.1016/j.ijrobp.2015.02.005.
93. Komatsu N, Hori S. Full restoration of peripheral Foxp3+ regulatory T cell pool by radioresistant host cells in scurfy bone marrow chimeras. Proc Natl Acad Sci U S A. 2007;104(21):8959–64. doi:10.1073/pnas.0702004104.
94. Kondo K, Okuma K, Tanaka R, Matsuzaki G, Ansari AA, Tanaka Y. Rapid induction of OX40 ligand on primary T cells activated under DNA-damaging conditions. Hum Immunol. 2008;69(9):533–42. doi:10.1016/j.humimm.2008.07.001.
95. Lamers CH, Sleijfer S, van Steenbergen S, van Elzakker P, van Krimpen B, Groot C, Vulto A, den Bakker M, Oosterwijk E, Debets R, Gratama JW. Treatment of metastatic renal cell carcinoma with CAIX CAR-engineered T cells: clinical evaluation and management of on-target toxicity. Mol Ther: J Am Soc Gene Ther. 2013;21(4):904–12. doi:10.1038/mt.2013.17.
96. Leary RJ, Kinde I, Diehl F, Schmidt K, Clouser C, Duncan C, Antipova A, Lee C, McKernan K, De La Vega FM, Kinzler KW, Vogelstein B, Diaz Jr LA, Velculescu VE. Development of personalized tumor biomarkers using massively parallel sequencing. Sci Transl Med. 2010;2(20):20ra14. doi:10.1126/scitranslmed.3000702.
97. Lechleider RJ, Arlen PM, Tsang KY, Steinberg SM, Yokokawa J, Cereda V, Camphausen K, Schlom J, Dahut WL, Gulley JL. Safety and immunologic response of a viral vaccine to prostate-specific antigen in combination with radiation therapy when metronomic-dose interleukin 2 is used as an adjuvant. Clin Cancer Res: Off J Am Assoc Cancer Res. 2008;14(16):5284–91. doi:10.1158/1078-0432.CCR-07-5162.
98. Lee RC, Feinbaum RL, Ambros V. The C. elegans heterochronic gene lin-4 encodes small RNAs with antisense complementarity to lin-14. Cell. 1993;75(5):843–54.
99. Lee Y, Kim M, Han J, Yeom KH, Lee S, Baek SH, Kim VN. MicroRNA genes are transcribed by RNA polymerase II. EMBO J. 2004;23(20):4051–60. doi:10.1038/sj.emboj.7600385.
100. Lesterhuis WJ, Salmons J, Nowak AK, Rozali EN, Khong A, Dick IM, Harken JA, Robinson BW, Lake RA. Synergistic effect of CTLA-4 blockade and cancer chemotherapy in the induction of anti-tumor immunity. PLoS ONE. 2013;8(4), e61895. doi:10.1371/journal.pone.0061895.
101. Lewis BP, Burge CB, Bartel DP. Conserved seed pairing, often flanked by adenosines, indicates that thousands of human genes are microRNA targets. Cell. 2005;120(1):15–20. doi:10.1016/j.cell.2004.12.035.
102. Li H, Liu G, Xia L, Zhou Q, Xiong J, Xian J, Du M, Zhang L, Liao L, Su X, Li Z, Luo Q, Cheng Y, Zhang T, Wang D, Yang ZZ. A polymorphism in the DNA repair domain of APEX1 is associated with the radiation-induced pneumonitis risk among lung cancer patients after radiotherapy. Br J Radiol. 2014;87(1040):20140093. doi:10.1259/bjr.20140093.
103. Li SE, Guo F, Wang P, Han L, Guo Y, Wang XA, Li J, Lyu YM. X-ray-induced expression changes of TNFSF4 gene in human peripheral blood. Biomed Environ Sci: BES. 2014;27(9):729–32. doi:10.3967/bes2014.107.
104. Lim SH, Chua W, Cheng C, Descallar J, Ng W, Solomon M, Bokey L, Wong K, Lee MT, de Souza P, Shin JS, Lee CS. Effect of neoadjuvant chemoradiation on tumor-infiltrating/associated lymphocytes in locally advanced rectal cancers. Anticancer Res. 2014;34(11):6505–13.
105. Lin GH, Edele F, Mbanwi AN, Wortzman ME, Snell LM, Vidric M, Roth K, Hauser AE, Watts TH. Contribution of 4-1BBL on radioresistant cells in providing survival signals through 4-1BB expressed on CD8(+) memory T cells in the bone marrow. Eur J Immunol. 2012;42(11):2861–74. doi:10.1002/eji.201242503.

106. Lu J, Getz G, Miska EA, Alvarez-Saavedra E, Lamb J, Peck D, Sweet-Cordero A, Ebert BL, Mak RH, Ferrando AA, Downing JR, Jacks T, Horvitz HR, Golub TR. MicroRNA expression profiles classify human cancers. Nature. 2005;435(7043):834–8. doi:10.1038/nature03702.
107. Mak RH, Alexander BM, Asomaning K, Heist RS, Liu CY, Su L, Zhai R, Ancukiewicz M, Napolitano B, Niemierko A, Willers H, Choi NC, Christiani DC. A single-nucleotide polymorphism in the methylene tetrahydrofolate reductase (MTHFR) gene is associated with risk of radiation pneumonitis in lung cancer patients treated with thoracic radiation therapy. Cancer. 2012;118(14):3654–65. doi:10.1002/cncr.26667.
108. Mansfield AS, Roden AC, Peikert T, Sheinin YM, Harrington SM, Krco CJ, Dong H, Kwon ED. B7-H1 expression in malignant pleural mesothelioma is associated with sarcomatoid histology and poor prognosis. J Thorac Oncol. 2014;9(7):1036–40. doi:10.1097/JTO.0000000000000177.
109. Marks LB, Bentzen SM, Deasy JO, Kong FM, Bradley JD, Vogelius IS, El Naqa I, Hubbs JL, Lebesque JV, Timmerman RD, Martel MK, Jackson A. Radiation dose-volume effects in the lung. Int J Radiat Oncol Biol Phys. 2010;76(3 Suppl):S70–6. doi:10.1016/j.ijrobp.2009.06.091.
110. Masuya D, Huang C, Liu D, Nakashima T, Kameyama K, Haba R, Ueno M, Yokomise H. The tumour-stromal interaction between intratumoral c-Met and stromal hepatocyte growth factor associated with tumour growth and prognosis in non-small-cell lung cancer patients. Br J Cancer. 2004;90(8):1555–62. doi:10.1038/sj.bjc.6601718.
111. Michael A, Bajracharya SD, Yuen PS, Zhou H, Star RA, Illei GG, Alevizos I. Exosomes from human saliva as a source of microRNA biomarkers. Oral Dis. 2010;16(1):34–8. doi:10.1111/j.1601-0825.2009.01604.x.
112. Mikuriya S, Saito T, Matsuba T, Torii A, Sato O, Adachi H, Yokohari R, Matsumura K, Seto T. Pathologic and immunologic analysis for a case with carcinoma of aberrant breast of the axilla showed "abscopal effect" after the radiotherapy (author's transl). Nihon Gan Chiryo Gakkai Shi. 1978;13(4):406–13.
113. Moeller BJ, Cao Y, Li CY, Dewhirst MW. Radiation activates HIF-1 to regulate vascular radiosensitivity in tumors: role of reoxygenation, free radicals, and stress granules. Cancer Cell. 2004;5(5):429–41.
114. Mole RH. Whole body irradiation; radiobiology or medicine? Br J Radiol. 1953;26(305):234–41. doi:10.1259/0007-1285-26-305-234.
115. Morgensztern D, Politi K, Herbst RS. EGFR mutations in non-small-cell lung cancer: find, divide, and conquer. JAMA Oncol. 2015;1(2):146–8. doi:10.1001/jamaoncol.2014.278.
116. Muenst S, Soysal SD, Tzankov A, Hoeller S. The PD-1/PD-L1 pathway: biological background and clinical relevance of an emerging treatment target in immunotherapy. Expert Opin Ther Targets. 2015;19(2):201–11. doi:10.1517/14728222.2014.980235.
117. Nagaraj AB, Joseph P, DiFeo A. miRNAs as prognostic and therapeutic tools in epithelial ovarian cancer. Biomark Med. 2015;9(3):241–57. doi:10.2217/bmm.14.108.
118. Nagaraj NS, Datta PK. Targeting the transforming growth factor-beta signaling pathway in human cancer. Expert Opin Investig Drugs. 2010;19(1):77–91. doi:10.1517/13543780903382609.
119. Nakajima G, Hayashi K, Xi Y, Kudo K, Uchida K, Takasaki K, Yamamoto M, Ju J. Non-coding MicroRNAs hsa-let-7g and hsa-miR-181b are associated with chemoresponse to S-1 in colon cancer. Cancer Genomics Proteomics. 2006;3(5):317–24.
120. Nakamura Y, Niki T, Goto A, Morikawa T, Miyazawa K, Nakajima J, Fukayama M. c-Met activation in lung adenocarcinoma tissues: an immunohistochemical analysis. Cancer Sci. 2007;98(7):1006–13. doi:10.1111/j.1349-7006.2007.00493.x.
121. Nakanishi M, Chuma M, Hige S, Asaka M. Abscopal effect on hepatocellular carcinoma. Am J Gastroenterol. 2008;103(5):1320–1. doi:10.1111/j.1572-0241.2007.01782_13.x.
122. Newcomb EW, Demaria S, Lukyanov Y, Shao Y, Schnee T, Kawashima N, Lan L, Dewyngaert JK, Zagzag D, McBride WH, Formenti SC. The combination of ionizing radiation and peripheral vaccination produces long-term survival of mice bearing established invasive GL261 gliomas. Clin Cancer Res: Off J Am Assoc Cancer Res. 2006;12(15):4730–7. doi:10.1158/1078-0432.CCR-06-0593.

123. Newman AM, Bratman SV, To J, Wynne JF, Eclov NC, Modlin LA, Liu CL, Neal JW, Wakelee HA, Merritt RE, Shrager JB, Loo Jr BW, Alizadeh AA, Diehn M. An ultrasensitive method for quantitating circulating tumor DNA with broad patient coverage. Nat Med. 2014;20(5):548–54. doi:10.1038/nm.3519.
124. Niki Karachaliou R, Nilsson JA, Berenguer J, Capitan AG, Schellen P, Teixido C, Kuiper JL, Drees E, Grabowska M, van Keulen M, Tannous JM, Heideman D, Thunnissen E, Dingemans A-MC, Ramirez SV, Tannous BA, Drozdowskyj A, Smit EF, Wurdinger T, Rosell R. EML4-ALK rearrangement in blood platelets and outcome to crizotinib in non-small-cell lung cancer patients. 2015 ASCO Annual Meeting. J Clin Oncol. 2015;33(suppl; abstr 8082)
125. Ogden CA, deCathelineau A, Hoffmann PR, Bratton D, Ghebrehiwet B, Fadok VA, Henson PM. C1q and mannose binding lectin engagement of cell surface calreticulin and CD91 initiates macropinocytosis and uptake of apoptotic cells. J Exp Med. 2001;194(6):781–95.
126. Ohba K, Omagari K, Nakamura T, Ikuno N, Saeki S, Matsuo I, Kinoshita H, Masuda J, Hazama H, Sakamoto I, Kohno S. Abscopal regression of hepatocellular carcinoma after radiotherapy for bone metastasis. Gut. 1998;43(4):575–7.
127. Okwan-Duodu D, Pollack BP, Lawson D, Khan MK. Role of radiation therapy as immune activator in the era of modern immunotherapy for metastatic malignant melanoma. Am J Clin Oncol. 2015;38(1):119–25. doi:10.1097/COC.0b013e3182940dc3.
128. Ott PA, Hodi FS, Robert C. CTLA-4 and PD-1/PD-L1 blockade: new immunotherapeutic modalities with durable clinical benefit in melanoma patients. Clin Cancer Res: Off J Am Assoc Cancer Res. 2013;19(19):5300–9. doi:10.1158/1078-0432.CCR-13-0143.
129. Pang Q, Wei Q, Xu T, Yuan X, Lopez Guerra JL, Levy LB, Liu Z, Gomez DR, Zhuang Y, Wang LE, Mohan R, Komaki R, Liao Z. Functional promoter variant rs2868371 of HSPB1 is associated with risk of radiation pneumonitis after chemoradiation for non-small cell lung cancer. Int J Radiat Oncol Biol Phys. 2013;85(5):1332–9. doi:10.1016/j.ijrobp.2012.10.011.
130. Papageorgis P, Stylianopoulos T. Role of TGFbeta in regulation of the tumor microenvironment and drug delivery (review). Int J Oncol. 2015;46(3):933–43. doi:10.3892/ijo.2015.2816.
131. Pasquinelli AE, Reinhart BJ, Slack F, Martindale MQ, Kuroda MI, Maller B, Hayward DC, Ball EE, Degnan B, Muller P, Spring J, Srinivasan A, Fishman M, Finnerty J, Corbo J, Levine M, Leahy P, Davidson E, Ruvkun G. Conservation of the sequence and temporal expression of let-7 heterochronic regulatory RNA. Nature. 2000;408(6808):86–9. doi:10.1038/35040556.
132. Perrot I, Blanchard D, Freymond N, Isaac S, Guibert B, Pacheco Y, Lebecque S. Dendritic cells infiltrating human non-small cell lung cancer are blocked at immature stage. J Immunol. 2007;178(5):2763–9.
133. Pigati L, Yaddanapudi SC, Iyengar R, Kim DJ, Hearn SA, Danforth D, Hastings ML, Duelli DM. Selective release of microRNA species from normal and malignant mammary epithelial cells. PLoS ONE. 2010;5(10), e13515. doi:10.1371/journal.pone.0013515.
134. Piotrowska Z, Niederst MJ, Karlovich CA, Wakelee HA, Neal JW, Mino-Kenudson M, Fulton L, Hata AN, Lockerman EL, Kalsy A, Digumarthy S, Muzikansky A, Raponi M, Garcia AR, Mulvey HE, Parks MK, DiCecca RH, Dias-Santagata D, Iafrate AJ, Shaw AT, Allen AR, Engelman JA, Sequist LV. Heterogeneity underlies the emergence of EGFRT790 wild-type clones following treatment of T790M-positive cancers with a third-generation EGFR inhibitor. Cancer Discov. 2015;5(7):713–22. doi:10.1158/2159-8290.CD-15-0399.
135. Piroozmand A, Hassan ZM. Evaluation of natural killer cell activity in pre and post treated breast cancer patients. J Cancer Res Ther. 2010;6(4):478–81. doi:10.4103/0973-1482.77110.
136. Porter DL, Levine BL, Kalos M, Bagg A, June CH. Chimeric antigen receptor-modified T cells in chronic lymphoid leukemia. N Engl J Med. 2011;365(8):725–33. doi:10.1056/NEJMoa1103849.
137. Postow MA, Callahan MK, Barker CA, Yamada Y, Yuan J, Kitano S, Mu Z, Rasalan T, Adamow M, Ritter E, Sedrak C, Jungbluth AA, Chua R, Yang AS, Roman RA, Rosner S, Benson B, Allison JP, Lesokhin AM, Gnjatic S, Wolchok JD. Immunologic correlates of the abscopal effect in a patient with melanoma. N Engl J Med. 2012;366(10):925–31. doi:10.1056/NEJMoa1112824.

138. Puyol M, Martin A, Dubus P, Mulero F, Pizcueta P, Khan G, Guerra C, Santamaria D, Barbacid M. A synthetic lethal interaction between K-Ras oncogenes and Cdk4 unveils a therapeutic strategy for non-small cell lung carcinoma. Cancer Cell. 2010;18(1):63–73. doi:10.1016/j.ccr.2010.05.025.
139. Qinfeng S, Depu W, Xiaofeng Y, Shah W, Hongwei C, Yili W. In situ observation of the effects of local irradiation on cytotoxic and regulatory T lymphocytes in cervical cancer tissue. Radiat Res. 2013;179(5):584–9. doi:10.1667/RR3155.1.
140. Qu Y, Zhang B, Liu S, Zhang A, Wu T, Zhao Y. 2-Gy whole-body irradiation significantly alters the balance of CD4+ CD25- T effector cells and CD4+ CD25+ Foxp3+ T regulatory cells in mice. Cell Mol Immunol. 2010;7(6):419–27. doi:10.1038/cmi.2010.45.
141. Kurzrock R, Schwaederle MC, Husain H, Schwab RB, Nagy RJ, Lanman RB, Talasaz AA. Detection rate of actionable mutations in diverse cancers using a biopsy-free (blood) circulating tumor DNA assay. In: 2015 ASCO Annual Meeting. J Clin Oncol. 2015;33(suppl; abstr 11004).
142. Rees GJ. Abscopal regression in lymphoma: a mechanism in common with total body irradiation? Clin Radiol. 1981;32(4):475–80.
143. Rees GJ, Ross CM. Abscopal regression following radiotherapy for adenocarcinoma. Br J Radiol. 1983;56(661):63–6. doi:10.1259/0007-1285-56-661-63.
144. Reinhart BJ, Slack FJ, Basson M, Pasquinelli AE, Bettinger JC, Rougvie AE, Horvitz HR, Ruvkun G. The 21-nucleotide let-7 RNA regulates developmental timing in Caenorhabditis elegans. Nature. 2000;403(6772):901–6. doi:10.1038/35002607.
145. Reits EA, Hodge JW, Herberts CA, Groothuis TA, Chakraborty M, Wansley EK, Camphausen K, Luiten RM, de Ru AH, Neijssen J, Griekspoor A, Mesman E, Verreck FA, Spits H, Schlom J, van Veelen P, Neefjes JJ. Radiation modulates the peptide repertoire, enhances MHC class I expression, and induces successful antitumor immunotherapy. J Exp Med. 2006;203(5): 1259–71. doi:10.1084/jem.20052494.
146. Restifo NP, Kawakami Y, Marincola F, Shamamian P, Taggarse A, Esquivel F, Rosenberg SA. Molecular mechanisms used by tumors to escape immune recognition: immunogenetherapy and the cell biology of major histocompatibility complex class I. J Immunother Emphasis Tumor Immunol: Off J Soc Biol Ther. 1993;14(3):182–90.
147. Robbins PD, Morelli AE. Regulation of immune responses by extracellular vesicles. Nat Rev Immunol. 2014;14(3):195–208. doi:10.1038/nri3622.
148. Robert L, Harview C, Emerson R, Wang X, Mok S, Homet B, Comin-Anduix B, Koya RC, Robins H, Tumeh PC, Ribas A. Distinct immunological mechanisms of CTLA-4 and PD-1 blockade revealed by analyzing TCR usage in blood lymphocytes. Oncoimmunology. 2014;3, e29244. doi:10.4161/onci.29244.
149. Rodriguez PC, Quiceno DG, Zabaleta J, Ortiz B, Zea AH, Piazuelo MB, Delgado A, Correa P, Brayer J, Sotomayor EM, Antonia S, Ochoa JB, Ochoa AC. Arginase I production in the tumor microenvironment by mature myeloid cells inhibits T-cell receptor expression and antigen-specific T-cell responses. Cancer Res. 2004;64(16):5839–49. doi:10.1158/0008-5472. CAN-04-0465.
150. Rolfo C, Castiglia M, Hong D, Alessandro R, Mertens I, Baggerman G, Zwaenepoel K, Gil-Bazo I, Passiglia F, Carreca AP, Taverna S, Vento R, Peeters M, Russo A, Pauwels P. Liquid biopsies in lung cancer: the new ambrosia of researchers. Biochim Biophys Acta. 2014;1846(2):539–46. doi:10.1016/j.bbcan.2014.10.001.
151. Schreiber RD, Old LJ, Smyth MJ. Cancer immunoediting: integrating immunity's roles in cancer suppression and promotion. Science. 2011;331(6024):1565–70. doi:10.1126/science.1203486.
152. Schuler PJ, Harasymczuk M, Schilling B, Saze Z, Strauss L, Lang S, Johnson JT, Whiteside TL. Effects of adjuvant chemoradiotherapy on the frequency and function of regulatory T cells in patients with head and neck cancer. Clin Cancer Res: Off J Am Assoc Cancer Res. 2013;19(23):6585–96. doi:10.1158/1078-0432.CCR-13-0900.

153. Sconocchia G, Eppenberger S, Spagnoli GC, Tornillo L, Droeser R, Caratelli S, Ferrelli F, Coppola A, Arriga R, Lauro D, Iezzi G, Terracciano L, Ferrone S. NK-cells and T cells cooperate during the clinical course of colorectal cancer. Oncoimmunology. 2014;3(8), e952197. doi:10.4161/21624011.2014.952197.
154. Shaw AT, Kim DW, Nakagawa K, Seto T, Crino L, Ahn MJ, De Pas T, Besse B, Solomon BJ, Blackhall F, Wu YL, Thomas M, O'Byrne KJ, Moro-Sibilot D, Camidge DR, Mok T, Hirsh V, Riely GJ, Iyer S, Tassell V, Polli A, Wilner KD, Janne PA. Crizotinib versus chemotherapy in advanced ALK-positive lung cancer. N Engl J Med. 2013;368(25):2385–94. doi:10.1056/NEJMoa1214886.
155. Shi W, Siemann DW. Augmented antitumor effects of radiation therapy by 4-1BB antibody (BMS-469492) treatment. Anticancer Res. 2006;26(5A):3445–53.
156. Shi Y, Evans JE, Rock KL. Molecular identification of a danger signal that alerts the immune system to dying cells. Nature. 2003;425(6957):516–21. doi:10.1038/nature01991.
157. Shibamoto Y, Okamoto M, Kobayashi M, Ayakawa S, Iwata H, Sugie C, Mitsuishi Y, Takahashi H. Immune-maximizing (IMAX) therapy for cancer: combination of dendritic cell vaccine and intensity-modulated radiation. Mol Clin Oncol. 2013;1(4):649–54. doi:10.3892/mco.2013.108.
158. Sinha P, Clements VK, Bunt SK, Albelda SM, Ostrand-Rosenberg S. Cross-talk between myeloid-derived suppressor cells and macrophages subverts tumor immunity toward a type 2 response. J Immunol. 2007;179(2):977–83.
159. Siva S, Callahan J, MacManus MP, Martin O, Hicks RJ, Ball DL. Abscopal [corrected] effects after conventional and stereotactic lung irradiation of non-small-cell lung cancer. J Thorac Oncol: Off Publ Int Assoc Stud Lung Cancer. 2013;8(8):e71–2. doi:10.1097/JTO.0b013e318292c55a.
160. Smalheiser NR. Exosomal transfer of proteins and RNAs at synapses in the nervous system. Biol Direct. 2007;2:35. doi:10.1186/1745-6150-2-35.
161. Snyder A, Makarov V, Merghoub T, Yuan J, Zaretsky JM, Desrichard A, Walsh LA, Postow MA, Wong P, Ho TS, Hollmann TJ, Bruggeman C, Kannan K, Li Y, Elipenahli C, Liu C, Harbison CT, Wang L, Ribas A, Wolchok JD, Chan TA. Genetic basis for clinical response to CTLA-4 blockade in melanoma. N Engl J Med. 2014;371(23):2189–99. doi:10.1056/NEJMoa1406498.
162. Sperduto PW, Wang M, Robins HI, Schell MC, Werner-Wasik M, Komaki R, Souhami L, Buyyounouski MK, Khuntia D, Demas W, Shah SA, Nedzi LA, Perry G, Suh JH, Mehta MP. A phase 3 trial of whole brain radiation therapy and stereotactic radiosurgery alone versus WBRT and SRS with temozolomide or erlotinib for non-small cell lung cancer and 1 to 3 brain metastases: Radiation Therapy Oncology Group 0320. Int J Radiat Oncol Biol Phys. 2013;85(5):1312–8. doi:10.1016/j.ijrobp.2012.11.042.
163. Srivastava P. Roles of heat-shock proteins in innate and adaptive immunity. Nat Rev Immunol. 2002;2(3):185–94. doi:10.1038/nri749.
164. Sun Y, Nowak KA, Zaorsky NG, Winchester CL, Dalal K, Giacalone NJ, Liu N, Werner-Wasik M, Wasik MA, Dicker AP, Lu B. ALK inhibitor PF02341066 (crizotinib) increases sensitivity to radiation in non-small cell lung cancer expressing EML4-ALK. Mol Cancer Ther. 2013;12(5):696–704. doi:10.1158/1535-7163.MCT-12-0868.
165. Sundaresan TK, Sequist LV, Heymach JV, Riely GJ, Janne PA, Koch WH, Sullivan JP, Fox DB, Maher R, Muzikansky A, Webb A, Tran HT, Giri U, Fleisher M, Yu H, Wei W, Johnson BE, Barber TA, Walsh JR, Engelman JA, Stott SL, Kapur R, Maheswaran S, Toner M, Haber DA. Detection of T790M, the acquired resistance EGFR mutation, by tumor biopsy versus noninvasive blood-based analyses. Clin Cancer Res: Off J Am Assoc Cancer Res. 2015. doi:10.1158/1078-0432.CCR-15-1031.
166. Takaya M, Niibe Y, Tsunoda S, Jobo T, Imai M, Kotani S, Unno N, Hayakawa K. Abscopal effect of radiation on toruliform para-aortic lymph node metastases of advanced uterine cervical carcinoma – a case report. Anticancer Res. 2007;27(1B):499–503.

167. Tamura K, Shibata Y, Matsuda Y, Ishida N. Isolation and characterization of an immunosuppressive acidic protein from ascitic fluids of cancer patients. Cancer Res. 1981; 41(8):3244–52.
168. Tonn T, Schwabe D, Klingemann HG, Becker S, Esser R, Koehl U, Suttorp M, Seifried E, Ottmann OG, Bug G. Treatment of patients with advanced cancer with the natural killer cell line NK-92. Cytotherapy. 2013;15(12):1563–70. doi:10.1016/j.jcyt.2013.06.017.
169. Topalian SL, Drake CG, Pardoll DM. Targeting the PD-1/B7-H1(PD-L1) pathway to activate anti-tumor immunity. Curr Opin Immunol. 2012;24(2):207–12. doi:10.1016/j.coi.2011.12.009.
170. Townsend SE, Allison JP. Tumor rejection after direct costimulation of CD8+ T cells by B7-transfected melanoma cells. Science. 1993;259(5093):368–70.
171. Tseng CW, Trimble C, Zeng Q, Monie A, Alvarez RD, Huh WK, Hoory T, Wang MC, Hung CF, Wu TC. Low-dose radiation enhances therapeutic HPV DNA vaccination in tumor-bearing hosts. Cancer Immunol Immunother: CII. 2009;58(5):737–48. doi:10.1007/s00262-008-0596-0.
172. Tucker SL, Li M, Xu T, Gomez D, Yuan X, Yu J, Liu Z, Yin M, Guan X, Wang LE, Wei Q, Mohan R, Vinogradskiy Y, Martel M, Liao Z. Incorporating single-nucleotide polymorphisms into the Lyman model to improve prediction of radiation pneumonitis. Int J Radiat Oncol Biol Phys. 2013;85(1):251–7. doi:10.1016/j.ijrobp.2012.02.021.
173. Twyman-Saint Victor C, Rech AJ, Maity A, Rengan R, Pauken KE, Stelekati E, Benci JL, Xu B, Dada H, Odorizzi PM, Herati RS, Mansfield KD, Patsch D, Amaravadi RK, Schuchter LM, Ishwaran H, Mick R, Pryma DA, Xu X, Feldman MD, Gangadhar TC, Hahn SM, Wherry EJ, Vonderheide RH, Minn AJ. Radiation and dual checkpoint blockade activate non-redundant immune mechanisms in cancer. Nature. 2015;520(7547):373–7. doi:10.1038/nature14292.
174. Valadi H, Ekstrom K, Bossios A, Sjostrand M, Lee JJ, Lotvall JO. Exosome-mediated transfer of mRNAs and microRNAs is a novel mechanism of genetic exchange between cells. Nat Cell Biol. 2007;9(6):654–9. doi:10.1038/ncb1596.
175. Vanpouille-Box C, Diamond JM, Pilones KA, Zavadil J, Babb JS, Formenti SC, Barcellos-Hoff MH, Demaria S. TGFbeta is a master regulator of radiation therapy-induced antitumor immunity. Cancer Res. 2015;75(11):2232–42. doi:10.1158/0008-5472.CAN-14-3511.
176. Vatner RE, Formenti SC. Myeloid-derived cells in tumors: effects of radiation. Semin Radiat Oncol. 2015;25(1):18–27. doi:10.1016/j.semradonc.2014.07.008.
177. Vey N, Bourhis JH, Boissel N, Bordessoule D, Prebet T, Charbonnier A, Etienne A, Andre P, Romagne F, Benson D, Dombret H, Olive D. A phase 1 trial of the anti-inhibitory KIR mAb IPH2101 for AML in complete remission. Blood. 2012;120(22):4317–23. doi:10.1182/blood-2012-06-437558.
178. Vinogradskiy Y, Tucker SL, Bluett JB, Wages CA, Liao Z, Martel MK. Prescribing radiation dose to lung cancer patients based on personalized toxicity estimates. J Thorac Oncol: Off Publ Int Assoc Stud Lung Cancer. 2012;7(11):1676–82. doi:10.1097/JTO.0b013e318269410a.
179. Vivier E, Ugolini S, Blaise D, Chabannon C, Brossay L. Targeting natural killer cells and natural killer T cells in cancer. Nat Rev Immunol. 2012;12(4):239–52. doi:10.1038/nri3174.
180. Voets AM, Oberije C, Struijk RB, Reymen B, De Ruyck K, Thierens H, Vandecasteele K, De Neve W, Houben R, De Ruysscher D, Smeets HJ, Lambin P. No association between TGF-beta1 polymorphisms and radiation-induced lung toxicity in a European cohort of lung cancer patients. Radiother Oncol: J Eur Soc Ther Radiol Oncol. 2012;105(3):296–8. doi:10.1016/j.radonc.2012.09.016.
181. Voo KS, Bover L, Harline ML, Vien LT, Facchinetti V, Arima K, Kwak LW, Liu YJ. Antibodies targeting human OX40 expand effector T cells and block inducible and natural regulatory T cell function. J Immunol. 2013;191(7):3641–50. doi:10.4049/jimmunol.1202752.
182. Walter S, Weinschenk T, Stenzl A, Zdrojowy R, Pluzanska A, Szczylik C, Staehler M, Brugger W, Dietrich PY, Mendrzyk R, Hilf N, Schoor O, Fritsche J, Mahr A, Maurer D, Vass V, Trautwein C, Lewandrowski P, Flohr C, Pohla H, Stanczak JJ, Bronte V, Mandruzzato S,

Biedermann T, Pawelec G, Derhovanessian E, Yamagishi H, Miki T, Hongo F, Takaha N, Hirakawa K, Tanaka H, Stevanovic S, Frisch J, Mayer-Mokler A, Kirner A, Rammensee HG, Reinhardt C, Singh-Jasuja H. Multipeptide immune response to cancer vaccine IMA901 after single-dose cyclophosphamide associates with longer patient survival. Nat Med. 2012;18(8):1254–61. doi:10.1038/nm.2883.

183. Walunas TL, Lenschow DJ, Bakker CY, Linsley PS, Freeman GJ, Green JM, Thompson CB, Bluestone JA. CTLA-4 can function as a negative regulator of T cell activation. Immunity. 1994;1(5):405–13.
184. Wang L, Bi N. TGF-beta1 gene polymorphisms for anticipating radiation-induced pneumonitis in non-small-cell lung cancer: different ethnic association. J Clin Oncol: Off J Am Soc Clin Oncol. 2010;28(30):e621–2. doi:10.1200/JCO.2010.31.0458.
185. Wang YS, Tsang YW, Chi CH, Chang CC, Chu RM, Chi KH. Synergistic anti-tumor effect of combination radio- and immunotherapy by electro-gene therapy plus intra-tumor injection of dendritic cells. Cancer Lett. 2008;266(2):275–85. doi:10.1016/j.canlet.2008.02.063.
186. Weiss GJ, Bemis LT, Nakajima E, Sugita M, Birks DK, Robinson WA, Varella-Garcia M, Bunn Jr PA, Haney J, Helfrich BA, Kato H, Hirsch FR, Franklin WA. EGFR regulation by microRNA in lung cancer: correlation with clinical response and survival to gefitinib and EGFR expression in cell lines. Ann Oncol: Off J Eur Soc Med Oncol/ESMO. 2008;19(6): 1053–9. doi:10.1093/annonc/mdn006.
187. Welsh JW, Komaki R, Amini A, Munsell MF, Unger W, Allen PK, Chang JY, Wefel JS, McGovern SL, Garland LL, Chen SS, Holt J, Liao Z, Brown P, Sulman E, Heymach JV, Kim ES, Stea B. Phase II trial of erlotinib plus concurrent whole-brain radiation therapy for patients with brain metastases from non-small-cell lung cancer. J Clin Oncol. 2013;31(7): 895–902. doi:10.1200/JCO.2011.40.1174.
188. Weng D, Song B, Koido S, Calderwood SK, Gong J. Immunotherapy of radioresistant mammary tumors with early metastasis using molecular chaperone vaccines combined with ionizing radiation. J Immunol. 2013;191(2):755–63. doi:10.4049/jimmunol.1203286.
189. Wheatley-Price P, Ding K, Seymour L, Clark GM, Shepherd FA. Erlotinib for advanced non-small-cell lung cancer in the elderly: an analysis of the National Cancer Institute of Canada Clinical Trials Group Study BR.21. J Clin Oncol. 2008;26(14):2350–7. doi:10.1200/JCO.2007.15.2280.
190. Wightman B, Ha I, Ruvkun G. Posttranscriptional regulation of the heterochronic gene lin-14 by lin-4 mediates temporal pattern formation in C. elegans. Cell. 1993;75(5):855–62.
191. Willimsky G, Blankenstein T. Sporadic immunogenic tumours avoid destruction by inducing T-cell tolerance. Nature. 2005;437(7055):141–6. doi:10.1038/nature03954.
192. Wu L, Yun Z, Tagawa T, Rey-McIntyre K, de Perrot M. CTLA-4 blockade expands infiltrating T-cells and inhibits cancer cell repopulation during the intervals of chemotherapy in murine mesothelioma. Mol Cancer Ther. 2012;11(8):1809–19. doi:10.1158/1535-7163.MCT-11-1014.
193. Xiong H, Liao Z, Liu Z, Xu T, Wang Q, Liu H, Komaki R, Gomez D, Wang LE, Wei Q. ATM polymorphisms predict severe radiation pneumonitis in patients with non-small cell lung cancer treated with definitive radiation therapy. Int J Radiat Oncol Biol Phys. 2013;85(4): 1066–73. doi:10.1016/j.ijrobp.2012.09.024.
194. Xu J, Escamilla J, Mok S, David J, Priceman S, West B, Bollag G, McBride W, Wu L. CSF1R signaling blockade stanches tumor-infiltrating myeloid cells and improves the efficacy of radiotherapy in prostate cancer. Cancer Res. 2013;73(9):2782–94. doi:10.1158/0008-5472.CAN-12-3981.
195. Yin M, Liao Z, Liu Z, Wang LE, Gomez D, Komaki R, Wei Q. Functional polymorphisms of base excision repair genes XRCC1 and APEX1 predict risk of radiation pneumonitis in patients with non-small cell lung cancer treated with definitive radiation therapy. Int J Radiat Oncol Biol Phys. 2011;81(3):e67–73. doi:10.1016/j.ijrobp.2010.11.079.
196. Yin M, Liao Z, Liu Z, Wang LE, O'Reilly M, Gomez D, Li M, Komaki R, Wei Q. Genetic variants of the nonhomologous end joining gene LIG4 and severe radiation pneumonitis in

nonsmall cell lung cancer patients treated with definitive radiotherapy. Cancer. 2012;118(2):528–35. doi:10.1002/cncr.26214.
197. Yuan X, Liao Z, Liu Z, Wang LE, Tucker SL, Mao L, Wang XS, Martel M, Komaki R, Cox JD, Milas L, Wei Q. Single nucleotide polymorphism at rs1982073:T869C of the TGFbeta 1 gene is associated with the risk of radiation pneumonitis in patients with non-small-cell lung cancer treated with definitive radiotherapy. J Clin Oncol: Off J Am Soc Clin Oncol. 2009;27(20):3370–8. doi:10.1200/JCO.2008.20.6763.
198. Zhang L, Yang M, Bi N, Fang M, Sun T, Ji W, Tan W, Zhao L, Yu D, Lin D, Wang L. ATM polymorphisms are associated with risk of radiation-induced pneumonitis. Int J Radiat Oncol Biol Phys. 2010;77(5):1360–8. doi:10.1016/j.ijrobp.2009.07.1675.
199. Zou W, Chen L. Inhibitory B7-family molecules in the tumour microenvironment. Nat Rev Immunol. 2008;8(6):467–77. doi:10.1038/nri2326.
200. Zschenker O, Raabe A, Boeckelmann IK, Borstelmann S, Szymczak S, Wellek S, Rades D, Hoeller U, Ziegler A, Dikomey E, Borgmann K. Association of single nucleotide polymorphisms in ATM, GSTP1, SOD2, TGFB1, XPD and XRCC1 with clinical and cellular radiosensitivity. Radiother Oncol: J Eur Soc Ther Radiol Oncol. 2010;97(1):26–32. doi:10.1016/j.radonc.2010.01.016.

Esophageal Cancer

13

Ugur Selek, Yasemin Bolukbasi, Erkan Topkan,
and Zhongxing Liao

Epidemiology

For squamous cell carcinoma (SCC), lifestyle risk predisposing factors include dose-dependent smoking and alcohol consumption; alcohol consumption could be synergistic with smoking. Dietary risk factors include low intake of vegetables, fruits, fish, poultry, and vitamins but high in take of red meat and processed foods. Tylosis and Plummer-Vinson syndromes are predisposing genetic factors for SCC of the esophagus. Gastroesophageal reflux disease and Barrett's esophagitis are known risk factors for dysplasia leading to invasive adenocarcinoma, mainly at the distal esophagus or gastroesophageal junction (GEJ). Human papillomavirus is an infectious contributing factor; *Helicobacter pylori* is a risk factor for gastric cancer, but not for esophageal cancer. Injury from lye ingestion, achalasia, and esophageal diverticuli are other possible risk factors.

U. Selek, MD
Department of Radiation Oncology, Faculty of Medicine, Koc University, Istanbul, Turkey
e-mail: uselek@ku.edu.tr; ugurselek@yahoo.com

Y. Bolukbasi, MD
Department of Radiation Oncology, Koc University, School of Medicine, Istanbul, Turkey

Department of Radiation Oncology, Faculty of Medicine, Baskent University, Adana, Turkey
e-mail: yaseminb@amerikanhastanesi.org; ybolukbasi@mdanderson.org

E. Topkan, MD
Department of Radiation Oncology, Baskent University, Adana, Turkey
e-mail: docdretopkan@gmail.com

Z. Liao, MD (✉)
Division of Radiation Oncology, The University of Texas, MD Anderson Cancer Center,
1422 Pressler St, Unit 1422, Houston, TX, 77030, USA
e-mail: zliao@mdanderson.org

G. Ozyigit et al. (eds.), *Principles and Practice of Radiotherapy Techniques in Thoracic Malignancies*, DOI 10.1007/978-3-319-28761-4_13

Pathological and Biological Features

SCC and adenocarcinoma are the two major types of esophageal cancer. Over the past 3 decades, the proportions have shifted from about 90 % being SCC to about 50 % being adenocarcinoma [2]. Adenocarcinoma arises mostly at the distal esophagus or GEJ, and SCC arises mostly at the mid-esophagus or above.

Staging

The esophagus has an endoscopic length of approximately 40 cm from the upper incisor teeth and the cricoid cartilage at the level of vertebra C7 and extending past the diaphragm to join with the stomach (generally at the lower border of vertebra T11). Workup for the initial evaluation and disease staging is summarized in Table 13.1. The tumor location affects classification, lymphatic drainage, and options for management [3, 4]: general sections are the cervical esophagus (from the level of the cricopharyngeus muscle to the level of the sternal notch), the upper thoracic esophagus (to the azygos arch inferiorly), the middle thoracic esophagus (to the level of the inferior pulmonary vein), and the lower thoracic esophagus (to the lower esophageal sphincter at the esophagogastric junction). According to the seventh edition of the AJCC staging system (Table 13.2), the tumor position is determined by the upper edge of the tumor in the esophagus, not where the tumor volume is largest. Tumors at the esophagogastric junction are staged as esophageal cancer when the tumor's epicenter is within the lower thoracic esophagus, at the esophagogastric junction, or within the proximal 5 cm of the stomach with extension into the esophagus [4, 5].

The length of the primary tumor, although critical for target delineation, is not included in the current staging system. The seventh edition has the same T1–T3 classifications, but the T4 classification has been changed to either resectable T4a (invasion of the pleura, pericardium, or diaphragm) or unresectable T4b (invasion of the aorta, carotid vessels, azygos vein, left main bronchus, vertebral body, or trachea) [4]. The revised manual defines regional lymph nodes to include any paraesophageal lymph nodes, from cervical to celiac, owing to the longitudinal nature of lymphatic drainage. The N classification is also based on the number of involved nodes (N1, one or two; N2, three to six; N3, seven or more). Besides the communication of the caval and the portal venous systems within the submucosa of the esophagus [6], a rich network links the lymphatics in the lamina propria and submucosa and the lymphatics in the muscularis propria and adventitia. Therefore, extensive intramucosal and submucosal spread beyond a grossly visible tumor is not surprising and should be an important consideration in defining the clinical target volume (CTV) in esophageal cancer. Generally all three groups of upper, middle, and lower lymphatic trunks drain into the paraesophageal lymph nodes adjacent to the esophagus; the cervical nodes drain into the internal jugular and upper tracheal nodes; the thoracic nodes into the superior, middle, and lower mediastinal nodes; and

Table 13.1 Workup at initial evaluation

Workup		
History	Screen for family history	
Physical examination		
Complete blood count and comprehensive blood chemistry		
Upper GI endoscopy	Biopsy	
Chest/abdominal CT with oral and IV contrast	If M0	If M1
	Positron emission tomography-computed tomography (PET-CT)	Biopsy of metastatic focus
		HER2–neu testing if adenocarcinoma
	Endoscopic ultrasound (EUS)	
	Endoscopic resection (ER) if early stage	
	Bronchoscopy for tumors at or above the carina	
Assign Siewert category for esophagogastric junction (EGJ) adenocarcinomas	Type I: distal esophageal tumor centered within 1–5 cm above the anatomic EGJ	
	Type II: cardia tumor centered within 1 cm above and 2 cm below the EGJ	
	Type III: subcardial carcinoma centered between 2 and 5 cm below the EGJ, infiltrating the EGJ and the distal esophagus from below	
Smoking cessation	Advice, counseling, pharmacotherapy	
Nutritional assessment and counseling	Consider nutritional support with nasogastric or J-tube but not percutaneous endoscopic gastrostomy (PEG)	

the abdominal nodes into the superior gastric artery, celiac axis, common hepatic artery, and splenic artery nodes.

The revised seventh edition manual also defined separate stage groupings based on the histology of the tumor (Table 13.3) [4, 5].

Evidence-Based Treatment Approaches

The tumor histology (squamous or adenocarcinoma) currently does not influence the choice of therapy, but it does influence the location of the tumor. Epidemiological evidence suggests that adenocarcinoma tends to arise from Barrett's dysplasia in the lower esophagus or GEJ, whereas most SCC arises in the upper esophagus.

Table 13.2 Comparison of changes in sixth and seventh editions of AJCC

	Comparison of TNM staging system	
	Sixth edition	Seventh edition
Tumor	Tis: carcinoma in situ	Tis: high-grade dysplasia
	T1: invasion of lamina propria, muscularis mucosae, or submucosa	T1a: tumor invades lamina propria or muscularis mucosae
		T1b: tumor invades submucosa
	T2: invasion of muscularis propria	Same
	T3: invasion of adventitia	Same
	T4: invasion of adjacent structures	T4a: resectable (pleura, pericardium, or diaphragm)
		T4b: unresectable (aorta, vertebral body, or trachea)
Node	N0: absent	Same
	N1: present	N1: 1–2 regional LNs
		N2: 3–6 regional LNs
		N3: ≥7 regional LNs
	M0: absent	Same
Metastasis	M1a: cervical LN (in upper esophageal cancer) or celiac LN (in lower esophageal cancer)	M1: present
	M1b: all other distant metastases	
LN: lymph node		

Standard treatment options in clude esophagectomy for surgically resectable tumors or concurrent chemoradiotherapy for surgically unresectable tumors. However, the rates of local-regional failure after surgery (37–59 %), radiotherapy (68 %), preoperative chemotherapy and surgery (27–58 %), chemoradiotherapy (46–58 %), and preoperative chemoradiotherapy and surgery (23 %) all remain high, as does the rate of distant metastasis; indeed, the 5-year overall survival (OS) rates are low at 20–27 % [7, 8].

Because radiotherapy is a vital part of the overall management strategy, clinicians must understand the natural course of tumor dissemination to accurately delineate the treatment target for precise delivery of the dose so as to eradicate the tumor and yet spare the surrounding organs at risk. Radiotherapy has evolved greatly over time, from two-dimensional external beam radiotherapy, which had major uncertainties in dose distribution and lack of normal tissue sparing, to three-dimensional conformal radiotherapy and on to intensity-modulated radiotherapy, which has much more desirable dose conformality, which minimizes irradiation of critical normal structures and reduces toxicity. This form of radiotherapy has shown promise for improving treatment efficacy by providing better tumor coverage and reducing toxic effects on normal tissue, possibly allowing escalation of the radiation dose.

The major goal of treatment is to provide the longest possible OS and disease-free survival (DFS), by R0 resection if surgery is used and by complete pathological response if nonsurgical methods such as chemoradiotherapy are used. Summarized

Table 13.3 Stage groupings for squamous cell carcinoma and adenocarcinoma

Stage groupings for squamous cell carcinoma					
TM category	N0		N1	N2	N3
	G1	G2–G3			
T1M0	IA	IB	IIB	IIIA	IIIC
T2M0			IIB	IIIA	IIIC
LE	IB	IIA			
UME	IIA	IIB			
T3M0			IIIA	IIIB	IIIC
LE	IB	IIA			
UME	IIA	IIB			
T4M0			IIIC		
T4a	IIIA				
T4b	IIIC				
IIIC					
Any T, M1	IV				

G histologic grade, *LE* lower esophagus, *UME* upper and middle esophagus

Stage groupings for adenocarcinoma					
TM category	N0		N1	N2	N3
	G1–G2	G3			
T1M0	IA	IB	IIB	IIIA	IIIC
T2M0	IB	IIA	IIB	IIIA	IIIC
T3M0	IIB		IIIA	IIIB	IIIC
T4M0			IIIC		
T4a	IIIA				
T4b	IIIC				
Any T, M1	IV				

below is current evidence supporting the choice of treatment according to the type and extent of the tumor.

Superficial Tumors

The advent of routine endoscopic surveillance for patients with Barrett's esophagus has led to an increase in the global incidence of superficial (T1) esophageal cancer. The two major treatment options for early esophageal cancer, balancing the risk of nodal metastases and procedural risk based on the depth of tumor invasion into the esophageal wall are surgical esophagectomy and endoscopic resection. Submucosa invasion or muscularis mucosa invasion with lymphovascular invasion increases nodal metastasis risk which precludes pure eligibility for endoscopic therapy alone [9, 10]. For fit patients with submucosal (T1b) cancer, esophagectomy will maximize the chance for cure. Evidence on the use of radio therapy or chemoradiotherapy as definitive treatment for superficial esophageal cancer is very limited, and therefore such treatment should be reserved for patients with medical contraindications for surgery or patients who are ineligible for endoscopic therapy because of varices, previous perforation, or severe cervical spine disease.

Locoregional Cancer (Stages I–III)

All patients with potentially resectable localized thoracic esophageal cancer (>5 cm from the cricopharyngeus) and intra-abdominal esophageal or EGJ cancer should be evaluated in a multidisciplinary setting for to consider esophagectomy. Esophagectomy should be done by experienced surgeons, and nodal dissection must be adequate (at least 15 lymph nodes, ≥30 if possible) for a significant reduction in mortality [11, 12].

Only an R0 resection provides substantial long-term survival for patients treated surgically for localized esophageal cancer because of the risk of microscopically positive margins, which confer a disappointing prognos is, even when preoperative chemotherapy is used (Table 13.4) [13]. The Radiation Therapy Oncology Group trial 8911 (Intergroup 113) compared chemotherapy plus surgery (216 patients) versus surgery alone (227 patients) for localized esophageal cancer. The rates of R0

Table 13.4 Perioperative chemotherapy trials

Preoperative chemotherapy plus surgery versus surgery trials						
Trials and References		Median Survival (months)	1 year OS Rate (%)	2 year OS Rate (%)	3 year OS Rate (%)	5 year OS Rate (%)
Kelsen et al.; RTOG 8911 (INT-0113) [7]	Surgery alone	14.9 m	60	37		R0 32 vs R1 5
Preoperative chemotherapy	Cisplatin and fluorouracil ×3 pre- and ×2 post-op	16.1 m	59	35		
MRC trial [14]	Surgery alone	13.3		34		
Preoperative chemotherapy	Cisplatin 80 mg/m^2 + fluorouracil 1,000 mg/m^2 ×2 cycles	16.8		43		
Cunningham et al.; MAGIC [8]	Surgery alone					23
Preoperative chemotherapy	Epirubicin, cisplatin, and infused fluorouracil					36
Ando et al.; JCOG 9907 [15]	Surgery alone					
Preoperative chemotherapy	Two courses of cisplatin plus fluorouracil					55
Postoperative chemotherapy						43

resection were 59 % for the surgery-only group and 63 % for the neoadjuvant chemotherapy group ($P = 0.5137$); 32 % of patients with R0 resections were alive and free of disease at 5 years in comparison with only 5 % of those with an R1 resection [13]. Thus RTOG 8911 showed that postoperative chemoradiotherapy could offer the possibility of long-term disease-free survival to a small percentage of patients, even after an R1 resection.

For cervical or cervicothoracic tumors less than 5 cm from the cricopharyngeus, the recommended treatment is definitive chemoradiation. Preoperative chemoradiotherapy is recommended (41.4–50.4 Gy + concurrent chemotherapy) for non-cervical T1b, N+ and T2–T4a, N0–N+ esophageal cases [16–21], and definitive chemoradiotherapy is the recommended treatment for cervical esophageal cancer and T4b cases, and is an option for patients with non-cervical esophageal cancer who decline surgery (50–50.4 Gy + concurrent chemotherapy) [22, 23]. Radiotherapy alone produces inferior results for both SCC and adenocarcinoma histology relative to chemoradiotherapy according to RTOG 85-01, a randomized trial of chemoradiotherapy (four cycles of fluorouracil and cisplatin given concurrently with 50 Gy in 2 Gy/fraction/day) versus radiotherapy alone (64 Gy in 2 Gy/fraction/day), each without resection [24, 25]. Median survival times were 14 vs 9 months; 5-year OS rates were 27 % (projected 8- and 10-year OS rates of 22 % and 20 %) vs 0%. Local failure as the first site of failure was also higher in the radiotherapy-only group (47 % vs 65 %). The subsequent INT 0123 (RTOG 94-05) trial assessed radiotherapy dose escalation with the same concurrent cisplatin-fluorouracil regimen (64.8 Gy vs 50.4 Gy) and reported no significant difference between the high-dose or standard-dose groups in median survival times (13 vs 18 months), in 2-year OS rates (31 % vs 40 %), and in rates of locoregional persistence or failure (56 % vs 52 %) [26]. The value and efficacy of definitive chemoradiotherapy for locally advanced esophageal cancer have been confirmed in subsequent trials [27–29], in which overall response rates were higher to docetaxel and cisplatin for SCC (71 % complete response) [27] and favorable but not significantly different for FOLFOX4 (fluorouracil, leucovorin, and oxaliplatin) compared with CF [29].

Although preoperative chemoradiotherapy followed by surgery is generally agreed to be the most appropriate treatment for resectable esophageal cancer (Table 13.5), debate is continuing in light of the challenging results of the phase III CROSS and FFCD 9901 trials [19, 30]. CROSS, the largest trial of esophageal cancer (368 patients with T2–3, N0–1, M0 esophageal or EGJ cancer in which the length and width of the primary tumor ≤8 cm; 75 % adenocarcinoma and 23 % SCC), revealed that preoperative chemoradiotherapy with concurrent carboplatin and paclitaxel produced significantly improved OS (median survival times 49 vs 24 months; 1-, 2-, 3-, and 5-year OS rates 82 %, 67 %, 58 %, and 47 % vs 70 %, 50 %, 44 %, and 34 %) and DFS versus surgery alone, in addition to higher R0 resection rates (92 % vs 69 %), higher pathologic complete response rates in SCC than in adenocarcinoma (49 % vs 23 %; $P = 0.008$), and lower rates of locoregional recurrence (14 % vs 34 %; $P = <0.001$) [19, 20]. On the other hand, FFCD 9901 showed higher rates of postoperative mortality (11.1 % vs 4 %; $P = 0.049$) from preoperative chemoradiotherapy with concurrent cisplatin-fluorouracil versus surgery alone, and no improvement in

Table 13.5 Preoperative chemoradiotherapy trials

Trial and Reference	Median Survival (months)	1 year OS (%)	2 year OS (%)	3 year OS (%)	5 year OS (%)
Urba et al. [62]	17.6	58		16	
Surgery alone					
Preoperative chemoradiotherapy schedule: cisplatin 20 mg/m^2/day on days 1 through 5 and 17 through 21, fluorouracil 300 mg/m^2/day on days 1 through 21, and vinblastine 1 mg/m^2/day on days 1 through 4 and 17 through 20; concurrent with 45 Gy as 1.5 Gy/fraction twice daily in 15 weekdays	16.9	72		30	
Walsh et al.[63]	11	42	26	6	
Surgery alone					
Preoperative chemoradiotherapy schedule: two courses of chemotherapy in weeks 1 and 6 (fluorouracil 15 mg/kg/day for 5 days, and cisplatin 75 mg/m^2 on day 7); concurrent with 40 Gy, as 2.66 Gy/fraction in 15 weekdays	16	57	37	32	
Tepper J; CALGB 9781 [21]	1.79				16
Surgery alone					
Preoperative chemoradiotherapy schedule: cisplatin 100 mg/m^2 and fluorouracil 1,000 mg/m^2/d for 4 days on weeks 1 and 5; concurrent with 50.4 Gy as 1.8 Gy/fraction in 28 weekdays	4.48				39
Mariette et al.; FFCD 9901 [30]				47.5	
Surgery alone					
Preoperative chemoradiotherapy schedule: two courses of fluorouracil 800 mg/m^2 and cisplatin 75 mg/m^2; concurrent with 45 Gy as 1.8 Gy/fraction in 25 weekdays				53	
Van Hagen et al.; Dutch CROSS [19]	24	70	50	44	34
Surgery alone					
Preoperative chemoradiotherapy schedule: weekly carboplatin (area under curve of 2 mg/ml/min) and paclitaxel (50 mg/m^2) for 5 weeks; concurrent with 41.4 Gy as 1.8 Gy/fraction in 23 weekdays	49.4	82	67	58	47

OS rates (3 years, 47.5 % vs 53 %; $P=0.94$) or R0 resection rates (93.8 % vs 92.1 %), for patients with localized stage I-II esophageal cancer [30, 31]. The prospective randomized trial CALGB 9781 enrolled only 56 patients, but also concluded from an intent-to-treat analysis that trimodality therapy (chemoradiotherapy with cisplatin-fluorouracil) versus surgery alone for stage I–III esophageal cancer showed a significant survival advantage favoring trimodality therapy (median 4.5 vs 1.8 years; 39 % vs 16 % at 5 years) [21]. Recent meta-analyses confirmed that preoperative chemoradiotherapy plus surgery led to significant reductions in mortality and locoregional recurrence at 3 years [16, 17]; the hazard ratio (HR) for all-cause mortality for neoadjuvant chemoradiotherapy versus surgery alone was found to be 0.78 (95 % confidence interval [CI] 0.70–0.88; $P < 0.0001$), 0.80 ($P = 0.004$) for SCC and 0.75 ($P = 0.02$) for adenocarcinoma, whereas the HR for neoadjuvant chemotherapy was 0.87 (0.79–0.96; $P = 0.005$), 0.92 ($P = 0.18$) for SCC and 0.83 ($P = 0.01$) for adenocarcinoma [18]. The poorly accruing POET has been the only phase III trial to compare neoadjuvant chemotherapy with chemoradiotherapy. This trial enrolled only 126 patients with Siewert I or II/III adenocarcinoma of the GEJ [32]; preoperative chemoradiotherapy was found to produce higher complete response rates (15.6 % vs 2.0 %), lower local recurrence rates (59.0 % vs 76.5 %; $P = 0.06$), and longer absolute survival rates (3-year OS, 47.7 % vs 27.7 %) but none of these apparent differences reached statistical significance.

Esophagectomy is the preferred next step after preoperative chemoradiotherapy, but close surveillance is appropriate for selected cases with no evidence of residual disease [33]. Salvage esophagectomy is recommended for disease that persists after definitive chemoradiotherapy [33, 34]. Preoperative chemotherapy is another option [7, 8, 14, 15]. Esophagectomy for patients with non-cervical esophageal cancer without preoperative treatment may be an option for low-risk, well-differentiated lesions smaller than 2 cm [35]. For patients who underwent esophagectomy without preoperative treatment, fluoropyrimidine-based chemotherapy is recommended for R1 or R2 resection, or no adjuvant treatment for R0 resection [35]. For patients who undergo preoperative chemotherapy followed by esophagectomy, fluoropyrimidine-based is also recommended for R1 or R2 resection, or surveillance for an R0 resection [7, 8, 14, 15, 35].

Postoperative chemoradiotherapy for node-positive or T3–T4 resectable adenocarcinoma of the stomach or EGJ (20 % of 556 stage IB–IV, M0 patients, 1988 AJCC) was investigated in the SWOG 9008/INT-0116 trial [36]. Compared with surgery alone, postoperative chemoradiotherapy with fluorouracil and lecovorin led to significantly improved OS (median survival times, 36 vs 27 months, $P = 0.005$; and OS rates 50 % vs 41 % at 3 years) and relapse-free survival rates (48 % vs 31 % at 3 years) without any increase in late toxicity [37]. Postoperative CRT was also shown retrospectively to be associated with survival benefit for patients with node-positive locoregional esophageal cancer [38, 39]. A DFS benefit was also found (37 % vs 24 % at 3 years for patients with node-positive EGJ adenocarcinoma who did not receive neoadjuvant chemotherapy) [40].

The potential effect of postoperative radiotherapy after radical surgery for esophageal carcinoma was investigated by Xiao et al. in their pre-PET-CT staging era cohort of 495 patients with SCC (200 got postoperative radiotherapy and 275 got surgery alone) [41]. The postoperative radiotherapy covered the entire mediastinum and bilateral supraclavicular areas (midplane dose 50–60 Gy, 25–30 fractions, 5–6 weeks) and led to a nonsignificant benefit in OS at 5 years (31.7 % for surgery alone vs 41.3 % for postoperative radiotherapy, $P = 0.4474$) at with a highly significant survival benefit for stage III patients (13.1 % vs 35.1 %, $P = 0.0027$) [41]. This group also retrospectively analyzed the role of postoperative radiotherapy for 549 patients (274 got postoperative radiotherapy and 275 got surgery alone) based on nodal positivity (269 with N0 159 with 1–2 positive nodes and 121 with ≥3 positive nodes) [42]. Both nodal positivity and receipt of postoperative radiotherapy significantly affected OS [42]; postoperative RT reduced the incidence of intrathoracic recurrence and supraclavicular lymph node metastasis in all patients. For patients with T3 tumors, the 5-year survival rates were 50.6 % for those with N0 disease, 29.3 % for those with 1–2 positive nodes, and 11.7 % for those with 3 or more positive nodes ($P=0.0000$); OS rates for node-positive patients were 17.6 % for 1–2 nodes and 34.1 % for 3 or more nodes ($P=0.0378$) [42]. Schreiber et al. used the Surveillance, Epidemiology, and End Results database to analyze the effect of adjuvant radiotherapy on 1,046 patients (683 with surgery alone and 363 with postoperative radiotherapy) [43]. For patients with stage III disease, postoperative radiotherapy conferred significant improvement in median OS time and 3-year OS rates ($P<0.001$) and disease-specific survival rates regardless of tumor histology ($P<0.001$). On the other hand, other series have found no survival benefit from postoperative radiotherapy, one in 221 patients (102 surgery only, 119 surgery with postoperative radiotherapy) with SCC of the middle to lower third of the esophagus [44], and the other with 30 surgery and 30 surgery and postoperative radiotherapy [45].

For patients who are medically unfit for surgery but can tolerate chemotherapy or chemoradiation, definitive chemoradiotherapy is the preferred option (50–50.4 Gy + fluoropyrimidine-based chemotherapy) [46–49], but single-modality chemotherapy or radiotherapy could be used for patients with poor performance status [50–53]. Palliative radiotherapy and best supportive care are viable options for patients who are medically unfit for surgery and cannot tolerate chemotherapy or chemoradiation [50, 54–56].

For inoperable locally advanced or recurrent or metastatic adenocarcinoma of the esophagus or EGJ, adding trastuzumab therapy in addition to chemotherapy is being considered for patients with HER2-neu overexpression in the ToGA trial [57].

Should Every Patient Undergo Esophagectomy? Selecting Patients Best Suited for Chemoradiotherapy Alone

Two randomized trials, both almost exclusively with patients with SCC, have been done to evaluate the necessity of surgery after definitive chemoradiotherapy [58, 59]; neither found any survival advantage from adding surgery after definitive chemoradiotherapy. One trial tested trimodality therapy consisting of induction chemotherapy (3 cycles of fluorouracil, leucovorin, etoposide, and cisplatin), followed by chemoradiotherapy (40 Gy with cisplatin and etoposide), followed by surgery and compared that with the same induction chemotherapy, followed by chemoradiotherapy with dose escalation to at least 65 Gy without surgery [58]. Adding surgery to chemoradiotherapy improved local tumor control (2-year progression-free survival rates were 64.3 % for trimodality with surgery vs 40.7 % for chemoradiotherapy, HR] 2.1, $P=0.003$) but not survival. Treatment-related mortality rates were significantly higher for the surgery group (12.8 % vs 3.5 %), $P=0.03$), and response to induction chemotherapy was a favorable prognostic factor for both groups of high-risk patients (HR 0.30, 95 % CI, 0.19–0.47; $P<0.0001$). The other trial, FFCD 9102 (89 % SCC) randomized 259 of 444 eligible patients with T3N0-1M0 thoracic esophageal cancer to receive surgery or continuation of chemoradiation (three cycles of fluorouracil/cisplatin with either conventional [20 Gy] or split-course [15 Gy] radiotherapy) if the patients responded to neoadjuvant chemoradiotherapy of (two cycles of fluorouracil/cisplatin on days 1–5 and 22–26 with concomitant conventional radiotherapy (46 Gy in 4.5 weeks) or split-course radiotherapy (15 Gy, days 1–5 and 22–26) [59]. Adding surgery to chemoradiotherapy improved local tumor control rates at 2 years (66.4 % for trimodality with surgery vs, 57 % for chemoradiotherapy, HR 2.1, $P=0.003$) and reduced the needs for stents (5 % for trimodality with surgery vs 32 % chemoradiotherapy, $P<0.001$) but did not improve survival (2-year survival rates 34 % for trimodality with surgery vs 40 % for chemoradiotherapy, $P=0.44$). Moreover, treatment-related mortality at 3 months was significantly higher in the surgery group (9.3 % vs 0.8 %, $P=0.002$).

SCOPE1, a multicenter UK phase II–III trial of 258 patients (65 adenocarcinoma, 188 SCC, and 5 undifferentiated pathology), tested intensification of treatment without surgery, as definitive chemoradiotherapy with 50 Gy in 25 fractions plus four cycles of cisplatin/capecitabine, with or without the epidermal growth factor receptor antagonist cetuximab [60]. No benefit was found from adding cetuximab to chemoradiotherapy, with more treatment failures at 24 weeks and shorter median survival (22.1 months vs 25.4 months, $P=0.035$). Chemoradiotherapy alone, with careful follow-up and salvage surgery, seems to be a sound approach for patients with SCC who achieve a pathologic complete response, but the lack of data on patients with adenocarcinoma suggests that nonsurgical approaches be avoided in such patients [61].

Surveillance Salvage

Surveillance, with salvage treatment as needed, is less common among patients undergoing trimodality therapy than among those treated with bimodality therapy [34]. In one analysis of 518 patients who received trimodality therapy (chemoradiotherapy followed by surgery), 27 patients (5 %) had local-only failure, but 188 (36 %) had distant failure, with or without local failure. Salvage therapy was ultimately beneficial to only 2 % of the 518 patients. On the other hand, salvage strategies were more effective for patients treated with definitive chemoradiotherapy without surgery [33]. In that analysis of 276 patients who did not have surgery within 6 months of chemoradiotherapy had local recurrence rates of 91 % within 2 years and 98 % within 3 years. First relapses were local only in 64 patients (23.2 %), distant (with or without local) in 120 patients (43.5 %), and 92 patients (33.3 %) had no relapses. Final relapse rates were 33.3 % none, 14.5 % local only, 15.9 % distant only, and 36.2 % distant and local. Among the 64 patients with local-only relapse, disease in 36 % could be salvaged with surgery (8 % of all patients), with corresponding median OS times of 58.6 months versus 9.5 months for those who did not have surgical salvage.

Recommended Algorithm for Treatment of Esophageal Cancer

The recommended treatment algorithm for esophageal cancer is summarized in Table 13.6.

Target Volume Determination and Delineation Guidelines

The normal anatomy of the esophagus, with its submucosal network and longitudinal direction of lymph drainage, tends to promote "skip" metastases. Which presents an ongoing challenge in defining the CTV, particularly in light of ongoing

Table 13.6 Recommended algorithm for treatment of esophageal cancer

Tis or T1a	ER ± ablation		
	Esophagectomy if extensive or nodular disease		
T1bN0	Medically fit for surgery	Esophagectomy	
	Medically unfit for surgery	ER ± ablation	
		ER ± ablation	
		Cervical esophagus	First choice: definitive CRT
			First choice:
	Medically fit for surgery		preop CRT + esophagectomy
T1b, N+		Non-cervical esophagus	Definitive CRT if declines surgery
Or			Preoperative C + esophagectomy (if adenocancer)
T2–T4a, N0–N+	Medically unfit for surgery		Esophagectomy if low-risk well-differentiated <2 cm tumors
		First choice: definitive CRT	
		Chemotherapy	
		RT	
		Palliative/best supportive care	
	First choice: definitive CRT		
	Chemotherapy alone if invasion of trachea, great vessels, heart		
T4b	Palliative/best supportive care		
Unresectable			

ER endoscopic resection, *CRT* concurrent chemoradiotherapy, *C* chemotherapy efforts to standardize contouring [64]. Our current recommendation is to create planning target volume that extend 5 cm proximally and distally, with a, 2-cm radial margin around the gross tumor (Table 13.7).

Radial invasion in esophageal cancer is common owing to the lack of serosa, which typically serves as a barrier of local extension. Local invasion of the adjacent organs and structures such as the pericardium, heart, great vessels, trachea, and vertebral bodies should be evaluated carefully.

Nodal spread mainly depends on tumor location; the paraesophageal nodes are the first-echelon nodal drainage stop. Regional nodes are the supraclavicular and cervical nodes for tumors of the cervical esophagus, mediastinal paratracheal and subcarinal nodes for tumors of the thoracic esophagus, and left gastric and celiac axis nodes for tumors of the distal esophagus.

Simulation

Simulation and treatment should be done while the patient's stomach is empty (i.e., nil per os for at least 3 h). The simulation procedure for esophageal cancer is similar to that for lung cancer, including the use of comfortable but strict immobilization for supine patients with their arms over their head (moving arms away from any possible beam

Table 13.7 Summary of site- and technique-specific coverage and treatment planning details

<table>
<tr><th>Tumor location</th><th>iGTV/GTV to CTV margin</th><th>ITV/CTV to PTV margin</th><th>Elective nodal coverage</th><th>Neoadjuvant dose</th><th>Definitive dose</th></tr>
<tr><td rowspan="3">Upper esophagus, above the carina</td><td rowspan="3">3 cm craniocaudally, 8 mm circumferentially</td><td>No 4DCT/motion management and daily IGRT: 1–1.5 cm</td><td rowspan="3">Supraclavicular and periesophageal</td><td rowspan="3">41.4–50.4 Gy in 23–28 fractions</td><td rowspan="3">50.4–66/70 (at the cervical esophagus) Gy in 1.8–2.0 Gy per fraction</td></tr>
<tr><td>4DCT/motion management or daily IGRT: 0.5–1 cm</td></tr>
<tr><td>Both 4DCT/motion management and daily IGRT: 0.5 cm</td></tr>
<tr><td>Distal esophagus and GEJ, below the carina</td><td>Same</td><td>Same</td><td>Periesophageal and celiac ± perigastric, splenic hilum, left gastric, porta hepatis, SMA due to extension into the stomach</td><td>41.4–50.4 Gy in 23–28 fractions</td><td></td></tr>
</table>

IGRT image-guided radiotherapy, *GEJ* gastroesophageal junction, *SMA* superior mesenteric artery angles), holding a T-bar if possible, and with the neck slightly extended and supported by a custom-made cushion for stability. The simulation computed tomography (CT) images should preferably be in ≤3-mm slices. Intravenous and oral contrast is recommended. Four-dimensional CT (4D-CT) is preferred for simulation [65, 66]. Because distal esophageal tumors have significantly greater superior-inferior and anteroposterior motion than do proximal or mid-esophageal tumors, procedures to estimate the internal motion of intrathoracic structures and total extent of motion of the target and critical structures are crucial (Fig. 13.1), particularly if 4D-CT is not available. Alternatives include maximal inspiration and expiration CT scans or slow helical CT scans [67].

Gross Tumor Volume The GTV should include the gross disease at the primary disease site including any extension through the wall, any part of the esophagus wall that is thicker than 0.5 cm, and any grossly involved lymph nodes (nodes that are >1 cm in diameter or have a necrotic center or are positive on PET), which should be delineated on CT, MRI, or PET-CT scans (highly recommended; see Fig. 13.2), as well as findings from clinical examinations, endoscopic ultrasonography, barium swallow, and endoscopy.

Internal Target Volume or Internal GTV Contouring for the GTV should be based on 4D-CT data (respiratory data sets are "binned" by phase: 0–100 % at 10 % interval) in addition to all previously gathered information, and the iGTV is contoured by using the maximum intensity projection (MIP) settings, with modifications based on visual verification of contours in individual respiratory phases (Fig. 13.3) [65].

The GTV can be subdivided into the primary [tumor] site (GTV-P) and the grossly involved lymph nodes (GTV-N). Thorough contouring of the GTV-P is required based on the exact pattern of spread:

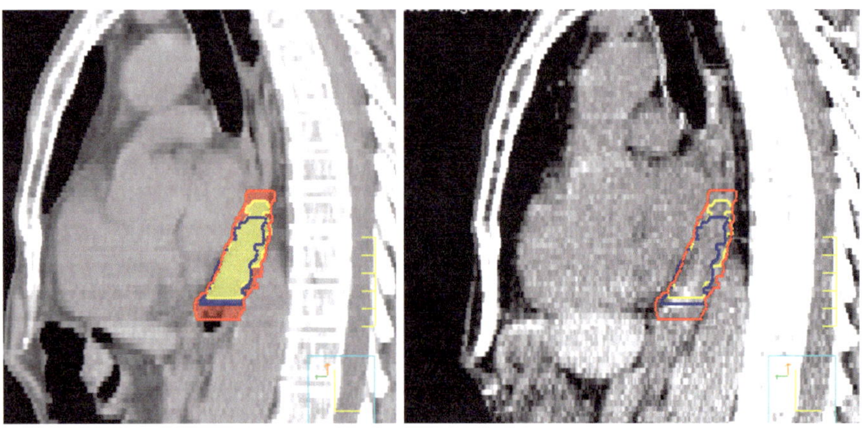

Fig. 13.1 4D-CT estimates internal motion in all extents, especially for the superior-inferior and anteroposterior motion of a distal esophageal tumor. *Blue* contours, conventional CT; *yellow* contours, PET-CT fusion; *red* contours, 4D-CT MIP-based delineation

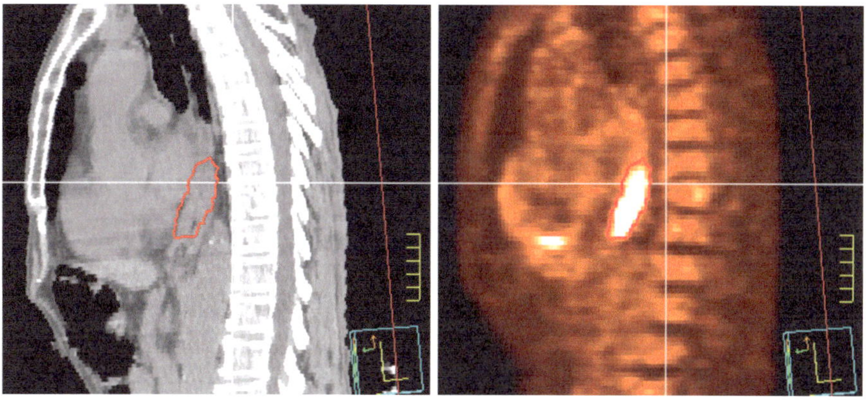

Fig. 13.2 Registering a PET-CT scan to a simulation CT scan can help with GTV delineation

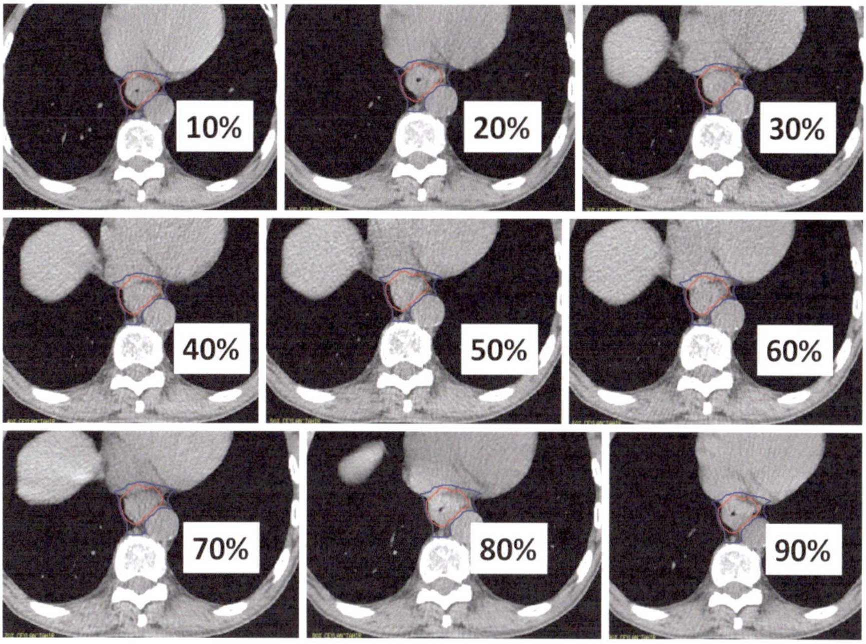

Fig. 13.3 iGTV contouring based on 4D-CT including respiratory data sets "binned" by phase (0–100 % at 10 % intervals); phase delineation at maximum intensity projection (MIP) also generally covers all movement in all phases

Radial and Local

- Is there pericardium invasion (T4a)?
- Is there pleural invasion (T4a)?
- Is there diaphragm invasion (T4a)?
- Is there tracheal invasion (T4b)?
- Is there lung invasion (T4b)?

- Is there great vessel/heart invasion (T4b)?
- Is there liver/pancreas/spleen invasion (T4b)?

Nodal

- What is the highest-echelon nodal disease?
- Is nodal disease regional or non-regional?
- Cervical esophagus: lower cervical and supraclavicular nodes
- Proximal third: paraesophageal and supraclavicular nodes
- Middle third: paraesophageal nodes
- Distal third: paraesophageal, perigastric lesser curvature and celiac axis nodes

Clinical Target Volume Because esophageal cancer can be multicentric or include submucosal "skip" metastases at considerable distances from the primary tumor [68], delineation of the CTV requires generous proximal and distal margins as well as confidence in knowing the extent of disease. Following the recommendations at the time to treat the entire esophagus because of the risk of marginal failure [25, 69, 70], RTOG 85-01 required that the entire esophagus be included in the radiotherapy portals, which led to severe toxicity when radiotherapy was given with concurrent chemotherapy [24]. The subsequent, RTOG 94-05 trial thus recommended 5-cm proximal and distal margins and a 2-cm lateral margin from the lateral border of the GTV [71], based on pathological evidence suggesting that microscopic spread within the esophagus was <3 cm about 94 % of cases except for distal microscopic spread in GEJ adenocarcinoma, which was generally <5 cm [72]. In current practice, most CTVs include an expansion of at least 3-cm following the esophageal mucosa. CTV margins should be modified to avoid irradiating nearby critical normal structures (Fig. 13.4). Whether the radiotherapy is to given before surgery or as

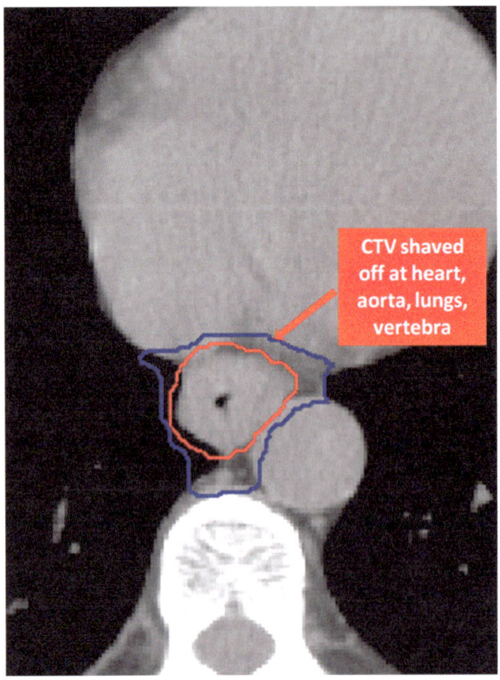

Fig. 13.4 The CTV is generated with an 8-mm expansion radially along the esophagus, which should be modified of "shaved off" to avoid irradiating critical normal structures

definitive treatment, the CTV should include the primary tumor and involved nodes, plus elective primary and nodal regions at risk:

- *Cervical esophageal tumors*: The CTV should encompass the lower cervical, supraclavicular, and superior mediastinal nodes, which generally extend from the laryngopharynx to the upper two-thirds of the esophagus, to cover submucosal spread longitudinally with a 3-cm expansion on the GTV craniocaudally and an 8-mm expansion radially along the esophagus.
- *Mid- and upper thoracic esophageal tumors*: The CTV should encompass the periesophageal and mediastinal lymph nodes plus any submucosal spread longitudinally, with a 3-cm expansion of the GTV craniocaudally and an 8-mm expansion radially along the esophagus. Supraclavicular lymph nodes should be included in the CTV for tumors above the carina.
- *Distal esophageal and GEJ tumors*: The CTV should include the periesophageal and the celiac lymph nodes plus the submucosal spread longitudinally, with a 3-cm expansion of the GTV craniocaudally at the distal esophagus, a 3-cm expansion cranially, and a 5-cm expansion caudally at the GEJ, and an 8-mm expansion radially. Regardless of the location of the primary tumor, the CTV expansion must not be a simple geometric expansion from the GTV; rather, it should follow the shape and course of the esophageal mucosa.

Planning Target Volume The PTV includes an extra margin around the CTV to compensate for variability and uncertainties in treatment setup (internal organ motion is handled with 4D-CT or alternatives). It is especially important to account for respiratory motion for tumors involving the distal esophagus or GEJ. Margins over the CTV are established in accordance with the techniques used for simulation (encompassing internal motion or not), and use of daily imaging (KV, cone beam CT, etc.). Using advanced modalities could allow some margins to be reduced. If the treating institution has not defined the appropriate magnitude of the PTV, a minimum of 5 mm in all directions should be used for each PTV. Acceptable margins for CTV to PTV are as follows:

- –1.5 cm if without 4D-CT or alternative simulation and without daily imaging
- 0.5–1.0 cm if with 4D-CT or alternative simulation and without daily imaging
- 0.5 cm if both with 4D-CT or alternative simulation and daily imaging

Contouring: A Case Example

Delineation of an iGTV and a CTV on a conventional CT scan for a patient with a T3N0M0 distal esophageal SCC is presented in Fig. 13.5.

Treatment Planning

Delineation guidelines for organs at risk have been standardized and are available in RTOG atlases; one exception is the larynx, which also needs to be delineated [73]. Normal tissue constraints can be based on the Quantitative Analysis of Normal Tissue Effects in the Clinic (QUANTEC) guidelines with normal tissue complication probability (NTCP) models (Figs. 13.6 and 13.7) (Table 13.8) [74].

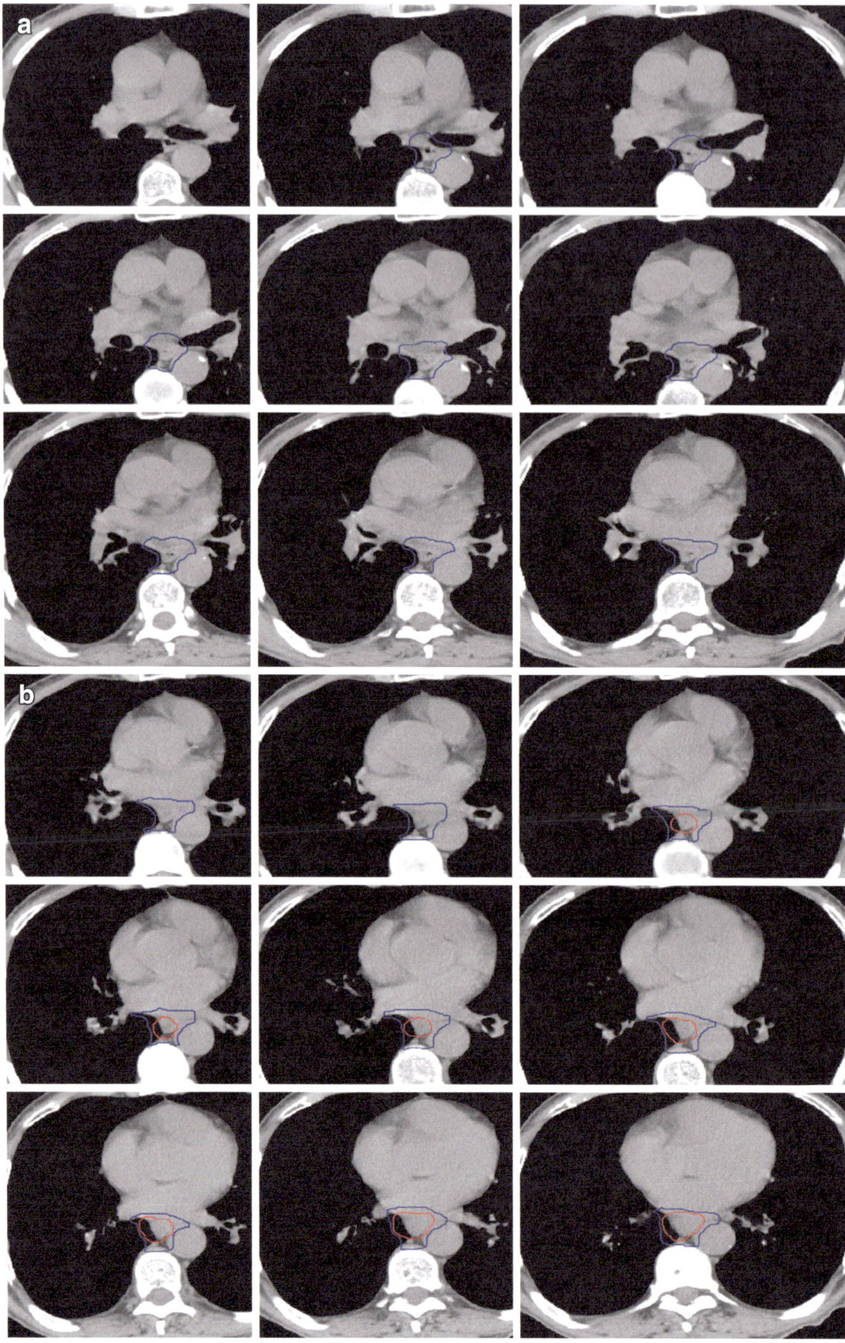

Fig. 13.5 Target delineation for a T3N0M0 SCC of the distal esophagus with coverage of the periesophageal nodes and elective coverage of the celiac nodes (*red*, iGTV; *blue*, CTV)

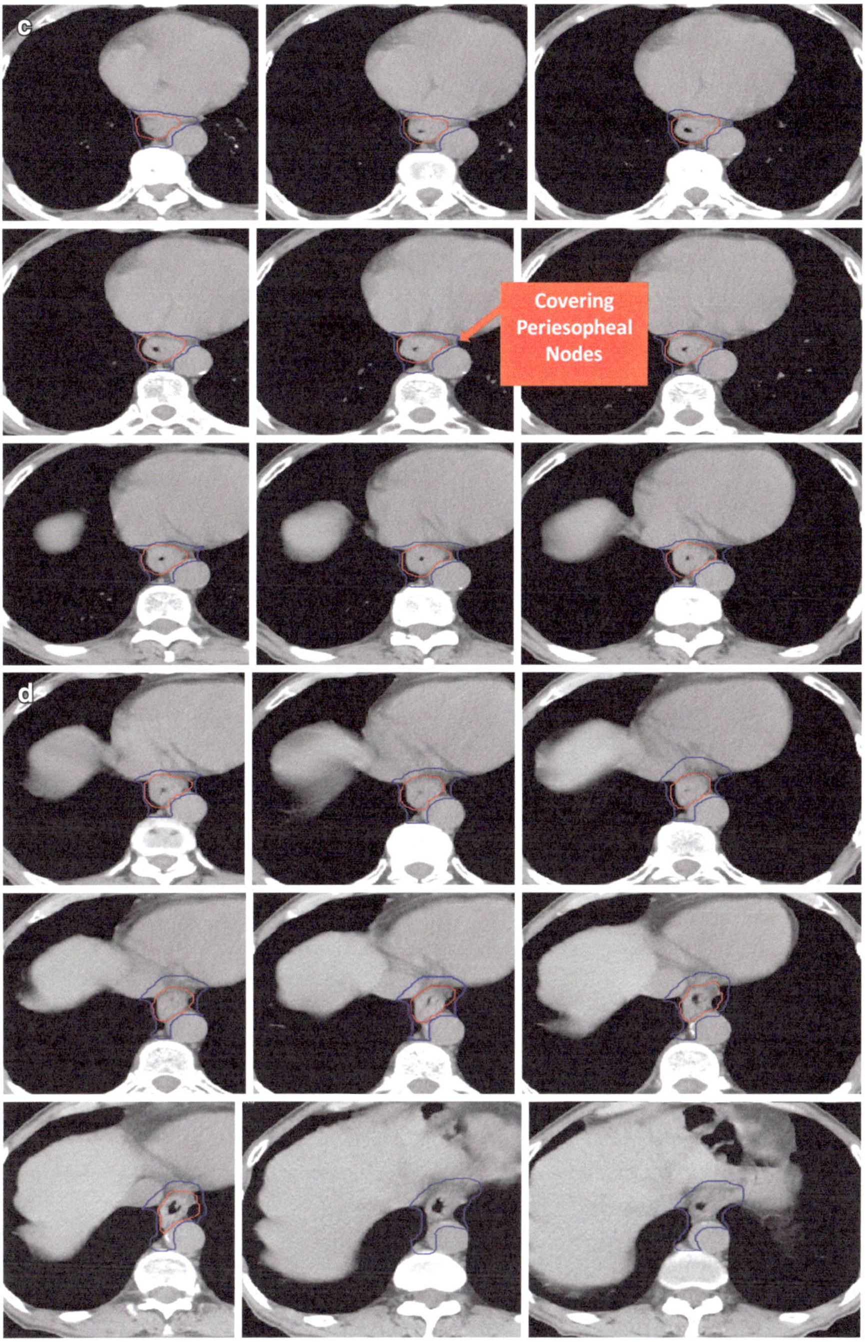

Fig. 13.5 (continued)

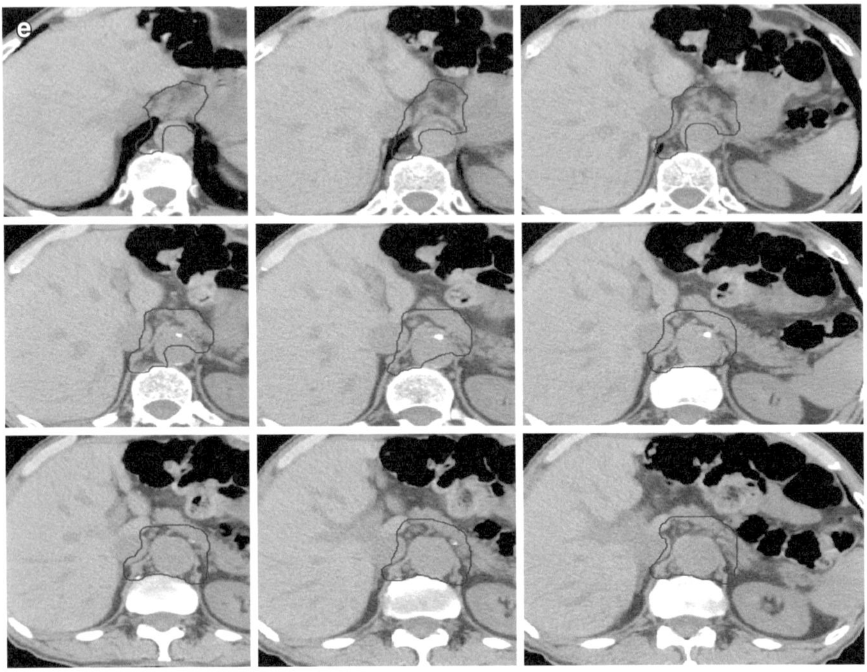

Fig. 13.5 (continued)

Treatment Planning Assessment

Our institutional standard is to deliver 100 % of the prescribed dose to the GTV and 95 % of the prescribed dose to the PTV:

- *Step 1*: Check whether the targets are adequately covered: All plans should be normalized to cover at least 95 % of the volume of the PTV by the prescribed isodose surface, and 99 % of the PTV needs to be at or above 93 % of prescribed dose.
- *Step 2*: Check for the presence of large hot spots: No more than 20 % of the PTV is to be at or above 107 % of prescribed dose, and no more than 5 % of PTV is to be at or above 114 % of the prescribed dose.
- *Step 3*: Check whether the normal tissue constraints are met.
- *Step 4*: Check the placement of any hot/cold spots (slide by slide by looking at isodose distribution): hot spots need to be located in the GTV.

Recommended Algorithm for Follow-Up Surveillance of Esophageal Cancer

The recommended algorithm for surveillance of esophageal cancer after treatment is summarized in Fig. 13.8 [20, 33, 34, 77].

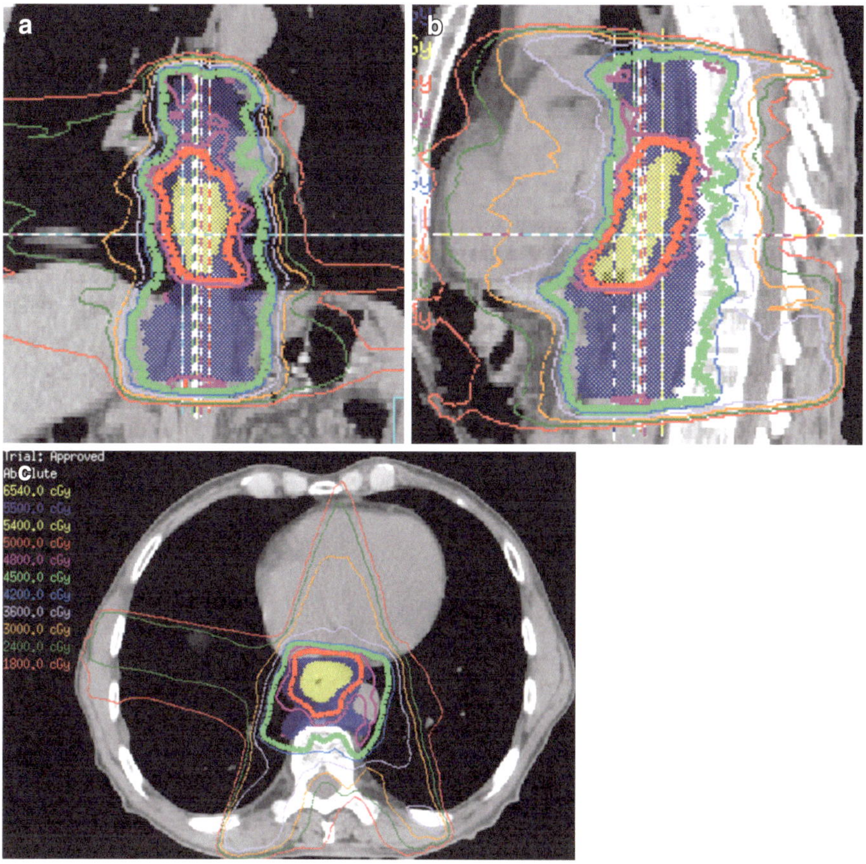

Fig. 13.6 A simultaneous integrated intensity-modulate radiotherapy plan for a distal esophageal tumor. The prescribed dose was 50 Gy (2 Gy/fraction/day) to the iGTV and 45 Gy (1.8 Gy/fraction/day) to the PTV; (**a**) coronal, (**b**) sagittal, and (**c**) axial images

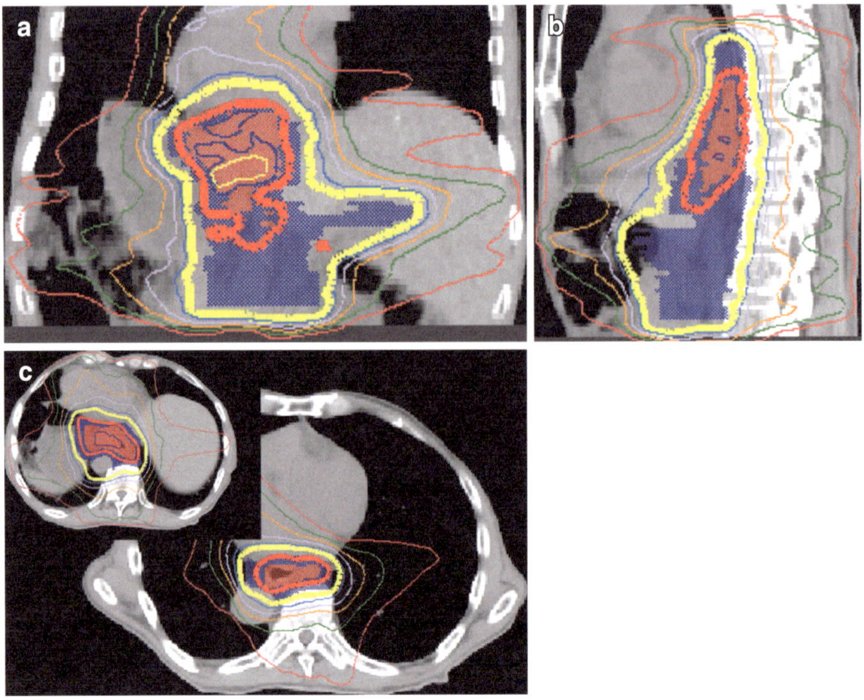

Fig. 13.7 A simultaneous integrated volumetric modulated arc therapy plan for an esophagogastric tumor with situs inversus totalis; the prescribed dose was 50 Gy (2 Gy/fraction/day) to the iGTV and 45 Gy (1.8 Gy/fraction/day) to the PTV; (**a**) coronal, (**b**) sagittal, and (**c**) axial images

Table 13.8 Guidelines for normal tissue constraints

Organ	Constraints [74]		
Larynx	Mean dose <44 Gy		
	D_{max} <66 Gy		
	V_{50} <27 %[75]		
Spinal cord	D_{max} <45 Gy		
	D_{max} <40 Gy if 3 Gy/fraction		
	Even the tumor too close, D_{max} should be <60 Gy		
Lung	Mean dose <20 Gy		
	Mean dose <8 Gy if post-pneumonectomy		
	RT alone	RT with concurrent chemotherapy	Neoadjuvant treatment before surgery [76]
	$V_{20} \leq 40$ %	$V_{20} \leq 35$ %	$V_{20} \leq 30$ %
		$V_{10} \leq 45$ %	$V_{10} \leq 40$ %
		$V_5 \leq 65$ %	$V_5 \leq 55$ %
	V20 <10 % and V5 <60 % if post-pneumonectomy		

Table 13.8 (continued)

Organ	Constraints [74]
Heart	Mean dose <26 Gy
	V_{30} ≤45 %
Esophagus	Mean dose <34 Gy
	D_{max} ≤80 Gy
	V_{70} <20 %
	V_{50} <50 %
Kidney	20 Gy <32 % of bilateral kidney
Liver	Mean dose <30 Gy
	V30 <40 %

Dmax maximal dose, *GTV* gross tumor volume, *RT* radiotherapy

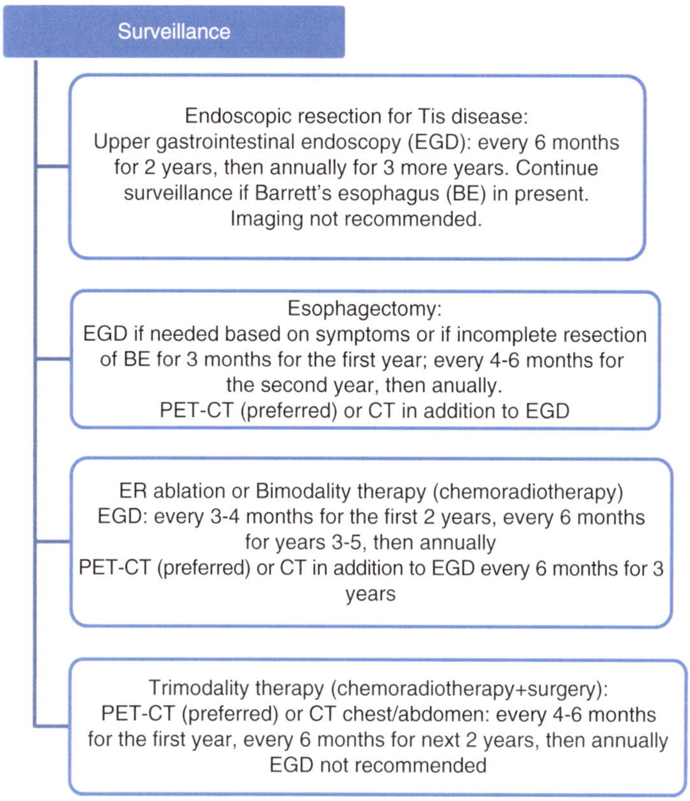

Fig. 13.8 Recommended algorithm for follow-up

References

1. Siewert J, Fink U, Beckurts K, Roder J. Surgery of squamous cell carcinoma of the esophagus. Ann Oncol. 1994;5:1–7.
2. Devesa S, Blot W, Fraumeni JF. Changing patterns in the incidence of esophageal and gastric carcinoma in the United States. Cancer. 1998;83:2049–53.
3. Hong SJ, Kim TJ, Nam KB, Lee IS, Yang HC, Cho S, Kim K, Jheon S, Lee KW. New TNM staging system for esophageal cancer: what chest radiologists need to know. Radiographics. 2014;34(6):1722–40.
4. Rice TW, Blackstone EH, Rusch VW. 7th edition of the AJCC cancer staging manual: esophagus and esophagogastric junction. Ann Surg Oncol. 2010;17(7):1721–4.
5. Sobin LH, Compton CC. TNM seventh edition: what's new, what's changed: communication from the International Union Against Cancer and the American Joint Committee on Cancer. Cancer. 2010;116(22):5336–9.
6. DeNardi FG, Riddell RH. The normal esophagus. Am J Surg Pathol. 1991;15(3):296–309.
7. Kelsen DP, Ginsberg R, Pajak TF, Sheahan DG, Gunderson L, Mortimer J, Estes N, Haller DG, Ajani J, Kocha W, et al. Chemotherapy followed by surgery compared with surgery alone for localized esophageal cancer. N Engl J Med. 1998;339(27):1979–84.
8. Cunningham D, Allum WH, Stenning SP, Thompson JN, Van de Velde CJ, Nicolson M, Scarffe JH, Lofts FJ, Falk SJ, Iveson TJ, et al. Perioperative chemotherapy versus surgery alone for resectable gastroesophageal cancer. N Engl J Med. 2006;355(1):11–20.
9. Eguchi T, Nakanishi Y, Shimoda T, Iwasaki M, Igaki H, Tachimori Y, Kato H, Yamaguchi H, Saito D, Umemura S. Histopathological criteria for additional treatment after endoscopic mucosal resection for esophageal cancer: analysis of 464 surgically resected cases. Mod Pathol. 2006;19(3):475–80.
10. Akutsu Y, Uesato M, Shuto K, Kono T, Hoshino I, Horibe D, Sazuka T, Takeshita N, Maruyama T, Isozaki Y, et al. The overall prevalence of metastasis in T1 esophageal squamous cell carcinoma: a retrospective analysis of 295 patients. Ann Surg. 2013;257(6):1032–8.
11. Groth SS, Virnig BA, Whitson BA, DeFor TE, Li ZZ, Tuttle TM, Maddaus MA. Determination of the minimum number of lymph nodes to examine to maximize survival in patients with esophageal carcinoma: data from the Surveillance Epidemiology and End Results database. J Thorac Cardiovasc Surg. 2010;139(3):612–20.
12. Rizk NP, Ishwaran H, Rice TW, Chen LQ, Schipper PH, Kesler KA, Law S, Lerut TE, Reed CE, Salo JA, et al. Optimum lymphadenectomy for esophageal cancer. Ann Surg. 2010;251(1):46–50.
13. Kelsen DP, Winter KA, Gunderson LL, Mortimer J, Estes NC, Haller DG, Ajani JA, Kocha W, Minsky BD, Roth JA, et al. Long-term results of RTOG trial 8911 (USA Intergroup 113): a random assignment trial comparison of chemotherapy followed by surgery compared with surgery alone for esophageal cancer. J Clin Oncol. 2007;25(24):3719–25.
14. Surgical resection with or without preoperative chemotherapy in oesophageal cancer: a randomised controlled trial. Lancet. 2002; 359(9319):1727–33.
15. Ando N, Kato H, Igaki H, Shinoda M, Ozawa S, Shimizu H, Nakamura T, Yabusaki H, Aoyama N, Kurita A, et al. A randomized trial comparing postoperative adjuvant chemotherapy with cisplatin and 5-fluorouracil versus preoperative chemotherapy for localized advanced squamous cell carcinoma of the thoracic esophagus (JCOG9907). Ann Surg Oncol. 2012;19(1):68–74.
16. Urschel JD, Vasan H. A meta-analysis of randomized controlled trials that compared neoadjuvant chemoradiation and surgery to surgery alone for resectable esophageal cancer. Am J Surg. 2003;185(6):538–43.
17. Fiorica F, Di Bona D, Schepis F, Licata A, Shahied L, Venturi A, Falchi AM, Craxi A, Camma C. Preoperative chemoradiotherapy for oesophageal cancer: a systematic review and meta-analysis. Gut. 2004;53(7):925–30.

18. Sjoquist KM, Burmeister BH, Smithers BM, Zalcberg JR, Simes RJ, Barbour A, Gebski V. Survival after neoadjuvant chemotherapy or chemoradiotherapy for resectable oesophageal carcinoma: an updated meta-analysis. Lancet Oncol. 2011;12(7):681–92.
19. van Hagen P, Hulshof MC, van Lanschot JJ, Steyerberg EW, van Berge Henegouwen MI, Wijnhoven BP, Richel DJ, Nieuwenhuijzen GA, Hospers GA, Bonenkamp JJ, et al. Preoperative chemoradiotherapy for esophageal or junctional cancer. N Engl J Med. 2012;366(22): 2074–84.
20. Oppedijk V, van der Gaast A, van Lanschot JJ, van Hagen P, van Os R, van Rij CM, van der Sangen MJ, Beukema JC, Rutten H, Spruit PH, et al. Patterns of recurrence after surgery alone versus preoperative chemoradiotherapy and surgery in the CROSS trials. J Clin Oncol. 2014;32(5):385–91.
21. Tepper J, Krasna MJ, Niedzwiecki D, Hollis D, Reed CE, Goldberg R, Kiel K, Willett C, Sugarbaker D, Mayer R. Phase III trial of trimodality therapy with cisplatin, fluorouracil, radiotherapy, and surgery compared with surgery alone for esophageal cancer: CALGB 9781. J Clin Oncol. 2008;26(7):1086–92.
22. Kleinberg L, Forastiere AA. Chemoradiation in the management of esophageal cancer. J Clin Oncol. 2007;25(26):4110–7.
23. Suntharalingam M. Definitive chemoradiation in the management of locally advanced esophageal cancer. Semin Radiat Oncol. 2007;17(1):22–8.
24. Cooper JS, Guo MD, Herskovic A, Macdonald JS, Martenson Jr JA, Al-Sarraf M, Byhardt R, Russell AH, Beitler JJ, Spencer S, et al. Chemoradiotherapy of locally advanced esophageal cancer: long-term follow-up of a prospective randomized trial (RTOG 85-01). Radiation Therapy Oncology Group. JAMA. 1999;281(17):1623–7.
25. Herskovic A, Martz K, al-Sarraf M, Leichman L, Brindle J, Vaitkevicius V, Cooper J, Byhardt R, Davis L, Emami B. Combined chemotherapy and radiotherapy compared with radiotherapy alone in patients with cancer of the esophagus. N Engl J Med. 1992;326(24):1593–8.
26. Minsky BD, Pajak TF, Ginsberg RJ, Pisansky TM, Martenson J, Komaki R, Okawara G, Rosenthal SA, Kelsen DP. INT 0123 (Radiation Therapy Oncology Group 94-05) phase III trial of combined-modality therapy for esophageal cancer: high-dose versus standard-dose radiation therapy. J Clin Oncol. 2002;20(5):1167–74.
27. Li QQ, Liu MZ, Hu YH, Liu H, He ZY, Lin HX. Definitive concomitant chemoradiotherapy with docetaxel and cisplatin in squamous esophageal carcinoma. Dis Esophagus. 2010;23(3):253–9.
28. Ruppert BN, Watkins JM, Shirai K, Wahlquist AE, Garrett-Mayer E, Aguero EG, Sherman CA, Reed CE, Sharma AK. Cisplatin/Irinotecan versus carboplatin/paclitaxel as definitive chemoradiotherapy for locoregionally advanced esophageal cancer. Am J Clin Oncol. 2010;33(4):346–52.
29. Conroy T, Galais MP, Raoul JL, Bouche O, Gourgou-Bourgade S, Douillard JY, Etienne PL, Boige V, Martel-Lafay I, Michel P, et al. Definitive chemoradiotherapy with FOLFOX versus fluorouracil and cisplatin in patients with oesophageal cancer (PRODIGE5/ACCORD17): final results of a randomised, phase 2/3 trial. Lancet Oncol. 2014;15(3):305–14.
30. Mariette C, Dahan L, Mornex F, Maillard E, Thomas PA, Meunier B, Boige V, Pezet D, Robb WB, Le Brun-Ly V, et al. Surgery alone versus chemoradiotherapy followed by surgery for stage I and II esophageal cancer: final analysis of randomized controlled phase III trial FFCD 9901. J Clin Oncol. 2014;32(23):2416–22.
31. Czito BG, Palta M, Willett CG. Results of the FFCD 9901 trial in early-stage esophageal carcinoma: is it really about neoadjuvant therapy? J Clin Oncol. 2014;32(23):2398–400.
32. Stahl M, Walz MK, Stuschke M, Lehmann N, Meyer HJ, Riera-Knorrenschild J, Langer P, Engenhart-Cabillic R, Bitzer M, Konigsrainer A, et al. Phase III comparison of preoperative chemotherapy compared with chemoradiotherapy in patients with locally advanced adenocarcinoma of the esophagogastric junction. J Clin Oncol. 2009;27(6):851–6.

33. Sudo K, Xiao L, Wadhwa R, Shiozaki H, Elimova E, Taketa T, Blum MA, Lee JH, Bhutani MS, Weston B, et al. Importance of surveillance and success of salvage strategies after definitive chemoradiation in patients with esophageal cancer. J Clin Oncol. 2014;32(30):3400–5.
34. Sudo K, Taketa T, Correa AM, Campagna MC, Wadhwa R, Blum MA, Komaki R, Lee JH, Bhutani MS, Weston B, et al. Locoregional failure rate after preoperative chemoradiation of esophageal adenocarcinoma and the outcomes of salvage strategies. J Clin Oncol. 2013;31(34):4306–10.
35. Stahl M, Mariette C, Haustermans K, Cervantes A, Arnold D. Oesophageal cancer: ESMO Clinical Practice Guidelines for diagnosis, treatment and follow-up. Ann Oncol. 2013;24 Suppl 6:vi51–6.
36. Macdonald JS, Smalley SR, Benedetti J, Hundahl SA, Estes NC, Stemmermann GN, Haller DG, Ajani JA, Gunderson LL, Jessup JM, et al. Chemoradiotherapy after surgery compared with surgery alone for adenocarcinoma of the stomach or gastroesophageal junction. N Engl J Med. 2001;345(10):725–30.
37. Smalley SR, Benedetti JK, Haller DG, Hundahl SA, Estes NC, Ajani JA, Gunderson LL, Goldman B, Martenson JA, Jessup JM, et al. Updated analysis of SWOG-directed intergroup study 0116: a phase III trial of adjuvant radiochemotherapy versus observation after curative gastric cancer resection. J Clin Oncol. 2012;30(19):2327–33.
38. Bedard EL, Inculet RI, Malthaner RA, Brecevic E, Vincent M, Dar R. The role of surgery and postoperative chemoradiation therapy in patients with lymph node positive esophageal carcinoma. Cancer. 2001;91(12):2423–30.
39. Rice TW, Adelstein DJ, Chidel MA, Rybicki LA, DeCamp MM, Murthy SC, Blackstone EH. Benefit of postoperative adjuvant chemoradiotherapy in locoregionally advanced esophageal carcinoma. J Thorac Cardiovasc Surg. 2003;126(5):1590–6.
40. Kofoed SC, Muhic A, Baeksgaard L, Jendresen M, Gustafsen J, Holm J, Bardram L, Brandt B, Breno J, Svendsen LB. Survival after adjuvant chemoradiotherapy or surgery alone in resectable adenocarcinoma at the gastro-esophageal junction. Scand J Surg. 2012;101(1):26–31.
41. Xiao ZF, Yang ZY, Liang J, Miao YJ, Wang M, Yin WB, Gu XZ, Zhang DC, Zhang RG, Wang LJ. Value of radiotherapy after radical surgery for esophageal carcinoma: a report of 495 patients. Ann Thorac Surg. 2003;75(2):331–6.
42. Xiao ZF, Yang ZY, Miao YJ, Wang LH, Yin WB, Gu XZ, Zhang DC, Sun KL, Chen GY, He J. Influence of number of metastatic lymph nodes on survival of curative resected thoracic esophageal cancer patients and value of radiotherapy: report of 549 cases. Int J Radiat Oncol Biol Phys. 2005;62(1):82–90.
43. Schreiber D, Rineer J, Vongtama D, Wortham A, Han P, Schwartz D, Choi K, Rotman M. Impact of postoperative radiation after esophagectomy for esophageal cancer. J Thorac Oncol. 2010;5(2):244–50.
44. Teniere P, Hay JM, Fingerhut A, Fagniez PL. Postoperative radiation therapy does not increase survival after curative resection for squamous cell carcinoma of the middle and lower esophagus as shown by a multicenter controlled trial. French University Association for Surgical Research. Surg Gynecol Obstet. 1991;173(2):123–30.
45. Fok M, Sham JS, Choy D, Cheng SW, Wong J. Postoperative radiotherapy for carcinoma of the esophagus: a prospective, randomized controlled study. Surgery. 1993;113(2):138–47.
46. Blum MA, Taketa T, Sudo K, Wadhwa R, Skinner HD, Ajani JA. Chemoradiation for esophageal cancer. Thorac Surg Clin. 2013;23(4):551–8.
47. Shiozaki H, Sudo K, Xiao L, Wadhwa R, Elimova E, Hofstetter WL, Skinner HD, Lee JH, Weston B, Bhutani MS, et al. Distribution and timing of distant metastasis after local therapy in a large cohort of patients with esophageal and esophagogastric junction cancer. Oncology. 2014;86(5–6):336–9.
48. Pottgen C, Stuschke M. Radiotherapy versus surgery within multimodality protocols for esophageal cancer – a meta-analysis of the randomized trials. Cancer Treat Rev. 2012;38(6):599–604.

49. Amini A, Ajani J, Komaki R, Allen PK, Minsky BD, Blum M, Xiao L, Suzuki A, Hofstetter W, Swisher S, et al. Factors associated with local-regional failure after definitive chemoradiation for locally advanced esophageal cancer. Ann Surg Oncol. 2014;21(1):306–14.
50. Prasad NR, Karthigeyan M, Vikram K, Parthasarathy R, Reddy KS. Palliative radiotherapy in esophageal cancer. Indian J Surg. 2015;77(1):34–8.
51. Berger AK, Zschaebitz S, Komander C, Jager D, Haag GM. Palliative chemotherapy for gastroesophageal cancer in old and very old patients: a retrospective cohort study at the National Center for Tumor Diseases, Heidelberg. World J Gastroenterol. 2015;21(16):4911–8.
52. Murray LJ, Din OS, Kumar VS, Dixon LM, Wadsley JC. Palliative radiotherapy in patients with esophageal carcinoma: a retrospective review. Pract Radiat Oncol. 2012;2(4):257–64.
53. Freeman RK, Ascioti AJ, Mahidhara RJ. Palliative therapy for patients with unresectable esophageal carcinoma. Surg Clin N Am. 2012;92(5):1337–51.
54. Yamashita M, Yamashita H, Shibata S, Okuma K, Nakagawa K. Symptom relief effect of palliative high dose rate intracavitary radiotherapy for advanced esophageal cancer with dysphagia. Oncol Lett. 2015;9(4):1747–52.
55. Hingorani M, Dixit S, Johnson M, Plested V, Alty K, Colley P, Beavis AW, Roy R, Maraveyas A. Palliative radiotherapy in the presence of well-controlled metastatic disease after initial chemotherapy may prolong survival in patients with metastatic esophageal and gastric cancer. Cancer Res Treat. 2015;47:706–17.
56. Nieman DR, Peters JH. Treatment strategies for esophageal cancer. Gastroenterol Clin N Am. 2013;42(1):187–97.
57. Bang YJ, Van Cutsem E, Feyereislova A, Chung HC, Shen L, Sawaki A, Lordick F, Ohtsu A, Omuro Y, Satoh T, et al. Trastuzumab in combination with chemotherapy versus chemotherapy alone for treatment of HER2-positive advanced gastric or gastro-oesophageal junction cancer (ToGA): a phase 3, open-label, randomised controlled trial. Lancet. 2010;376(9742):687–97.
58. Stahl M, Stuschke M, Lehmann N, Meyer HJ, Walz MK, Seeber S, Klump B, Budach W, Teichmann R, Schmitt M, et al. Chemoradiation with and without surgery in patients with locally advanced squamous cell carcinoma of the esophagus. J Clin Oncol. 2005;23(10):2310–7.
59. Bedenne L, Michel P, Bouche O, Milan C, Mariette C, Conroy T, Pezet D, Roullet B, Seitz JF, Herr JP, et al. Chemoradiation followed by surgery compared with chemoradiation alone in squamous cancer of the esophagus: FFCD 9102. J Clin Oncol. 2007;25(10):1160–8.
60. Crosby T, Hurt CN, Falk S, Gollins S, Mukherjee S, Staffurth J, Ray R, Bashir N, Bridgewater JA, Geh JI, et al. Chemoradiotherapy with or without cetuximab in patients with oesophageal cancer (SCOPE1): a multicentre, phase 2/3 randomised trial. Lancet Oncol. 2013;14(7):627–37.
61. Jang R, Darling G, Wong RK. Multimodality approaches for the curative treatment of esophageal cancer. J Natl Compr Cancer Netw. 2015;13(2):229–38.
62. Urba SG, Orringer MB, Turrisi A, Iannettoni M, Forastiere A, Strawderman M. Randomized trial of preoperative chemoradiation versus surgery alone in patients with locoregional esophageal carcinoma. J Clin Oncol. 2001;19(2):305–13.
63. Walsh TN, Noonan N, Hollywood D, Kelly A, Keeling N, Hennessy TP. A comparison of multimodal therapy and surgery for esophageal adenocarcinoma. N Engl J Med. 1996;335(7):462–7.
64. Wu AJ, Bosch WR, Chang DT, Hong TS, Jabbour SK, Kleinberg LR, Mamon HJ, Thomas Jr CR, Goodman KA. Expert consensus contouring guidelines for intensity modulated radiation therapy in esophageal and gastroesophageal junction cancer. Int J Radiat Oncol Biol Phys. 2015;92(4):911–20.
65. Pan X, Zhang X, Li Y, Mohan R, Liao Z. Impact of using different four-dimensional computed tomography data sets to design proton treatment plans for distal esophageal cancer. Int J Radiat Oncol Biol Phys. 2009;73(2):601–9.
66. Patel AA, Wolfgang JA, Niemierko A, Hong TS, Yock T, Choi NC. Implications of respiratory motion as measured by four-dimensional computed tomography for radiation treatment planning of esophageal cancer. Int J Radiat Oncol Biol Phys. 2009;74(1):290–6.

67. Keall PJ, Mageras GS, Balter JM, Emery RS, Forster KM, Jiang SB, Kapatoes JM, Low DA, Murphy MJ, Murray BR, et al. The management of respiratory motion in radiation oncology report of AAPM Task Group 76. Med Phys. 2006;33(10):3874–900.
68. Mauer AM, Weichselbaum RR, Steele GD, Phillips TL, Chabner BA. Multimodality therapy for carcinoma of the esophagus. In: Steele GD, Phillips TL, Chabner BA, editors. American Cancer Society Atlas of Clinical Oncology Cancer of the Upper Gastrointestinal Tract. Chicago: BC Decker; 2002.
69. Miller C. Carcinoma of the esophagus and gastric cardia. Br J Surg. 1962;49:507–22.
70. Elkon D, Lee MS, Hendrickson FR. Carcinoma of the esophagus: sites of recurrence and palliative benefits after definitive radiotherapy. Int J Radiat Oncol Biol Phys. 1978; 4:615–20.
71. Kachnic LA, Winter K, Wasserman T, Kelsen D, Ginsberg R, Pisansky TM, Martenson J, Komaki R, Okawara G, Rosenthal SA, et al. Longitudinal quality-of-life analysis of RTOG 94-05 (Int 0123): a phase III trial of definitive chemoradiotherapy for esophageal cancer. Gastrointest Cancer Res. 2011;4(2):45–52.
72. Gao XS, Qiao X, Wu F, Cao L, Meng X, Dong Z, Wang X, Gao G, Wu TT, Komaki R, et al. Pathological analysis of clinical target volume margin for radiotherapy in patients with esophageal and gastroesophageal junction carcinoma. Int J Radiat Oncol Biol Phys. 2007; 67(2):389–96.
73. Radiation Therapy Oncology Group Core Lab. Organs at risk and target atlases. http://www.rtog.org/CoreLab/ContouringAtlases/LungAtlas.aspx
74. Marks LB, Yorke ED, Jackson A, Ten Haken RK, Constine LS, Eisbruch A, Bentzen SM, Nam J, Deasy JO. Use of normal tissue complication probability models in the clinic. Int J Radiat Oncol Biol Phys. 2010;76(3 Suppl):S10–9.
75. Rancati T, Schwarz M, Allen AM, Feng F, Popovtzer A, Mittal B, Eisbruch A. Radiation dose-volume effects in the larynx and pharynx. Int J Radiat Oncol Biol Phys. 2010;76(3 Suppl):S64–9.
76. Lee HK, Vaporciyan AA, Cox JD, Tucker SL, Putnam Jr JB, Ajani JA, Liao Z, Swisher SG, Roth JA, Smythe WR, et al. Postoperative pulmonary complications after preoperative chemoradiation for esophageal carcinoma: correlation with pulmonary dose-volume histogram parameters. Int J Radiat Oncol Biol Phys. 2003;57(5):1317–22.
77. Dorth JA, Pura JA, Palta M, Willett CG, Uronis HE, D'Amico TA, Czito BG. Patterns of recurrence after trimodality therapy for esophageal cancer. Cancer. 2014;120(14):2099–105.

Systemic Treatment of Esophageal Cancer

14

Sevil Bavbek

Introduction

The National Comprehensive Cancer Network (NCCN) provides guidelines for the treatment of esophageal cancer [1–3]. Treatment options include local mucosal resection or ablation therapies, esophagectomy, chemotherapy, and radiation therapy. Treatment is primarily dictated by stage, tumor location, and patients' medical fitness for receiving a particular therapeutic modality. However, we lack definitive data from randomized trials for many clinical situations. Outcomes also generally are relatively poor, so establishing optimal treatment for different clinical situations remains an area of active research [4]. The NCCN guidelines often display a spectrum of potential treatments for many clinical situations, reflecting the lack of clear-cut level 1 evidence. Given both the generally poor overall prognosis and the potential morbidity associated with therapy, multidisciplinary evaluation by surgery, medical oncology, and radiation oncology should be considered for all patients before a treatment strategy is initiated. Treatment that does not follow guidelines should probably only be used in the context of clinical trials.

Patients can be categorized even more simply when considering treatment. When considering treatment for esophageal cancer patients, the approach is initially dictated by whether the patients have been determined to have early-stage superficial cancers, cancers that are locally advanced with locoregional disease but no distant metastases, and cancers with distant disease. Systemic therapy plays a palliative role in the management of metastatic cancer. It remains adjunctive to radiation and surgery in the management of locally advanced operable and inoperable esophageal cancers [5].

S. Bavbek, MD
Department of Medical Oncology, American Hospital,
Guzelbahce Sokak, No. 20, Tesvikiye, Istanbul, Turkey
e-mail: sbavbek@yahoo.com

G. Ozyigit et al. (eds.), *Principles and Practice of Radiotherapy Techniques in Thoracic Malignancies*, DOI 10.1007/978-3-319-28761-4_14

Table 14.1 Single-agent efficacy of chemotherapy in esophageal cancer

Agent	Histology	Pts	RR%	95 % CI	Reference
Cisplatin	SCC	152	28	20–35	[12–15]
	AC	12	8	0–26	[16]
Bleomycin	SCC	80	15	7–23	[17–19]
Mitomycin	SCC	58	26	15–37	[20, 21]
5-FU	SCC	26	15	1–26	[22]
Etoposide	SCC	26	19	7–41	[23]
Vindesine	SCC	86	22	3–32	[24]
Vinorelbine	SCC	30	20	8–39	[25]
Paclitaxel	SCC	18	28	8–48	[26]
	AC	32	34	15–51	
Docetaxel	SCC	27	30	NA	[27]
	SCC+AC	38	23	NA	[11]
Irinotecan	AC	21	14	3–36	[28]

Modified from Enzinger et al. [139]
AC adenocancer, *CI* confidence interval, *NA* not available, *5-FU* fluorouracil

Approximately 50 % of patients have evidence of distant metastatic disease at the time of diagnosis [6, 7]. Palliative therapy is recommended for these patients and can include chemotherapy, clinical trial enrollment if available, or best supportive care. Best supportive care is often the most appropriate treatment option. Patients' performance status should determine whether chemotherapy is added to best supportive care [8].

Chemotherapy in Metastatic Esophageal Cancer

Chemotherapy for esophageal cancer was initially used in the setting of recurrent and metastatic disease. The common patient with esophageal cancer is aged 60 or older, with major tumor-related symptoms and additional comorbidities. They are thus poor candidates for clinical trials. In addition, the majority of patients present with advanced disease, poor performance status, weight loss, and complications which limit patient's tolerance for toxic chemotherapy. Response to chemotherapy is around 50–60 % in locally advanced disease but decreases to 30 % in metastatic esophageal cancer. The activity of single agents is listed in Table 14.1. Responses are generally short lived, lasting 2–4 months, and are usually associated with little palliative and no survival benefit. Cisplatin and taxanes are the most active agents, and carboplatin has been disappointing in both SCC and adenocarcinomas [9, 10]. Docetaxel 100 mg/m^2 every 3 weeks has been active in second line [11].

Newer agents have also been tested in esophagogastric cancer, the most promising have been capecitabine, as well as premetrexate, taxanes, and irinotecan [29]. Response rates and mechanisms of action have been listed in Table 14.2.

Table 14.2 New agents in esophagogastric cancer [29]

Class	Agent	Mechanism of action	RR%
Antimetabolite	Capecitabine	Reduces thymidine production	30
	Premetrexate	Inhibits TS	21
	S-1	TS and CDHP inhibition	26
Heavy metal	Oxaliplatin	Intrastrand and interstrand platinum DNA cross-links	na
Taxane	Paclitaxel	Microtubule inhibition	13
	Docetaxel		21
Topoisomerase inhibitor	Irinotecan	Inhibits topoisomerase I	21

Table 14.3 Cisplatin-5-FU-based combinations in locally advanced or metastatic esophageal cancer

Tx	Dose	Histology	Stage	Pts	RR%	Med OS (mo)	Reference
CDDP/FU	100	SCC	M1	37	43	NA	[31]
	1,000×5						
CDDP/FU	100	SCC	LAD+M1	34	35	8	[32]
	1,000×5						
CDDP/FU	70	SCC	LAD+M1	36	36	NA	[33]
	700×5						
CDDP/	100	SCC	LAD+M1	17	23	6+	[34]
FU/	370×5						
FA	200×5						
CDDP/	20×5	SCC	LAD+M1	31	58	11	[35]
FU/	600×5						
FA	200×5						

Modified from Stahl [140]
CDDP cisplatin, *FA* folinic acid, *IFN* interferon alpha, *LAD* locally advanced disease, *M1* metastatic disease

Combination chemotherapy is generally cisplatin based in esophageal cancer. The first regimens combined cisplatin with bleomycin or methotrexate in two to three or four drug regimens. The regimen of cisplatin-bleomycin and vindesine was introduced by Kelsen and Ilson in patients with unresectable or metastatic SCC esophageal cancer [30]. Response rates of 30–35 % showed a durability for 5–6 months; median survival was 6–8 months. Despite the toxicity, initial combinations did not prove better than single agents in terms of survival. The common regimen of cisplatin-infusional fluorouracil (5-FU) was introduced in the late 1980s (Table 14.3). Cisplatin was given as 100 mg/m^2 on day 1 or in divided doses for 5 days. 5-FU was given 1 g/m^2/day for 5 days in a continuous infusion. Response rates climbed to 47–64 % in locoregional or locally advanced disease.

The combination of cisplatin-5-FU was tested in unresectable/metastatic SCC in a randomized phase II EORTC trial against single-agent cisplatin [32]. The RR of the combination was 35 %, significantly higher than 19 % for single-agent cisplatin;

this did not translate into a survival benefit (8 months for the combination vs. 7 months for cisplatin only, 1-year survival 34 % vs. 27 %, 2-year survival 18 % vs. 9 %). The lack of survival benefit was interpreted as due to the higher level of treatment-related deaths in the combination arm. The results of this study cast doubt on the use of combination therapy in advanced disease.

The addition of paclitaxel to cisplatin or cisplatin+5-FU produced superior response rates but no significant survival benefit. In a randomized phase II study, paclitaxel 175 mg/m^2 over 3 h was added to cisplatin 20 mg/m^2 × 5 days and 5-FU 750 mg/m^2 ci (continuous infusion) × 5 days, in recurrent or metastatic esophageal cancer [36]. Major responses were seen in 48 %, with complete response in 7 out of 60 patients evaluable. The median duration of response was 5.7 months, and the median survival 10.8 months. Toxicity was severe, but manageable; the prominence of sensory neuropathy was of special interest. Irinotecan was combined with cisplatin in a phase II study of 35 patients with metastatic esophageal cancer [37]. The response rate was 57 % with a complete response rate of 6 %, and similar response rates were seen for both squamous and adenocancer.

Oxaliplatin-based therapy has modest reported activity in the metastatic setting [38], although it is considered equivalent to cisplatin, given the equivalence in the locally advanced treatment setting [39]. In the phase II trial of oxaliplatin, 5-FU, and leucovorin (FOLFOX) in metastatic disease, the overall response rate was 23.2 % with a disease control rate of 67.9 %. The median progression-free survival (PFS) was 4.4 months, and the median overall survival (OS) was 7.7 months; these results were not very impressive [38]. The FOLFOX regimen proved equal to cisplatin-5-FU in the PRODIGE5/ACCORD17 trial, where definitive chemoradiotherapy with FOLFOX versus fluorouracil and cisplatin was compared in patients with localized or locally advanced esophageal cancer [39]. Median progression-free survival was 9.7 months (95 % CI 8.1–14.5) in the FOLFOX group and 9.4 months (8.1–10.6) in the fluorouracil and cisplatin group (HR 0.93, 95 % CI 0.70–1.24; $p=0.64$). Toxicity was similar in both treatment arms.

Pure chemotherapy trials of metastatic esophageal cancer are few; most of the chemotherapy data is either from or combined with locally advanced disease. The combination of cisplatin and infusional fluorouracil is still the accepted treatment standard for metastatic SCC of the esophagus, although taxanes, oxaliplatin, and irinotecan are also felt to be active [40]. Given the fact that combination therapy does not improve survival significantly in the metastatic setting, palliative treatment of the common, poor performance status, malnourished esophageal cancer patient should be single-agent chemotherapy, while combination regimens should be reserved for the occasional young patient with good performance status and low metastatic burden.

Second-Line Chemotherapy in Esophageal Cancer

Patients with esophageal cancer often have significant comorbidities, including obesity, heart disease, and emphysema, which, when coupled with progressive dysphagia and malnutrition, often limit therapeutic opportunities after first-line therapy.

Performance status generally worsens significantly following chemotherapy, rendering second-line chemotherapy inaccessible to many patients.

Thallinger et al. have reported a critical analysis of second-line chemotherapy in esophageal SCC and AC [41]. Computerized (MEDLINE) and manual searches were performed to identify articles published on this topic between 1996 and 2011. Twenty-five published trials and four abstracts presented at scientific meetings were identified. A total of 10 trials included only patients with squamous cell carcinomas (SCCs), 4 focused exclusively on adenocarcinoma (AC); the remaining 15 studies included both SCC and AC. The majority of trials (17 of 29) used docetaxel in combination with platinum analogs, 8 used single-agent cytotoxic chemotherapy, and 6 evaluated targeted therapies.

Response rates are generally low in these small studies, ranging between 0 % and 39 %. Response duration is also short; time to progression ranges from 1.4 to 6.2 months, and the overall survival is 4.0–11.4 months. Only 30–40 % of patients are able to move from first- to second-line treatment. Single-agent vinorelbine, irinotecan, and taxanes have all proved weak in the second-line setting, and standard use of single agents is not justified by these small-scale studies.

Combination regimens have a different range of activity in second-line systemic treatment. The combination of docetaxel and capecitabine [42] and several different regimens of docetaxel and irinotecan [43, 44] have shown low response rates, unimpressive survival rates at the expense of significant toxicity. A phase II trial of cisplatin 75 mg/m^2 and docetaxel 70 mg/m^2 every 3 weeks in 35 patients who have previously received cisplatin/infusional fluorouracil resulted in a 34.2 % response rate with 2.6 % complete response (CR) [45]. Progression-free and overall survival were disappointing at 4.5 and 7.4 months, respectively, and grade 3–4 toxicities were seen in half of the patients. Another platinum compound, nedaplatin, was combined with docetaxel or vindesine in a number of studies. All of these were confined to Asian patients only, and response rates ranged between 11 % and 39 % [46–51]. The combination of docetaxel, nedaplatin, and fluorouracil resulted in a RR of 63 % in a small pilot study. All nedaplatin regimens were well tolerated; however, PFS was modest in the range of 1.8–6.5 months.

Another combination is the DCF (docetaxel, cisplatin, infusional fluorouracil) regimen, also proven active in other cancers. A phase II trial of patients pretreated with cisplatin received DCF (docetaxel 60 mg/m^2 day 1, cisplatin 10 mg/m^2 and 5-FU 500 mg/m^2 days 1–5 every 21 days) [52]. Overall response rate was 35 %, with one CR and six PRs; time to progression was 4 months and overall survival was 8 months. Another trial using a similar regimen in patients previously treated with nedaplatin or cisplatin resulted in a response rate of 50 % [53]. Both studies showed quite severe neutropenia, making the use of this regimen difficult in the advanced palliative setting.

The combination of mitomycin 6 mg/m^2, ifosfamide 3 g/m^2, and cisplatin 50 mg/m^2 every 3 weeks was tested in patients with SCC and prior platinum/5-FU chemotherapy [54]. Response rate was 12.5 %, and SD rate was 37.5 %. WHO grades 3–4 neutropenia was observed in 21 % of patients. Progression-free survival was 2.0 months (95 % CI, 1.4–2.5 months), and overall survival was 5.2 months (95 % CI, 3.3–7.0 months).

Chemotherapy in Localized/Locally Advanced Esophageal Cancer

In locoregionally advanced esophageal cancer, combination chemotherapy has been investigated in combination with radiation or surgery to try to reduce the high rate of systemic relapse noted when surgery or radiotherapy alone is used. Trials of neoadjuvant/adjuvant chemotherapy, definitive chemoradiotherapy, and preoperative chemoradiation have been extensively discussed in the previous chapter. Chemotherapy has been used both preoperatively and postoperatively, usually with cisplatin-based multi-agent regimens. Randomized trials of preoperative chemotherapy usually consist of two or three cycles followed by resection; some studies have also added postoperative chemotherapy. The safety of preoperative chemotherapy is demonstrated by the lack of increase in perioperative morbidity if surgery is performed in experienced hands. All of the preoperative chemotherapy regimens are cisplatin based, the majority of which are cisplatin and infusional 5-FU. Preoperative chemotherapy provides no consistent survival benefit, compared with resection alone except in one recent study which enrolled over 800 patients [55]. The lack of survival advantage in neoadjuvant chemotherapy trials may be due in part to the small number of patients enrolled or alternatively to the poor locoregional control obtained with standard esophageal resection. In the large randomized trial by the MRC (Medical Research Council) Esophageal Cancer Study Group, median survival increased from 13 months in the surgery arm to 17 months in the preoperative chemotherapy arm ($p<0.05$) [55]; the chemotherapy regimen was cisplatin and infusional 5-FU.

Postoperative chemotherapy has not proven to be of any benefit after surgery and has been shown to increase postoperative complications [56].

Chemoradiation has also been used in the treatment of esophageal cancer. The concurrent use of chemotherapy and radiotherapy is theoretically appealing because, in addition to the systemic effects of chemotherapy, certain agents behave as radiosensitizers. Trials of chemoradiation vs. radiation alone generally include either cisplatin/5-FU or mitomycin/5-FU regimens [56–59]. Definitive chemoradiation with occasional salvage surgery is a feasible approach in squamous cell esophageal cancer. Chemoradiation is also used pre- or postoperatively [60–63]. Preoperative chemoradiation has not been consistently proven to increase survival, but trails are short on power due to insufficiently small patient numbers. A survival benefit for combined therapy is evident in patients who are found to have a complete pathologic response in the surgical specimen. Since surgery or radiation therapy alone has poor outcomes, definitive chemoradiotherapy alone or preoperative chemoradiation and surgery is usually prescribed for non-metastatic, locoregionally advanced esophageal cancer. The treatment regimen of choice for chemoradiation remains cisplatin/5-FU. One recent trial of definitive chemoradiation (PRODIGE5/ACCORD17) has shown the FOLFOX regimen to be equal to cisplatin/5-FU, but more convenient in terms of serious adverse events [39].

Chemotherapy for Esophageal Adenocarcinoma

Several drug therapy classes, including platinum, fluoropyrimidines, topoisomerase inhibitors, taxanes, and anthracyclines, are active in both gastric and gastroesophageal junction adenocarcinomas. Chemotherapy combinations seem to be equally active in both cancers (Table 14.4) [64]. It is clear that some disease subtypes may need more specific types of treatment as we enter the era of targeted therapy.

Chemotherapy vs. best supportive care trials show a survival advantaging metastatic GE adenocancer in both the first- [65–67] and second-line settings [68–70]. A meta-analysis of first-line chemotherapy studies reported a hazard ratio (HR) of 0.39 (95 % CI, 0.28–0.52; $P<0.001$) for overall survival (OS) in favor of chemotherapy, translating to a benefit in weighted median average survival of approximately 6 months [71]. The standard chemotherapy regimen in the first line is either cisplatin-infusional 5-FU or a three-drug combination. Oxaliplatin and capecitabine have been found as noninferior to cisplatin and fluorouracil, respectively, with perhaps a more manageable toxicity profile, and both of these agents are now established in combination chemotherapy regimens for metastatic disease [74, 76, 77]. The so-called DCF regimen definitely shows a significant survival advantage when compared to cisplatin-FU [72]; however, this comes at the price of significant toxicity, mainly myelosuppression and mucositis [78]. Further studies aimed at decreasing the toxicity of this regimen by weekly, biweekly administrations [79–81]. In general, response rates of chemotherapy in advanced gastric/gastroesophageal cancer exceed 40 %, but most patients still have a median survival <1 year, and survival >2 years is rare. This unimpressive survival is an indication for looking at targeted therapies to increase success in the treatment of this disease.

Table 14.4 Larger randomized trials of combination chemotherapy in esophageal adenocarcinoma

Trial	Year	Treatment	Patients	RR%	1 year OS	Reference
Van Cutsem et al.	2006	CF	224	25	32	[72]
		DCF	221	37	40	
Gimbaud et al.	2014	FOLFOXIRI	207	39.2	11.2	[73]
		ECX	209	37.8	10.7	
Cunningham et al.	2008	ECF	263	40.7	37.7	[74]
		ECX	250	46.4	40.8	
		EOF	245	42.4	40.4	
		EOX	244	47.9	46.8	
Ajani et al.	2010	CS	527	29.1	NR	[75]
		CF	526	31.9	NR	

CF cisplatin-FU, *DCF* docetaxel-cisplatin-FU, *FOLFOXIRI* FU-oxaliplatin-folinic acid-irinotecan, *ECX* epirubicin-cisplatin-capecitabine, *ECF* epirubicin-cisplatin-FU, *EOF* epirubicin-oxaliplatin-FU. *EOX* epirubicin-oxaliplatin-capecitabin, *CS* cisplatin-S1, *RR* response rate, *OS* overall survival

Second-Line Chemotherapy

Following the first-line failure with clinical progression, performance status unfortunately declines considerably. Patients with esophageal cancer frequently face malnutrition and dietary problems, resulting in major weight loss. Especially in case of peritoneal carcinomatosis, with insufficient bowel function, significant GI symptoms deteriorate functional status and limit treatment options [82]. Nevertheless, second-line therapy has been a standard care approach in selected patients, based on three randomized trials demonstrating a significant survival benefit with chemotherapy over the best supportive care alone [68–70]. Moreover, a subsequent meta-analysis of them concluded on a survival HR of 0.73 (95 % CI, 0.58–0.96), where the second-line setting improved the survival with the HR of 0.57 (95 % CI, 0.36–0.91) in highly functioning patients with performance status of 0–1 [83].

Molecular Biology of Esophageal SCC and Adenocarcinoma

Chromosomal aberrations have been documented in esophageal cancer resulting in gene dysregulation, such as the *C-MYC* and *ERBB2* (*HER-2*) oncogenes related with amplifications on 8q and 17q [84, 85].

EGFR overexpression in association with poor prognosis in esophageal or GEJ cancer has encouraged many studies of relevant EGFR-targeting agents, such as tyrosine kinase inhibitors (TKIs) and monoclonal antibodies (mAbs). However, EGFR TKIs in esophageal cancer unfortunately caused relatively high toxicity besides lower activity due to the low incidence of activating mutations of EGFR. On the other hand, *HER-2* targeting has been the current standard option in *HER*-2 amplification confirmed stage IV gastroesophageal cancer [86]. The pathogenesis of *MYC* in esophageal cancer has not been decrypted yet. Loss of TP53 heterozygosity is present in more than half of the cases which is a viable predictor of poor prognosis and disease progression [87–89]. Goh et al. analyzed an array comparative genomic hybridization matching the gene expression profiling in order to find possible original genes for significant prognosis in esophageal adenocarcinomas [90]. The authors revealed 17 common regions of gain and 11 common regions of losses with unique 2 deletions (p16/*CDKN2*, *MBNL1*) and 4 gains (EGFR, *WT1*, *NEIL2*, *MTMR9*) which had individual and collective prognostic significance.

Inactivating mutations of *NOTCH1* were demonstrated in 21 % of squamous cell esophageal carcinomas while none in adenocarcinomas [91]. Another study used high-density genomic profiling arrays. Amplified genes including *ERBB2*, *FGFR1*, *FGFR2*, *EGFR*, and *MET* were defined in 37 % of tumors, more prevalent in gastric cancers, in 296 esophageal and gastric cancer patients [92].

Targeted Therapies in Esophageal SCC and Adenocarcinoma

Trastuzumab and ramucirumab have been approved in the last 5 years both in the first- and second-line settings of the treatment of advanced or metastatic gastroesophageal adenocarcinoma [93]. Randomized clinical trials to evaluate novel treatments will expectantly improve outcomes in the natural course of esophageal cancer.

EGFR

EGFR overexpression by immunohistochemistry indicating poor prognosis is present in 32–65 % of esophageal or GEJ tumors [94–97], whereas EGFR mutations are uncommon with rates of 0 % in European studies to 12–14 % in Asian studies [98]. Therefore, both tyrosine kinase inhibitors (TKIs) and monoclonal antibodies (mAbs) in esophageal or GEJ cancer were not successful due to just overexpression of EGFR without activating mutations.

Two phase II trials in advanced esophageal cancer with single-agent gefitinib documented infrequent partial responses of 2.8 % and 11.1 %, respectively, with poor median PFS [99, 100]. The combination of gefitinib with CF for the neoadjuvant treatment did not significantly improve 3-year OS (40 % vs. 28 %, p 0.06) in locally advanced esophageal cancer [101]. Phase II Southwest Oncology Group (SWOG) study with erlotinib also showed only objective response rate of 9 % in 44 advanced GEJ patients [102].

Cetuximab has been the mostly studied monoclonal antibody targeting EGFR in esophageal cancer; however, the final phase II and III studies were disappointing despite early good results (Table 14.5). Cetuximab in second line as a single agent in advanced esophageal cancer has no role [108]. There is no improved survival data for cetuximab in the palliative use in esophageal cancer [107]. There are conflicting results in phase II trials of cetuximab for locally advanced esophageal cancer in addition to chemoradiotherapy. For example, SWOG 0414 was closed early due to poor accrual which combined cisplatin/irinotecan/cetuximab and radiation [109]. Phase III RTOG study randomizing patients to preoperative cisplatin/paclitaxel/radiation with or without cetuximab has recently closed the adenocarcinoma arm because of futility, while it has been continuing for squamous histology. Phase II studies of FOLFOX-cetuximab-radiotherapy and cisplatin-paclitaxel-cetuximab-radiotherapy have documented very promising median PFS and OS in addition to favorable RR of 77.2 and 97.7 %, respectively [104, 105]. However, English phase II/III study has demonstrated increased toxicity and poorer survival with cetuximab for patients unfit for surgery in addition to concurrent radiotherapy with cisplatin and capecitabine [106]. A biological agent might display a great range from poor to perfect response and low to fatal toxicity in different and complex clinical scenarios.

Table 14.5 Cetuximab trials in esophageal cancer

Phase	NCT identifier	Patients	Regimen	Outcome
IB/II	NCT00445861	Stage IIB–IIIC resectable esophageal/GEJ tumor	Preoperative cisplatin/docetaxel/cetuximab	pCR and near pCR 68 %
II	NCT00551759 (E2205)	Stage IA–IIIC resectable esophageal/GEJ adenocarcinoma	Preoperative cetuximab/5-FU/oxaliplatin/radiation	Closed; excess lung toxicity
			Postoperative cetuximab/docetaxel	
II	NCT00544362	Stage II–III esophageal/GEJ tumors	Cisplatin/5-FU/cetuximab	pCR not increased [103]
II	NCT00578201	Stage III esophageal squamous tumors	Preoperative 5-FU/leucovorin/oxaliplatin/cetuximab for 2 cycles followed by 5-FU/leucovorin/oxaliplatin/cetuximab/radiation plus or minus surgery	ORR 77.2 %, median PFS 13.8 months, OS 21.6 months [104]
II	NCT00815308	Stage II–III esophageal squamous tumors not candidates for surgery	Cisplatin/paclitaxel/radiation/cetuximab	ORR 97.7 %, median PFS 13.9 months, median OS 16.8 months [105]
II	NCT00109850 (SWOG0414)	Stage III esophageal/GEJ tumors not candidates for surgery	Cisplatin/irinotecan/cetuximab/radiation	Closed early of poor accrual
				Toxic deaths
III	NCT01107639	Stage IIB–IIIC resectable esophageal/GEJ tumors	Preoperative cisplatin/docetaxel/cetuximab/radiation followed by postoperative cetuximab versus CRT alone	Accruing
III	NCT00655876	Stage IIA–IV (M1a) esophageal/GEJ tumors	Preoperative paclitaxel/cisplatin/radiation plus or minus cetuximab	Adeno arm closed for futility, squamous arm recruiting
II/III	NCT00509561	Stage IA–IIIC esophageal/GEJ (type 1) tumors not candidates for surgery	Cisplatin/capecitabine/radiation plus or minus cetuximab	Completed; increased toxicity and decreased survival in cetuximab arm (22 months vs 25 months) [106]
II	NCT00381706 (CALGB 80,403/ECOG 1206)	First-line stage IV esophageal/GEJ tumors	Epirubicin/cisplatin/fluorouracil-cetuximab, 5-FU/leucovorin/oxaliplatin plus cetuximab, irinotecan/cisplatin-cetuximab	RR: ECF+cetuximab 58 %; FOLFOX+cetuximab 51 %; irinotecan/cisplatin – cetuximab, 38 % [107]
II	NCT00096031 (SWOG 0415)	Second-line stage IV esophageal/GEJ adenocarcinoma	Single-agent cetuximab	ORR 2 %, median PFS 1.8 months [108]

Phase II ACOSOG study showed promising pCR and near pCR rates with panitumumab (fully human mAb against EGFR); on the other hand, phase III REAL-3 trial could not demonstrate efficacy which blurred its use in esophageal cancer [110]. Overall, both cetuximab and panitumumab studies in the treatment of esophageal cancer failed to give hope for EGFR mAbs at current setup.

HER-2

Besides the HER1 (human epidermal growth factor receptor 1), HER2 is also expressed in gastroesophageal cancers, involved in critical steps for malignancy. Since trastuzumab (humanized monoclonal antibody blocking HER2 activation) in landmark ToGA (Trastuzumab in Combination with Chemotherapy Versus Chemotherapy Alone for Treatment of HER2-Positive Advanced Gastric or Gastro-oesophageal Junction Cancer) trial was used in combination with capecitabine and cisplatin [86], and significantly improved median OS (13.5 vs. 11.1 months; HR, 0.74; $P=0.0048$) with greater benefit in HER2-overexpressed subpopulation (OS, 16.1 vs. 11.8 months; $P=0.0046$), combination of trastuzumab with chemotherapy for HER2-positive gastric and gastroesophageal junction adenocarcinomas is the current standard. Whether a high tumor burden requires a higher maintenance, trastuzumab dosing is being tested in the HELOISE trial (Herceptin in Combination with Cisplatin/Capecitabine Chemotherapy in Patients with HER2-Positive Metastatic Gastric or Gastro-esophageal Junction Cancer). HER2 is significantly more prevalently positive in proximal gastric and esophageal tumors [111, 112].

Trastuzumab emtansine (T-DM1) is the combination of the antibody with a cytotoxic anti-microtubule macrolide, binding HER2 and disrupting of the PI3K/AKT pathway [113]. Comparison of T-DM1 with single-agent taxane is ongoing in previously treated metastatic gastric cancer in GATSBY study. Pertuzumab blocks HER2 dimerization by targeting the extracellular dimerization domain and acts independently of trastuzumab [114], and both pertuzumab to trastuzumab are combined with cisplatin plus capecitabine in the first-line setting in HER2-positive gastric cancer in JACOB study. Lapatinib has been examined in first-line LOGIC trial [115] and second-line TyTAN trial [116], but have not improved survival.

Targeting Angiogenesis

VEGF (vascular endothelial growth factor) family of VEGF-A to VEGF-E and placental growth factors 1 and 2 besides their receptor tyrosine kinases are important in cancer angiogenesis [117]. Ramucirumab (fully human immunoglobulin G1 monoclonal antibody) targets VEGFR-2 and improved survival as monotherapy in REGARD study in previously treated advanced gastric and GEJ adenocarcinoma [118]. Ramucirumab was combined with paclitaxel versus placebo and paclitaxel as second-line treatment in RAINBOW study [119]. Ramucirumab significantly improved survival, with an HR of 0.78 ($P=0.047$) in double-blind, placebo-controlled REGARD trial. A larger study, RAINBOW, randomly assigned paclitaxel with or without ramucirumab, and addition of ramucirumab demonstrated an improved median survival of 9.6 months versus 7.4 months with paclitaxel alone (HR of 0.81, $P=0.017$) and progression-free survival of (HR of 0.635, $P<0.001$) 4.4 months versus 2.9 months with paclitaxel alone [119]. However, ramucirumab could not improve the outcome in the first-line setting of advanced gastroesophageal adenocarcinoma [120].

AVAGAST randomized phase III trial of first-line chemotherapy with or without bevacizumab, in advanced gastric cancer, was negative for survival (HR, 0.87; $P=0.1$, median survival, 12.1 versus 10.1 months) but positive for PFS (HR, 0.80; $P=0.0032$, 6.7 vs. 5.3 months) [121], while improved survival was noted in patients with plasma VEGF-A levels > the median (HR, 0.72) or neuropilin 1 expression < the median (HR, 0.75) [122].

Apatinib, VEGFR-2 inhibitor, demonstrated an improvement in OS in a phase III study of apatinib versus placebo in the third-line setting of 270 patients (HR, 0.71; $P<0.016$) [123].

Anti-VEGFR trials failed in esophageal cancer. A phase II study of sunitinib combined with chemoradiotherapy prior for resectable cases and adjuvant sunitinib was in progress [124]. In a recent phase II trial, sorafenib had inadequate activity as a single agent for metastatic esophageal and GEJ tumors, with a median PFS of 3.7 months and OS of 8.9 months [125].

Immune Checkpoint Inhibition

Immunosurveillance is demonstrated to significantly alter in esophageal cancers [126–128]. PD-L1 is the first identified for the prevention of autoimmunity [129]. Engagement of PD-L1 on dendritic cells with the programmed death 1 (PD-1) receptor on T cells sends an inhibitory signal that activates T-cell anergy or apoptosis [130]. In esophageal cancer, expression of PD-L1 and PD-L2 is correlated with poor survival in esophageal cancers [126, 127]. It is noteworthy that 43 % of esophageal SCCs and 70 % of esophageal adenocarcinomas express PD-L1 [127], and its expression is independently correlated with poor survival [126].

Pembrolizumab successfully blocks the negative regulatory signaling of the PD-1 receptor expressed on T cell. It has been reported that pembrolizumab have substantial activity in patients with advanced gastric cancer expressing PD-L1 [131].

MET and Hepatocyte Growth Factor

Activation of the MET pathway causes a stimulation of cell detachment, migration, and invasion [132]. MET interacts with EGFR family receptor tyrosine kinases [133]. *MET* is amplified in nearly 2–10 % of GEJ adenocarcinomas [6].

In a recent trial, survival for EGFR-amplified tumors was 11.2 months; for HER-2-amplified tumors, survival was 16.9 months; for without amplification of

MET/EGFR/HER-2, survival was 16.9 months [134]. Tivantinib is a selective inhibitor of the receptor TK, c-Met. Tivantinib has preliminary activity in phase I trials with GEJ and gastric tumors [135]. Ongoing trials are combining tivantinib with 5-FU/leucovorin/oxaliplatin for advanced esophageal and GEJ or gastric tumors.

Fibroblast Growth Factor Receptor

Fibroblast growth factor receptor (FGFR)-2 is amplified in nearly 4 % of esophageal cancers and was correlated with higher grade, advanced stage, and poor prognosis [104, 136–138]. Cediranib is a potent inhibitor of FGFR-2, of multiple VEGF receptors, and of c-Kit. Cediranib in esophageal or gastric cancer requires further studies [104]. AZD4547 is a potent, selective inhibitor of FGFR1, FGFR2, and FGFR3 and is currently being studied in second-line systemic therapy for FGFR-amplified advanced esophageal cancers in a randomized phase II study [104].

Conclusion

Targeted therapy has potential to cure more patients when used in combination with multimodality treatment of esophageal SCC and adenocancer. Conducting large, randomized trials with multi-institutional efforts, where patients have been molecularly selected for treatment, will hopefully improve our understanding of therapy and clinical outcome.

References

1. Devesa SS, Blot WJ, Fraumeni Jr JF. Changing patterns in the incidence of esophageal and gastric adenocarcinoma in the U.S. Cancer. 1998;83:2049–53.
2. Stein SJ, Sendler A, Fink U, et al. Multidisciplinary approach to esophageal and gastric cancer. Surg Clin North Am. 2000;80:659–82.
3. Ajani JA, Barthel JS, Bentrem DJ, et al. Esophageal and esophagogastric junction cancers. J Natl Compr Canc Netw. 2011;9:830–87.
4. D'Amico TA. Surgery for esophageal cancer. Gastrointest Cancer Res. 2008;2:S6–9.
5. Graham AJ, Shrive FM, Ghali WA, et al. Defining the optimal treatment of locally advanced esophageal cancer: a systematic review and decision analysis. Ann Thorac Surg. 2007;83:1257–64.
6. Enzinger PC, Mayer RJ. Esophageal cancer. N Engl J Med. 2003;349:2241–52.
7. Horner M, Ries L, Krapcho M, et al. SEER cancer statistics review, 1975–2006, National Cancer Institute. Bethesda. Available online: http://seer.cancer.gov/csr/1975_2006/, based on November 2008 SEER data submission, posted to the SEER web site. 2009.
8. Berry MF. Esophageal cancer: staging system and guidelines for staging and treatment. J Thorac Dis. 2014;6 Suppl 3:S289–97.
9. Mannell A, Winters Z. Carboplatin in the treatment of esophageal cancer. S Afr Med J. 1989;76:213–4.
10. Sternberg C, Kelsen D, Dukeman M, et al. Carboplatin: a new platin analog in the treatment of epidermoid carcinoma of the esophagus. Cancer Treat Rep. 1985;69:1305–7.
11. Albertsson M, Fagerberg J, Jacobsen A, et al. Preliminary results of a phase 2 study with Taxotere (docetaxel) in patients with primary untreated or recurrent esophagus cancer. Proc ASCO. 2000;19:A1218. abst.

12. Panettiere FJ, Leichman L, O'Bryan R, et al. Cis-diam-minedichloride platinum (II), an effective agent in the treatment of epidermoid carcinoma of the esophagus. A preliminary report of an ongoing SWOG study. Cancer Clin Trials. 1981;4:29–31.
13. Ravry MJ, Moore MR, Omura GA, et al. Phase II evaluation of cisplatin in squamous carcinoma of the esophagus: a Southeastern Cancer Study Group trial. Cancer Treat Rep. 1985;69:1457–8.
14. Davis S, Shanmugathasa M, Kessler W. Cis-diam-minedichloride platinum (II)in the treatment of esophageal carcinoma. Cancer Treat Rep. 1980;69:709–11.
15. Murthy SK, Prabkaharan PS, Chandrashekar M, et al. Neoadjuvant Cis-DDP in esophageal cancers: an experience at a regional cancer center, India. J Surg Oncol. 1990;45:173–6.
16. Ajani J, Kantarjian H, Kanojia M, et al. Phase II trial of cis-platinum in advanced upper gastrointestinal cancer. Proc ASCO. 1984;2, C-573.
17. Stephens FO. Bleomycin-a new approach in cancer chemotherapy. Med J Aust. 1973;1:1277–83.
18. Bonadonna G, De Lena M, Monfardini S, et al. Clinical trials with bleomycin in lymphomas and in solid tumors. Eur J Cancer. 1972;8:205–15.
19. Ravry M, Moertel CG, Schutt AJ, et al. Treatment of advanced SCC of the gastrointestinal tract with bleomycin. Cancer Chemother Rep. 1973;57:493–5.
20. Engstrom PF, Lavin PT, Klaassen DJ, et al. phase II evaluation of mitomycin and cisplatin in advanced esophageal carcinoma. Cancer Treat Rep. 1983;67:713–5.
21. Whittington RM, Close HP. Clinical experience with mitomycin C. Cancer Chemother Rep. 1970;54:195–8.
22. Ezdinli EZ, Gelber R, Desai DV, et al. Chemotherapy of advanced esophageal carcinoma: ECOG experience. Cancer. 1980;46:2149–53.
23. Harstrick A, Bokemayer C, Preusser P, et al. Phase II study of single agent etoposide in patients with metastatic SCC of the esophagus. Cancer Chemother Pharmacol. 1992;29:321–2.
24. Kelsen DP, Bains M, Cvitkovic E, et al. Vindesine in the treatment of esophageal carcinoma: a phase II study. Cancer Treat Rep. 1979;63:2019–21.
25. Conroy T, Etienne PL, Adenis A, et al. Phase II trial of vinorelbine in metastatic squamous cell esophageal carcinoma. EORTC Gastrointestinal Cancer Cooperative Group. J Clin Oncol. 1996;14:164–70.
26. Ajani JA, Ilson DH, Daugherty K, et al. Activity of taxol in patients with SCC and AC of the esophagus. J Natl Cancer Inst. 1994;86:1086–91.
27. Slabber CF, Falkson CI, Musi NNM, et al. A phase II study of docetaxel in advanced, inoperable squamous carcinoma of the esophagus. Proc ASCO. 1999;18, A1151.
28. Lin L, Hecht J. A phase II trial of irinotecan in patients with advanced adenocarcinoma of the GE junction. Proc ASCO. 2000;19, 1130.
29. National Cancer Institute. http.www.cancer.gov/drugdictionary.
30. Ilson DH, Kelsen DP. Chemotherapy in esophageal cancer. Anticancer Drugs. 1993;4:287–99.
31. De Besi P, Sileni VC, Salvagno L, et al. Phase II study of cisplatin, 5-FU and allopurinol in advanced esophageal cancer. Cancer Treat Rep. 1986;70:909–10.
32. Bleiberg H, Conroy T, Paillot B, et al. Randomized phase II study of cisplatin and 5-FU vs cisplatin alone in advanced squamous cell oesophageal cancer. Eur J Cancer. 1997;33:1216–20.
33. Iizuka T, Kakegawa T, Ide H, et al. Phase II evaluation of cisplatin and 5-FU in advanced squamous cell carcinoma of the esophagus: A Japanese Esophageal Oncology Group Trial. Jpn J Clin Oncol. 1992;22:172–6.
34. Zaniboni A, Simoncini E, Tonini G, et al. Cisplatin, high-dose folinic acid and 5-FU in squamous cell carcinoma of the esophagus. A pilot study. Chemioterapia. 1987;6:387–9.
35. Feliu J, Gonzales BM, Garcia GC, et al. Phase II study of cisplatin, 5-FU, and leukovorin in inoperable squamous cell carcinoma of the esophagus. ONCOPAZ Cooperative Group, Spain. Am J Clin Oncol. 1996;19:577–80.

36. Ilson DH, Ajani J, Bhalla K, et al. Phase II trial of paclitaxel, 5-FU, and cisplatin in patients with advanced carcinoma of the esophagus. J Clin Oncol. 1998;16:1826–34.
37. Ilson DH, Saltz L, Enzinger P, et al. Phase II trial of weekly irinotecan plus cisplatin in advanced esophageal cancer. J Clin Oncol. 1999;17:3270–5.
38. Wang J, Chang J, Yu H, et al. A phase II study of oxaliplatin in combination with leucovorin and fluorouracil as first-line chemotherapy in patients with metastatic squamous cell carcinoma in esophagus. Cancer Chemother Pharmacol. 2013;71:905–11.
39. Conroy T, Galais MP, Raoul JL, et al. Definitive chemoradiotherapy with FOLFOX versus fluorouracil and cisplatin in patients with esophageal cancer (PRODIGE5/ ACCORD17): Final results of a randomized, phase 2/3 trial. Lancet Oncol. 2014;15:305–14.
40. Ilson DH. Esophageal cancer chemotherapy: recent advances. Gastrointest Cancer Res. 2008;2:85–92.
41. Thallinger CMR, Raderer M, Hejna M. Esophageal cancer: a critical evaluation of systemic second-line therapy. J Clin Oncol. 2011;29:4709–14.
42. Lorenzen S, Duyster J, Lersch C, et al. Capecitabine plus docetaxel every 3 weeks in first- and second-line metastatic oesophageal cancer: final results of a phase II trial. Br J Cancer. 2005;92:2129–33.
43. Lordick F, von Schilling C, Bernhard H, et al. Phase II trial of irinotecan plus docetaxel in cisplatin-pretreated relapsed or refractory oesophageal cancer. Br J Cancer. 2003; 89:630–3.
44. Burtness B, Gibson M, Egleston B, et al. Phase II trial of docetaxel-irinotecan combination in advanced esophageal cancer. Ann Oncol. 2009;20:1242–8.
45. Shim HJ, Cho SH, Hwang JE, et al. Phase II study of docetaxel and cisplatin chemotherapy in 5-fluorouracil/cisplatin pretreated esophageal cancer. Am J Clin Oncol. 2010;33:624–8.
46. Mafune K, Yamada K, Imamura K, et al. Docetaxel, 5-fluorouracil and nedaplatin as second-line chemotherapy for patients with esophageal cancer after esophagectomy: a pilot study. J Clin Oncol. 2006;24(suppl):635s. abstr 14140.
47. Yoshioka T, Sakayori M, Kato S, et al. Dose escalation study of docetaxel and nedaplatin in patients with relapsed or refractory squamous cell carcinoma of the esophagus pretreated using cisplatin, 5-fluorouracil, and radiation. Int J Clin Oncol. 2006;11:454–60.
48. Nakajima Y, Suzuki T, Haruki S, et al. A pilot trial of docetaxel and nedaplatin in cisplatin-pretreated relapsed or refractory esophageal squamous cell cancer. Hepatogastroenterology. 2008;55:1631–5.
49. Jin J, Xu X, Wang F, et al. Second-line combination chemotherapy with docetaxel and nedaplatin for cisplatin-pretreated refractory metastatic/recurrent esophageal squamous cell carcinoma. J Thorac Oncol. 2009;4:1017–21.
50. Osaka Y, Takagi Y, Hoshino S, et al. Combination chemotherapy with docetaxel and nedaplatin for recurrent esophageal cancer in an outpatient setting. Dis Esophagus. 2006; 19:473–6.
51. Kanai M, Matsumoto S, Nishimura T, et al. Retrospective analysis of 27 consecutive patients treated with docetaxel/nedaplatin combination therapy as a second-line regimen for advanced esophageal cancer. Int J Clin Oncol. 2007;12:224–7.
52. Tanaka T, Fujita H, Sueyoshi S, et al. Second-line combination chemotherapy with docetaxel for cisplatin-pretreated refractory metastatic esophageal cancer: a preliminary report of initial experience. Chemotherapy. 2007;53:449–53.
53. Minamide J, Aoyama N, Takada K, et al. Evaluation of docetaxel, CDDP and 5-FU combined therapy as second-line chemotherapy for esophagus cancer [In Japanese]. Gan To Kagaku Ryoho. 2007;34:49–52.
54. Park BB, Im YH, Hwang IG, et al. Salvage chemotherapy with mitomycin C, ifosfamide, and cisplatin (MIC) for previously treated metastatic or recurrent esophageal squamous cell carcinoma. Invest New Drugs. 2008;26:387–92.
55. Medical Research Council Oesophageal Cancer Working Party. Surgical resection with or without preoperative chemotherapy in oesophageal cancer: a randomised controlled trial. Lancet. 2002;359:1727–33.

56. Le Prise E, Etienne PL, Meunier B, et al. A randomized study of chemotherapy, radiation therapy, and surgery versus surgery for localized squamous cell carcinoma of the esophagus. Cancer. 1994;73:1779–84.
57. Smith TJ, Ryan LM, Douglass Jr HO, et al. Combined chemoradiotherapy vs. radiotherapy alone for early stage squamous cell carcinoma of the esophagus: a study of the Eastern Cooperative Oncology Group. Int J Radiat Oncol Biol Phys. 1998;42:269–76.
58. Cooper JS, Guo MD, Herskovic A, et al. Chemoradiotherapy of locally advanced esophageal cancer. JAMA. 1999;281:1623–7.
59. Slabber CF, Nel JS, Schoeman L, et al. A randomized study of radiotherapy alone versus radiotherapy plus 5-fluorouracil and platinum in patients with inoperable, locally advanced squamous cancer of the esophagus. Am J Clin Oncol. 1998;21:462–5.
60. Walsh TN, Noonan N, Hollywood D, et al. A comparison of multimodal therapy and surgery for esophageal adenocarcinoma. N Engl J Med. 1996;335:462–7.
61. Bosset J-F, Gignoux M, Triboulet J-P, et al. Chemoradiotherapy followed by surgery compared with surgery alone in squamous-cell cancer of the esophagus. N Engl J Med. 1997;337:161–7.
62. Urba S, Orringer M, Turrisi A, et al. Randomized preoperative locoregional chemoradiation versus surgery alone in patients with resectable esophageal cancer. J Clin Oncol. 2001;19:305–13.
63. Burmeister BH, Smithers BM, Fitzgerald L, et al. A randomized phase III trial of preoperative chemoradiation followed by surgery *CR-S) versus surgery alone (S) for localized resectable cancer of the esophagus [abstract]. Proc Am Soc Clin Oncol. 2002;21:130a.
64. Chau I, Norman AR, Cunningham D, et al. The impact of primary tumour origins in patients with advanced oesophageal, oesophago-gastric junction and gastric adenocarcinoma: individual patient data from 1775 patients in four randomised controlled trials. Ann Oncol. 2009;20:885–91.
65. Glimelius B, Ekström K, Hoffman K, et al. Randomized comparison between chemotherapy plus best supportive care with best supportive care in advanced gastric cancer. Ann Oncol. 1997;8:163–8.
66. Murad A, Santiago F, Petroianu A, et al. Modified therapy with 5-fluorouracil, doxorubicin, and methotrexate in advanced gastric cancer. Cancer. 1993;72:37–41.
67. Pyrhönen S, Kuitunen T, Nyandoto P, et al. Randomised comparison of fluorouracil, epidoxorubicin and methotrexate (FEMTX) plus supportive care with supportive care alone in patients with non-resectable gastric cancer. Br J Cancer. 1995;71:587–91.
68. Ford HE, Marshall A, Bridgewater JA, et al. Docetaxel versus active symptom control for refractory oesophageal adenocarcinoma (COUGAR-02): an open-label, phase 3, randomised controlled trial. Lancet Oncol. 2014;15:78–86.
69. Kang JH, Lee SI, Lim dH, et al. Salvage chemotherapy for pretreated gastric cancer: a randomized phase III trial comparing chemotherapy plus best supportive care with best supportive care alone. J Clin Oncol. 2012;30:1513–8.
70. Thuss-Patience PC, Kretzschmar A, Deist T, et al. Irinotecan versus best supportive care (BSC) as second-line therapy in gastric cancer: a randomized phase III study of the Arbeitsgemeinschaft Internistische Onkologie (AIO). J Clin Oncol. 2009;27(suppl):211s. abstr 4540.
71. Wagner AD, Grothe W, Haerting J, et al. Chemotherapy in advanced gastric cancer: a systematic review and meta-analysis based on aggregate data. J Clin Oncol. 2006;24:2903–9.
72. Van Cutsem E, Moiseyenko VM, Tjulandin S, et al. Phase III study of docetaxel and cisplatin plus fluorouracil compared with cisplatin and fluorouracil as first-line therapy for advanced gastric cancer: a report of the V325 study group. J Clin Oncol. 2006;24:4991–7.
73. Guimbaud R, Louvet C, Ries P, et al. Prospective, randomized, multicenter phase III study of fluorouracil, leucovorin, and irinotecan versus epirubicin, cisplatin, and capecitabine in advanced gastric adenocarcinoma fluorouracil: a French intergroup (Federation Francophone de Cancerologie Digestive, Federation Nationale des Centres de Lutte Contre le Cancer, and Groupe Cooperateur Multidisciplinaire en Oncologie) study. J Clin Oncol. 2014;32:3520–6.

74. Cunningham D, Starling N, Rao S, et al. Capecitabine and oxaliplatin for advanced esophagogastric cancer. N Engl J Med. 2008;358:36–46.
75. Ajani JA, Rodriguez W, Bodoky G, et al. Multicenter phase III comparison of cisplatin/S-1 with cisplatin/infusional fluorouracil in advanced gastric or gastroesophageal adenocarcinoma study: the FLAGS trial. J Clin Oncol. 2010;28:1547–53.
76. Al-Batran SE, Hartmann JT, Probst S, et al. Phase III trial in metastatic gastroesophageal adenocarcinoma with fluorouracil, leucovorin plus either oxaliplatin or cisplatin: a study of the Arbeitsgemeinschaft Internistische Onkologie. J Clin Oncol. 2008;26:1435–42.
77. Kang YK, Kang WK, Shin DB, et al. Capecitabine/cisplatin versus 5-fluorouracil/cisplatin as first-line therapy in patients with advanced gastric cancer: a randomised phase III noninferiority trial. Ann Oncol. 2009;20:666–73.
78. Ilson DH. Docetaxel, cisplatin, and fluorouracil in gastric cancer: does the punishment fit the crime? J Clin Oncol. 2007;25:3188–90.
79. Lorenzen S, Hentrich M, Haberl C, et al. Split-dose docetaxel, cisplatin and leucovorin/fluorouracil as first-line therapy in advanced gastric cancer and adenocarcinoma of the gastroesophageal junction: results of a phase II trial. Ann Oncol. 2007;18:1673–9.
80. Tebbutt NC, Cummins MM, Sourjina T, et al. Randomised, non-comparative phase II study of weekly docetaxel with cisplatin and 5-fluorouracil or with capecitabine in oesophagogastric cancer: the AGITG ATTAX trial. Br J Cancer. 2010;102:475–81.
81. Shah MA, Stoller R, Shibata S, et al. Random assignment multicenter phase II study of modified docetaxel, cisplatin, fluorouracil (mDCF) versus DCF with growth factor support (GCSF) in metastatic gastroesophageal adenocarcinoma (GE). J Clin Oncol. 2010; 28(suppl):304s. abstr 4014.
82. Power DG, Kelsen DP, Shah MA. Advanced gastric cancer: slow but steady progress. Cancer Treat Rev. 2010;36:384–92.
83. Iacovelli R, Pietrantonio F, Farcomeni A, et al. Chemotherapy or targeted therapy as second-line treatment of advanced gastric cancer. A systemic review and meta-analysis of published studies. PLoS One. 2014;9, e108940.
84. Gu J, Ajani JA, Hawk ET, et al. Genome-wide catalogue of chromosomal aberrations in Barrett's esophagus and esophageal adenocarcinoma: a high-density single nucleotide polymorphism array analysis. Cancer Prev Res (Phila). 2010;3:1176–86.
85. Varis A, Puolakkainen P, Savolainen H, et al. DNA copy number profiling in esophageal Barrett adenocarcinoma: comparison with gastric adenocarcinoma and esophageal squamous cell carcinoma. Cancer Genet Cytogenet. 2001;127:53–8.
86. Bang YJ, Van Gutsem E, Feyereislova A, et al. Trastuzumab in combination with chemotherapy versus chemotherapy alone for treatment of HER2- positive advanced gastric or gastrooesophageal junction cancer (ToGA): a phase 3, open-label, randomised controlled trial. Lancet. 2010;376:687–97.
87. Reid BJ, Prevo LJ, Galipeau PC, et al. Predictors of progression in Barrett's esophagus II: baseline 17p (p53) loss of heterozygosity identifies a patient subset at increased risk for neoplastic progression. Am J Gastroenterol. 2001;96:2839–48.
88. Hollstein MC, Metcalf RA, Welsh JA, et al. Frequent mutation of the p53 gene in human esophageal cancer. Proc Natl Acad Sci U S A. 1990;87:9958–61.
89. Casson AG, Mukhopadhyay T, Cleary KR, et al. p53 gene mutations in Barrett's epithelium and esophageal cancer. Cancer Res. 1991;51:4495–9.
90. Goh XY, Rees JR, Paterson AL, et al. Integrative analysis of array-comparative genomic hybridisation and matched gene expression profiling data reveals novel genes with prognostic significance in oesophageal adenocarcinoma. Gut. 2011;60:1317–26.
91. Agrawal N, Jiao Y, Bettegowda C, et al. Comparative genomic analysis of esophageal adenocarcinoma and squamous cell carcinoma. Cancer Discov. 2012;2:899–905.
92. Dulak AM, Schumacher SE, van Lieshout J, et al. Gastrointestinal adenocarcinomas of the esophagus, stomach, and colon exhibit distinct patterns of genome instability and oncogenesis. Cancer Res. 2012;72:4383–93.

93. Shah MA. Gastrointestinal cancer: targeted therapies in gastric cancer—the dawn of a new era. Nat Rev Clin Oncol. 2014;11:10–1.
94. Hanawa M, Suzuki S, Dobashi Y, et al. EGFR protein overexpression and gene amplification in squamous cell carcinomas of the esophagus. Int J Cancer. 2006;118:1173–80.
95. Kitagawa Y, Ueda M, Ando N, et al. Further evidence for prognostic significance of epidermal growth factor receptor gene amplification in patients with esophageal squamous cell carcinoma. Clin Cancer Res. 1996;2:909–14.
96. Wang KL, Wu TT, Choi IS, et al. Expression of epidermal growth factor receptor in esophageal and esophagogastric junction adenocarcinomas: association with poor outcome. Cancer. 2007;109:658–67.
97. Yu WW, Guo YM, Zhu M, et al. Clinicopathological and prognostic significance of EGFR over-expression in esophageal squamous cell carcinoma: a meta-analysis. Hepatogastroenterology. 2011;58:426–31.
98. Gonzaga IM, Soares-Lima SC, de Santos PT, et al. Alterations in epidermal growth factor receptors 1 and 2 in esophageal squamous cell carcinomas. BMC Cancer. 2012;12:569.
99. Janmaat ML, Gallegos-Ruiz MI, Rodriguez JA, et al. Predictive factors for outcome in a phase II study of gefitinib in second-line treatment of advanced esophageal cancer patients. J Clin Oncol. 2006;24:1612–9.
100. Ferry DR, Anderson M, Beddard K, et al. A phase II study of gefitinib monotherapy in advanced esophageal adenocarcinoma: evidence of gene expression, cellular, and clinical response. Clin Cancer Res. 2007;13:5869–75.
101. Rodriguez CP, Adelstein DJ, Rice TW, et al. A phase II study of perioperative concurrent chemotherapy, gefitinib, and hyperfractionated radiation followed by maintenance gefitinib in locoregionally advanced esophagus and gastroesophageal junction cancer. J Thorac Oncol. 2010;5:229–35.
102. Dragovich T, McCoy S, Fenoglio-Preiser CM, et al. Phase II trial of erlotinib in gastroesophageal junction and gastric adenocarcinomas: SWOG 0127. J Clin Oncol. 2006;24:4922–7.
103. Dahan L, Chibaudel F, Di Fiore P, et al. Chemoradiation with FOLFOX plus cetuximab in locally advanced cardia or esophageal cancer: final results of a GERCOR phase II trial (ERaFOX). Paper presented at: 2011 American Society of Clinical Oncology annual meeting; 3–7 Jun 2011; Chicago.
104. Gavine PR, Mooney L, Kilgour E, et al. AZD4547: an orally bioavailable, potent, and selective inhibitor of the fibroblast growth factor receptor tyrosine kinase family. Cancer Res. 2012;72:2045–56.
105. Dahan L, Mariette C, Ychou M, et al. Neoadjuvant chemoradiotherapy with 5-fluorouracil-cisplatin combined with cetuximab in patients with resectable locally advanced esophageal carcinoma: a prospective phase I/II trial (FFCD-PRODIGE 3) – preliminary phase II results. Paper presented at: 2012 American Society of Clinical Oncology annual meeting; 1–5 Jun 2012; Chicago.
106. Crosby T, Hurt C, Falk S, et al. SCOPE 1: a phase II/III trial of chemoradiotherapy in esophageal cancer plus or minus cetuximab. Paper presented at: American Society of Clinical Oncology 2013 gastrointestinal cancers symposium; 24–26 Jan 2013; San Francisco.
107. Enzinger PC, Burtness B, Hollis D, et al. CALGB 80403/ECOG 1206: a randomized phase II study of three standard chemotherapy regimens (ECF, IC, FOLFOX) plus cetuximab in metastatic esophageal and GE junction cancer. Paper presented at: 2010 ASCO annual meeting; 4–8 Jun 2010; Chicago. p. 74.
108. Gold PJ, Goldman B, Iqbal S, et al. Cetuximab as second-line therapy in patients with metastatic esophageal adenocarcinoma: A phase II Southwest Oncology Group Study (S0415). J Thorac Oncol. 2010;5:1472–6.
109. Tomblyn MB, Goldman BH, Thomas Jr CR, et al. Cetuximab plus cisplatin, irinotecan, and thoracic radiotherapy as definitive treatment for locally advanced, unresectable esophageal cancer: a phase-II study of the SWOG (S0414). J Thorac Oncol. 2012;7:906–12.

110. Reed CE, Decker PA, Schefter TE, et al. A phase II study of neoadjuvant therapy with cisplatin, docetaxel, panitumumab plus radiation therapy followed by surgery in patients with locally advanced adenocarcinoma of the distal esophagus (ACOSOG Z4051). Paper presented at: 2012 American Society of Clinical Oncology annual meeting; 1–5 June 2012; Chicago.
111. Rüschoff J, Dietel M, Baretton G, et al. HER2 diagnostics in gastric cancer: guideline validation and development of standardized immunohistochemical testing. Virchows Arch. 2010;457:299–307.
112. Tafe LJ, Janjigian YY, Zaidinski M, et al. Human epidermal growth factor receptor 2 testing in gastroesophageal cancer: correlation between immunohistochemistry and fluorescence in situ hybridization. Arch Pathol Lab Med. 2010;135:1460–5.
113. LoRusso PM, Weiss D, Guardino E, et al. Trastuzumab emtansine: a unique antibody-drug conjugate in development for human epidermal growth factor receptor 2-positive cancer. Clin Cancer Res. 2011;17:6437–47.
114. Lynce F, Swain SM. Pertuzumab for the treatment of breast cancer. Cancer Invest. 2014;32:430–8.
115. Hecht JR, Bang YJ, Qin S, et al. Lapatinib in combination with capecitabine plus Oxaliplatin (CapeOx) in HER2-positive advanced or metastatic gastric, esophageal, or gastroesophageal adenocarcinoma (AC): the TRIO-013/LOGiC trial. J Clin Oncol. 2013;31(suppl 15s):243s. abstr LBA4001.
116. Satoh T, Xu RH, Chung HC, et al. Lapatinib plus paclitaxel versus paclitaxel alone in the second-line treatment of HER2-amplified advanced gastric cancer in Asian populations: TyTAN—a randomized, phase III study. J Clin Oncol. 2014;32:2039–49.
117. Shibuya M. Differential roles of vascular endothelial growth factor receptor-1 and receptor-2 in angiogenesis. J Biochem Mol Biol. 2006;39:469–78.
118. Fuchs CS, Tomasek J, Yong CJ, et al. Ramucirumab monotherapy for previously treated advanced gastric or gastro-esophageal junction adenocarcinoma (REGARD): an international, randomized, multicentre, placebo-controlled, phase 3 trial. Lancet. 2014;383:31–9.
119. Wilke H, Muro K, Van Custem E, et al. Ramucirumab plus paclitaxel versus placebo plus paclitaxel in patients with previously treated advanced gastric or gastro-esophageal junction adenocarcinoma (RAINBOW): a double-blind randomised phase 3 trial. Lancet Oncol. 2014;15:1224–35.
120. Yoon HH, Bendell JC, Braiteh FS, et al. Ramucirumab (RAM) plus FOLFOX as front-line therapy (Rx) for advanced gastric or esophageal adenocarcinoma (GE-AC): randomized, double-blind, multicenter phase 2 trial. J Clin Oncol. 2014;32(suppl 15s):256s. abstr 4004.
121. Ohtsu A, Shah MA, Van Cutsem E, et al. Bevacizumab in combination with chemotherapy as first-line therapy in advanced gastric cancer: a randomized, double-blind, placebo-controlled phase III study. J Clin Oncol. 2011;29:3968–76.
122. Kang YK, Ohtsu A, Van Cutsem E, et al. AVAGAST: a randomized, double-blind, placebo-controlled, phase III study of first-line capecitabine and cisplatin plus bevacizumab or placebo in patients with advanced gastric cancer (AGC). J Clin Oncol. 2010;28(suppl):302s. abstr LBA4007.
123. Qin S. Phase III study of apatinib in advanced gastric cancer: a randomized, double-blind, placebo-controlled trial. J Clin Oncol. 2014;32(suppl 15s):255s. abstr 4003.
124. Knox JJ, Wong R, Darling GE, et al. Adjuvant sunitinib for locally advanced esophageal cancer: results of a phase II trial. Paper presented at: 2011 American Society of Clinical Oncology annual meeting; 3–7 June 2011; Chicago.
125. Ku GY, Janjigian YY, Shah MA, et al. Phase II trial of sorafenib in esophageal and gastro-esophageal junction cancer: response and prolonged stable disease observed in adenocarcinoma. Paper presented at: American Society of Clinical Oncology 2013 gastrointestinal cancers symposium; 24–26 Jan 2013; San Francisco.
126. Ohigashi Y, Sho M, Yamada Y, et al. Clinical significance of programmed death-1 ligand-1 and programmed death-1 ligand-2 expression in human esophageal cancer. Clin Cancer Res. 2005;11:2947–53.

127. Lu B, Chen L, Liu L, et al. T-cell-mediated tumor immune surveillance and expression of B7 co-inhibitory molecules in cancers of the upper gastrointestinal tract. Immunol Res. 2011;50:269–75.
128. Kono K, Kawaida H, Takahashi A, et al. CD4(+)CD25 high regulatory T cells increase with tumor stage in patients with gastric and oesophageal cancers. Cancer Immunol Immunother. 2006;55:1064–71.
129. Fife BT, Pauken KE. The role of PD-1 pathway in autoimmunity and peripheral tolerance. Ann NY Acad Sci. 2011;1217:45–59.
130. Keir ME, Butte MJ, Freeman GJ, et al. PD-1 and its ligands in tolerance and immunity. Annu Rev Immunol. 2008;26:677–704.
131. Muro K, Bang Y, Shankaran V, et al. A phase 1b study of pembrolizumab (Pembro; MK-3475) in patients with advanced gastric cancer. Ann Oncol. 2014;25(abstr LBA15).
132. Graziano F, Galluccio N, Lorenzini P, et al. Genetic activation of the MET pathway and prognosis of patients with high-risk, radically resected gastric cancer. J Clin Oncol. 2011;29:4789–95.
133. Bachleitner-Hofmann T, Sun MY, Chen CT, et al. HER kinase activation confers resistance to MET tyrosine kinase inhibition in MET oncogene-addicted gastric cancer cells. Mol Cancer Ther. 2008;7:3499–508.
134. Kato H, Arao T, Matsumoto K, et al. Gene amplification of EGFR, HER2, FGFR2 and MET in esophageal squamous cell carcinoma. Int J Oncol. 2013;42:1151–8.
135. Yap TA, Harris D, Barriuso J, et al. Phase I trial to determine the dose range for the c-Met inhibitor ARQ 197 that inhibits c-Met and FAK phosphorylation, when administered by an oral twice-a-day schedule. Paper presented at: 2008 American Society of Clinical Oncology annual meeting; 30 May–3 Jun 2008; Chicago.
136. Matsumoto K, Arao T, Hamaguchi T, et al. FGFR2 gene amplification and clinicopathological features in gastric cancer. Br J Cancer. 2012;106:727–32.
137. Yashiro M, Shinto O, Nakamura K, et al. Synergistic antitumor effects of FGFR2 inhibitor with 5-fluorouracil on scirrhous gastric carcinoma. Int J Cancer. 2010;126:1004–16.
138. Satoh T, Yamada Y, Muro K, et al. Phase I study of cediranib in combination with cisplatin plus fluoropyrimidine (S-1 or capecitabine) in Japanese patients with previously untreated advanced gastric cancer. Cancer Chemother Pharmacol. 2012;69:439–46.
139. Enzinger PC, Ilson DH, Kelsen DP. Chemotherapy in esophageal cancer. Semin Oncol. 1999;26:12–20.
140. Stahl M. Chemotherapy of esophageal carcinoma. Onkologie. 1999;22:98–104.

Advanced Surgical Approaches for the Management of Esophageal Carcinoma

15

Boris Sepesi and Wayne Hofstetter

One Hundred Years of Esophagectomy

Surgery has been used to manage various disease processes for hundreds of years. Advanced body cavity operations, however, did not become possible until the beginning of the twentieth century, when the discovery of ether anesthesia enabled surgeons to perform prolonged operations, organ extirpations, and reconstructive surgeries. Some of the major accomplishments of the early twentieth century included Billroth's pioneering of surgical techniques and strategies for the management of gastric cancer and Halsted's use of radical mastectomy with extensive lymph node dissection for breast cancer [1].

Early advances in esophageal and thoracic surgery trailed behind those in abdominal and breast surgery. Intrathoracic esophageal carcinoma was difficult to manage at that time. Single-lung ventilation did not exist, which complicated the management of pneumothorax during operation. Sauerbruch, an eminent surgeon of the time, considered carcinoma of the esophagus to be inoperable and advised against surgically removing the involved thoracic esophagus [2].

Despite Sauerbruch's recommendation, Torek, using chloroform and ether anesthesia, performed the first successful esophagectomy via right thoracotomy for an esophageal squamous cell carcinoma (SCC) in Germany in 1913. The patient's intrathoracic lung adhesions prevented the lung from collapsing during the operation, and Torek used an extracorporeal esophagogastrostomy to reconstruct enteral continuity. The patient survived for 12 years and ultimately died of pneumonia rather than cancer. Encouraged by this result, Torek continued to perform resections of the esophagus for cancer. He reported his esophagectomy series in 1929, citing a

B. Sepesi, MD (✉) • W. Hofstetter
Department of Thoracic and Cardiovascular Surgery, The University of Texas MD Anderson Cancer Center, 1515 Holcombe Blvd., Houston, TX 77030, USA
e-mail: bsepesi@mdanderson.org; WHofstetter@mdanderson.org

G. Ozyigit et al. (eds.), *Principles and Practice of Radiotherapy Techniques in Thoracic Malignancies*, DOI 10.1007/978-3-319-28761-4_15

postoperative mortality rate that would be considered prohibitively high by today's standards. However, through his experience, Torek recognized that surgery offered a potential cure for localized esophageal cancer. Anticipating improvements in overall perioperative care, he continued to advocate for surgical therapy for the disease [2].

With further progress in anesthesia and critical care, the surgical treatment of esophageal cancer evolved over the remainder of the twentieth century. Although perioperative morbidity and mortality improved, they still remained quite high relative to other surgical procedures. The major complications recognized as contributing to the high morbidity and mortality of esophagectomy were cardiopulmonary complications related to thoracotomy incisions and intrathoracic anastomotic leaks that caused mediastinitis. To avoid thoracotomy-associated complications, surgeons began resecting the esophagus via abdominal and left neck incisions and utilizing transhiatal dissection of the esophagus [3]. In addition, esophagus–stomach anastomoses were placed increasingly in the neck, which simplified the management of anastomotic leaks; rather than having to reoperate for mediastinitis due to thoracic anastomotic dehiscence, surgeons could simply reopen the initial incision to address the issue [4].

As esophagectomy itself became safer and perioperative outcomes continued to improve, some surgeons began performing more extensive lymphatic nodal dissections and wider local excisions. Similar to Halsted's radical mastectomy, more aggressive en bloc resection techniques with extensive lymphadenectomies in the abdomen, chest, and sometimes neck became favored in the hope that the disease would be extirpated in its entirety, resulting in a cure. This approach was a logical conclusion to the high rates of local regional failures experienced as a result of operating on more advanced disease. In time, it was discovered that although this approach might benefit a select group of patients, more extensive dissection does not universally equal better oncologic outcomes [5].

In the past several decades, surgical techniques have evolved rapidly. Nowadays, depending on the surgery center and the surgeon's expertise, esophageal cancer may be resected via minimally invasive techniques (including abdominal laparoscopy and video-assisted thoracoscopy) [6], robot-assisted techniques [7], or traditional open techniques [8]. A number of esophagectomy types, including vagal-sparing esophagectomy [9], inversion esophagectomy [10], abdominal esophagectomy [11], transthoracic (Ivor Lewis) esophagectomy [8], three-field (McKeown) esophagectomy [12], and left thoracoabdominal esophagectomy [13], have been developed. Depending on the tumor location and type of esophageal resection, anastomoses can be performed high in the abdomen, in the chest, or in the neck. The indications for a given type of esophagectomy depend on the circumstances. Arguments about the superiority of one approach over another are likely unjustified. Surgeons should choose the approach they are most comfortable with to achieve complete R0 resections with adequate lymph node dissection to maximize the oncologic benefit of surgery. In addition, patient selection, meticulous operation, and judicious postoperative care are all important to achieving excellent perioperative outcomes.

Since the first successful esophagectomy over 100 years ago, much has been learned about the surgical aspects of esophageal resections and reconstructions. Esophagectomy results have improved significantly, with perioperative mortality rates declining from nearly 90 % in the early 1900s to less than 5 % today [14]. Advancements in surgical and anesthesia techniques, along with improvements in patient selection and preparation for these extensive procedures, have played major roles in this significant improvement. In addition, an improved understanding of cancer biology has revealed that surgery alone benefits only a select group of patients who have early esophageal cancer.

Multimodality Therapy for Esophageal Cancer

The best oncologic outcomes in esophageal cancer patients, especially those with locally or regionally advanced disease, seem to be achieved with multimodality therapy consisting of chemotherapy, radiation therapy, and surgery [15].

Following the discovery of radium and its antitumor effects in the early twentieth century, radiation therapy became a frequently used modality for many diseases. Radiation therapy for esophageal cancer initially consisted primarily of treatment with radium bougies until the emergence of external beam radiation. Both techniques caused tumor regression and elicited the occasional complete tumor response.

Considering the high rates of local recurrence after surgical resection, preoperative radiation was added to surgery to decrease the local recurrence rate and improve survival. Most randomized trials tested this approach in esophageal SCC and utilized radiation doses of 20–40 Gy. This was not a biologically adequate dose, however, since none of the trials, including a meta-analysis of 1147 patients [16], showed that the regimen had a significant survival benefit [16]. Later trials, this time investigating radiation therapy in the postoperative setting to avoid worsening perioperative complications, used higher doses of 40–60 Gy. This approach showed benefit in some trials, but the overall data were too conflicting to support clear conclusions about its absolute value in prolonging patients' lives [17]. The data did indicate that the combination of surgery and radiation improved locoregional disease control, however.

Despite improvements in locoregional disease control, most esophageal cancer patients continued to die of metastatic disease. Thus, the administration of systemic chemotherapy prior to surgery became an appealing option in esophageal cancer patients: Chemotherapy would be given preoperatively to eliminate potential micrometastases and downstage the primary tumor, thus allowing for more frequent complete surgical resection. Administering chemotherapy preoperatively would also provide the opportunity to measure the treatment response radiographically and quantify the biologic response in pathologic specimens by assessing the viability of tumor cells. Biologic response has since been shown to correlate with overall patient outcome [18].

In one of the first trials of chemotherapy for esophageal cancer, Roth et al. compared chemotherapy followed by surgery with surgery alone [19]. The trial, which revealed that patients whose disease had a major or complete response to chemotherapy, had a significantly longer median survival duration and also provided the first insight into the biologic heterogeneity of esophageal carcinoma. Another trial conducted by Kelsen et al. (USA Intergroup 113), however, did not demonstrate a survival benefit of chemotherapy, perhaps owing to poor local disease control and inconsistencies in disease staging and response evaluation [20]. Later trials, such as the MRC (Medical Research Council) trial in 2002 and the MAGIC (Medical Research Council Adjuvant Infusion Chemotherapy) trial in 2006, showed that administering chemotherapy prior to surgery had a survival benefit in esophageal carcinoma patients [21, 22]. Current chemotherapeutic regimens for the treatment of esophageal cancer are based on a platinum compound, either cisplatin or carboplatin, combined with either 5-fluorouracil or taxanes.

Another common treatment combination for locally advanced esophageal cancer is concomitant chemotherapy and radiation therapy followed by surgical resection. This approach, known as trimodality therapy, is based on the observation that chemotherapy combined with radiation therapy has a synergistic anticancer effect and the fact that each therapy alone at high doses can cause excessive toxicity and thus treatment-related morbidity. As with the early trials of chemotherapy plus surgery, the early trials of trimodality therapy for esophageal cancer also had inconsistent disease staging and dissimilar perioperative outcomes between the study arms, factors that obscured the therapy's true potential oncologic benefit. However, one study would soon set the standard for all future randomized clinical trials in esophageal cancer. In 2012, van Hagen et al. published the results of the CROSS (Chemoradiotherapy for Oesophageal Cancer Followed by Surgery Study) trial, which analyzed the outcomes of 366 patients with esophageal adenocarcinoma (75 %) or SCC (22 %) randomized to surgery alone ($N = 188$) or trimodality therapy ($N = 178$). The trimodality regimen consisted of carboplatin plus paclitaxel with concurrent radiation (41.4 Gy) for 5 weeks followed by esophagectomy. In this randomized trial, the two study arms had similar perioperative outcomes, which allowed for the assessment of the effect of neoadjuvant chemoradiation on overall survival. This well-executed trial revealed that, compared with the surgery-alone arm, the trimodality therapy arm had a higher R0 resection rate and a longer overall median survival duration (49 months versus 24 months; hazard ratio [HR], 0.65 [95 % CI, 0.49–0.87]; $p = 0.003$). In addition, the estimated 5-year survival rate of the trimodality therapy group (47 %) was significantly higher than that of the surgery-alone group (34 %; HR, 0.65 [95 % CI, 0.49–0.87]; $p = 0.003$). Interestingly, the trimodality strategy seemed to have benefited mainly patients with squamous cell histology and node-negative status [15].

In spite of the results of the CROSS trial, debate continues as to whether chemotherapy combined with en bloc esophagectomy would achieve results similar to those achieved with chemoradiation and surgery. There are two trials comparing these therapies, one a randomized POET trial by Stahl et al. [23] and the other a phase II randomized trial by Burmeister et al. [24]. Although neither trial reached the targeted improvement in survival, there was a significant difference in DFS and a trend in OS favoring the CXRT arm of the POET trial.

Principles of Surgery for Esophageal Carcinoma

Timing of Esophagectomy

Esophagectomy is an extensive procedure, and appropriately timed surgery is of the utmost importance. Paramount to effective treatment planning is an accurate assessment of the patient's nutritional status. Most patients with esophageal cancer come to medical attention only after developing dysphagia, sometimes lasting weeks or months; weight loss often finally pushes them to seek help. Therefore careful assessment and optimization of nutritional status is a *sine qua non* for successful therapy. Patient's weight, but also serum levels of albumin and prealbumin, should be measured. Optimization of nutritional parameters via enteral route is preferred over parenteral route.

Upfront surgery for esophageal carcinoma is generally indicated only in patients with mucosal T1a or submucosal T1b disease. Patients with T2 cancers involving the muscularis propria are also candidates for upfront esophagectomy, as most have disease that is generally over-staged after evaluation with endoscopic ultrasonography. The timing of upfront surgery depends mainly on the patient's nutritional and physiologic status. If the patient has an albumin level of ≥3.5 g/dL and optimal cardiopulmonary function, proceeding with an esophagectomy is reasonable.

The decision of whether to use trimodality therapy for esophageal cancer should be made before initiating treatment. However, deciding when to perform surgery following neoadjuvant chemoradiation can be challenging. In general, the goal is to complete the surgical resection within 4–6 weeks after chemoradiation; however, many patients have not fully recovered from chemoradiation at that point. Occasionally, more time is required to prepare the patient for esophagectomy. Whether the timing of esophagectomy after chemoradiation influences outcomes such as complications, long-term survival, or pathologic complete response remains largely unclear, although at least one study's findings would seem to suggest that it does not. Kim et al. conducted a retrospective analysis comparing the outcomes of 150 patients who underwent esophagectomy within 8 weeks after chemoradiation and 116 patients who underwent esophagectomy more than 8 weeks after chemoradiation. The authors found that the operative time, operative blood loss amount, anastomotic leak rate, and other perioperative complications did not differ between the groups. Importantly, the groups' pathologic complete response and overall survival rates were not significantly different. Rather, the authors' multivariable analysis revealed that weight loss (HR, 1.84) was independently associated with complications; female gender (HR, 2.51), body mass index >25 (HR, 2.69), and squamous cell histology (HR, 4.87) were independently associated with pathologic complete response; and age (HR, 1.03), number of positive lymph nodes (HR, 1.11), and pathologic stage IV disease (HR, 5.10) were significantly associated with survival. Thus, the study's findings suggest that surgical resection can be delayed longer than 8 weeks after chemoradiation without compromising short- or long-term outcomes [25].

Salvage and Selective Esophagectomy

In the era of multimodality therapy, impeccable perioperative outcomes are necessary to demonstrate the oncologic benefit of surgery in patients with esophageal cancer. As mentioned previously, most randomized trials in esophageal cancer patients were hindered by significant discordance in surgical outcomes between study arms, thus obscuring the actual benefit of surgery for esophageal cancer in the multimodality setting. In high-risk patients or patients who require more than 12 weeks to recover from definitive chemoradiation, a strategy of selective or salvage esophagectomy may be applied. In this approach, surgery is performed only in the setting of disease persistence or recurrence after definitive chemoradiation. This treatment paradigm was the focus of the Radiation Therapy Oncology Group 0246 phase II trial by Swisher et al. The study was designed to detect an improvement in the 1-year survival rate from 60 % to 77.5 % in patients who underwent definitive chemoradiation followed by selective/salvage esophagectomy. More than 70 % of the patients enrolled in the trial had clinical stage T3 or N1 disease. Of the 41 patients included in the analysis, 21 (51 %) underwent salvage esophagectomy for residual or recurrent disease, and one patient requested resection. The overall survival rate was 53 % for patients with complete clinical response after definitive chemoradiation, 33 % for patients with clinical incomplete response, and 41 % for patients with clinical incomplete response salvaged by surgery. Following induction chemotherapy and chemoradiation, three patients died of treatment-related complications, underscoring the toxicity of this regimen, and one patient died of disease progression; in the surgery group, one patient died postoperatively [26]. The results of this study suggest that salvage esophagectomy following definitive chemoradiation is a feasible and safe treatment strategy and provides an additional survival benefit in patients with incomplete clinical response after definitive chemoradiation.

Esophageal Replacement Conduits

Following esophagectomy, the continuity of the gastrointestinal tract may be reestablished with a tabularized stomach, a free segment of the jejunum, a pedicle of jejunum in Roux-en-Y fashion, or colon interposition. Of these options, the stomach is the most reliable and most commonly used conduit for esophageal replacement.

Stomach

The stomach has an abundant blood supply, and after careful mobilization and a Kocher maneuver (i.e., mobilization of the duodenum), it easily reaches to the neck. For stomach mobilization, first, the lesser sac is entered, and the greater omentum is separated from the transverse colon and mesocolon. During this process, it is imperative to preserve the right gastroepiploic artery, which will provide the main blood supply to the created conduit, and the omental pedicle, which will be used for

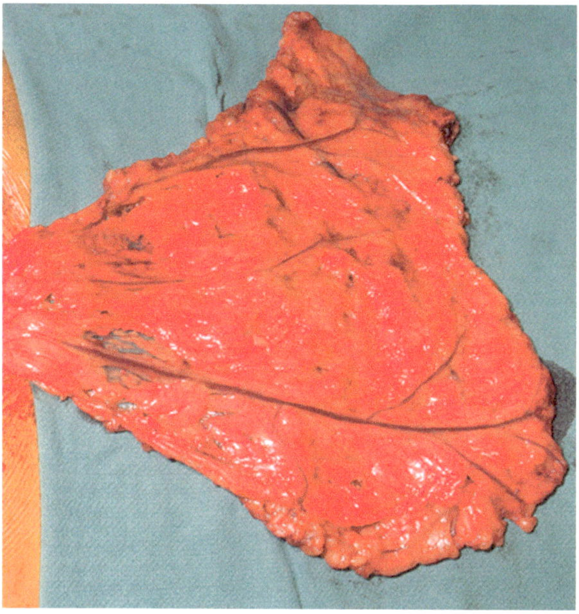

Fig. 15.1 Mobilized omental pedicle to be transposed to the chest for anastomotic reinforcement

anastomotic reinforcement. After omental mobilization (Fig. 15.1), the greater curvature of the stomach is mobilized by dividing the short gastric arteries. On the medial aspect of the stomach, the pars flaccida is opened, and the lesser curvature is mobilized to the level of the diaphragmatic crus, which is circumferentially dissected to expose the distal esophagus. If a distal esophageal tumor invades the crus or the diaphragm, a portion of the crus or the diaphragm can be resected en bloc with the esophagus and the proximal stomach to achieve negative radial margins. After the mobilization of the lesser and greater gastric curvatures, the left gastric artery is exposed and divided at its takeoff from the celiac trunk, and all nodal tissue along this artery is swept with the specimen. Starting at the incisura and continuing toward the angle of His, a linear stapler helps to create a gastric conduit approximately 4–5 cm in width which allows for optimal gastric emptying while minimizing leaks. This tubular gastric pedicle, with a blood supply based mainly on the right gastroepiploic artery, will serve as a neoesophagus.

Jejunum

If the stomach is not available—either because of previous gastric surgery or because it has already been used as a conduit of choice in an operation for previous esophageal replacement—the jejunum is used as the replacement conduit. The reestablishment of intestinal continuity with a free or pedicled jejunal graft is technically challenging and should be performed in centers experienced with this approach. The most critical part of this operation is selecting the blood supply to the long jejunal Roux limb to ensure that the pedicle will reach to the neck for the

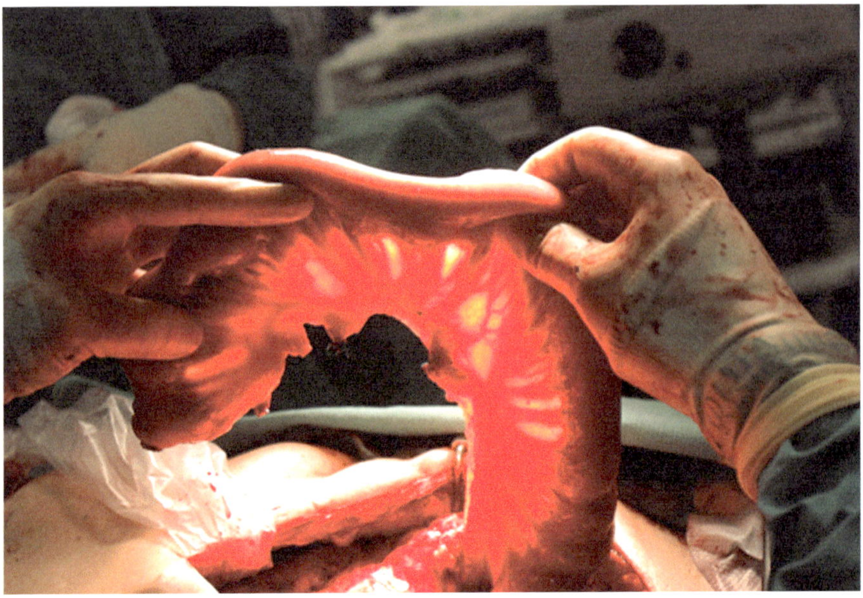

Fig. 15.2 Mobilized jejunum, prepared for transposition to the neck

anastomosis and the blood supply to the remaining small intestine will not be compromised. Generally, this type of reconstruction requires "supercharging" the conduit in the neck by anastomosing the mesenteric artery and vein to either the internal thoracic artery and vein or to other suitable blood vessels in the neck.

The mobilization of the jejunal conduit begins with careful transillumination of the vascular arcade within the mesentery. Vascular branches coming off the superior mesenteric artery are then counted. The first branch must be preserved in its native position, as it supplies the portion of the jejunum just distal to the ligament of Treitz, which will be anastomosed to the distal portion of the Roux limb. The second and third jejunal branches are then divided up to the level of the bridging mesenteric arcades. The fourth branch of the jejunal arteries is the main pedicle that supplies the conduit. Because the proximal portion of the conduit is under warm ischemia during its transposition to the neck and until it is anastomosed to the internal thoracic vessels, all dissection and preparation for both vascular and enteric anastomoses should be completed prior to the division of the vascular supply (Figs. 15.2 and 15.3). Even relatively trivial inaccuracies in the conduct of the operation may result in major postoperative complications.

When successfully performed, long jejunal limb interposition results in a good functional outcome. The dreaded complication of jejunal limb ischemia is fortunately rare; however, nonobstructing mesenteric ischemia in the distal small bowel is a well-recognized event. Therefore, the success of this operation depends not only on meticulous technical performance but also judicious postoperative care, which includes careful attention to the fluid balance and resuscitation.

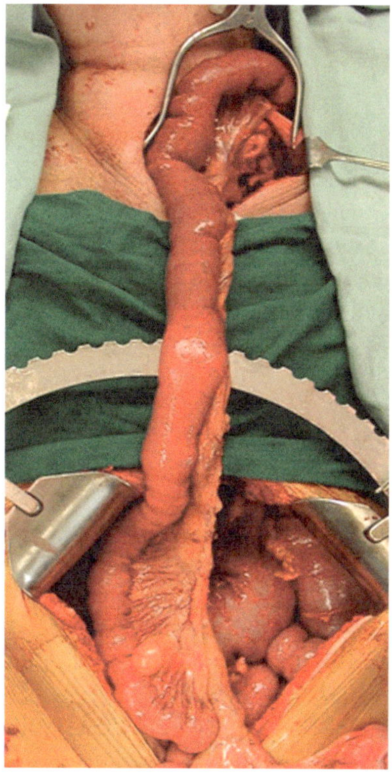

Fig. 15.3 Jejunal interposition to the neck (the length is measured here, and the conduit will ultimately lay in the retrosternal position)

Colon

The colon is the second most commonly used conduit for esophageal replacement. As in jejunal interposition, the success of colon interposition depends on judicious preoperative preparation, accurate delineation of vascular anatomy, and careful dissection and division of appropriate vascular structures. Unlike the jejunum, the colon is prone to having inherent pathologies such as colonic polyps, inflammatory colitis, or cancer. Therefore, before considering the colon as an esophageal replacement conduit, the surgeon must ensure that the colon is free of any inherent pathology.

Although the blood supply to the colon is generally consistent, anatomic variations, especially around the areas of hepatic and splenic flexure arcades, may exist; therefore, preoperative angiography is usually obtained to define the vascular anatomy. Computed tomography angiography with coronal and sagittal reconstructions is also useful in identifying atherosclerotic disease at the ostium of the inferior mesenteric artery, the presence of which could compromise blood flow to the colonic pedicle.

Right or left colon interposition is often referenced when discussing esophageal replacement, but actually, the transverse colon with a portion of the descending colon is used as a conduit most of the time. The "left colon" conduit is based on the ascending branch of the left colic artery, which is a branch of the inferior mesenteric artery and creates the arc of Riolan around the splenic flexure. The left colic artery communicates with the middle colic artery through collateral circulation with the artery of Drummond.

The mobilization of the colon begins with the division of the lateral abdominal wall attachments at the white line of Toldt. Both the ascending and descending colons are mobilized in this fashion, with careful mobilization of the hepatic and splenic flexures. The omentum is then detached from the transverse colon and mesocolon. After complete colonic mobilization, the mesocolon is transilluminated, and the vascular supply to the selected colonic pedicle is identified, dissected free, and tested for ischemia by temporarily clamping the vessels to be divided. One of the major technical challenges of this operation is the dissection of the middle colic artery and vein. These structures must be divided as close to their origin as possible to preserve collateral blood flow. Although it is uncommon, the middle colic vessels may also be anastomosed to internal thoracic vessels in the neck, thus supercharging the colonic conduit.

The advantages of "left" colon interposition are its generally reliable blood supply and isoperistaltic orientation. The downside of this approach is that it requires esophago-colostomy, colo-colostomy, and colo-gastrostomy or colo-jejunostomy anastomoses. Although technically nuanced, colon interposition can be performed successfully in the vast majority of cases after appropriate patient selection and preoperative evaluation. It provides satisfactory alimentation and has acceptable long-term gastrointestinal side effects.

Anastomoses: Locations, Types, and Complications

Creating the anastomosis between the esophageal remnant and replacement esophageal conduit is by far the most important aspect of esophagectomy. Anastomotic complications often determine both the short-term and long-term physiologic outcomes of this challenging procedure. Anastomotic dehiscence or leak is a rather common complication of esophagectomy and is mainly due to the relative ischemia of the gastric conduit. When the esophagogastrostomy is made in the cervical region, the rate of anastomotic leak is approximately 15 % [27]. Intrathoracic anastomotic leaks occur in approximately 8–10 % of patients [28]. Patients who undergo salvage esophagectomy have the highest anastomotic complication rate (15 %), likely owing to the chronic effect that radiation therapy has on esophageal tissue and its microvasculature [28].

In general, the lower in the chest the anastomosis is performed, the higher the likelihood of it healing successfully because of the more robust blood supply of the gastric body and antrum rather than the fundus. However, to achieve adequate proximal surgical margins and avoid debilitating gastroesophageal reflux, most surgeons elect to perform the anastomosis either at or above the level of the azygos arch in the chest or in the neck. The reason for performing the cervical anastomosis is the relative ease of the management of anastomotic complications in this region.

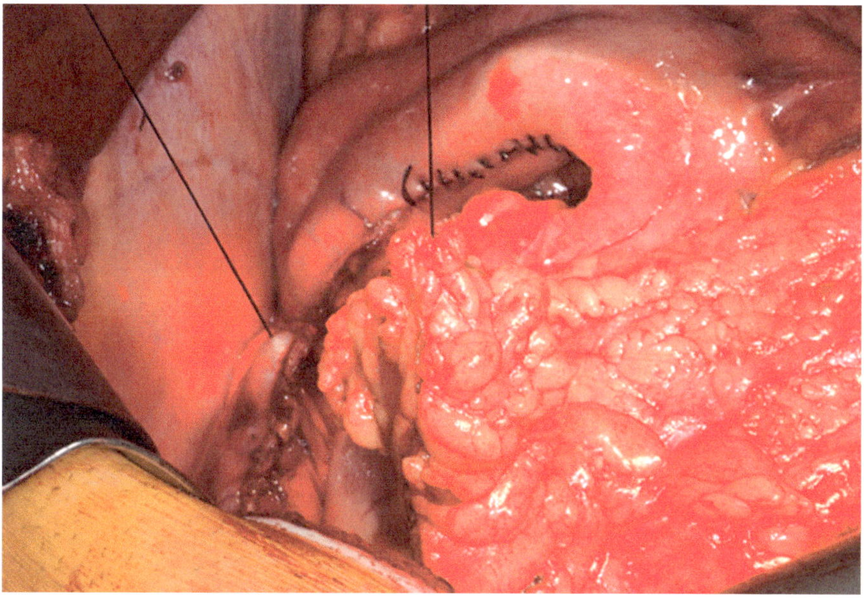

Fig. 15.4 The omental pedicle is sutured to the gastric conduit prior to transposition to the chest

Reopening the neck incision with adequate external drainage is usually all that is necessary to heal the anastomosis by secondary intention. Subsequent anastomotic stricture is common and requires serial dilation; in some instances of recurrent strictures, patients are taught self-dilation [27].

The leak rate of intrathoracic anastomoses is generally lower than that of cervical anastomoses. Historically, however, intrathoracic anastomotic complications have resulted in severe mediastinitis and high morbidity and mortality rates. This complication once usually required reoperation with anastomotic repair, buttressing of the repaired anastomosis with either a latissimus dorsi or serratus anterior muscle flap, and wide drainage [29]. To avoid this complication, surgeons began using the omentum to buttress the anastomosis. The omentum, whose blood supply depends on the right gastroepiploic artery, is mobilized with the greater curvature of the stomach. In our retrospective analysis, we reviewed the outcomes of 607 esophagectomy patients, of whom 215 (35 %) underwent anastomotic reinforcement with the omentum [27]. Anastomotic leak occurred in 51 (8.4 %) patients. The anastomotic leak rate of patients with omental wrapping of the anastomosis (4.7 %; odds ratio, 0.4) was significantly lower than that of patients without the omental wrapping (10.5 %). Patients who underwent salvage resection had the highest leak rate (15 %), but this rate declined to 4.6 % with the use of omental wrapping. Importantly, grade 3 leaks, defined by the necessity for reoperation, significantly declined when the omental pedicle was used (Figs. 15.4 and 15.5). Omental reinforcement of the intrathoracic esophagogastric anastomosis has since become a routine part of our clinical practice [27].

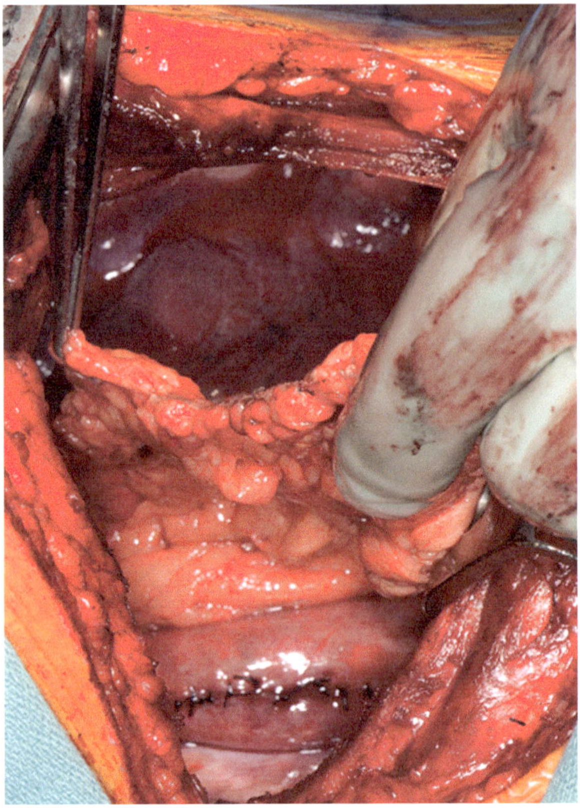

Fig. 15.5 The omentum is then enveloped around the anastomosis and gastric conduit

Surgeons often debate whether sewing or stapling results in fewer anastomotic complications. Whereas hand-sewn anastomoses are usually performed end-to-end, stapled anastomoses may be performed in a side-to-side fashion or end-to-end with a circular stapler. Blackmon et al. [30] compared the outcomes of patients in whom intrathoracic anastomoses were performed using these different techniques and found that the anastomotic leak rates of patients with side-to-side stapled anastomoses (8.7 %), circular "end-to-end stapled" anastomoses (4.3 %), and hand-sewn anastomoses (4.3 %) did not differ significantly ($p=0.78$). However, the postoperative dysphagia rate of patients with hand-sewn anastomoses (50 %) was twice that of patients with stapled anastomosis (25 %), which may have been due to a higher rate of stricture in the hand-sewn anastomosis group. Nevertheless, the type of anastomosis did not affect perioperative mortality or long-term oncologic outcomes [30].

Extent of Lymphadenectomy

Debate regarding the extent of lymphadenectomy in oncologic surgery has lasted decades and remains unsettled. How many lymph nodes draining a particular tumor site should be removed? Does the performance of extended lymphadenectomy actually influence survival? Is it necessary to remove a large number of lymph nodes if the patient already underwent neoadjuvant chemoradiation? These questions have not been answered completely in many epithelial malignancies, including esophageal carcinoma.

The idea that lymph nodes must be removed during oncologic surgery dates to the times of Halstead, who observed the sequential spread of breast cancer from the breast tissue to the axillary lymph nodes, then to the infraclavicular lymph nodes, then occasionally to the intramammary lymph nodes, and then throughout the body. This observation gave the impression that all solid tumors spread in an organized, consistent fashion, in which local disease progressively spreads to regional lymph nodes before spreading systemically. Based on this premise, sentinel lymph node biopsy became popularized in breast cancer surgery; if the sentinel lymph node was positive, complete axillary dissection was recommended in the hope of achieving both locoregional control and prolonged survival. However, mounting data suggest that this is not the case in all situations and that the risk of systemic disease is related much more to cancer biology rather than to local or regional disease burden, although the disease burden especially in the lymph nodes is a fairly consistent predictor for the risk of systemic disease. However, depending on its biology, even a small tumor may have the ability to metastasize systemically.

Performing lymphadenectomy for esophageal cancer is somewhat more challenging than performing it for breast or colorectal cancer, for example. This is mainly because the esophagus has haphazard—and extensive—lymphatic drainage; it spans from the neck to the abdomen and therefore drains into cervical, intrathoracic, and abdominal lymph nodes. Thus, tumor location plays an important role in choosing which nodal areas should be dissected during esophagectomy. The surgical approach also influences which nodal stations are dissected and how many lymph nodes are removed. Sentinel lymph node biopsy for esophageal cancer has not been developed and remains an area of ongoing research.

For distal and gastroesophageal junction esophageal cancers, which are mostly adenocarcinomas, abdominal D2 lymphadenectomy and intrathoracic lymphadenectomy are recommended. Abdominal D2 lymphadenectomy includes the resection of the perigastric lymph nodes and nodes along the branches of the celiac artery, and intrathoracic lymphadenectomy includes the resection of the periesophageal and subcarinal lymph nodes. Some surgeons advocate adding dissection of the paratracheal lymph nodes and skeletonization of the recurrent laryngeal nerves and adding cervical lymphadenectomy, even in the setting of distal esophageal adenocarcinoma [31]. For mid-esophageal tumors, which initially spread to the intrathoracic lymph nodes but may also involve either cervical or abdominal lymph nodes, lymphadenectomy is also generally restricted to thoracic and abdominal lymph nodes. (Cervical lymph node dissection may be indicated in select cases, however.) Cervical esophageal cancers, which are most commonly SCCs, are generally treated with definitive chemoradiation and thus are not treated surgically. In rare instances of surgical resection of these cancers, which may necessitate total laryngectomy with cervical esophagectomy, standard bilateral neck dissection is advocated.

The optimal lymphadenectomy for esophageal cancer and the influence of lymphadenectomy on patient survival have been difficult to define, mainly owing to stage migration (the "Will Rogers phenomenon"). Most data used to investigate these issues are from cases of esophageal resection in which surgery was the sole treatment modality. As a result, the appropriate extent of nodal harvest during esophagectomy following neoadjuvant chemoradiation has not yet been defined. Utilizing the Worldwide Esophageal Cancer Collaboration database, Rizk et al. studied the relationship between lymphadenectomy and survival and attempted to define optimal lymphadenectomy. The study cohort consisted of 4627 esophageal cancer patients who underwent esophagectomy alone. Five-year survival appeared to improve as the number of resected lymph nodes increased. For each pathologic stage, the authors identified a different target number of lymph nodes to resect: 10–12 nodes for pathologic pT1 disease, 15–22 nodes for pT2 disease, and 31–42 nodes for pT3/T4 disease [32]. These findings are consistent with the fact that tumors that penetrate deeper into the esophageal wall have a higher chance of nodal metastasis; therefore, the resection of more than 30 lymph nodes allows for more accurate pathologic staging. As expected, the authors found that the extent of lymphadenectomy was not associated with a survival benefit in patients with carcinoma in situ (whose chance of nodal disease is nearly 0 %) or in patients with more than seven positive lymph nodes (whose risk of systemic disease is almost 100 %). Thus, any additional lymph node resection in either group would not impact overall survival [32].

Lymphadenectomy is generally safe and does not add significant morbidity in most cases. The most dreaded complication of extended lymphadenectomy is uncontrolled chyle leak, which can be fatal if uncontrolled but is exceedingly rare.

Postoperative Care and Surveillance

In addition to optimal patient selection and the safe performance of esophageal resection, excellent postoperative care has also contributed to significant improvements in perioperative outcomes in patients who have undergone esophagectomy. Relationships between hospital volume and patient outcomes and between surgeon volume and patient outcomes have been well established. Given the complexity of the perioperative and postoperative care of patients with the disease, esophageal cancer should be managed only in centers specializing in this disease process. The conduct of anesthesia, fluid management, pain control, and early recognition and treatment of possible postoperative complications are all important factors that influence patients' overall outcome.

Nutritional support practices continue to vary among institutions. Although most institutions still employ enteral nutrition via feeding jejunostomy, some institutions allow early feeding by mouth, and others support patients with total parenteral nutrition until enteral feeding is possible. These practices, none of which have been subjected to rigorous randomized study, represent local treatment paradigms rather than the standard of care. Even if the anastomosis heals without complications, it generally takes a few weeks until patients are able to ingest enough calories by mouth to support their needs. Therefore, it is recommended that a feeding jejunostomy be placed to allow enteral nutrition, as it benefits patients in whom anastomotic complications arise or patients who experience delayed gastric emptying or a lack of appetite.

When esophageal cancer patients finally recover from trimodality therapy, the question of how frequently surveillance should be performed arises. Patients often live in fear that the disease will reappear as either locoregional or distant metastatic recurrence. The purpose of periodic surveillance is to identify such recurrence early enough that salvage therapy can be implemented. However, no evidence-based algorithms guiding surveillance in these patients are available. Most providers follow patients every 3–6 months with clinical examination and a variety of imaging and/or endoscopy studies. However, this strategy is often costly, provokes anxiety in patients, and may not ultimately change patient outcomes.

To determine the usefulness of frequent, rigorous surveillance, Sudo et al. retrospectively reviewed the outcomes of a surveillance strategy for patients who had undergone trimodality or bimodality therapy for esophageal cancer. The authors first identified 518 patients who underwent trimodality therapy for esophageal adenocarcinoma [33]. Surveillance was performed every 3 months for the first year, every 6 months for 2 more years, and then annually thereafter. Computed tomography or positron emission tomography–computed tomography was performed at each follow-up visit, and endoscopy with esophageal biopsy was performed every 6 months for the first 18 months and annually thereafter. As expected, the rate of distal recurrence (36 %) was higher than the rate of locoregional recurrence (5 %). Salvage chemoradiation or surgery was used in a very select group of patients with local recurrence. The median overall survival duration of patients who had local recurrence following trimodality therapy was 17 months, and only ten of these patients lived more than 2 years. Overall, rigorous surveillance benefitted only 2 % of the 518 patients, and the authors concluded that surveillance after trimodality therapy is unlikely to result in additional salvaged lives [33].

Sudo et al. then reviewed the outcomes of the surveillance and salvage treatment of 276 patients who underwent bimodality therapy for either esophageal adenocarcinoma or SCC. Contrary to the salvage therapy findings in patients who had trimodality therapy, 36 % of the patients who had locoregional recurrence after bimodality therapy—approximately 8 % of all patients—benefited from similarly frequent and rigorous surveillance. The median overall survival duration of the patients who underwent salvage surgery was an impressive 58.6 months, substantially higher than that of the patients who were unable to undergo salvage surgery (9.5 months). Considering the fact that the vast majority of local recurrences (>98 %) occurred in the first 36 months, the authors recommended that esophageal cancer patients undergoing bimodality therapy should receive vigilant surveillance during this period to potentially catch recurrences early enough to render salvage surgery feasible [34].

Conclusion

Much about our understanding of esophageal carcinoma has changed in the century since Torek performed the first successful esophagectomy for the disease. The etiology shifted from one of squamous cell histology to one of adenocarcinoma. Surgery improved from having nearly universal perioperative mortality to being relatively safe and requiring only a 1-week hospital stay. Early esophageal carcinoma is now managed with organ-sparing techniques, and multimodality therapy, offering survival outcomes that are better than those achieved with surgery alone, has become the standard of care for locally advanced disease. However, despite this exceptional progress, esophageal carcinoma continues to be a highly lethal malignancy. Further advancements will require novel therapies that target the cancer's biology and/or microenvironment. Immunotherapy or novel targeted therapies may improve upon the benefits of surgery, chemotherapy, and radiation in the management of advanced esophageal carcinoma. Surgeons who take on the challenge of treating patients with esophageal cancer should possess not only excellent technical operative skills but also a thorough knowledge of multimodality therapy and nuances in overall perioperative and long-term patient management.

References

1. Ravitch MM. Carcinoma of the breast: the place of the Halsted radical mastectomy. Johns Hopkins Med J. 1971;129(4):202–11.
2. Dubecz A, Schwartz SI. Franz John A. Torek. Ann Thorac Surg. 2008;85(4):1497–9.
3. Orringer MB. Transhiatal esophagectomy without thoracotomy for carcinoma of the thoracic esophagus. Ann Surg. 1984;200(3):282–8.
4. Peterson BE, Chissov VI, Mamontov AS, Pavlov IN. One-stage resection of the cardia and esophagus with delayed extracavitary neck anastomosis in cancer. Khirurgiia (Mosk). 1982;(5):29–32. Russian.
5. Altorki NK, Skinner DB. En bloc esophagectomy: the first 100 patients. Hepatogastroenterology. 1990;37(4):360–3.
6. Luketich JD, Alvelo-Rivera M, Buenaventura PO, Christie NA, McCaughan JS, Litle VR, Schauer PR, Close JM, Fernando HC. Minimally invasive esophagectomy: outcomes in 222 patients. Ann Surg. 2003;238(4):486–94.
7. Park SY, Kim DJ, Yu WS, Jung HS. Robot-assisted thoracoscopic esophagectomy with extensive mediastinal lymphadenectomy: experience with 114 consecutive patients with intrathoracic esophageal cancer. Dis Esophagus. 2015. doi:10.1111/dote.12335.
8. Mathisen DJ, Grillo HC, Wilkins Jr EW, Moncure AC, Hilgenberg AD. Transthoracic esophagectomy: a safe approach to carcinoma of the esophagus. Ann Thorac Surg. 1988;45(2):137–43.
9. Peyre CG, DeMeester TR. Vagal-sparing esophagectomy. Adv Surg. 2008;42:109–16.
10. Jobe BA, Reavis KM, Davis JJ, Hunter JG. Laparoscopic inversion esophagectomy: simplifying a daunting operation. Dis Esophagus. 2004;17(1):95–7.
11. Martin JT, Mahan A, Zwischenberger JB, McGrath PC, Tzeng CW. Should gastric cardia cancers be treated with esophagectomy or total gastrectomy? A comprehensive analysis of 4,996 NSQIP/SEER patients. J Am Coll Surg. 2015;220(4):510–20.
12. Baba M, Aikou T, Yoshinaka H, Natsugoe S, Fukumoto T, Shimazu H, Akazawa K. Long-term results of subtotal esophagectomy with three-field lymphadenectomy for carcinoma of the thoracic esophagus. Ann Surg. 1994;219(3):310–6.

13. Gillies RS, Simpkin A, Sgromo B, Marshall RE, Maynard ND. Left thoracoabdominal esophagectomy: results from a single specialist center. Dis Esophagus. 2011;24(3):138–44.
14. Rutegård M, Lagergren P, Johar A, Lagergren J. Time shift in early postoperative mortality after oesophagectomy for cancer. Ann Surg Oncol. 2015;22(9):3144–9.
15. van Hagen P, Hulshof MC, van Lanschot JJ, Steyerberg EW, van Berge Henegouwen MI, Wijnhoven BP, Richel DJ, Nieuwenhuijzen GA, Hospers GA, Bonenkamp JJ, Cuesta MA, Blaisse RJ, Busch OR, ten Kate FJ, Creemers GJ, Punt CJ, Plukker JT, Verheul HM, Spillenaar Bilgen EJ, van Dekken H, van der Sangen MJ, Rozema T, Biermann K, Beukema JC, Piet AH, van Rij CM, Reinders JG, Tilanus HW, van der Gaast A, CROSS Group. Preoperative chemoradiotherapy for esophageal or junctional cancer. N Engl J Med. 2012;366(22): 2074–84. doi:10.1056/NEJMoa1112088.
16. Arnott SJ, Duncan W, Gignoux M, Girling DJ, Hansen HS, Launois B, Nygaard K, Parmar MK, Roussel A, Spiliopoulos G, Stewart LA, Tierney JF, Mei W, Rugang Z. Preoperative radiotherapy in esophageal carcinoma: a meta-analysis using individual patient data (Oesophageal Cancer Collaborative Group). Int J Radiat Oncol Biol Phys. 1998;41: 579–83.
17. Teniere P, Hay JM, Fingerhut A, Fagniez PL. Postoperative radiation therapy does not increase survival after curative resection for squamous cell carcinoma of the middle and lower esophagus as shown by a multicenter controlled trial. Surg Gyn Obstet. 1991;173:123–30.
18. Francis AM, Sepesi B, Correa AM, Blum MA, Erasmus JJ, Lee JH, Maru DM, Mehran RJ, Rice DC, Roth JA, Vaporciyan AA, Walsh GL, Welsh JW, Swisher SG, Hofstetter WL, University of Texas MD Anderson Esophageal Cancer Group. The influence of histopathologic tumor viability on long-term survival and recurrence rates following neoadjuvant therapy for esophageal adenocarcinoma. Ann Surg. 2013;258(3):500–7.
19. Roth JA, Pass HI, Flanagan MM, Graeber GM, Rosenberg JC, Steinberg S. Randomized clinical trial of preoperative and postoperative adjuvant chemotherapy with cisplatin, vindesine, and bleomycin for carcinoma of the esophagus. J Thorac Cardiovasc Surg. 1988;96: 242–8.
20. Kelsen DP, Winter KA, Gunderson LI, Mortimer J, Norman CE, Haller DG, Ajani JA, Kocka W, Minsky BD, Roth JA, Willett CG. Long-term results of RTOG trial 8911 (USA intergroup 113): a random assignment trial comparison of chemotherapy followed by surgery compared with surgery alone for esophageal cancer. J Clin Oncol. 2007;25:3719–25.
21. Medical Research Council Oesophageal Cancer Working Party. Surgical resection with or without preoperative chemotherapy in oesophageal cancer: a randomized controlled trial. Lancet. 2002;359:1727–33.
22. Cunningham D, Allum WH, Stenning SP, Thompson JN, Van De Velde CJH, Nicholson M, Scarffe H, Lofts FJ, Falk SJ, Iveson TJ, Smith DB, Langley RE, Verma M, Weeden S, Chua YJ. Perioperative chemotherapy versus surgery alone for resectable gastroesophageal cancer. N Engl J Med. 2006;355:11–20.
23. Stahl M, Walz MK, Stuschke M, et al. Phase III comparison of preoperative chemotherapy compared with chemoradiotherapy in patients with locally-advanced adenocarcinoma of the esophagogastric junction. J Clin Oncol. 2009;27:851–6.
24. Burmeister BH, Smithers BM, Gebski V, Fitzgerald L, Simes RJ, Devitt P, Ackland S, Gotley DC, Joseph D, Millar J, North J, Walpole ET, Denham JW, Trans-Tasman Radiation Oncology Group, Australasian Gastro-Intestinal Trials Group. Surgery alone versus chemoradiotherapy followed by surgery for resectable cancer of the oesophagus: a randomised controlled phase III trial. Lancet Oncol. 2005;9:659–68.
25. Kim JY, Correa AM, Vaporciyan AA, Roth JA, Mehran RJ, Walsh GL, Rice DC, Ajani JA, Maru DM, Bhutani MS, Welsh J, Marom EM, Swisher SG, Hofstetter WL. Does the timing of esophagectomy after chemoradiation affect outcome? Ann Thorac Surg. 2012;93(1):207–12.
26. Swisher SG, Winter KA, Komaki RU, Ajani JA, Wu TT, Hofstetter WL, Konski AA, Willett CG. A phase II study of a paclitaxel-based chemoradiation regimen with selective surgical salvage for resectable locoregionally advanced esophageal cancer: initial reporting of RTOG 0246. Int J Radiat Oncol Biol Phys. 2012;82(5):1967–72. doi:10.1016/j.ijrobp.2011.01.043. Epub 2011 Apr 18.

27. Chang AC, Orringer MB. Management of cervical esophagogastric stricture. Semin Thorac Cardiovasc Surg. 2007;19(1):66–71. Review.
28. Sepesi B, Swisher SG, Walsh GL, Correa A, Mehran RJ, Rice D, Roth J, Vaporciyan A, Hofstetter WL. Omental reinforcement of the thoracic esophagogastric anastomosis: an analysis of leak and reintervention rates in patients undergoing planned and salvage esophagectomy. J Thorac Cardiovasc Surg. 2012;144(5):1146–50. doi:10.1016/j.jtcvs.2012.07.085. Epub 2012 Aug 28.
29. Martin LW, Swisher SG, Hofstetter W, Correa AM, Mehran RJ, Rice DC, Vaporciyan AA, Walsh GL, Roth JA. Intrathoracic leaks following esophagectomy are no longer associated with increased mortality. Ann Surg. 2005;242(3):392–9; discussion 399–402.
30. Blackmon SH, Correa AM, Wynn B, Hofstetter WL, Martin LW, Mehran RJ, Rice DC, Swisher SG, Walsh GL, Roth JA, Vaporciyan AA. Propensity-matched analysis of three techniques for intrathoracic esophagogastric anastomosis. Ann Thorac Surg. 2007;83(5):1805–13; discussion 1813.
31. Stiles BM, Mirza F, Port JL, Lee PC, Paul S, Christos P, Altorki NK. Predictors of cervical and recurrent laryngeal lymph node metastases from esophageal cancer. Ann Thorac Surg. 2010;90(6):1805–11.
32. Rizk NP, Ishwaran H, Rice TW, Chen LQ, Schipper PH, Kesler KA, Law S, Lerut TE, Reed CE, Salo JA, Scott WJ, Hofstetter WL, Watson TJ, Allen MS, Rusch VW, Blackstone EH. Optimum lymphadenectomy for esophageal cancer. Ann Surg. 2010;251(1):46–50.
33. Sudo K, Taketa T, Correa AM, Campagna MC, Wadhwa R, Blum MA, Komaki R, Lee JH, Bhutani MS, Weston B, Skinner HD, Maru DM, Rice DC, Swisher SG, Hofstetter WL, Ajani JA. Locoregional failure rate after preoperative chemoradiation of esophageal adenocarcinoma and the outcomes of salvage strategies. J Clin Oncol. 2013;31(34):4306–10. doi:10.1200/JCO.2013.51.7250. Epub 2013 Oct 21.
34. Sudo K, Xiao L, Wadhwa R, Shiozaki H, Elimova E, Taketa T, Blum MA, Lee JH, Bhutani MS, Weston B, Ross WA, Komaki R, Rice DC, Swisher SG, Hofstetter WL, Maru DM, Skinner HD, Ajani JA. Importance of surveillance and success of salvage strategies after definitive chemoradiation in patients with esophageal cancer. J Clin Oncol. 2014;32(30):3400–5. doi:10.1200/JCO.2014.56.7156. Epub 2014 Sept 15.

Radiotherapy in Thymic Tumors

16

Ugur Selek, Yasemin Bolukbasi, Erkan Topkan,
and Ritsuko Komaki

Pathological and Biological Features

The thymus normally has separate lobules, with a sharp distinction between the lymphocyte-rich cortex and the epithelial cell-rich medulla which also contains characteristic Hassall's corpuscles of concentric layers of mature epithelial cells [5]. Thymic neoplasms arising in the anterior mediastinum are rare, but, variations in migration of embryonic endodermal epithelium of the third pharyngeal pouches could account for findings of gross or microscopic thymic tissue anywhere between the hyoid bone and the diaphragm [6]. The thymus, primarily involved in the processing and maturation of lymphocytes to be released into circulation as T lymphocytes, is very small at birth (approximately 15 g), grows to 40–45 g around puberty, and continuously involutes in elderly to an atrophic state.

U. Selek, MD
Department of Radiation Oncology, Koc University, Faculty of Medicine, Istanbul, Turkey

Department of Radiation Oncology, The University of Texas, MD Anderson Cancer Center, Houston, TX, USA

Y. Bolukbasi
Department of Radiation Oncology, Koc University, Faculty of Medicine, Istanbul, Turkey

E. Topkan, MD
Department of Radiation Oncology, Baskent University, Adana, Turkey

R. Komaki, MD (✉)
Division of Radiation Oncology, The University of Texas, MD Anderson Cancer Center, 1515 Holcombe Blvd, B2.4451, Unit 97, Houston, TX, USA
e-mail: rkomaki@mdanderson.org

G. Ozyigit et al. (eds.), *Principles and Practice of Radiotherapy Techniques in Thoracic Malignancies*, DOI 10.1007/978-3-319-28761-4_16

Pathology

The World Health Organization (WHO) histological classification system for thymoma was announced in 1999 [7], and it has been shown to be reproducible for clinically distinct patient groups and have independent prognostic value for clinical management decisions [8]. The subgroups of primary epithelial thymic tumors, types A, AB, B1, B2, B3, and C (thymic carcinoma), are given in Table 16.1, accompanied with common terminology [9]. WHO type A and AB are generally encapsulated and clinically associated with stage I or II disease, whereas other histologies are frequently associated with invasive and disseminated disease (stage III or IV) [8, 10].

Staging

A workup revealing a well-defined anterior mediastinal mass in the thymic bed, with negative tumor markers and absence of continuity with the thyroid, indicates a thymic tumor and mandates multidisciplinary evaluation for tissue diagnosis and resectability (Table 16.2). The most often recommended imaging modality the

Table 16.1 The subgroups of primary epithelial thymic tumors

Epithelial thymoma type	Terminology	Frequency (%)	Composed of
A	Spindle cell; medullary thymoma	9	Few lymphocytes and bland spindle cells
AB	Mixed thymoma	24	Resembling type A plus predominant lymphocytic infiltrate and plump cells
B1	Predominantly cortical; organoid; lymphocytic; lymphocyte-rich thymoma	13	Predominant lymphocytic population and epithelial cells with vesicular and small nucleoli
B2	Cortical thymoma	24	Predominantly lymphocytic thymoma with scattered plump cells with vesicular nuclei
B3	Well-differentiated thymic carcinoma; epithelial; squamoid; atypical thymoma	15	Predominantly polygonal or round epithelial cells with mild atypia
C	Thymic carcinoma	15	Highly atypical cells which do not resemble the thymic organ and lack the immature T-cell lymphocytes: epidermoid keratinizing (squamous cell); epidermoid non-keratinizing; lymphoepithelioma-like; sarcomatoid; clear cell; basaloid; *mucoepidermoid*; papillary; undifferentiated carcinoma

Table 16.2 Workup at initial evaluation

Workup		
Physical examination for adenopathy		
Complete blood count		
Comprehensive blood chemistry (including serum beta-human chorionic gonadotropin and alpha-fetoprotein to rule out germ cell tumors)		
Chest CT with IV contrast detailed based on ITMIG-modified RECIST criteria [11, 15]	Overall tumor burden	Five lesions (two per organ)
	Target lesion measurement plane	Axial
	Target lesion axis to be measured	Long axis (except pleura and lymph nodes)
	Lymph node: measurement plane	Short axis
	Lymph node: minimum size to be included as target lesion	15 mm
	Pleura: measurement plane	Short axis
	Pleura considered as one organ: number of lesions allowed	Unidimensional measurement composed of six lesions: two sites at three different levels
MRI of the chest if pericardial or great vessel invasion		
Pulmonary function tests		
PET-CT, optional		

staging workup is computerized tomography (CT) because it is the most reproducible method to measure lesions at admission and at follow-up for response assessment [11]. A CT-controlled core biopsy is generally the first step to highlight the histology and differential diagnosis, especially between lymphomas, lung cancers, germ cell tumors, and soft tissue sarcomas [4]. A recent meta-analysis of the use of ^{18}F-FDG-PET-CT for predicting WHO grade of malignancy in thymic epithelial tumors (TETs) compared maximum standardized uptake values (SUVmax) in patients with low-risk thymomas (A, AB, B1), high-risk thymomas (B2, B3), and thymic carcinomas (C) and demonstrated a statistically significant difference that could appropriately predict the malignant nature of the different TETs [12]. Tumor size and imaging features on CT were shown to distinguish between stage I–II and III–IV to possibly identify candidates for surgery [13, 14].

As no official and scientifically validated stage classification system has been established for thymic malignancies, the Masaoka system with the modification proposed by Koga et al. was selected by the International Thymic Malignancy Interest Group (ITMIG) to be used until 2017; clinical staging of thymic epithelial tumors is described in Table 16.3 [16–19].

Evidence-Based Treatment Approaches

As the extent of malignancy is generally defined by microscopic or macroscopic invasion of the tumor capsule or surrounding organs, exploration at surgery is critical for establishing the malignant nature of a thymoma. Surgical series emphasize the

Table 16.3 Masaoka system, proposed modification of Koga, and Yamakawa-Masaoka TNM staging [10, 16, 17, 19]

Masaoka's clinical staging [16]			
Stage I: macroscopically completely encapsulated and microscopically no capsular invasion			
Stage II: macroscopic invasion into surrounding fatty tissue or mediastinal pleura or microscopic invasion into capsule			
Stage III: Macroscopic invasion into neighboring organs, i.e., pericardium, great vessels, or the lung			
Stage IVa: pleural or pericardial dissemination			
Stage IVb: lymphogenous or hematogenous metastasis			
Proposed modification of Koga's pathologic tumor extent [10, 17]			
Stage I: grossly and microscopically completely encapsulated			
Stage II: microscopic transcapsular invasion (IIa) or macroscopic invasion into thymic or surrounding fatty tissue or grossly adherent to but not breaking through mediastinal pleura or pericardium (IIb)			
Stage III: macroscopic invasion of neighboring organ (e.g., pericardium, great vessels, or the lung)			
Stage IVa: pleural or pericardial dissemination			
Stage IVb: lymphogenous or hematogenous metastasis			
Yamakawa-Masaoka TNM classification and staging [19]			
T factor			
T1: macroscopically completely encapsulated and microscopically no capsular invasion			
T2: macroscopically adhesion or invasion into surrounding fatty tissue or mediastinal pleura or microscopic invasion into capsule			
T3: invasion into neighboring organs, such as pericardium, great vessels, and the lung			
T4: pleural or pericardial dissemination			
N factor			
N0: no lymph node metastasis			
N1: metastasis to anterior mediastinal lymph nodes			
N2: metastasis to intrathoracic lymph nodes except anterior mediastinal lymph nodes			
N3: metastasis to extrathoracic lymph nodes			
M factor			
M0: mo hematogenous metastasis			
M1: hematogenous metastasis			
TNM stage			
Stage I	T1	N0	M0
Stage II	T2	N0	M0
Stage III	T3	N0	M0
Stage IVa	T4	N0	M0
Stage IVb	Any T	N1, 2, 3	M0
	Any T	Any N	M1

importance of en bloc and total resection of all invaded structures for significant disease-free and overall survival benefits in comparison to partial resection or biopsy alone, and the requirement of radiotherapy if complete resection it cannot be ensured [4, 20, 21]. The ITMIG also underlined the importance of en bloc complete resection in both open and minimally invasive resection procedures and suggests considering all thymomas potentially malignant because even stage I thymomas could recur if not resected according to surgical oncologic principles. Resection must also include the surrounding thymus and fatty tissue (not shelled out) in addition to parietal and visceral metastases in case of invasion into the pleural space [22]. Therefore, the main treatment of early- stage disease is surgery, but unresectable and advanced disease requires a multimodality approach.

The prognosis is directly related to WHO histological classification type, Masaoka clinical stage, and surgical resection status [10, 16, 21, 23–25]. The role of radiotherapy should be considered in light of these factors.

Stage I

A stage I thymoma is understood to have no transcapsular invasion [10]. Masaoka stage I disease with complete resection provides 100 % survival rates at 5 years, and radiotherapy has no role in treatment because of the low likelihood of recurrence [23, 26–28]. The only randomized trial of stage I disease had 29 patients and demonstrated that postoperative radiotherapy (PORT) is not necessary for Masaoka stage I [28]; overall survival rates at 10 years were 92 % for surgery alone and 82 % for PORT. The Surveillance, Epidemiology, and End Results (SEER) registry data from 1973 to 2005 identified 275 Masaoka stage I patients and revealed no benefit from PORT and a possible adverse effect on 5-year cancer-specific survival rates (91 % vs. 98 %, $p=0.03$) [23].

Stage II

A tumor with transcapsular invasion (IIa), or macroscopic invasion into thymic or surrounding fatty tissue, or gross adherence to but not breaking through mediastinal pleura or pericardium (IIb), is designated stage II [10]. Though surgery-alone series with complete R0 resection noted a 98 % survival rate at 5 years, retrospective series have shown supportive [26, 29–31] or contrary [32–35] findings from the use of adjuvant radiotherapy for aggressive tumor histologies or Masaoka stage II disease. In cases of R0 resection with no residual disease on imaging, a multidisciplinary evaluation is necessary to define the risk and need for adjuvant treatment. The most important factors for recommending postoperative adjuvant radiotherapy should be positive surgical margins (R1 or R2 resection) or histological B-C, with high recurrence risk as opposed to R0 resection or and low risk for type A or AB [34, 36].

Stage III–IV

Stage III disease is based on microscopic findings and evidence of macroscopic invasion into neighboring organ, either partially or penetrating (e.g., mediastinal pleura, pericardium, great vessel, or lung) [10]. Any pleural or pericardial tumor nodules separated from the primary tumor denote stage IVa, and involvement and hematogenous metastases denote stage IVb.

Preoperative radiological findings usually predict surgical resectability of thymoma; incomplete resections were found to be associated with ≥50 % abutment of an adjacent vessel and pleural nodularity as well as lobulated tumor contour, thoracic lymphadenopathy, and adjacent lung changes [14]. The length of contact between the tumor contour and the lung has been also considered a prognostic factor for pleural recurrence after surgery alone [37]. In general, locally advanced and bulky disease at preoperative staging justifies a neoadjuvant approach in an attempt to downstage disease before surgery, usually with cisplatin-based chemotherapy or less often with chemoradiotherapy [38, 39]. Locally invasive or unresectable thymoma or thymic carcinoma can be converted to resectable thymoma and thymic carcinoma with neoadjuvant chemotherapy consisting of cyclophosphamide, doxorubicin, cisplatin, and prednisone (CAPP) ×3 cycles, which has improved outcomes in a phase II study [40]. Patients all underwent thymectomy followed by PORT to the tumor bed to 50 Gy in 25 fractions and or to 60 Gy in 30 fractions if the microscopic margin was positive [40].

No consensus has been reached on the role and timing of radiotherapy for locally advanced disease. Kondo and Monden documented outcomes of 1320 patients with TET treated between 1990 and 1994 at 115 institutions and suggested that adjuvant radiotherapy could not effectively prevent local recurrences in Japanese patients with totally resected stage II or III Japanese patients; also, adjuvant radiation or chemotherapy did not improve the prognosis for patients with totally resected stage III–IV thymoma or thymic carcinoma [34]. In contrast, Curran et al. emphasized the importance of adjuvant radiotherapy for totally resected stage II or III disease; revealed mediastinal recurrence as the first site of failure in such cases after complete resection without radiotherapy, in addition to poor salvage; and noted a 5-year actuarial mediastinal relapse rate of 53 % after total resection without adjuvant radiotherapy, 0 % with radiotherapy, and 21 % after subtotal resection/biopsy plus radiotherapy [26]. Urgesi et al., reporting an experience with 59 stage III patients, also encouraged adjuvant radiotherapy [30]. SEER data suggested significant improvement with PORT for patients with Masaoka stage II–III disease, with at 5-year overall survival rates (76 % with PORT vs. 66 % for surgery alone, $p=0.01$) but not in cancer-specific survival at 5 years (91 % vs. 86 %, $p=0.12$); also, no benefit from PORT was found after extirpative surgery (defined as radical or total thymectomy) [23]. The conclusion of that study was that PORT had a possible benefit in overall survival in patients with Masaoka stage II–III disease, especially without R0 surgery. The Japanese Association for Research on the Thymus published their experience with 1110 Masaoka stage II or III thymoma cases and revealed no benefit from PORT on relapse-free or overall survival in these patients [41]. For stage III disease, PORT after even an R0 resection is usually recommended as adjuvant treatment regardless of histological type because the risk of local recurrence is high for this stage [42].

Thymic Carcinoma

Thymic carcinomas, with their aggressive clinical nature and poor prognosis, are distinct from the rest of the TETs [43].

The Japanese Association for Research on the Thymus recently emphasized the importance of PORT in a review of 155 stage II and III thymic carcinoma cases, as it improves relapse-free survival (hazard ratio, 0.48; 95 % confidence interval, 0.30–0.78; $p = 0.003$) but not overall survival, because patients with thymic carcinoma died of distant metastasis [41]. Another study of 1042 cases of thymic carcinoma also underlined the importance of PORT for an overall survival benefit [44]. The European Society of Thoracic Surgeons, reviewing 229 thymic carcinoma cases, found that PORT significantly prolonged overall survival [45]. Multimodality treatment is essential for prolonging survival. Molecular pathology of thymic carcinoma has been well documents; abnormalities of oncogenes and tumor suppressor genes in thymic carcinoma have led to significantly higher expression of EGFR, c-Kit, BCL2, and TP53 relative to thymoma [46]. Based on the clinical patterns of failures and the molecular pathology of thymoma versus thymic carcinoma, thymic carcinoma requires more aggressive systemic treatment, with PORT if the tumor is operable or aggressive chemoradiotherapy if it is not operable.

Target Volume Determination and Delineation Guidelines

The ITMIG initiative on radiation therapy definitions and reporting guidelines for radiation therapy for thymic malignancies has had greatly beneficial effects on documentation and global reproducibility (Table 16.4) [47].

Simulation

The simulation procedure for thymic tumors is similar to that for lung cancer, including the use of comfortable but strict immobilization for supine patients with their arms over their head (moving arms away from any possible beam angles), holding a T-bar if possible, and with the neck slightly extended, supported by a custom-made cushion for stability. The simulation CT images should preferably be in ≤ 3 mm slices; intravenous contrast is favored for better anatomical differentiation. A four-dimensional (4D) CT scan is preferred, if available to appropriately assess breathing-related internal motion during treatment planning [47, 48]; other motion-encompassing options could be slow CT scanning covering the whole breathing cycle or obtaining CT both at inspiratory and expiratory phases to define internal motion [49]. PET-CT can also be a good aid for tumor delineation.

Table 16.4 Short summary of technique-specific coverage and treatment planning details

Tumor GTV	iGTV/GTV to CTV margin	ITV/CTV to PTV margin	Neoadjuvant dose	Adjuvant dose R0	Adjuvant dose R1–2	Definitive dose
The gross disease and any macroscopic invasion into thymic or surrounding fatty tissue or surrounding organs (mediastinal pleura, pericardium, great vessels, lung, etc.) plus any grossly involved lymph nodes (>1 cm or nodes with a necrotic center or PET positive)	0.5–1 cm craniocaudally and circumferentially	No 4DCT/motion management and daily IGRT: 1–1.5 cm	40–64 Gy in 1.8–2.0 Gy/fraction	45–50 Gy in 1.8–2.0 Gy/fraction	54–64 Gy in 1.8–2.0 Gy/fraction	54–70 Gy in 1.8–2.0 Gy/fraction
	Make sure to cover postoperative bed including surgical clips	4DCT/motion management or daily IGRT: 0.5–1 cm				
		Both 4DCT/motion management and daily IGRT: 0.5 cm				

IGRT, image-guided radiation therapy

Gross Tumor Volume

An appropriate GTV should include the gross disease and any macroscopic invasion into thymic or surrounding fatty tissue or surrounding organs (mediastinal pleura, pericardium, great vessels, lung, etc.) plus any grossly involved lymph nodes (nodes that are >1 cm in diameter or have a necrotic center or are positive on PET) which should be delineated on determined from CT, MRI, or PET-CT scans. A joint ITMIG radiologist/radiation oncologist task force is working on a consensus atlas for delineation recommendations but this atlas has yet to be completed.

Internal Target Volume or Internal GTV

The GTV contouring is based on 4D CT data (respiratory data sets are "binned" by phase: 0–100 % at 10 % intervals) in addition to all previously gathered information, and the iGTV is contoured by using the maximum intensity projection (MIP) settings, with modifications based on visual verification of contours in individual respiratory phases.

The GTV can be subdivided into the primary [tumor] site (GTV-P) and involved gross lymph nodes (GTV-N). Thorough contouring of the GTV-P is required based on the exact pattern of spread:

Radial and Local

- Is there mediastinal pleural invasion (T2)?
- Is there pericardium invasion (T3)?
- Is there lung invasion (T3)?
- Is there great vessels/heart invasion (T3)?
- Is there any pleural or pericardial nodule (T4)?

Nodal

- Is there nodal disease in anterior mediastinum (N1)?
- Is there intrathoracic nodal disease aside from anterior mediastinum (N2)?
- Is there extrathoracic nodal disease (N3)?

Clinical Target Volume (CTV)

CTV is delineated as any possible microscopic spread and areas at risk for microscopic spread in addition to the iGTV of the primary tumor and involved nodes, plus the preoperative extent and operative bed if surgery has been done (Figs. 16.1 and 16.2). The previous approach was to cover the whole mediastinum, but the current recommendation, in the era of CT simulation, is to limit the CTV by using preoperative imaging and intraoperative findings and surgical clips. The margin over the iGTV is 0.5–1.0 cm.

Planning Target Volume (PTV)

The PTV includes an extra margin around the CTV to compensate for variability and uncertainties in treatment setup (internal organ motion is handled with 4DCT or alternatives). Margins over the CTV are established in accordance with the

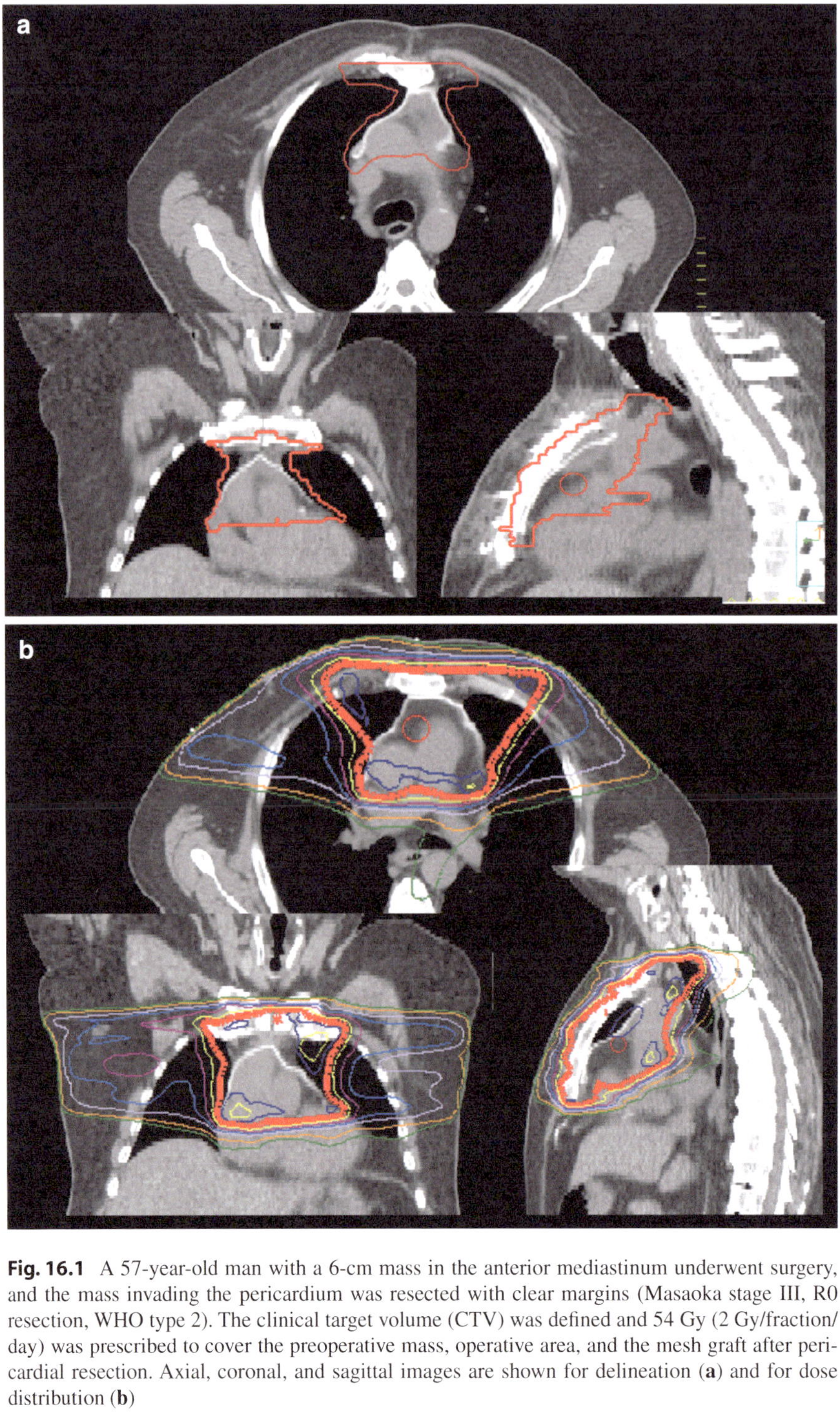

Fig. 16.1 A 57-year-old man with a 6-cm mass in the anterior mediastinum underwent surgery, and the mass invading the pericardium was resected with clear margins (Masaoka stage III, R0 resection, WHO type 2). The clinical target volume (CTV) was defined and 54 Gy (2 Gy/fraction/day) was prescribed to cover the preoperative mass, operative area, and the mesh graft after pericardial resection. Axial, coronal, and sagittal images are shown for delineation (**a**) and for dose distribution (**b**)

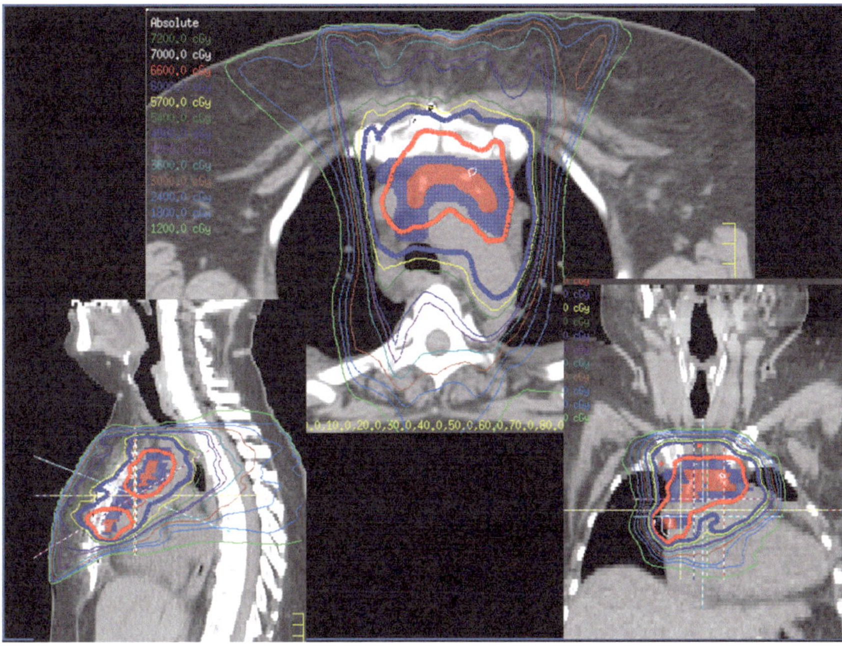

Fig. 16.2 A 59-year-old woman with an invasive mass located in the anterior mediastinum underwent biopsy revealing type B3 thymoma. She underwent four cycles of neoadjuvant chemotherapy (cisplatin, etoposide, ifosfamide) and then surgery with R2 resection. Radiation was prescribed as a simultaneous integrated boost with 59.4 Gy (1.8 Gy/fraction/day) covering the operative bed and 66 Gy (2 Gy/fraction/day) covering the grossly positive surgical margin; axial, coronal, and sagittal images are shown

techniques used for simulation (encompassing internal motion or not), and use of daily image guidance (kV, cone beam CT, etc.). Using advanced modalities could allow some margins to be reduced. If the treating institution has not defined the appropriate magnitude of the PTV, a minimum of 5 mm in all directions should be used for each PTV. Acceptable margins for CTV to PTV are as follows:

- −1.5 cm if without 4D CT or alternative simulation and without daily imaging
- 0.5–1.0 cm if with 4D CT or alternative simulation and without daily imaging
- 0.5 cm if both with 4D CT or alternative simulation and daily imaging

Case Contouring: A Case Example

A 47-year-old woman with a 5-cm mass located in the anterior mediastinum underwent surgery, and the mass invading the pericardium was resected with clear margins (Masaoka stage III disease, R0 resection, WHO type 2). The CTV was defined and 54 Gy (1.8 Gy/fraction/day) was prescribed to cover the preoperative mass and operative area; axial slice-by-slice images used for CTV delineation are shown in Fig. 16.3.

Treatment Planning

No randomized trial data exist to support the choice of radiotherapy doses for thymoma and thymic carcinoma but a general consensus comes from the studies shown in Table 16.5 [42, 47]. Kundel et al. reported that PORT to doses above 45 Gy improved disease-free and overall survival in their patients with invasive stage II thymoma [50]. Zhu et al. pointed out the prognostic importance of doses above 50 Gy for 5-year overall survival for patients with unresectable disease [51], and Fuller et al. underlined the significance of doses above 60 Gy for unresectable or local residual disease [24]. ITMIG guidelines outline the minimum postoperative adjuvant dose for patients with R0 resection for thymoma should be 40 Gy, in

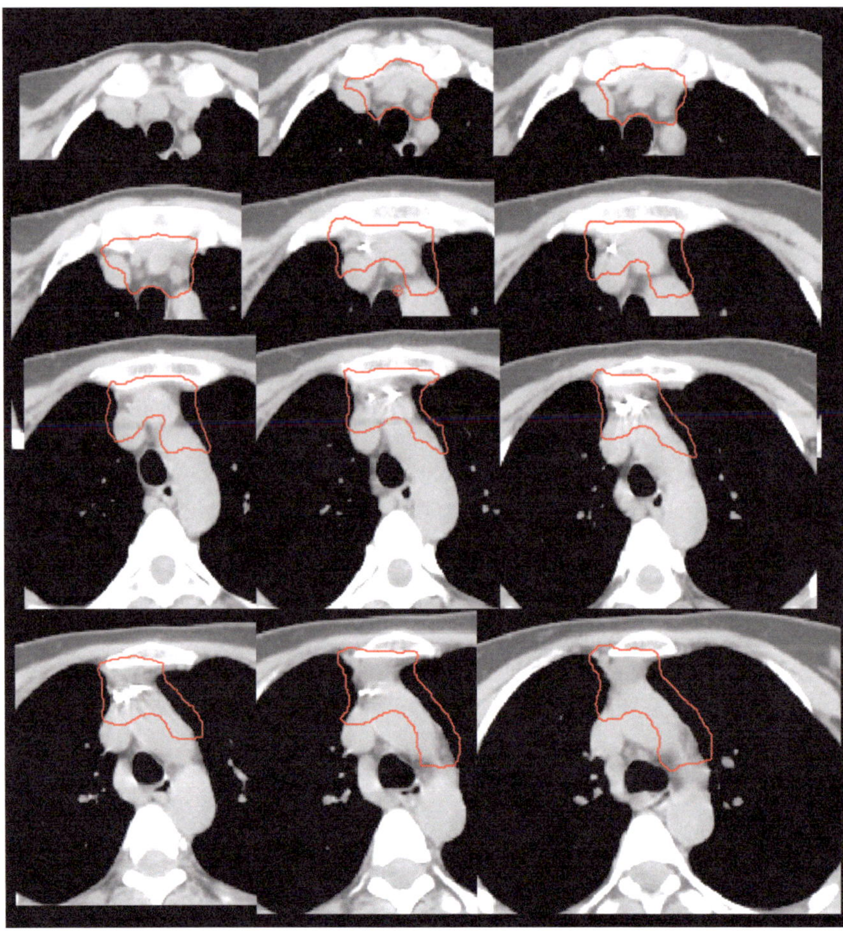

Fig. 16.3 A 47-year-old woman with a 5-cm mass located in the anterior mediastinum underwent surgery, and the mass invading the pericardium was resected with clear margins (Masaoka stage III, R0 resection, WHO type 2). The CTV was delineated and 54 Gy (1.8 Gy/fraction/day) prescribed to cover the preoperative mass and operative area. Shown are axial slice-by-slice images of tumor borders

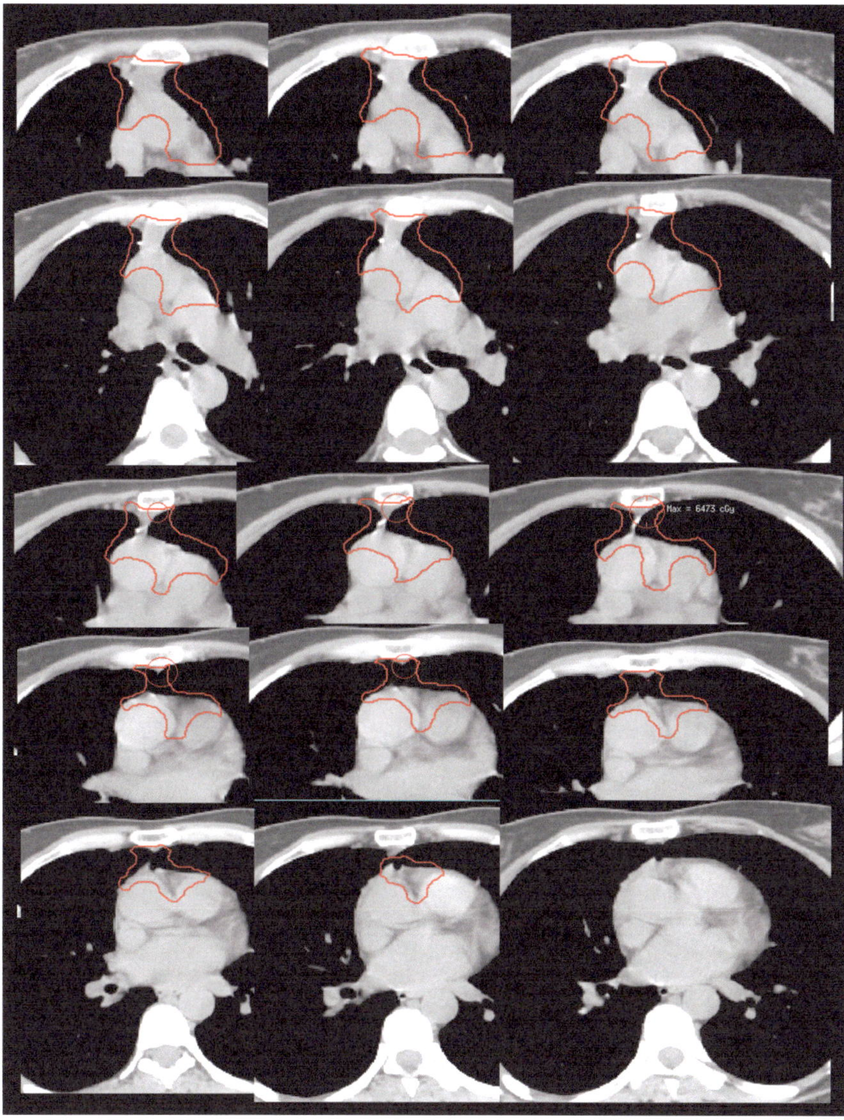

Fig. 16.3 (continued)

1.8–2 Gy fractions; doses below 54 Gy are not recommended for gross residual disease in case of R1/R2 resection; and doses above 64 Gy are not considered appropriate in the postoperative setting [47]. Because patients given PORT for invasive thymoma could live long enough to manifest late effects of cardiac toxicity such as coronary artery disease or myocardial infarcts, PORT needs to be given within dose volume constraints [47]. It is very important to use proton treatment – if available – to reduce cardiac dose in cases in which the treatment volume is very large [48] (Fig. 16.4).

Table 16.5 Summary of thymoma trials from different centers

Author, year	Center	#	Dose	5-year local control	5-year disease-free survival	5-year overall survival
Nakahara 1988 [52]	Osaka University	141	Postoperative 30 Gy in 3 weeks to 50 Gy in 6 weeks	–	–	100 %, stage I; 91.5 %, stage II; 87.8 %, stage III; 46.6 %, stage IV
Curran 1988 [26]	Fox Chase Cancer Center	103	Postoperative 32–60 Gy	100 % for R0 stage II and III; 79 % for R1–2 stage II and III	100 %, stage I; 58 %, stage II; 53 %, stage III	67 %, stage I; 86 %, stage II; 69 %, stage III
Urgesi 1990 [30]	University of Torino	77	Postoperative 39.6 and 46 Gy whole mediastinum plus 10–16 Gy boost. Preoperative 30 Gy followed by a postoperative boost of 16–24 Gy	–	–	70.9 %, stage III; 26.3 %, stage IVa
Jackson 1991 [53]	Peter MacCallum Cancer Institute	28	Postoperative 40–50 Gy	61 %	–	53 %
Haniuda 1992 [54, 55]	Shinshu University	70	Postoperative 40–50 Gy	100 %, stage I and stage II p0 with or without RT; 100 %, stage II p1 with RT and 63.6 % without RT	–	74 % for stage II
Pollack 1992 [56]	U. T. M. D. Anderson Cancer Center	36	Postoperative median dose 50 Gy (40–60)	–	4 %, stage I;71 %, stage II; 50 %, stage III; 29 %, stage IVA	74 %, stage I; 71 %,stage II; 50 %, stage III, 29 %, stage IV

Cowen 1995 [57]	10 French centers	149	Preoperative 22–50 Gy; postoperative 30–70 Gy	100 %, stage I; 98 %, stage II;69 %, stage III;59 % stage IVa	59.5 %	–
Mornex,1995 [29]	10 French cancer centers	90	Postoperative 30–70 Gy	66 %, stage III and IV; 84 %, after partial resection vs. 55 % after biopsy	–	51 %
Regnard 1996 [58]	Marie Lannelongue Hospital	307	Postoperative in invasive or metastatic cases	–	55 %, surgery; 59 PORT at 15 years	–
Latz 1997 [33]	University of Heidelberg	43	Postoperative 10–72 Gy	81 % within the radiation field	–	90 %,stage II; 67 %, stage III; 30 %, stage IV
Gripp 1998 [59]	Heinrich-Heine-University	70	Postoperative 45 (20–60) Gy	50 %, surgery; 80 %, PORT for R0	–	–
Myojin 2000 [60]	Massachusetts General Hospital	32	Preoperative 40 Gy; postoperative 45–50 Gy for close resection margins, 54 Gy for R1, and 60 Gy for R2	62.5 %	–	71 %
Mangi 2002 [32]	Massachusetts General Hospital	49 (stage II)	Postoperatively 45.5 (30–61) Gy	–	–	84 %, surgery; 100 %, PORT at 15 years
Kondo 2003 [34]	115 Japanese institutes	1320	Postoperatively 40 Gy	99.1 %, stage I; 95.9 %, stage II; 71.6 %, stage III; 65.7 %, stage IV	–	93 %, total resection; 64 %, subtotal resection; 36 %, inoperable for stage III and IV thymoma
Singhal 2003 [36]	Pennsylvania	70	Postoperatively 45–55 Gy	–	–	91 %

(continued)

Table 16.5 (continued)

Author, year	Center	#	Dose	5-year local control	5-year disease-free survival	5-year overall survival
Eralp 2003 [61]	University of Istanbul, Capa	36	Postoperatively 50.4–60 Gy	–	–	56.9 months, surgery; 106.3 months, PORT
Zhu 2004 [51]	Cancer Hospital of Fudan University	175	Postoperative 50–55 if R0, 60–65 if R1/R2	99.6 %, stage I; 56.4 %, stage II; 42.7 %, stage III; 21.6 %, stage IV	–	96 %, stage I; 77.8 %, stage II; 56.6 %, stage III; 35.6 % stage IV
Kim 2004 [40]	University of Texas, M. D. Anderson Cancer Center	22, trimodality	Postoperative 50 Gy if R0, 60 if R1	–	77 %	20/22 alive at analysis
Mangi 2005 [62]	Massachusetts General Hospital	45	–	–	–	Disease-specific survival at 5 years: 75 %, surgery; 79 %, PORT
Rena 2007 [63]	University of Eastern Piedmont "A. Avogadro"	58 stage II	Postoperative 50 (45–54) Gy	–	94 %	No difference
Utsumi 2009 [64]	Osaka University	324	Postoperative 10–50 Gy	–	92.8 % with RT; 94.4 % without RT. 10 years for patients without RT, Masaoka stage I and II, WHO A, AB, or B1, was 100 %	10 years, 77.3 % stage I, 85 % stage II, 79.9 % stage III, 62.5 % stage IV
Vasiliou 2009 [65]	University of Patras	41	Postoperative 50.7 (39–58) Gy	–	90.5 months, surgery; 43 months, PORT	–

Fernandes 2010	SEER	1334	–	–	–	PORT does not increase the risk of cardiac mortality or secondary malignancy
Forquer 2010 [23]	SEER	901	–	–	–	76 %, PORT; 66 %, surgery alone, Masaoka stage II and III (cancer-specific survival 91 % PORT; 86 %, surgery alone)
Chen 2010 [66]	Tianjin Medical University Cancer Hospital	142	Postoperative 60 (22–60) Gy	–	97.6 %, surgery; 92.3 %, PORT	Disease-specific survival at 5 years: 97.5 %, surgery; 96.4 %, PORT
Chang 2011 [67]	Seoul National University	76	Postoperative 50 Gy (range: 43.2–66 Gy)	The median time to recurrence; 37.4, surgery; 50.6 months, PORT	80 %, surgery; 97.8 %, PORT	–
Berman 2011 [68]	University of Pennsylvania	62	Postoperative 50.4 Gy (range:45–74.6 Gy)	Proportion of recurrences: 8 %, surgery; 0 %, PORT	–	One death occurred in each group, observation, and radiation
Oh 2012 [69]	Samsung Medical Center, Sungkyunkwan University	110, stage I–II	Postoperative 54 (44–60) Gy	–	98.1 %, surgery; 94.5 %, PORT at 10 years	Disease-specific survival: 100 %, surgery; 93.5 %, PORT at 10 years
Weksler 2012 [70]	SEER	476 stage III	Postoperatively	–	–	105 months, surgery; 127 months, PORT
Fan 2013 [71]	–	65 stage III	Postoperative 56 (28–60) Gy	–	–	81.5 %, surgery; 91.7 %, PORT

(continued)

Table 16.5 (continued)

Author, year	Center	#	Dose	5-year local control	5-year disease-free survival	5-year overall survival
Gao 2013 [72]	Chest Hospital of Jiao Tong University, Sixth Hospital of Jiao Tong University	105 type B3	Postoperative 49 (36–66) Gy	–	–	Masaoka stage and adjuvant radiation are prognostic factors for stage III and IV
Yan 2014 [73]	University of Washington Medical Center	40	Postoperative 50.4 (45–55) Gy for stage II; 59.4 (45–70) Gy for stage III	–	–	72.9 %, surgery; 88.4 %, PORT, potential OS benefit in positive margin
Song 2014 [74]	Zhejiang Cancer Hospital	42 type B2	Postoperative 40–60 Gy	–	62.8 %	84.9 %, PORT had no effect in type B2
Rathod 2014 [75]	Tata Memorial Hospital	62	50–60 Gy, radical; 39 Gy, palliative	–	–	90 % at 3 years. Resectable, 94 %; non-resectable, 81 %
Häfner 2015 [76]	Heidelberg University Hospital	41	Postoperative 51.7 (49–60) Gy	–	100 %, WHO A/AB/B1/B2; 63.6 %, B3/C	100 %, stages I + II; 80 %, stage III; 66.7 %, stage IV
Omasa 2015 [41]	32 Japanese institutions	155 thymic carcinoma and 1110 thymoma	–	–	PORT for stage II and III thymic carcinoma: hazard ratio, 0.48; $P=0.003$. PORT for stage II and III thymoma: not significant	For stage II and III thymic carcinoma: hazard ratio, 0.94; 95 %; $P=0.536$. PORT for stage II and III thymoma: not significant
Perri 2015 [77]	Italy	22	Postoperative 50 (range 44–60) Gy	68 %		74 %

PORT postoperative radiotherapy, *RT* radiotherapy, *SEER* the Surveillance, Epidemiology, and End Results registry data, *p0* no adhesion to the mediastinal pleura, *p1* fibrous adhesion to the mediastinal pleura without microscopic invasion, and *p2* microscopic invasion of the mediastinal pleura

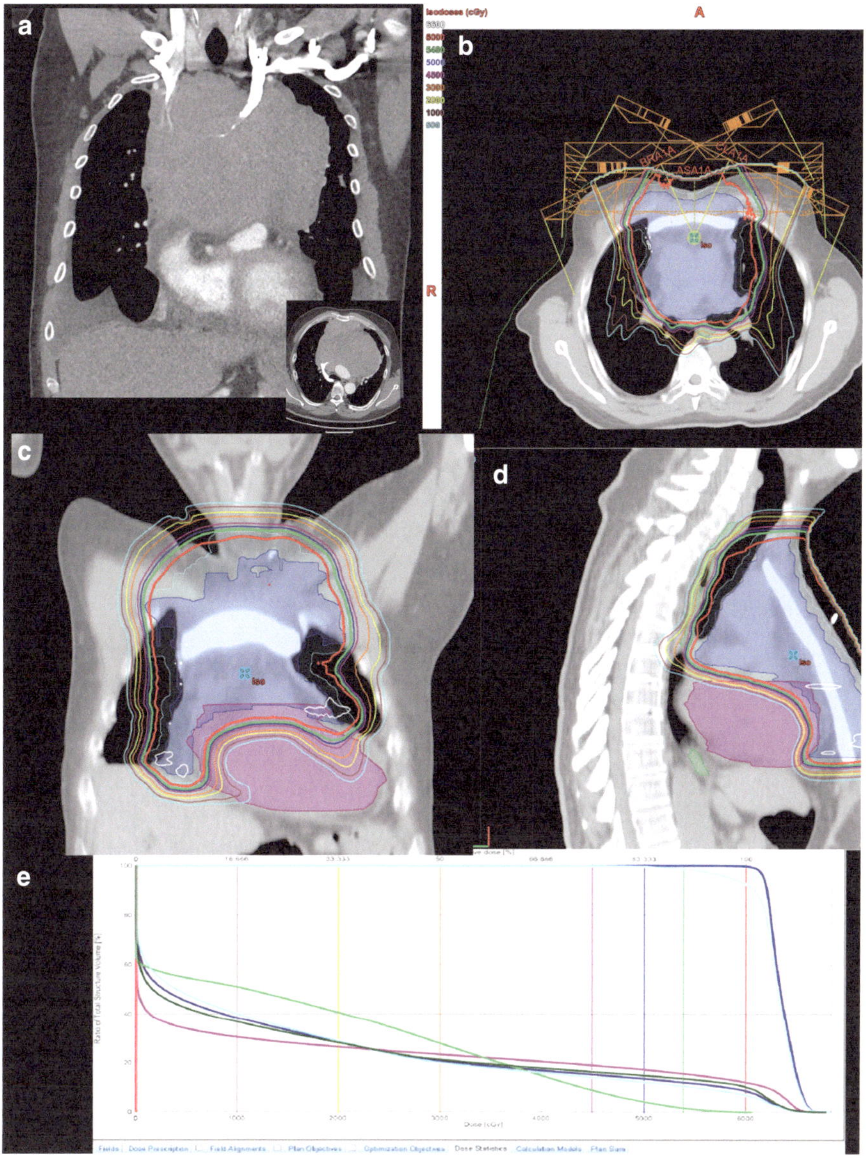

Fig. 16.4 A 51-year-old man with Masaoka stage IVA invasive thymoma. He underwent neoadjuvant chemotherapy consisting of 4 cycles of cyclophosphamide, doxorubicin vincristine, and cisplatin with minimal response. Because the tumor still measured 23 cm, a neoadjuvant radiotherapy approach was not possible, and he underwent second-line chemotherapy with gemcitabine, which he could not tolerate. (**a**) coronal and axial after chemotherapy. He then underwent a very extensive radical thymectomy with reconstruction of the sternum after resection of the medial portion of the 1st through 10th medial ribs bilaterally in addition to removal of the phrenic nerve and pericardium. Because of the positive margins were still evident after surgery, PORT, was prescribed with protons (60 Gy, in 30 fractions of 2 Gy/fraction/day). axial (**b**), coronal (**c**), sagittal (**d**), and dose volume histogram (**e**) images are shown

Guidelines for delineating organs at risk have been standardized in RTOG atlases [78]; normal tissue constraints can be based on quantitative analysis of normal tissue effects in the clinic (QUANTEC) guidelines with normal tissue complication probability models (Table 16.6) [47, 79].

Treatment Planning Assessment

Our institutional standard is to deliver 100 % prescribed dose to the GTV and 95 % of the prescribed dose to the PTV.

- Step 1: Check whether the targets are adequately covered: All plans should be normalized to cover at least 95 % of the volume of PTV by the prescribed isodose surface and 99 % of the PTV needs to be at or above 93 % of the prescribed dose.
- Step 2: Check whether a large hot spot: is present. No more than 20 % of the PTV is at or above 107 % of the prescribed dose, and no more than 5 % of the PTV is at or above 114 % of the prescribed dose.

Table 16.6 Guidelines for normal tissue constraints [47, 79]

Organ	Constraints		
Spinal cord	D_{max} <45 Gy		
	D_{max} <40 Gy if 3 Gy/fraction		
	Even the tumor too close, D_{max} should be <60 Gy		
Lung (total lung GTV; solely total lung for postoperative cases without GTV)	Mean dose < 20 Gy		
	Mean dose < 8 Gy if post-pneumonectomy		
	RT Alone	RT with concurrent chemotherapy	Neoadjuvant treatment before surgery
	V_{20} ≤40 %	V_{20} ≤35 %	V_{20} ≤30 %
		V_{10} ≤45 %	V_{10} ≤40 %
		V_5 ≤65 %	V_5 ≤55 %
	V20 <10 % and V5 <60 % if post-pneumonectomy		
Heart	Mean dose <26 Gy		
	V_{30} ≤45 %		
Esophagus	Mean dose <34 Gy		
	D_{max} ≤80 Gy		
	V_{70} <20 %		
	V_{50} <50 %		
Kidney	20 Gy <32 % of bilateral kidney		
Liver	Mean dose <30 Gy		
	V30 <40 %		

Dmax maximal dose, *GTV* gross tumor volume, *RT* radiotherapy

- Step 3: Check whether the normal tissue constraints are met.
- Step 4: Check whether the placement of the hot/cold spots is correct (slide by slide, by looking at isodose distribution): hot spots need to be located in the GTV.

Recommended Treatment Algorithm for Treatment of Thymoma

The recommended algorithm for the treatment of thymoma is summarized in Table 16.7.

Recommended Algorithm for Follow-Up

The recommended algorithm for follow-up is summarized in Fig. 16.5.

Table 16.7 Recommended treatment algorithm for treatment of thymoma

	Masaoka I		Masaoka II		Masaoka III		Masaoka IV
WHO pathology	R0	R1–2	R0	R1–2	R0	R1–2	R1–2
A, AB, B1	Ø	RT	Ø	RT	RT	RT	CRT
B2, B3, TC	Ø	RT	RT	CRT	RT/CRT	CRT	CRT

R0 complete resection, *R1–R2* microscopic/gross residual disease, *RT* postoperative radiotherapy, *CRT* concurrent or sequential chemotherapy and radiotherapy

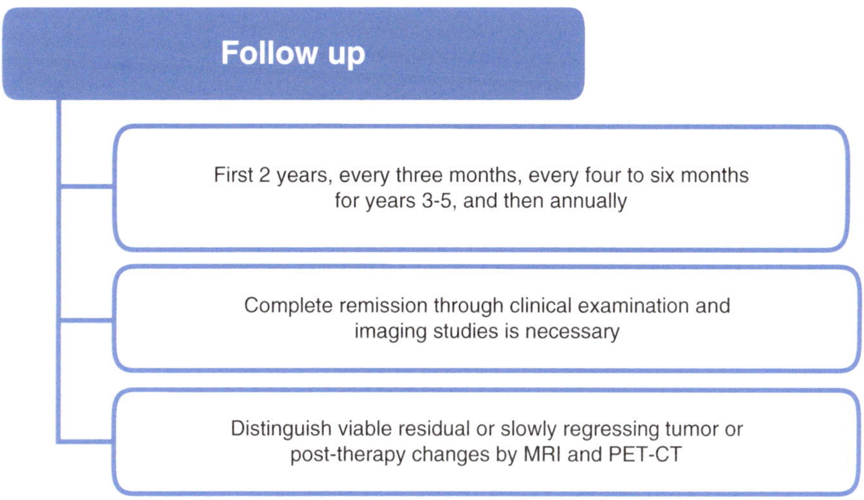

Fig. 16.5 Recommended algorithm for follow-up

References

1. Lewis JE, Wick MR, Scheithauer BW, Bernatz PE, Taylor WF. Thymoma. A clinicopathologic review. Cancer. 1987;60(11):2727–43.
2. Safieddine N, Liu G, Cuningham K, Ming T, Hwang D, Brade A, Bezjak A, Fischer S, Xu W, Azad S, et al. Prognostic factors for cure, recurrence and long-term survival after surgical resection of thymoma. J Thorac Oncol. 2014;9(7):1018–22.
3. Muller-Hermelink HK, Marx A, Geuder K, Kirchner T. The pathological basis of thymoma-associated myasthenia gravis. Ann N Y Acad Sci. 1993;681:56–65.
4. Detterbeck FC, Parsons AM. Thymic tumors. Ann Thorac Surg. 2004;77(5):1860–9.
5. Marino M, Muller-Hermelink HK. Thymoma and thymic carcinoma. Relation of thymoma epithelial cells to the cortical and medullary differentiation of thymus. Virchows Arch A Pathol Anat Histopathol. 1985;407(2):119–49.
6. Jaretzki 3rd A, Wolff M. "Maximal" thymectomy for myasthenia gravis. Surgical anatomy and operative technique. J Thorac Cardiovasc Surg. 1988;96(5):711–6.
7. Rosai J, Sabin LH. Histological typing of tumors of the thymus. Berlin: Springer; 1999.
8. Detterbeck FC. Clinical value of the WHO classification system of thymoma. Ann Thorac Surg. 2006;81(6):2328–34.
9. Travis WD, Brambilla E, Muller-Hermelink HK, Harris CC. Pathology & genetics: tumours of the lung, pleura, thymus and heart. In: World Health Organization Classification of Tumours edn. Lyon: IARC Press; 2004.
10. Detterbeck FC, Nicholson AG, Kondo K, Van Schil P, Moran C. The Masaoka-Koga stage classification for thymic malignancies: clarification and definition of terms. J Thorac Oncol: 2011;6(7 Suppl 3):S1710–6.
11. Benveniste MF, Korst RJ, Rajan A, Detterbeck FC, Marom EM. A practical guide from the International Thymic Malignancy Interest Group (ITMIG) regarding the radiographic assessment of treatment response of thymic epithelial tumors using modified RECIST criteria. J Thorac Oncol. 2014;9(9 Suppl 2):S119–24.
12. Treglia G, Sadeghi R, Giovanella L, Cafarotti S, Filosso P, Lococo F. Is (18)F-FDG PET useful in predicting the WHO grade of malignancy in thymic epithelial tumors? A meta-analysis. Lung Cancer. 2014;86(1):5–13.
13. Marom EM, Milito MA, Moran CA, Liu P, Correa AM, Kim ES, Komaki R, Erasmus JJ, Hofstetter WL, Rice DC, et al. Computed tomography findings predicting invasiveness of thymoma. J Thorac Oncol. 2011;6(7):1274–81.
14. Hayes SA, Huang J, Plodkowski AJ, Katzen J, Zheng J, Moskowitz CS, Ginsberg MS. Preoperative computed tomography findings predict surgical resectability of thymoma. J Thorac Oncol. 2014;9(7):1023–30.
15. Benveniste MF, Rosado-de-Christenson ML, Sabloff BS, Moran CA, Swisher SG, Marom EM. Role of imaging in the diagnosis, staging, and treatment of thymoma. Radiographics: Rev Publ Radiol Soc N Am Inc. 2011;31(7):1847–61. discussion 1861–1843.
16. Masaoka A, Monden Y, Nakahara K, Tanioka T. Follow-up study of thymomas with special reference to their clinical stages. Cancer. 1981;48(11):2485–92.
17. Koga K, Matsuno Y, Noguchi M, Mukai K, Asamura H, Goya T, Shimosato Y. A review of 79 thymomas: modification of staging system and reappraisal of conventional division into invasive and non-invasive thymoma. Pathol Int. 1994;44(5):359–67.
18. Huang J, Detterbeck FC, Wang Z, Loehrer Sr PJ. Standard outcome measures for thymic malignancies. J Thorac Oncol. 2010;5(12):2017–23.
19. Yamakawa Y, Masaoka A, Hashimoto T, Niwa H, Mizuno T, Fujii Y, Nakahara K. A tentative tumor-node-metastasis classification of thymoma. Cancer. 1991;68(9):1984–7.
20. Detterbeck FC, Zeeshan A. Thymoma: current diagnosis and treatment. Chin Med J. 2013;126(11):2186–91.
21. Wright CD. Management of thymomas. Crit Rev Oncol Hematol. 2008;65(2):109–20.
22. Toker A, Sonett J, Zielinski M, Rea F, Tomulescu V, Detterbeck FC. Standard terms, definitions, and policies for minimally invasive resection of thymoma. J Thorac Oncol. 2011;6 (7 Suppl 3):S1739–42.

23. Forquer JA, Rong N, Fakiris AJ, Loehrer Sr PJ, Johnstone PA. Postoperative radiotherapy after surgical resection of thymoma: differing roles in localized and regional disease. Int J Radiat Oncol Biol Phys. 2010;76(2):440–5.
24. Fuller CD, Ramahi EH, Aherne N, Eng TY, Thomas Jr CR. Radiotherapy for thymic neoplasms. J Thorac Oncol. 2010;5(10 Suppl 4):S327–35.
25. Kondo K, Yoshizawa K, Tsuyuguchi M, Kimura S, Sumitomo M, Morita J, Miyoshi T, Sakiyama S, Mukai K, Monden Y. WHO histologic classification is a prognostic indicator in thymoma. Ann Thorac Surg. 2004;77(4):1183–8.
26. Curran Jr WJ, Kornstein MJ, Brooks JJ, Turrisi 3rd AT. Invasive thymoma: the role of mediastinal irradiation following complete or incomplete surgical resection. J Clin Oncol. 1988;6(11):1722–7.
27. Maggi G, Casadio C, Cavallo A, Cianci R, Molinatti M, Ruffini E. Thymoma: results of 241 operated cases. Ann Thorac Surg. 1991;51(1):152–6.
28. Zhang H, Lu N, Wang M, Gu X, Zhang D. Postoperative radiotherapy for stage I thymoma: a prospective randomized trial in 29 cases. Chin Med J. 1999;112(2):136–8.
29. Mornex F, Resbeut M, Richaud P, Jung GM, Mirabel X, Marchal C, Lagrange JL, Rambert P, Chaplain G, Nguyen TD. Radiotherapy and chemotherapy for invasive thymomas: a multicentric retrospective review of 90 cases. The FNCLCC trialists. Federation Nationale des Centres de Lutte Contre le Cancer. Int J Radiat Oncol Biol Phys. 1995;32(3):651–9.
30. Urgesi A, Monetti U, Rossi G, Ricardi U, Casadio C. Role of radiation therapy in locally advanced thymoma. Radiother Oncol. 1990;19(3):273–80.
31. Ogawa K, Uno T, Toita T, Onishi H, Yoshida H, Kakinohana Y, Adachi G, Itami J, Ito H, Murayama S. Postoperative radiotherapy for patients with completely resected thymoma: a multi-institutional, retrospective review of 103 patients. Cancer. 2002;94(5):1405–13.
32. Mangi AA, Wright CD, Allan JS, Wain JC, Donahue DM, Grillo HC, Mathisen DJ. Adjuvant radiation therapy for stage II thymoma. Ann Thorac Surg. 2002;74(4):1033–7.
33. Latz D, Schraube P, Oppitz U, Kugler C, Manegold C, Flentje M, Wannenmacher MF. Invasive thymoma: treatment with postoperative radiation therapy. Radiology. 1997;204(3):859–64.
34. Kondo K, Monden Y. Therapy for thymic epithelial tumors: a clinical study of 1,320 patients from Japan. Ann Thorac Surg. 2003;76(3):878–84. discussion 884–875.
35. Chen YD, Feng QF, Lu HZ, Mao YS, Zhou ZM, Ou GF, Wang M, Zhao J, Zhang HX, Xiao ZF, et al. Role of adjuvant radiotherapy for stage II thymoma after complete tumor resection. Int J Radiat Oncol Biol Phys. 2010;78(5):1400–6.
36. Singhal S, Shrager JB, Rosenthal DI, LiVolsi VA, Kaiser LR. Comparison of stages I-II thymoma treated by complete resection with or without adjuvant radiation. Ann Thorac Surg. 2003;76(5):1635–41. discussion 1641–1632.
37. Kato T, Iwano S, Taniguchi T, Kawaguchi K, Fukui T, Ishiguro F, Fukumoto K, Nakamura S, Hirakawa A, Yokoi K. The contact length between the tumor contour and the lung on computed tomography is a risk factor for pleural recurrence after complete resection of thymoma. Gen Thorac Cardiovasc Surg. 2015;63(6):343–8.
38. Spaggiari L, Casiraghi M, Guarize J. Multidisciplinary treatment of malignant thymoma. Curr Opin Oncol. 2012;24(2):117–22.
39. Wright CD, Choi NC, Wain JC, Mathisen DJ, Lynch TJ, Fidias P. Induction chemoradiotherapy followed by resection for locally advanced Masaoka stage III and IVA thymic tumors. Ann Thorac Surg. 2008;85(2):385–9.
40. Kim ES, Putnam JB, Komaki R, Walsh GL, Ro JY, Shin HJ, Truong M, Moon H, Swisher SG, Fossella FV, et al. Phase II study of a multidisciplinary approach with induction chemotherapy, followed by surgical resection, radiation therapy, and consolidation chemotherapy for unresectable malignant thymomas: final report. Lung Cancer. 2004;44(3):369–79.
41. Omasa M, Date H, Sozu T, Sato T, Nagai K, Yokoi K, Okamoto T, Ikeda N, Tanaka F, Maniwa Y. Postoperative radiotherapy is effective for thymic carcinoma but not for thymoma in stage II and III thymic epithelial tumors: the Japanese Association for Research on the Thymus Database Study. Cancer. 2015;121(7):1008–16.
42. Komaki R, Gomez DR. Radiotherapy for thymic carcinoma: adjuvant, inductive, and definitive. Front Oncol. 2014;3:330.

43. Suster S, Rosai J. Thymic carcinoma. A clinicopathologic study of 60 cases. Cancer. 1991;67(4):1025–32.
44. Ahmad U, Yao X, Detterbeck F, Huang J, Antonicelli A, Filosso PL, Ruffini E, Travis W, Jones DR, Zhan Y, et al. Thymic carcinoma outcomes and prognosis: results of an international analysis. J Thorac Cardiovasc Surg. 2015;149(1):95–100. 101 e101-102.
45. Ruffini E, Detterbeck F, Van Raemdonck D, Rocco G, Thomas P, Weder W, Brunelli A, Guerrera F, Keshavjee S, Altorki N, et al. Thymic carcinoma: a cohort study of patients from the European society of thoracic surgeons database. J Thorac Oncol. 2014;9(4):541–8.
46. Kuhn E, Wistuba II. Molecular pathology of thymic epithelial neoplasms. Hematol Oncol Clin N Am. 2008;22(3):443–55.
47. Gomez D, Komaki R, Yu J, Ikushima H, Bezjak A. Radiation therapy definitions and reporting guidelines for thymic malignancies. J Thorac Oncol. 2011;6(7 Suppl 3):S1743–8.
48. Gomez D, Komaki R. Technical advances of radiation therapy for thymic malignancies. J Thorac Oncol. 2010;5(10 Suppl 4):S336–43.
49. Keall PJ, Mageras GS, Balter JM, Emery RS, Forster KM, Jiang SB, Kapatoes JM, Low DA, Murphy MJ, Murray BR, et al. The management of respiratory motion in radiation oncology report of AAPM Task Group 76. Med Phys. 2006;33(10):3874–900.
50. Kundel Y, Yellin A, Popovtzer A, Pfeffer R, Symon Z, Simansky DA, Oberman B, Sadezki S, Brenner B, Catane R, et al. Adjuvant radiotherapy for thymic epithelial tumor: treatment results and prognostic factors. Am J Clin Oncol. 2007;30(4):389–94.
51. Zhu G, He S, Fu X, Jiang G, Liu T. Radiotherapy and prognostic factors for thymoma: a retrospective study of 175 patients. Int J Radiat Oncol Biol Phys. 2004;60(4):1113–9.
52. Nakahara K, Ohno K, Hashimoto J, Maeda H, Miyoshi S, Sakurai M, Monden Y, Kawashima Y. Thymoma: results with complete resection and adjuvant postoperative irradiation in 141 consecutive patients. J Thorac Cardiovasc Surg. 1988;95(6):1041–7.
53. Jackson MA, Ball DL. Post-operative radiotherapy in invasive thymoma. Radiother Oncol. 1991;21(2):77–82.
54. Haniuda M, Morimoto M, Nishimura H, Kobayashi O, Yamanda T, Iida F. Adjuvant radiotherapy after complete resection of thymoma. Ann Thorac Surg. 1992;54(2):311–5.
55. Haniuda M, Miyazawa M, Yoshida K, Oguchi M, Sakai F, Izuno I, Sone S. Is postoperative radiotherapy for thymoma effective? Ann Surg. 1996;224(2):219–24.
56. Pollack A, Komaki R, Cox JD, Ro JY, Oswald MJ, Shin DM, Putnam Jr JB. Thymoma: treatment and prognosis. Int J Radiat Oncol Biol Phys. 1992;23(5):1037–43.
57. Cowen D, Richaud P, Mornex F, Bachelot T, Jung GM, Mirabel X, Marchal C, Lagrange JL, Rambert P, Chaplain G, et al. Thymoma: results of a multicentric retrospective series of 149 non-metastatic irradiated patients and review of the literature. FNCLCC trialists. Federation Nationale des Centres de Lutte Contre le Cancer. Radiother Oncol. 1995;34(1):9–16.
58. Regnard JF, Magdeleinat P, Dromer C, Dulmet E, de Montpreville V, Levi JF, Levasseur P. Prognostic factors and long-term results after thymoma resection: a series of 307 patients. J Thorac Cardiovasc Surg. 1996;112(2):376–84.
59. Gripp S, Hilgers K, Wurm R, Schmitt G. Thymoma: prognostic factors and treatment outcomes. Cancer. 1998;83(8):1495–503.
60. Myojin M, Choi NC, Wright CD, Wain JC, Harris N, Hug EB, Mathisen DJ, Lynch T, Carey RW, Grossbard M, et al. Stage III thymoma: pattern of failure after surgery and postoperative radiotherapy and its implication for future study. Int J Radiat Oncol Biol Phys. 2000;46(4):927–33.
61. Eralp Y, Aydiner A, Kizir A, Kaytan E, Oral EN, Topuz E. Resectable thymoma: treatment outcome and prognostic factors in the late adolescent and adult age group. Cancer Investig. 2003;21(5):737–43.
62. Mangi AA, Wain JC, Donahue DM, Grillo HC, Mathisen DJ, Wright CD. Adjuvant radiation of stage III thymoma: is it necessary? Ann Thorac Surg. 2005;79(6):1834–9.
63. Rena O, Papalia E, Oliaro A, Ruffini E, Filosso P, Novero D, Maggi G, Casadio C. Does adjuvant radiation therapy improve disease-free survival in completely resected Masaoka stage II thymoma? Eur J Cardio-Thorac Surg. 2007;31(1):109–13.

64. Utsumi T, Shiono H, Kadota Y, Matsumura A, Maeda H, Ohta M, Yoshioka Y, Koizumi M, Inoue T, Okumura M. Postoperative radiation therapy after complete resection of thymoma has little impact on survival. Cancer. 2009;115(23):5413–20.
65. Vassiliou V, Tsamandas A, Katodritis N, Charoulis N, Koukouma A, Andreopoulos D, Salakou S, Zolota V, Papathanassopoulos P, Christodoulides G, et al. The role of postoperative radiotherapy in the management of patients with thymic tumors – a retrospective study. In Vivo. 2009;23(5):843–52.
66. Chen J, Wang P. Assessment of multimodality therapy for thymoma. Chin Med J. 2010; 123(10):1295–8.
67. Chang JH, Kim HJ, Wu HG, Kim JH, Kim YT. Postoperative radiotherapy for completely resected stage II or III thymoma. J Thorac Oncol. 2011;6(7):1282–6.
68. Berman AT, Litzky L, Livolsi V, Singhal S, Kucharczuk JC, Cooper JD, Friedberg JR, Evans TL, Stevenson JP, Metz JM, et al. Adjuvant radiotherapy for completely resected stage 2 thymoma. Cancer. 2011;117(15):3502–8.
69. Oh D, Ahn YC, Kim K, Kim J, Shim YM, Han J. Is there a role of postoperative radiation therapy in completely resected stage I/II thymic epithelial tumor? Cancer Res Treat. 2012;44(3):166–72.
70. Weksler B, Shende M, Nason KS, Gallagher A, Ferson PF, Pennathur A. The role of adjuvant radiation therapy for resected stage III thymoma: a population-based study. Ann Thorac Surg. 2012;93(6):1822–8. discussion 1828–1829.
71. Fan C, Feng Q, Chen Y, Zhai Y, Zhou Z, Chen D, Xiao Z, Zhang H, Li J, Hui Z, et al. Postoperative radiotherapy for completely resected Masaoka stage III thymoma: a retrospective study of 65 cases from a single institution. Radiat Oncol. 2013;8:199.
72. Gao L, Wang C, Fang W, Zhang J, Lv C, Fu S. Outcome of multimodality treatment for 188 cases of type B3 thymoma. J Thorac Oncol. 2013;8(10):1329–34.
73. Yan J, Liu Q, Moseley JN, Baik CS, Chow LQ, Goulart BH, Zlotnick D, Papanicolau-Sengos A, Gallaher I, Knopp JM, et al. Adjuvant radiotherapy for stages II and III resected thymoma: a single-institutional experience. Am J Clin Oncol. 2014.
74. Song Z, Jin X, Zhang Y. Treatment and prognosis of type B2 thymoma. World J Surg Oncol. 2014;12:291.
75. Rathod S, Munshi A, Paul S, Ganesh B, Prabhash K, Agarwal JP. Thymoma: first large Indian experience. Indian J Cancer. 2014;51(2):109–12.
76. Hafner MF, Roeder F, Sterzing F, Krug D, Koerber SA, Kappes J, Hoffmann H, Slynko A, Debus J, Bischof M. Postoperative radiotherapy of patients with thymic epithelial tumors (TET): a retrospective analysis of outcome and toxicity. Strahlenther Onkol. 2015;191(2):133–40.
77. Perri F, Pisconti S, Conson M, Pacelli R, Della Vittoria Scarpati G, Gnoni A, D'Aniello C, Cavaliere C, Licchetta A, Cella L, et al. Adjuvant treatment in patients at high risk of recurrence of thymoma: efficacy and safety of a three-dimensional conformal radiation therapy regimen. OncoTargets Ther. 2015;8:1345–9.
78. http://www.rtog.org/CoreLab/ContouringAtlases/LungAtlas.aspx.
79. Marks LB, Yorke ED, Jackson A, Ten Haken RK, Constine LS, Eisbruch A, Bentzen SM, Nam J, Deasy JO. Use of normal tissue complication probability models in the clinic. Int J Radiat Oncol Biol Phys. 2010;76(3 Suppl):S10–9.

Surgical Staging and Advanced Surgical Techniques in Thymic Cancers

17

Serhan Tanju, Suat Erus, and Sukru Dilege

Introduction

Thymoma and thymic carcinoma are the most frequent anterior mediastinal neoplasms that originates from epithelial tissue of the thymic gland. Histologic classification of thymomas has been under debate for many years until the World Health Organization (WHO) published and updated the histologic classification of thymomas in 1999 and 2004, respectively [1, 2]. In updated version, type C thymomas were classified in to separate type of thymic tumors as thymic carcinomas (Table 17.1). The widely used staging system, Masaoka classification published in 1981 and further refined with little modifications as the Masaoka-Koga staging system in 1994 (Table 17.2), was proved to be a significant factor for survival [3, 4].

Surgery in Thymic Malignancies

The treatment of thymic tumors depends on clinical stage; however, it is widely accepted that surgical resection is the mainstay of treatment [5]. Complete surgical resection which is proved to be one of the most important prognostic factors should be the goal even in advanced stage [6]. Patients with clinical stage III thymoma may require extended surgery to achieve complete resection.

S. Tanju, MD (✉) • S. Dilege, MD
Department of Thoracic Surgery, Faculty of Medicine, Koc University Hospital, Davutpasa Caddesi, No: 4, Topkapi, Istanbul 34010, Turkey
e-mail: stanju@ku.edu.tr; sdilege@gmail.com

S. Erus
Department of Thoracic Surgery, Koc University Hospital, Davutpasa Caddesi, No: 4, Topkapi, Istanbul 34010, Turkey
e-mail: serus@kuh.ku.edu.tr

G. Ozyigit et al. (eds.), *Principles and Practice of Radiotherapy Techniques in Thoracic Malignancies*, DOI 10.1007/978-3-319-28761-4_17

Table 17.1 WHO classification of thymic tumors

Thymoma	Thymic carcinoma	Neuroendocrine tumors
Type A, spindle cell; medullary	Squamous cell, epidermoid keratinizing	Well-differentiated neuroendocrine tumor/ carcinomas, including typical and atypical carcinoids
Type AB, mixed	Epidermoid nonkeratinizing	Poorly differentiated neuroendocrine carcinomas, including large and small cell neuroendocrine carcinoma
Type B1, lymphocyte-rich; lymphocytic; predominantly cortical; organoid	Basaloid	
Type B2 cortical	Lymphoepithelioma-like	
Type B3 epithelial; atypical; squamoid; well-differentiated thymic carcinoma	Mucoepidermoid carcinoma	
Micronodular thymoma	Sarcomatoid	
Metaplastic, sclerosing, microscopic thymoma	Clear cell	
Lipofibroadenoma	Mucoepidermoid	
	Papillary	
	Undifferentiated	
	Combined	

Table 17.2 The Masaoka-Koga staging system

Tumor stage	Description
I	Grossly and microscopically completely encapsulated tumor
II	(a) Microscopic transcapsular invasion
	(b) Macroscopic invasion into the thymic or surrounding fatty tissue or grossly adherent but not breaking through the mediastinal pleura or pericardium
III	Macroscopic invasion of neighboring organs (pericardium, great vessels, or lung)
IV	(a) Pleural or pericardial dissemination
	(b) Lymphatic or hematogenous metastasis

Clinical staging of thymic masses is crucial to determine appropriate treatment. A retrospective study published in 2014 showed that CT imaging had some features that were significantly correlated with the WHO classification, the Masaoka-Koga clinical staging and the completeness of resection; however, authors concluded that CT has no definite role to predict the survival rate of thymoma patients. CT features correlated with the WHO classification were tumor contours, homogeneity, degree of enhancement, fat plane obliteration with adjacent structures, the presence of mediastinal lymphadenopathy, irregular infiltration into the lung, and tumor shape. Lobulated or irregular tumor contours, the presence of calcifications, infiltration of surrounding fat, irregular infiltration into the lung, irregular infiltration into vasculature, more abutment of vessels, and pulmonary changes adjacent to the tumor were associated with the more advanced Masaoka-Koga clinical stage [7].

Thymic type A tumors are more likely to have round shapes and smooth contours on CT images when comparing with other types of thymic epithelial tumors. Besides, thymic carcinomas had a higher prevalence of irregular contours, and calcification was more frequently seen in type B tumors [8]. To predict incomplete resection in patients with thymic tumors preoperatively by CT images is a key point for surgeons. Hayes et al. in 2014, reported on 133 patients underwent surgical resection for thymoma. In this study, lobulated tumor contour ($p=0.016$), ≥ 50 % abutment of the circumference of an adjacent vessel ($p<0.001$), thoracic lymphadenopathy ($p=0.029$), adjacent lung changes ($p=0.005$), and pleural nodularity ($p=0.001$) were found to be significantly correlated with incomplete resection [9].

The recommended treatment option is surgery alone for stage I thymic tumors with a nearly 80 % 10-year survival rate [10]. Median sternotomy (MS) is widely used surgical incision that allows a maximal exposure of the anterior mediastinum to radical surgical removal of the thymoma along with the entire thymus and the mediastinal fat; thus, MS is a gold standard for surgical treatment of thymomas [6]. Moreover, minimally invasive techniques including conventional VATS and robotic-assisted thoracic surgery (RATS) become increasingly popular for anterior mediastinal procedures such as thymectomy in patients with myasthenia gravis and mediastinal mass resection. However, minimally approach to thymoma is still controversial. The main concern is the possibility of damage at the tumor capsule which may increase the risk of spreading tumor cells during the minimally invasive procedure. There are several studies about comparison between open and minimally invasive techniques in early stage thymoma (Table 17.3).

Pennathur et al. reported on a retrospective review of 40 patients who underwent surgical resection of early stage thymoma with open or minimally invasive thymectomy. This study showed that no significant differences were found in the estimated recurrence-free and overall 5-year survival rates (83–100 %) between the two groups [14].

More recently, RATS have been a surgery of choice for mediastinal malignancies. A multicenter study, aimed to evaluate the safety and feasibility of robotic thymectomy with analyzing the oncologic outcomes, was published in 2012. A total of 79 patients who underwent RATS for early stage thymoma was analyzed in terms of perioperative data and oncological outcome. One patient (1.3 %) required conversion to an open approach because of a large diameter tumor interfering with a safe dissection. Ten patients (12.7 %) had postoperative complications. Median hospital stay was 3 days (range, 2–15 days). Median diameter of the resected tumors was 3 cm and 5-year thymoma-related survival was 97 %. The authors concluded that RATS for thymoma was a technically sound and safe procedure with acceptable oncologic outcome [15].

A comparison study of 74 patients between RATS and open approach for early stage thymoma, published in 2014, showed that the duration of surgery and the intraoperative blood loss was significantly less (61.3 ± 21.8 vs. 466.1 ± 91.4) and the postoperative hospital stay significantly shorter days in the RATS group than in the open approach group (3.7 ± 1.1 vs. 11.6 ± 10.4 days) ($p<0.01$). Within the

Table 17.3 Comparison studies between VATS and median sternotomy (VATS vs MS)

Author	n	MG (%)	MBL (ml)	LOD (days)	LHS (days)	C (n)	MS I (n)	MS II (n)	R (n)	Median FU (months)	Study design
Chao et al. (2015) [11]	48 vs 48	26 vs 26	40 ± 66 vs 75 ± 96	4.4 ± 1.5 vs 4.9 ± 1.9	5.8 ± 2 vs 7 ± 2.2	2 vs 6	17 vs 17	31 vs 31	2 vs 3	75.5	R
Maniscalco et al. (2015) [12]	13 vs 14	39 vs 36	NA	NA	2.6 vs 5.4	2 vs 3	8 vs 10	5 vs 4	0	123	R
Jurado et al. (2012) [13]	10 vs 62	NA	7.5 vs 200	NA	4 vs 5	NA	4 vs 16	6 vs 41	0	24.2 vs 81	R
Pennathur et al. (2011) [14]	18 vs 22	40 vs 19	NA	NA	3 vs 5	NA	5 vs 9	13 vs 13	NA	27 vs 58	R

MG myasthenia gravis, *MBL* mean blood loss, *LOD* length of drainage, *LHS* length of hospital stay, *C* complication, *MS I* Masaoka stage I, *MS II* Masaoka stage II, *R* recurrence, *FU* follow-up, *R* retrospective postoperative follow-up period of 16.9 months (range, 1–48 months) in the RATS group and 18.1 months (range, 1–48 months) in the open approach group, no recurrence was observed [16].

RATS seems to be a good alternative for minimally invasive approach in early stage thymoma; however, thymoma requires longer follow-up data, such as more than 5 years, to determine the oncologic outcome of minimally invasive approaches; thus, additional randomized studies with a large number of patients are essential.

In case of clinically locally advance disease at Masaoka stage III, en bloc resection is essential; thus, resectability with tumor-free margins should be evaluated with contrast-enhanced spiral computerized tomography of the chest. If the patients have findings that suggested extensive invasion, large tumors with indistinct borders, or evidence of great vessel invasion, complete resection may not be achieved. In these circumstances, tru-cut biopsy followed by induction chemotherapy or chemoradiotherapy should be considered to increase the chance of complete resection. Along with CT, fluorine-18-fluorodeoxyglucose positron emission tomography (^{18}F-FDG PET) may provide additional data to predict the WHO grade of malignancy [17] and Masaoka stage.

A phase II, multi-institutional clinical trial was conducted in 2014 to determine the response rate, toxicity, and rate of complete resection after induction chemoradiotherapy for locally advanced thymic tumors. In this study, the induction therapy consisted of cisplatin, etoposide, and concurrent radiotherapy $\leq$4,500 cGy. Among 22 patients, a total of ten patients had a partial response, and 11 had stable disease detected with computerized tomography. Of the 21 patients who completed induction therapy, 17 (77 %) underwent an R0 resection, three (14 %) underwent R1 resection, and one (5 %) underwent debulking. The complication and mortality rate were 36 % and 9 %, respectively. No patient had a complete pathologic response, but five specimens (24 %) had <10 % viable tumor [18]. Ruffini et al. [19] reported the results of database developed by European Society of Thoracic Surgeons in 2014. A total of 2,030 patients including 1,798 thymomas, 191 thymic carcinoma (TC), and 41 neuroendocrine thymic tumor (NETT) were analyzed. Recurrence occurred in 141 patients (8 %) among 1,709 patients with complete resection. Authors showed that risk of recurrence increased with stage (IV 40 %) and histology (TC 30 %, NETT 37 %). The probability of an incomplete resection was higher in male patients and increased with tumor size, whereas decreased with the presence of myasthenia gravis. When comparing with A-AB-B1 thymoma, the probability of an incomplete resection is higher in B2-B3 thymoma, TC, and NETT. Five- and 10-year OS and DFS rates were 85 % and 73 % and 84 % and 70 %, respectively.

The role of surgery in stage IV is still controversial; nevertheless, multimodality treatment including surgical resection should be considered as the treatment of choice in patients with stage IV thymic malignancies. There are several studies reported a wide range of survival rates between 0 % and 71 % at 5 years [20–22]. Hamaji reported on a population-based analysis of 282 patients with stage IV thymoma. Among 282 patients, 110 patients underwent surgical resection and 172 were managed nonsurgically. The 5- and 10-year cancer-specific survival (CSS) rates were 78.8 % and 53.8 %, respectively; however, CSS rates were 51.9 % and

35.9 %, respectively, in patients with nonsurgical management. Even though this database did not include detailed data on chemoradiotherapy, multimodality treatment including surgery at stage IV may improve overall survival [23].

Surgery in Recurrent Thymic Malignancies

Recurrence after surgery is another critical issue on the treatment of thymic malignancies. Published guidelines recommend surgery for recurrent thymoma in case of a localized recurrence after apparently successful initial therapy [24, 25]. In one of the largest series published by Kondo et al., recurrence rates for stages I, II, III, and IV were 0.9 %, 4.1 %, 28.4 %, and 34.3 %, respectively [22]. Okumura et al. reported on 67 patients with recurrence after resections for thymic epithelial tumors. Among 67 patients, 27 had re-resection for recurrence. The 10-year survival rate was 70 % for patients who underwent a re-resection and 35 % for those who did not. There was a significant difference between the two groups ($p=0.002$). In addition, study showed that 5-year survival rate after the re-resection was 100 % in patients with type B1 tumors, 56 % in those with type B2 tumors, and 60 % in those with type B3 tumors. Authors concluded that recurrence following resection of type AB and type B1 tumors demonstrated a greater chance of treatment by re-resection surgery [26].

Case 1

A 37-year-old female patient presented with chest pain. Chest computed tomography (CT) revealed anterior mediastinal mass (Fig. 17.1). Tru-cut biopsy of the anterior mediastinal mass revealed the diagnosis as thymoma type B1. The patient underwent anterior mediastinal mass resection with median sternotomy. Histopathologic examination confirmed the diagnosis. The patient was staged as Masaoka-Koga stage I. CT revealed pleuroparenchymal metastatic nodules with

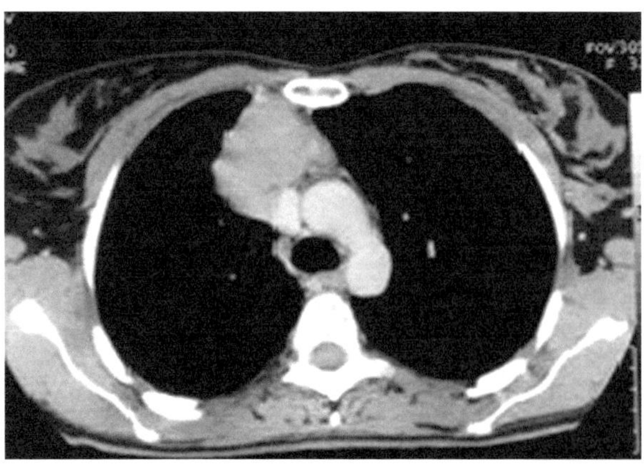

Fig. 17.1 CT revealed anterior mediastinal mass

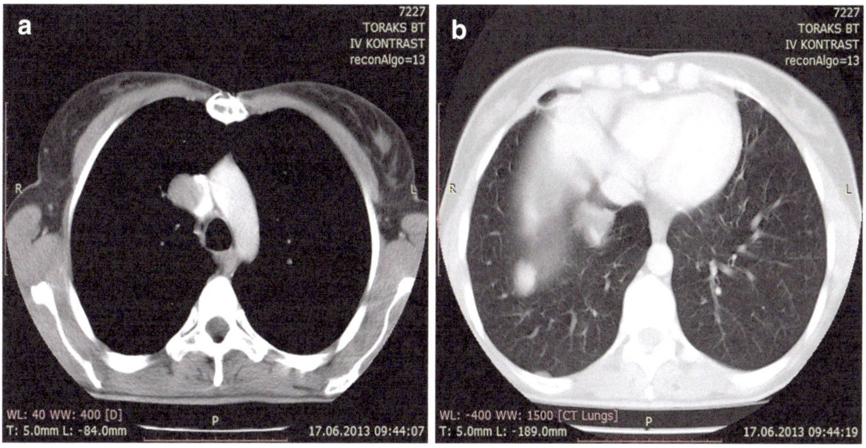

Fig. 17.2 (**a**, **b**) Pleuroparenchymal metastatic nodules with superior vena cava invasion

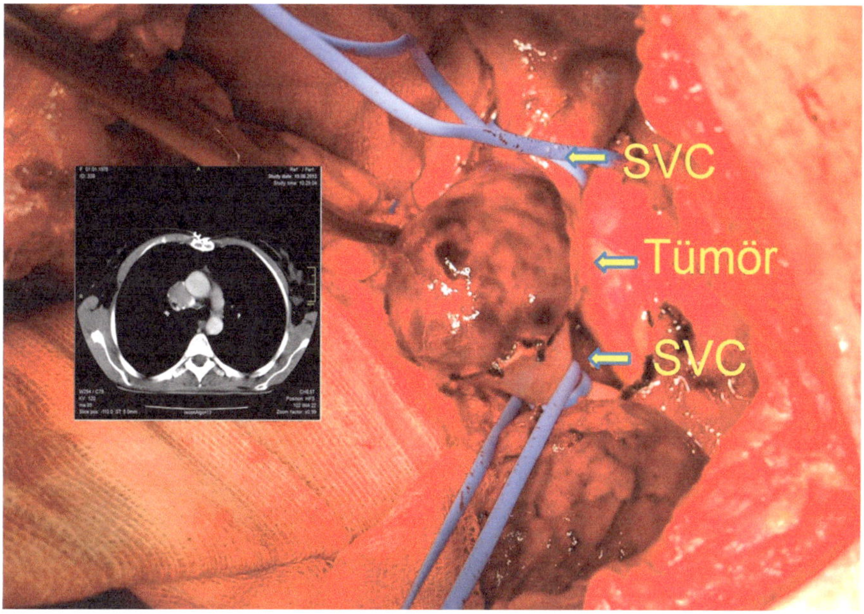

Fig. 17.3 Intraoperative view of tumor invading the superior vena cava

superior vena cava invasion at 3 years after the operation (Fig. 17.2a, b). Superior vena cava resection with graft interposition and resection of pleuroparenchymal nodules was performed following three courses of chemotherapy (cisplatin, cyclophosphamide, adriamycin) (Fig. 17.3). The patient underwent pleural implant resection at 1 year after the second operation. There is no recurrence detected on CT during the follow-up period of 1 year.

Case 2

A 47-year-old male patient presented with anterior mediastinal mass and right pleural nodular implants (Fig. 17.4). Tru-cut biopsy of the mass showed thymoma type B2. After four courses of cisplatin, cyclophosphamide, and adriamycin, CT revealed partial response. The patient underwent mediastinal mass resection with partial pericardial resection and right total parietal pleurectomy (Fig. 17.5a, b). The patient is in first year of follow-up without recurrence.

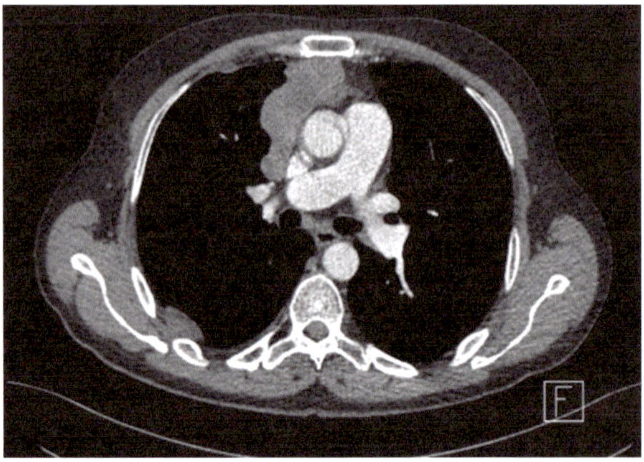

Fig. 17.4 Mediastinal mass with pleural implant

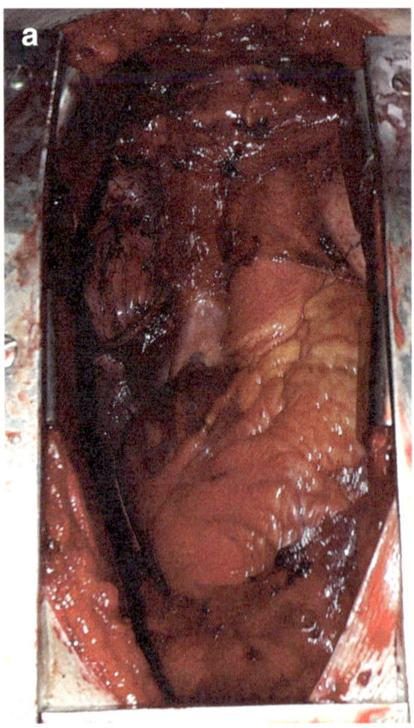

Fig. 17.5 (**a**) Intraoperative view of anterior mediastinum after resection. (**b**) Mediastinal mass and parietal pleura

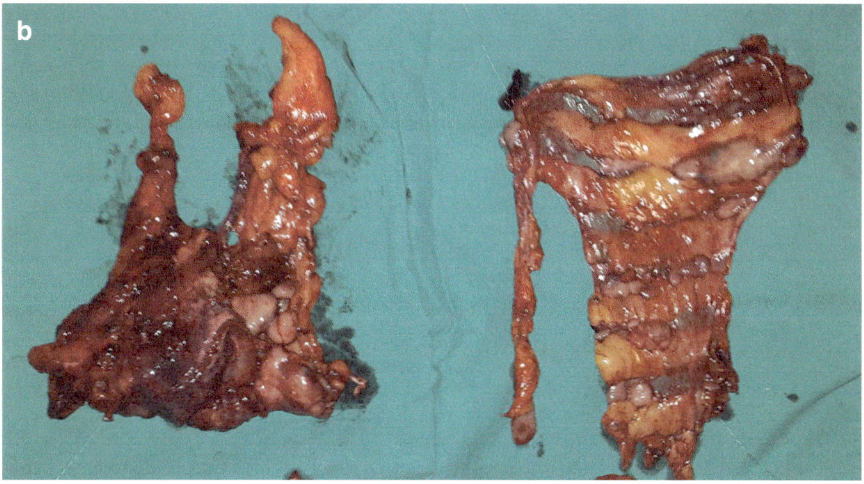

Fig. 17.5 (continued)

References

1. Rosai J, Sobin L. Histological typing of tumours of the thymus. In: Rosai J, Sobin L, editors. World Health Organization, International classification of tumours. Berlin: Springer; 1999. p. 9–14.
2. Travis WD, Brambilla E, Muller-Hermelink HK, et al. Pathology and genetics of tumours of the lung, pleura, thymus and heart. In: Kleihues P, Sobin LH, editors. WHO classification of tumours. 2nd ed. Lyon: IARC Press; 2004. p. 145–97.
3. Masaoka A, Monden Y, Nakahara K, et al. Follow-up study of thymomas with special reference to their clinical stages. Cancer. 1981;48:2485e92.
4. Koga K, Matsuno Y, Noguchi M, et al. A review of 79 thymomas: modification of staging system and reappraisal of conventional division into invasive and non-invasive thymoma. Pathol Int. 1994;44:359–67.
5. Ruffini E, Venuta F. Management of thymic tumors: a European perspective. J Thorac Dis. 2014;6:228–37.
6. Davenport E, Malthaner RA. The role of surgery in the management of thymoma: a systematic review. Ann Thorac Surg. 2008;86:673e84.
7. Yang Zhao, Haiquan Chen, Jianxin Shi, Limin Fan, Dingzhong Hu and Heng Zhao. The correlation of morphological features of chest computed tomographic scans with clinical characteristics of thymoma. Eur J Cardiothorac Surg. 2015;48:698–704.
8. Tomiyama N, Johkoh T, Mihara N, et al. Using the World Health Organization classification of thymic epithelial neoplasms to describe CT findings. AJR Am J Roentgenol. 2002;179(4):881e6.
9. Hayes SA, Huang J, Plodkowski AJ, Katzen J, Zheng J, Moskowitz CS, Ginsberg MS. Preoperative computed tomography findings predict surgical resectability of thymoma. J Thorac Oncol. 2014;9:1023–30.
10. Singhal S, Shrager JB, Rosenthal DI, Livolsi VA, Kaiser LR. Comparison of stages I-II thymoma treated by complete resection with or without adjuvant radiation. Ann Thorac Surg. 2003;76:51635–42.
11. Chao Y, Liu YH, Hsieh MJ, Wu YC, Chen TP, Lu MS, Lu HI, Liu HP. Long-term outcomes after thoracoscopic resection of stage I and II thymoma: a propensity-matched study. Ann Surg Oncol. 2015;22:1371–6.

12. Maniscalco P, Tamburini N, Quarantotto F, Grossi W, Garelli E, Cavallesco G. Long-term outcome for early stage thymoma: comparison between thoracoscopic and open approaches. Thorac Cardiovasc Surg. 2015;63:201–5.
13. Jurado J, Javidfar J, Newmark A, Lavelle M, Bacchetta M, Gorenstein L, D'Ovidio F, Ginsburg ME, Sonett JR. Minimally invasive thymectomy and open thymectomy: outcome analysis of 263 patients. Ann Thorac Surg. 2012;94:974–82.
14. Pennathur A, Qureshi I, Schuchert MJ, Dhupar R, Ferson PF, Gooding WE, Christie NA, Gilbert S, Shende M, Awais O, Greenberger JS, Landreneau RJ, Luketich JD. Comparison of surgical techniques for early-stage thymoma: feasibility of minimally invasive thymectomy and comparison with open resection. J Thorac Cardiovasc Surg. 2011;141:694–701.
15. Marulli G, Rea F, Melfi F, Schmid TA, Ismail M, Fanucchi O, Augustin F, Swierzy M, Di Chiara F, Mussi A, Rueckert JC. Robot-aided thoracoscopic thymectomy for early-stage thymoma: a multicenter European study. J Thorac Cardiovasc Surg. 2012;144:1125–32.
16. Ye B, Li W, Ge X, Feng J, Ji CY, Cheng M, Tantai JC, Zhao H. Surgical treatment of early-stage thymomas: robot-assisted thoracoscopic surgery versus transsternal thymectomy. Surg Endosc. 2014;28:122–6.
17. Tregliaa G, Sadeghib R, Giovanellaa L, Cafarotti S, Filosso P, Lococoe F. Is 18F-FDG PET useful in predicting the WHO grade of malignancy in thymic epithelial tumors? A meta-analysis. Lung Cancer. 2014;86:5–13.
18. Korst RJ, Bezjak A, Blackmon S, Choi N, Fidias P, Liu G, Marx A, Wright C, Mock S, Rutledge JR, Keshavjee S. Neoadjuvant chemoradiotherapy for locally advanced thymic tumors: a phase II, multi-institutional clinical trial. J Thorac Cardiovasc Surg. 2014;147:36–46.
19. Ruffini E, Detterbeck, Van Raemdonck D, Rocco G, Thomas P, Weder W, Brunelli A, Evangelista A, Venuta F. On behalf of the European Association of Thoracic Surgeons (ESTS) Thymic Working Group Tumours of the thymus: a cohort study of prognostic factors fromthe European Society of Thoracic Surgeons database. Eur J Cardiothorac Surg. 2014;46:361–8.
20. Yagi K, Hirata T, Fukuse T, et al. Surgical treatment for invasive thymoma, especially when the superior vena cava is invaded. Ann Thorac Surg. 1996;61:521–4.
21. Murakawa T, Nakajima J, Kohno T, et al. Results from surgical treatment for thymoma: 43 years of experience. J Thorac Cardiovasc Surg. 2000;48:89–95.
22. Kondo K, Monden Y. Therapy for thymic epithelial tumors: a clinical study of 1,320 patients from Japan. Ann Thorac Surg. 2003;76:878–84.
23. Hamaji M, Burt BM. Long-term outcomes of surgical and nonsurgical management of stage IV thymoma: a population-based analysis of 282 patients. Semin Thorac Cardiovasc Surg. 2015;27(1):1–3. doi:10.1053/j.semtcvs.2015.02.005.
24. Falkson CB, Bezjak A, Darling G, et al. The management of thymoma: a systematic review and practice guideline. J Thorac Oncol. 2009;4:911–9.
25. Thymomas and thymic carcinomas. NCCN clinical practice guidelines in oncology. Version I.2015.
26. Okumura M, Shiono H, Inoue M, et al. Outcome of surgical treatment for recurrent thymic epithelial tumors with reference to world health organization histologic classification system. J Surg Oncol. 2007;95:40–4.

Systemic Therapies in Thymic Malignancies

18

Kerim Kaban

Introduction

There are several types of neoplasms that can originate in the thymus gland such as germ cell tumors, lymphomas, or neuroendocrine cancers, but here, we will be discussing systemic treatment of only the most common types, thymoma (T) and thymic carcinoma (TC). These neoplasms are thymic epithelial tumors (TETs) and they form the most common histologic type of thymic neoplasms.

TETs are rare tumors. According to the National Cancer Institute's Surveillance, Epidemiology, and End Results (SEER) data, there are approximately 13 new cases of thymoma every year for every ten million people. However, it is very likely that cases of thymoma are underreported in the SEER database. That is because, when there is no capsule invasion, cases of thymoma are frequently considered as "benign" and therefore not captured by the SEER cancer registries [1]. Thymoma incidence is similar in males and females, and its incidence rises with increasing age and peaks in the seventh decade of life. Accordingly, thymoma is very uncommon in children and young adults. Interestingly, thymoma incidence is higher in African Americans and particularly in Asians/Pacific Islanders. The incidence rate in Asian/Pacific Islanders is almost three times that of whites, and the reason for that is unknown. Thymic carcinoma represents about 5 % of TETs, and therefore it is the "rarest of a rare disease" with worse prognosis [2].

K. Kaban, MD
Department of Medical Oncology, American Hospital,
Güzelbahçe Sokak, No: 20, Tesvikiye, Istanbul 34365, Turkey
e-mail: kabankerim@gmail.com

G. Ozyigit et al. (eds.), *Principles and Practice of Radiotherapy Techniques in Thoracic Malignancies*, DOI 10.1007/978-3-319-28761-4_18

ITMIG

Until recently, the information on TETs was mostly based on small retrospective series, majority of them with <50 patients, when the International Thymic Malignancy Interest Group (ITMIG) [3] was formed in 2010 to combine forces to create a database of all thymic malignancies. Initially, multiple workgroups of experts collectively created standards for reporting on these tumors so that everybody can speak the same "language" (http://journals.lww.com/jto/toc/2011/07001) [4–11]. Afterward, a new staging proposal and clinical guidelines were formed (http://journals.lww.com/jto/toc/2014/09002). These series of articles can both be accessed for free by anyone interested in the treatment of thymic malignancies, and they definitely form the starting point of the state-of-the-art treatment of TETs. They address a wide range of interrelated issues such as common definitions of mediastinal compartments and radiological response to therapy, guides for clinicians and radiologists evaluating patients with anterior mediastinal masses, for pathologists in classifying thymomas, as well as reviews on genetic abnormalities, paraneoplastic syndromes, and immunologic disorders in thymic malignancies [12–20].

This is a colossal undertake uniting the worldwide community involved in treating TETs with the common goal of overcoming the innate difficulties in improving the treatment of a rare cancer and sets an excellent example for other rare cancers, too. As of 2015, the retrospective database contains more than 7,000 cases from over 50 institutions. This database is already giving rise to many publications, but it naturally has some shortcomings due to its retrospective and multinational nature arching over a period of many decades. A prospective database is also now collecting predefined patient information since 2012, which will become an invaluable resource in the very near future.

Presentation and Diagnosis

Thymoma and thymic carcinoma are very different diseases (Table **18.1**), yet due to their rarity, they are frequently reported together in clinical studies.

There are three ways thymomas and thymic carcinomas are diagnosed.

First, anterior mediastinal masses are discovered incidentally during imaging tests done for other purposes in asymptomatic patients.

Second, there could be signs and symptoms due to the local progression of the disease or much less commonly due to distant metastasis. Mass effect and invasion into surrounding tissues can cause chest pain, cough, and shortness of breath. Superior vena cava syndrome and signs and symptoms due to damage to neighboring nerves can occur. Particularly, hoarseness due to recurrent laryngeal nerve damage and hemidiaphragmatic palsy due to the involvement of the phrenic nerve can happen. Shortness of breath could also be induced by pleural or pericardial effusions due to the spread of the tumor.

Table 18.1 Common features of thymoma and thymic carcinoma [96]

Associated characteristic feature	Thymoma	Thymic carcinoma
Histologic features resembling normal thymus[a]	Almost always	Not present
CD5, CD70, and CD117 expression in epithelial cells	No	Frequent (60 %)
Invasion	Not frequent but possible	Almost always
Myasthenia gravis and other autoimmune diseases	Common	Rare
Clinical correlation	Rarely metastasize. Often curable by surgery. Usually survival is long with an indolent clinical course	Usually locally advanced. Frequently metastatic. Survival is much worse than thymoma

[a]Lobular pattern, perivascular spaces, immature and TdT+/CD1a+/CD99+ T-cells

Any patient diagnosed with these conditions should be screened for thymoma, and worsening of these in a previously treated patient may suggest recurrence.

Third, patients commonly have signs and symptoms of thymic malignancy-related paraneoplastic disorders (PND) [20]. The most frequently encountered neurological PNDs are myasthenia gravis (MG), acquired neuromyotonia (Isaacs' syndrome), encephalitis, Morvan's syndrome, and myositis. MG is by far the most common of the PNDs. Around 15–20 % of MG patients have a thymoma, and 25–40 % of thymoma patients develop MG. MG is rarely seen in patients with thymic carcinoma. Other non-neurological common PNDs include pure red cell aplasia which occurs in up to 15 % of patients with thymoma and seen more commonly in older women and with spindle cell morphology. Surgery may not be curative for this PND. Finally, immunodeficiency, particularly hypogammaglobulinemia, occurs in less than 5 % of patients with thymoma. Conversely, up to 10 % of patients with acquired hypogammaglobulinemia have in fact thymoma, most commonly with spindle cell histology, and this is called Good syndrome.

Any patient diagnosed with these conditions should be screened for thymoma, and worsening of these in a previously treated patient may suggest recurrence.

Imaging and Differential Diagnosis

Compartments of the Mediastinum

Compartments of the mediastinum, as defined by ITMIG, are prevascular compartment (red), visceral compartment (green), and paravertebral compartment (yellow).

It is important to note that the prevascular compartment, where we encounter TETs, wraps around the pericardium in the visceral compartment [21] (Fig. 18.1).

It is important to note that the prevascular compartment, where we encounter TETs, wraps around the pericardium in the visceral compartment.

Differential Diagnosis of Prevascular Compartment Mass

The most common masses in the prevascular compartment include [21]:

- Thymic masses (cysts, hyperplasia, TETs, and neuroendocrine tumors)
- Germ cell neoplasms
- Lymphoma
- Metastatic lymphadenopathy
- Intrathoracic goiter

Approach for Diagnosis

Once a mass in the prevascular compartment is detected, there are three essential components of a reliable diagnostic approach:

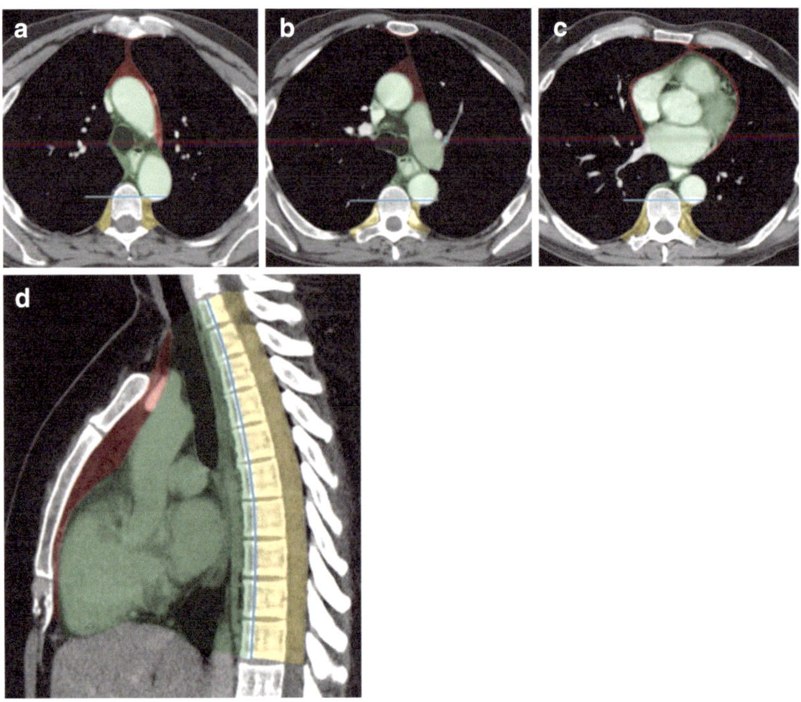

Fig. 18.1 CT images of transverse sections at three different levels (**a**–**c**) and sagittal section (**d**), depicting the prevascular (*red*), visceral (*green*), and paravertebral compartments (*yellow*). The *blue line* is the boundary between visceral and paravertebral compartments [21]

Be Aware of Demographics

First, the clinician should be aware that the most common types of masses encountered in the prevascular area change by age (Fig. 18.2). In younger patients, lymphoma, germ cell tumors, and teratoma are much more common, but by advancing age, the probability of thymoma increases gradually. As a rule of thumb, around 50 % or more of prevascular compartment masses in women over the age of 40 years are thymomas. Among men, the same holds true between the ages of 40–69 years. A less appreciated fact is that gender also plays an important role. For example, in women older than 80 years of age, about half of all prevascular compartment masses are thymomas, forming the most common type, whereas among men in the same age group, thyroid-related masses are the most common type, and only around 20 % of prevascular compartment masses are thymomas. Similarly, between the ages of 20–29 years, approximately 40 % of masses in the prevascular compartment are lymphoma in women, but in men, less than 25 % of such masses will be lymphoma, and the majority will be germ cell tumor [22].

The differential diagnosis of a prevascular compartment mass changes by gender and age.

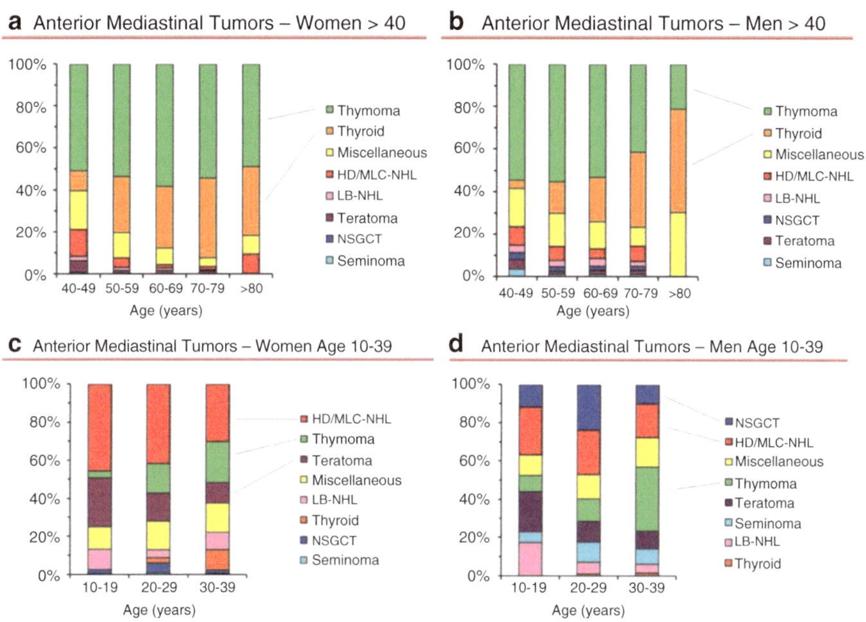

Fig. 18.2 Tumors of the prevascular compartment in patients over 40 years of age (**a**, men; **b**, women) and under 40 years of age (**c**, men; **d**, women). *HD* Hodgkin disease, *MLC-NHL* mediastinal large cell non-Hodgkin's lymphoma, *LB-NHL* lymphoblastic non-Hodgkin's lymphoma, *NSGCT* non-seminomatous germ cell tumor (used with permission from Detterbeck FC [22, 119])

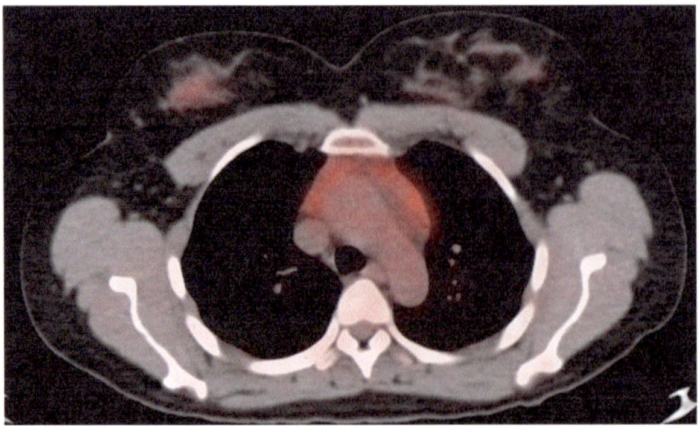

Fig. 18.3 Patient with thymic hyperplasia, 6 months after the completion of chemotherapy. Unless the history of chemotherapy is given, a misdiagnosis is possible

Communicate Clinical Information

Second, the clinician should communicate certain clinical information to the radiologist, for example, if it is known that the patient was treated with chemotherapy or steroids that could raise the possibility of thymic hyperplasia (Fig. 18.3). The signs and symptoms of a paraneoplastic syndrome such as myasthenia gravis make thymoma extremely likely, or the presence of "B" symptoms and an elevated LDH level suggest lymphoma. A large heterogeneous mass with the presence of lung metastases in a young man with a rapid onset of symptoms suggests germ cell tumor. Tumor markers, such as beta-HCG and AFP, should always be checked.

Radiological Appearance

Third, clearly, radiological appearance itself needs to be considered [23]:

- Lobular, homogeneous, or slightly heterogeneous mass with smooth contours located at the prevascular compartment suggests thymoma.
- Irregular contours with invasion into surrounding tissues in a heterogeneous mass with cystic and necrotic areas and calcifications inside, and surrounding enlarged lymph nodes, and possibly multiple pleural implants might suggest thymic carcinoma.
- The presence of visible areas of intralesional fat within a heterogeneous mass in the prevascular compartment is highly suggestive of a benign teratoma.
- A hyperdense lesion, which highly enhances with intravenous contrast and in continuity with the thyroid gland, is typical for a mediastinal goiter. However, it should be noted that connection to the thyroid gland may not always be visible.

In summary, correct diagnosis of a prevascular compartment mass relies on the demographic information, clinical presentation, and radiological appearance. A very useful algorithm for the differential diagnosis of prevascular compartment masses was published by Carter et al. as part of the ITMIG clinical guides, and it takes into account all of these three components of decision-making [23].

Other Imaging Studies

PET/CT

18-Fluorodeoxyglucose (FDG) positron emission tomography (PET) is *not* routinely recommended to assess thymic masses [24]. Still, the intensity of the FDG uptake on the initial PET scan correlates with the WHO histologic subtype [25]. Patients with thymic carcinoma have the highest intensity of FDG uptake, and that is followed by those with WHO type B3 and then low-risk thymomas with WHO histologic subtypes A, AB, B1, or B2, which tend not to show any increased FDG uptake in PET scan. Thymic hyperplasia may instead show increased uptake [26].

Radionuclide Scan

Scintigraphy, done with octreotide which is labeled with ^{111}indium-diethylenetriamine pentaacetic acid (^{111}In-DTPA), also known as OctreoScan®, was evaluated in patients with TETs. Increased uptake was seen in the majority of TETs, including thymic carcinomas [27, 28]. Tumor-to-lung (T/L) ratios were as high as 7.6-fold (range 1.7–7.6). Importantly, untreated tumors showed higher T/L ratios (4.34) than treated ones (2.68). Patients with thymic hyperplasia did not show any increased uptake. In a larger series of 20 patients with TETs (11 TC; five with non-neuroendocrine TC and six with neuroendocrine TC), once again the majority of tumors were detected by ^{111}In-DTPA-octreotide SPECT, and tumor-to-background ratios ranged between 1.67 and 10.10 [29].

The PET radiotracer, ^{68}Ga-DOTA-Tyr-octreotide (DOTATOC), is used for the PET/CT detection of the same tumor types detected by OctreoScan. Another radiotracer, ^{68}Ga-DOTATATE, is also reported to be sensitive for TETs [30, 31].

Need for Biopsy

If the clinical and radiological judgment highly suggests a thymic malignancy, and upfront surgery is possible, then a biopsy prior to surgery is not required [24]. In all other situations, biopsy, preferably a core-needle biopsy without violating the pleural space, is indicated. In patients older than 40 years of age, given that a mediastinal goiter is excluded, a lobulated and homogeneous, or slightly heterogeneous mass in the prevascular compartment should be considered to be highly consistent with a thymoma. The presence of PNDs such as MG makes the diagnosis almost certain [23]. The threshold to request a biopsy should be lower in the absence of MG for younger patients, particularly younger than 30 years of age even if the radiological appearance strongly suggests thymoma. In such patients, the frequency of TETs is much lower, and lymphoma, teratoma, and germ cell tumors are higher.

The threshold to request a biopsy should be lower in the absence of MG for younger patients, particularly younger than 30 years of age even if the radiological appearance strongly suggests thymoma.

Pathology

Currently, the World Health Organization (WHO) pathological classification is used for TETs. This classification system is discussed in detail elsewhere in this book, but in short, it entails five main subtypes (A, AB, B1, B2, and B3) for thymoma and thymic carcinoma, also known as type C [17, 32, 33]. Thymoma-specific 10-year survival is 100 % with WHO type A thymoma in almost all studies and slowly goes down to an average of 62 % (range 33–92 %, in different series) in WHO type B3 thymoma. The largest drop in survival is with thymic carcinoma, with a 10-year cancer-specific survival of 29 %.

Thymic carcinomas are similar to carcinomas seen in other organs and could come in many different subtypes such as squamous cell, mucoepidermoid, basaloid, or clear cell carcinomas among the many possible.

Staging

Staging for TETs (Table **18.2**) is discussed separately elsewhere in this book, but in summary, there are three distinct characteristics of staging for TETs:

- First, staging of TETs is primarily based upon the degree of invasion of adjacent structures and the presence of distant metastases.
- Second, lymph node involvement is not a component of stepwise staging, and when there are lymphatic metastases, just as it is the case with hematogenous metastases, the disease is staged as stage IVB.
- Third, all TETs, whether it is thymoma or thymic carcinoma, are staged similarly.

Application of this staging system in a large retrospective study involving 273 cases of thymoma and 20-year survival rates (as defined by freedom from tumor-related death) according to the Masaoka staging system was reported to be 89 % for stage I disease, 91 % for stage II disease, 49 % for stage III disease, and 0 % for stage IV disease [34]. Of note, multivariate analysis revealed that the WHO histologic classification system was also a significant independent prognostic factor. The 20-year survival rates for patients with type A, AB, B1, B2, and B3 tumors were 100 %, 87 %, 91 %, 59 %, and 36 %, respectively.

Treatment

The Difficulty of Interpreting Studies for the Treatment of TETs

One needs to be cautioned about the inherent difficulties of interpreting and comparing the results of multiple small studies for the treatment of TETs.

Table 18.2 Masaoka-Koga staging system with ITMIG description of details [6]

Stage		Definition
		With ITMIG description of details
I		Grossly and microscopically completely encapsulated tumor
		Includes tumors with invasion into but *not through* the capsule
		Tumors in which *capsule is missing* but *without invasion* into surrounding tissues
II	a	Microscopic transcapsular invasion
		Invasion not grossly appreciated
	b	Macroscopic invasion into thymic or surrounding fatty tissue, or grossly adherent to, but not breaking through mediastinal pleura or pericardium
		Gross visual tumor extension into normal thymus or perithymic fat surrounding the thymoma (microscopically confirmed)
		Adherence to pleura or pericardium making removal of these structures necessary during resection, with microscopic confirmation of perithymic invasion (but *without microscopic extension* into or through the mediastinal pleura or into the fibrous layer of pericardium)
III		*Macroscopic* invasion into neighboring organ (i.e., the pericardium, great vessel, or lung)
		This includes extension of the primary tumor to any of the following tissues:
		Microscopic involvement of mediastinal pleura (either partial or penetrating the elastin layer)
		Microscopic involvement of the pericardium (either partial in the fibrous layer or penetrating through to the serosal layer)
		Microscopically confirmed direct penetration into the outer elastin layer of the visceral pleura or into the lung parenchyma
		Invasion into the phrenic or vagus nerves (microscopically confirmed, adherence alone is not sufficient)
		Invasion into or penetration through major vascular structures (microscopically confirmed)
		Adherence (i.e., fibrous attachment) of the lung or adjacent organs *only if* there is mediastinal pleural or pericardial invasion (microscopically confirmed)
IV	a	Pleural or pericardial metastases
		Microscopically confirmed nodules, *separate from the primary tumor*, involving the visceral or parietal pleural surfaces, or the pericardial or epicardial surfaces
	b	Lymphogenous or hematogenous metastasis
		Any nodal involvement (e.g., anterior mediastinal, intrathoracic, low or anterior cervical nodes, any other extrathoracic nodes)
		Distant metastases (i.e., extrathoracic and outside the cervical perithymic region) or pulmonary parenchymal nodules (*not a pleural implant*)

Clearly, there are no randomized trials, and there will be none in the near future (though this could change now, with the establishment of ITMIG). It is difficult to compare results from the previous studies that are spread over a long period of decades, most with a handful of patients, using different techniques of radiotherapy, different chemotherapy protocols, and, for the case of neoadjuvant therapy, different and, perhaps even more importantly, subjective criteria such as "unresectable disease" to select patients for preoperative therapy. Furthermore, thymoma, and even thymic carcinoma, has a relatively long survival time, and comparing survival times from multiple different studies to judge the efficacy of a particular treatment type could be very misleading for two reasons: First, TETs are chemosensitive tumors and subsequent treatments can change the median survival time significantly, whereas progression-free survival is perhaps a better measure of treatment efficacy in advanced disease. The effect of treatment on median survival time will inevitably be diluted by further lines of different treatments. Second, TETs are not only rare tumors but a heterogeneous group of tumors as well. The composition of the histologic subtypes among any given study population will dramatically alter even the natural history of the disease without treatment. In addition, response to various treatments will differ based on the WHO subtype such that, for example, a WHO histologic subtype A thymoma is likely to respond to treatment differently than a WHO histologic type B3 thymoma. Finally, when we attempt to compare the results of neoadjuvant therapy trials, another difficulty we face is the surgical nature of the staging system. Indeed, the traditional staging of TETs is mostly based on the Masaoka staging system which relies upon the findings at the time of the surgery and under the microscope of the pathologist. Therefore, at times, depending on the diligence of the initial evaluation and imaging, and particularly in studies of previous decades, preoperative staging may not be as reliable. This is particularly true for Masaoka stage III patients.

Therefore, like most rare tumors, treatment recommendations are made by expert panels "inspired" by the results of the studies and pure experience [24, 35–37].

Surgery is the most important component of treatment and should be performed whenever complete resection (R0 resection) is possible.

Upfront Resectable Disease

Surgery is the most important step of treatment for TETs as long as a complete resection can be achieved, for it is the most significant prognostic factor determining the outcome [8, 38]. For this reason, any TET deemed resectable should undergo surgery. The decision for resectability is, on the other hand, a subjective one and strongly depends on the expertise of the surgeon. In most cases, direct invasion of the aorta, arch vessels, the main pulmonary artery, the myocardium, the trachea, or the esophagus is considered to be unresectable.

Importance of Lymph Nodes

Resection of TETs should always include nodal sampling.

In a series of thymoma reported by Weksler et al. [39], 442 patients who underwent resection with pathologic evaluation of at least 1 lymph node, 13 % had lymph node metastasis. Patients with positive nodes were younger and *had smaller tumors* than node-negative patients. Median survival of the node-positive patients was 98 months, compared with 144 months in node-negative patients ($p=0.013$). In multivariate analysis, the presence of positive nodes had a significant, independent, adverse impact on survival (hazard ratio 1.945, 95 % confidence interval 1.296–2.919, $P=0.001$).

The same group analyzed the impact of lymph node sampling in thymic carcinoma and thymic neuroendocrine tumors in a series of 92 patients [39]. A metastasis to at least one lymph node was detected in 40 % of the patients, which was more common in patients with thymic neuroendocrine tumors than in patients with thymic carcinoma (62 % vs 34 %). The presence of nodal metastases had significant, independent, adverse impact on survival (HR 2.933, 95 % CI 1.903–4.521, $p=0.001$). Median survival was 47 months in patients with nodal metastasis and 124 months in patients without nodal metastases ($p<0.001$).

Potentially Resectable Disease

Is There a Role of Surgery in Locally Advanced Thymoma?

Every effort should be made to achieve a complete resection even in patients with stage III or IVa thymoma. If complete resection is not deemed possible at the time of initial presentation, neoadjuvant treatment should be administered to make the tumor resectable.

In a series of 310 patients from Japan analyzing the surgical outcome of stage III patients with thymoma, it was possible to achieve R0 resection in 80 % of the cases. This was possible in the presence of involvement of the lung in 63 %, the pericardium in 49 %, the great vessels in 41 %, and the phrenic nerve in 27 % of the patients. Only 14 % of the patients received neoadjuvant therapy, and 47 % received adjuvant therapies. In the event of R0 resection, only 28 % experienced recurrence, mostly in the pleural space. The 10-year overall and disease-free survival in R0 resection group was 80 % and 52 %, respectively [40].

Is There a Role for Debulking Surgery for Thymoma or Thymic Carcinoma?

The available evidence, though conflicting, suggests that in selected patients, it may be considered.

JCOG 9606 was a phase II study of induction chemotherapy in 21 patients with stage III unresectable thymoma. Induction chemotherapy was followed by surgery, if the tumor became resectable, and then by adjuvant radiotherapy [41]. After the 9-week chemotherapy with the CODE regimen, R0 resection became possible in 43 % of the patients, and R1 and R2 resection was done in 5 % of the patients, respectively. Adjuvant radiotherapy was given to 63 % of those who could not undergo surgery and 44 % of those with R0 resection. Interestingly, the progression-free survival and overall survival were quite similar for those who had some sort of surgery (mostly R0) and those who could not have any surgery at all, which constituted almost half of the patients. The 8-year PFS and OS were 36 % and 26 %, and 73 % and 63 %, with or without surgery, respectively. When R0 resection was achieved, these rates were slightly better (44 % for PFS and 78 % for OS). This suggests that debulking surgery (R2 resection) is most likely not particularly helpful.

However, subtotal resection may be beneficial in selected cases of thymoma, particularly when it can be followed by definitive radiotherapy. In an analysis from SEER database exploring the outcomes of 282 patients with stage IV thymomas treated surgically and nonsurgically, the 10-year OS for surgical patients was 35 %, while for nonsurgical patients, it was 19 %. Interestingly, the difference in OS or cancer-specific survival between patients undergoing radical and lesser resection was not statistically significant suggesting that decreasing the tumor burden with debulking surgery might help in selected patients and supports a tailored surgical approach [42]. A meta-analysis of debulking surgery versus surgical biopsy for stage IV thymoma reached similar conclusions. The pooled HR was 0.451 (95 % confidence interval 0.336–0.605, $P<0.001$), in favor of debulking surgery [43].

ESMO Clinical Practice Guidelines note that partial resection is generally not recommended for thymic carcinoma [24]. However, in carefully selected cases, particularly if it can be followed by other effective treatments, debulking surgery could still be considered. In a database analysis from Japan, R0 resection was associated with most improved OS; however, both R1 and R2 (≥80 % tumor resection) subtotal resections resulted in superior OS compared with no resection [HR (95 % confidence interval) for R0, R1, and R2: 0.27 (0.15–0.48), 0.40 (0.22–0.74), and 0.38 (0.20–0.72), respectively]. Postoperative radiotherapy was associated with improved RFS after R0 resection [44].

Is There a Role of Neoadjuvant Concurrent Chemoradiotherapy?

It is difficult to compare the results of previous studies using subjective criteria such as "unresectable disease" to select the patients for preoperative therapy. In addition, the traditional staging of TETs uses the Masaoka staging system which relies upon the findings at the time of the surgery and under the microscope of the pathologist. Therefore, at times, depending on the diligence of the initial evaluation, preoperative staging may not be as reliable, particularly for Masaoka stage III patients.

Keeping all these valid concerns in mind, Korst et al. [25] recently undertook a small multi-institutional phase II study to determine the response rate, and the rate of complete resection after induction chemotherapy with cisplatin and etoposide, and concomitant radiotherapy for locally advanced thymic tumors. They clearly defined the radiological criteria for the high-risk patients to be included in the study:

- >8 cm in the greatest axial diameter
- 5–8 cm in the greatest axial diameter with at least one of the following:

  - Irregular or scalloped borders
  - Heterogeneous appearance
  - Ectopic calcification
  - Obvious great vessel and/or adjacent organ invasion or encirclement
- <5 cm in the greatest axial diameter with obvious great vessel and/or adjacent organ invasion or encirclement

The treatment that is used in the study mirrored the intergroup 0139 trial which tested neoadjuvant chemoradiotherapy in patients with locally advanced lung cancer:

Radiotherapy (IMRT or 3D conformal, 45 Gy) concurrent with two cycles of the PE chemotherapy protocol (cisplatin 50 mg/m^2 days 1, 8, 29, and 36 plus etoposide 50 mg/m^2 days 1–5, and 29–33) followed by surgical resection. Postoperatively, further treatment decisions were based on histologic subtype, postoperative stage, and completeness of resection as follows:

- If the resection was complete:
  - No additional chemotherapy

    WHO types A, AB, B1, and B2 *and* stage I or II
    - Additional chemotherapy with two cycles of chemotherapy with PE

      WHO type B3 and thymic carcinomas at any stage

      Masaoka stage III or IV, regardless of histologic subtype
- If the resection was incomplete, all patients were to receive additional concurrent RT (boost up to 60 Gy) with two cycles of PE chemotherapy.

Complete resection rate was 77 %. There was no pathologic complete remission (pCR), and only 48 % of the patients achieved PR, though most of the patients had some degree of response. Interestingly, of the seven patients with thymic carcinoma, four of them had a near pCR. Five years after the resection, the freedom from progression and overall actuarial survival of the entire 22-patient cohort was 83 % and 71 %, respectively. The impressive near pCRs seen in TC patients is encouraging, and while the patient numbers are certainly small to make a binding recommendation, in the absence of better data, one could consider multimodality treatment for unresectable patients with TC.

> Concurrent chemoradiotherapy may be preferred for TC when induction therapy is indicated. For thymoma, only induction chemotherapy might be more suitable. After the resection, if the margins are positive, then radiotherapy could be added.

What Is the Role of Induction Chemotherapy Alone?

NCCN and ESMO guidelines recommend induction chemotherapy alone (Table **18.3**), without concurrent radiotherapy for locally advanced unresectable thymoma and thymic carcinoma [24, 37]. However, as noted above, the recent results by Korst et al. suggests that, for thymic carcinoma, neoadjuvant concurrent

Table 18.3 Prospective neoadjuvant chemotherapy trials in locally advanced TETs

Chemotherapy regimen	N (T/TC)	RR (CR) %	R0 %	pCR %	OS %	PFS
Cisplatin + epirubicin + etoposide [97]	7 (4/3)	100 (29)	57	29	80 (2 years)	80 (2 years)
ADOC [98]	16 (16/0)	100 (43)	69	31	70 (3 years)	NA
PAC-P [99]	12 (12/0)	93 (25)	82	NA	100 (7 years)	73 (7 years)
PAC-P (CI) [100]	22 (22/0)	77 (14)	73	NA	95 (5 years) 79 (7 years)	53 (10 years)
Cisplatin + docetaxel [101]	27 (9/18)	63 (0)	56	NA	93 (4 years)	50 (4 years)

N number of patients; *T* thymoma; *TC* thymic carcinoma; *RR* response rate (complete + partial response); *CR* complete response; *OS* overall survival; *PFS* progression-free survival; *P* prospective; *D* day; *ADOC* cisplatin, doxorubicin, vincristine, cyclophosphamide; *PAC-P* cisplatin, doxorubicin, cyclophosphamide, prednisone; *PAC* cisplatin, doxorubicin, cyclophosphamide; *CI* continuous infusion; *NA* not available

chemoradiotherapy could be considered, too [25, 45]. Any platinum containing regimen could be used. PAC is commonly used for the relative ease of administration, but ADOC, PAC-P, PE, VIP, and carboplatin/paclitaxel are all acceptable alternatives [24, 37].

Adjuvant Therapy

Stage-Based Adjuvant Treatment Summary

It is important to note that resectable thymoma has such an excellent prognosis that there is little or nothing that adjuvant treatments can add as long as a complete resection is carried out (Table **18.4**). In accordance with that, a retrospective series of 262 patients with thymoma were reported by Safieddine et al. revealing adverse prognostic factors as incomplete resection, large tumor size (>7 cm), and higher Masaoka stage. In this series, 75 % of the patients had Masaoka stage II or more advanced disease. Sixty-five percent of the patients received adjuvant radiotherapy. Overall survival was 91 % at 15 years. Distant recurrence occurred only in 3 % of the patients and disease-related death occurred only in four patients (1.5 %) [46].

Chemotherapy

In the current guidelines for thymoma (Table **18.4**), chemotherapy after R0 resection (complete resection) is *not recommended* for any histologic subgroup. The same holds true even after an R1 resection (microscopic residual tumor). The only situation where the guidelines suggest chemotherapy may be *considered* is in the event of an R2 resection (macroscopic residual tumor) as an addition to definitive radiotherapy.

For thymic carcinoma (Table **18.5**), if the resection is R0, chemotherapy is only recommended by the ESMO guidelines and only for stage III patients. The guidelines suggest that, for R1 resection, chemotherapy could be *considered* even for stage I patients [37], but it is *recommended* for stage II and more advanced thymic carcinoma patients [24]. In every situation, chemotherapy is added to radiotherapy.

Radiotherapy

The role of radiotherapy in adjuvant therapy for thymoma is discussed separately elsewhere in this book, but in summary, radiotherapy is not recommended for Masaoka stage I patients. Even if there is transcapsular invasion, radiotherapy is recommended only for WHO histologic subtype B3 when the invasion is microscopic (Masaoka stage IIA) and, for subtypes B2 and B3, if the invasion is macroscopic (Masaoka stage IIB). Both ESMO and NCCN guidelines consider or recommend using radiotherapy starting from stage II patients (Table **18.4**).

Postoperative chemotherapy may be considered (Table **18.5**) as an option in stage II/III/IV thymic carcinomas, especially if not delivered as induction treatment [24].

Table 18.4 Thymoma – treatment recommendations after R0 surgery [24, 37]

Stage	Subtype	Treatment ESMO	NCCN
I	All	None	None
IIA	All but B3	None	Consider RT
	B3	RT	Consider RT
IIB	All but B2, B3	None	Consider RT
	B2, B3	RT	Consider RT
III	All	RT	Consider RT

R1 at any stage → RT (both ESMO and NCCN guidelines); R2 at any stage → definitive RT ± CT (NCCN guidelines)

CT chemotherapy, *ESMO* European Society of Medical Oncology, *NCCN* National Comprehensive Cancer Network, *R0* complete resection, *R1* microscopic residual tumor, *R2* macroscopic residual tumor, *RT* radiotherapy

Table 18.5 Thymic carcinoma – treatment recommendations after surgery [24, 37]

Resection	Stage	Treatment ESMO	NCCN
R0	I	RT	None
	IIA–IIB	RT	Consider RT
	III	CT → RT	Consider RT
R1	St I	RT	RT ± CT
	IIA–III	CT → RT	RT ± CT
R2	All stages	–	RT (definitive) + CT

CT chemotherapy, *ESMO* European Society of Medical Oncology, *NCCN* National Comprehensive Cancer Network, *R0* complete resection, *R1* microscopic residual tumor, *R2* macroscopic residual tumor, *RT* radiotherapy

Table 18.6 Carboplatin and paclitaxel in thymic carcinoma

Chemotherapy regimen	Drugs	Dose	Timing	Frequency
First line				
ADOC [47]	Cisplatin	50 mg/m^2	D1	q4 weeks
	Doxorubicin	40 mg/m^2	D1	
	Vincristine	0.6 mg/m^2	D3	
	Cyclophosphamide	700 mg/m^2	D4	
PAC [48]	Cisplatin	50 mg/m^2	D1	q3 weeks
	Doxorubicin	50 mg/m^2	D1	
	Cyclophosphamide	500 mg/m^2	D1	
PAC-P [49]	Cisplatin	30 mg/m^2/d	D1-3	q3 weeks
	Doxorubicin	20 mg/m^2/d CI	D1-3	
	Cyclophosphamide	500 mg/m^2	D1	
	Prednisone	100 mg/d	D1-5	
PE [50]	Cisplatin	60 mg/m^2	D1	q3 weeks
	Etoposide	120 mg/m^2/d	D1-3	
VIP [51]	Cisplatin	20 mg/m^2/d	D1-4	q3 weeks
	Etoposide	75 mg/m^2/d	D1-4	
	Ifosfamide	1.2 g/m^2/d	D1-4	
CODE [102]	Cisplatin	25 mg/m^2/w	Week 1–9	For 9 weeks
	Vincristine	1 mg/m^2/w	Week 1, 2, 4, 6, 8	
	Doxorubicin	40 mg/m^2/w	Week 1, 3, 5, 7, 9	
	Etoposide	80 mg/m^2/d D1-3	Week 1, 3, 5, 7, 9	
CbP [52, 103, 104]	Carboplatin	AUC 6	D1	q3 weeks
	Paclitaxel	200–225 mg/m^2	D1	
CisDoc [101]	Cisplatin	75 mg/m^2	D1	q3 weeks
	Docetaxel	75 mg/m^2	D1	
After first-line chemotherapy				
Cap-Gem [58]	Capecitabine	650 mg/m^2 per dose b.i.d	D1–14	q3 weeks
	Gemcitabine	1,000 mg/m^2/d	D1, D8	
Pemetrexed [55]	Pemetrexed	500 mg/m^2	D1	q3 weeks

Advanced Disease

Chemotherapy

Platinum-based combinations of chemotherapy are accepted as the standard first-line treatment of TETs requiring systemic therapy (Table **18.6**). In combination with platinum compounds, chemotherapy drugs such as doxorubicin, etoposide, cyclophosphamide, ifosfamide, and paclitaxel are among the most commonly used drugs

Table 18.7 Commonly used chemotherapy regimens

Chemotherapy	Type	N	Line	RR	DCR	DFS	MST	
CbP [104]	R	11	1st	36 (0+36)	82 (45)	8	22.7	From Japan
CbP [59]	R	16	1st	38 (13+25)	88 (50)	9	49	From Japan
CbP [52] B3 and C grouped together as TC!	P	23	1st	22 (0+22)	74 (52)	5	20	f/u 59 m. 44 pts, 23 with TC
CbP [103]	P	39	1st	36 (3+33)	95 (59)	7.5	NR	OS 1 year and 2 years: 85 and 71 %. WJOG4207L study

N number of patients, *RR* response rate, *DCR* disease control rate, *DFS* disease-free survival, *MST* median survival time, *CbP* carboplatin/paclitaxel, *R* retrospective, *P* prospective, *OS* overall survival

forming regimens such as ADOC [47], PAC [48], PAC-P [49], PE [50], VIP [51], and CbP [52] tested as first-line treatment for thymomas and thymic carcinomas (Tables **18.7**, **18.8**, **18.9**, and **18.10**) with response rates within the range of 43–56 % and progression-free survival of 17–26 months.

The ADOC regimen has been one of the earliest and most effective chemotherapy combinations used in patients with advanced thymoma [47]. The response rate of first-line treatment was an impressive 92 %, with 43 % of the patients achieving CR. This regimen has also been used for induction therapy in patients with thymic carcinoma in a small study with 8 patients. The response rate was slightly lower but still impressive: 75 % of the patients achieved PR [53]. In a retrospective analysis of ADOC regimen in thymic carcinoma, ORR was 50 % and DCR 88 %. Median survival was 21 months. Nearly 90 % of the patients were treatment naïve. Initial data suggest that carboplatin may not be interchangeable with cisplatin. Only one patient responded out of five patients who received carboplatin in place of cisplatin.

The response of TETs to chemotherapy varies depending on the histologic subtype. Thymomas may respond better to first-line platinum-based chemotherapy than do TCs. In addition, TCs do not respond to anthracyclines as well as thymomas [54]. Therefore, in the first-line setting, cisplatin and doxorubicin combinations are preferred for thymoma, and carboplatin/paclitaxel combination is frequently used for TCs [55].

Can We Replace Cisplatin with Carboplatin?

There is no definitive answer to this question, but until there is more data on this issue, it may be preferable not to make such a switch in regimens other than carboplatin and paclitaxel for now, at least in thymic carcinoma. Agatsuma et al. analyzed 29 patients with thymic carcinoma who received the ADOC regimen which consists of cisplatin, doxorubicin, vincristine, and cyclophosphamide and 5 patients who received carboplatin AUC instead. Median survival was 23.8 months with the standard cisplatin-containing ADOC regimen, whereas when cisplatin

Table 18.8 Efficacy of commonly used systemic treatments in advanced thymoma

Regimen	N	RR (CR) %	PFS (month)	MST (month)	Notes
First line					
Prospective					
ADOC [47]	37	92 (43)	12 (3–96+)	15 (5–96+)	From Padova, Italy
ADOC [98]	16	100 (43)	n/a	NR	3-year OS 70 %. pCR 31 %
PAC [48]	30	50 (10)	18.4	37.7 (2–91.9+)	5-year OS 32 %. 50 % with prior RT. 1 patient with TC
PE [50]	16	56 (31)	26.4	51.6	f/u 7 years. Survival at 5 years, 50 %; at 7 years, 42 %. Median duration of response among responders: 41 months
PAC → XRT → PAC [105]	23	70 (22)	93.2	93	A multimodality treatment study. 2 patients with TC
PAC-P [99]	12	93 (25)	NR	NR	7-year PFS and OS were 73 %, and 100 %, respectively
PAC-P (CI) [100]	22	77 (14)	NR	NR	10-year PFS was 53 %. 7-year OS was 79 %
VIP [51]	28	32 (0)	11.9 (<1–26)	31.6	f/u 43 m. 1-year OS and 2-year OS 89 % and 70 %
CODE [106]	27	59 (0)	9.5	73.2	PFS at 1 year 37 % and at 2 years 15 %. OS 2 years 89 % and at 5 years 65 %
CODE + XRT [41]	21	62 (0)	PFS 4.5 years		R0 39 %. PFS at 2, 5, and 8 years 80, 43, 32 %. OS at 2, 5, and 8 years 100, 85, 69 %. PFS and OS were similar in those who underwent surgery and those who did not (5- and 8-year PFS 46 and 36 % and OS 91 and 73 %)
Retrospective					
PE +/– RT [107]	11	73 (9)	37.7	128.1	RT was given whenever possible
Ifosfamide [108]	13	46 (38)	66+	5 year OS 57 %	1 patient received prior CT. Med CR duration 66+

N number of patients, *RR* response rate, *CR* complete remission, *PFS* progression free survival, *MST* median survival time, *OS* overall survival, see Table 18.6 for chemotherapy acronyms, *n/a* not available, *NR* not reached, *pCR* pathologic complete remission, *RT* radiotherapy, *TC* thymic carcinoma, *f/u* follow up, *CI* continuous infusion, *m* month, *CT* chemotherapy

50 mg/m^2 was switched with carboplatin AUC 3, median survival time was 7.7 months [56]. Admittedly, selection bias is almost certainly contributing to these results since patients received carboplatin in place of cisplatin due to poor renal function, advanced age, or poor performance status, and therefore, replacing cisplatin with carboplatin is not the only factor contributing to the worse median survival time.

Table 18.9 Efficacy of commonly used systemic treatments in advanced thymic carcinoma

Regimen	N	RR (CR) (%)	PFS (month)	MST (month)	Notes
First line					
Prospective					
CbP [103]	39	36 (3)	7.5	NR	Median OS not reached. OS 1 year and 2 years 85 and 71 %
Retrospective					
ADOC [53]	8	75	–	19	
CODE [109]	12	42 (0)	5.6	46	Estimated 1-year and 2-year OS 80 % and 58 %. Med f/u 14 months
CbP [104]	11	36 (0)	7.9	22.7	From Japan
CbP [59]	16	38 (13)	8.6	49.4	From Japan
ADOC [56]	34	50 (0)	–	21.3	OS 1 year 73 % and 3 years 34 %. 5 pts received carboplatin instead of cisplatin
Cisplatin + irinotecan [110]	9	56 (0)	7.9	33.8	1-year and 2-year OS 77.7 % and 55.6 %
CODE [102]	7	71 (0)			R0 % 86. OS 5 years and 10 years both 80 %
					RFS 5 years and 10 years 69 and 54 %
After first-line chemotherapy					
CbP [111]	3	66 (0)	n/a	n/a	1st-line ADOC in all with SD. 2nd-line irinotecan/cisplatin with SD as best response. 2nd + (33 % 2nd, 66 % 3rd)
CbP [112]	3	33 (0)	6.7	>36	1st-line ADOC
CbP [113]	12	25	3.5	24	Previous CT: 1st-line CAP 58 %, VIP 25 %, EP 17 %. No. of previous CT 58 % 2nd, 42 % 3rd
Platinum + irinotecan [114]	7	29 (0)	n/a	17.5	After ADOC. 2-year survival 43 %
Amrubicin + cisplatin or nedaplatin [115]	6	33 (0)	n/a	n/a	
Amrubicin [116]	9	44 (0)	4.9	6.4	
Docetaxel [60]	13	31	5.5	24	

N number of patients, *RR* response rate, *CR* complete remission, *PFS* progression free survival, *MST* median survival time, see Table 18.6 for chemotherapy acronyms, *OS* overall survival, med median, *f/u* follow up, *RFS* reccurence free survival, *n/a* not available, *SD* stable disease, *CT* chemotherapy

In another approach to this question, Okuma et al. reported that for advanced thymic carcinoma, cisplatin-based chemotherapy may be superior to carboplatin-based chemotherapy based on an analysis of 206 patients from ten studies. Response rates favored cisplatin-based chemotherapy (53.6 vs. 32.8 %; $p = 0.0029$) [54].

Table 18.10 Efficacy of commonly used systemic treatments in advanced TETs (mixed studies)

Regimen	N – T – TC	RR (CR) % – T – TC	PFS (month) – T – TC	MST (month) – T – TC	Notes
First line					
Prospective					
Cisplatin, epirubicin, etoposide [97]	7	100 (29)	NR	NR	OS and PFS at 2 years both 80 %
	–4				
	–3				
PACE [117]	14	43 (0)	n/a	14.7	14 % of patients previously received CT
	–7	–43 (0)		–	
	–7	–43 (0)		–	
VIP [51]	28	32 (0)	11.9	31.6	Median follow-up 43 months. 1-year OS 89 %, 2-year OS 70 %
	–20	–	–	–	
	–8	–	–	–	
VIP [118]	16	25 (6)	13.1	NR	Follow-up 32.6 months. Median OS not reached. 1-year OS 93.8, 2-year OS 78.1, and 3-year OS 58.6 %. Not reported separately for T and TC
	–12	–25 (8)	–	–	
	–4	–25 (0)	–	–	
CbP [52]	44				Median follow-up 59.4 months for thymoma and 63.8 months for thymic carcinoma
	–21	–(14)	–16.7	–NR	
	–23	–22 (0)	–5	–20	
Cis/Doc [101]	27	63 (0)	4-year 40.6	NR	4-year PFS 40.6 and OS 79.4 %. Median follow-up 42.6 months. Includes 2 patients with neuroendocrine carcinoma
	–9	–56 (0)	–		
	–18	–67 (0)	–		
Belinostat + PAC [83]	25	40 (4)	9	28.5	
	–11	–64 (9)	- NR	- NR	
	–14	–21 (0)	–7.2	–21.4	
PE + XRT [25]	21	48 (0)	NR	NR	77 % underwent R0, and 14 % R1 resection. Median follow-up 27 months. 5-year PFS and actuarial survival 83 % and 71 %
	–14				
	–7				
After first-line chemotherapy					
Prospective					
Octreotide, lanreotide + prednisone [66]	16	38 (6)	14	15	Patients were CT refractory. Median follow-up 43 months. 3 patients had small cell neuroendocrine carcinoma (1 PR, 1 SD)
	–10	–40 (10)	- n/a	- n/a	
	–6	–33 (0)	- n/a	- n/a	

Table 18.10 (continued)

Octreotide + prednisone [67]	38			46.3	
	–32	–38 (6)	–8.8	- NR	
	–6	–0 (0)	–4.5	–23.4	
Long-acting octreotide [68]	12	25 (0)	8	n/a	Median duration of clinical benefit was 47 months
	–9	–33 (0)	- n/a		
	–3	–0 (0)	- n/a		
Cap-Gem [58]	30	40 (10)	11	2-year OS 67	Median number of previous lines of CT was 3
	–22	–41 (14)	–11	- n/a	
	–8	–38 (0)	–6	- n/a	
Cixutumumab [82]	49	10 (0)	8.2	16.2	Median number of previous systemic treatment was 3
	–37	–14 (0)	–9.9	–27.5	
	–12	–0 (0)	–1.7	–8.4	
Everolimus [74]	35	11 (3)	12.1	24	Stable disease in 42 % of TC and 70 % of T
	–23	–4 (0)	- n/a	- n/a	
	–12	–25 (8)	- n/a	- n/a	
Belinostat [84]	40	5	5.8	19.2	
	–24	–8	–11.4	- NR	
	–16	–0	–2.7	–12.4	
Sunitinib [77]	39	18 (7)	–	–	Patients were CT refractory. Median follow-up 17 months. DCR 91 % in TC and 81 % in T. OS 1 year for TC 78 % and for T 86 %
	–16	–6 (0)	–8.5	–15.5	
	–23	–26 (0)	–7.2	- NR	
Retrospective					
Pemetrexed [55]	16	17 (0+17)	13.8	20.1	From Stanford. 2nd + (31 % 2nd, 69 % 3rd+) 12.5 % also received carboplatin
	6/10	10 (0+10)	6.5	12.7	

N number of patients, *T* thymoma, *TC* thymic carcinoma, *RR* response rate, *CR* complete remission, *PFS* progression free survival, *MST* median survival time, see Table 18.6 for chemotherapy acronyms, NR not reached, *OS* overall survival, *PFS* progression free survival, *CT* chemotherapy, *n/a* not availabile, *PR* partial response, *SD* stable disease, *DCR* disease control rate

NCCN guidelines, however, report that carboplatin/paclitaxel is recommended, because it has the highest response rate among thymic carcinomas in clinical trials [37]. The ADOC regimen is also effective, but it is more toxic than carboplatin/paclitaxel.

Previously Treated

Cap-Gem

Capecitabine plus gemcitabine (Table **18.10**) was tested in a phase II trial from Italy. Initial results [57] were encouraging and revealed 40 % response rate in previously treated patients with TETs and half of those were CRs. The 1- and 2-year survival rates were 80 % and 67 %, respectively. Final results were reported after 30 patients (thymoma, $n=22$; thymic carcinoma, $n=8$). Overall response rate was again 40 % and median progression-free survival was 11 months [58]. This combination was tolerated very well in cisplatin-pretreated patients and can certainly be considered as a second-line treatment.

Paclitaxel (or Nab-Paclitaxel) and Platinum Compounds

In a phase II study (Table **18.10**), carboplatin (AUC6) and paclitaxel (225 mg/m^2) were tested on previously untreated advanced TETs (21 thymoma, 23 thymic carcinomas). For the thymoma cohort, objective response rate was 43 % and a third of these were complete responses. For the thymic carcinoma group, overall response rate was 22 %, and there were no complete remissions. Progression-free survival was 17 months for thymomas and 5 months for thymic carcinomas [52].

In a retrospective series of 16 patients from Japan with recurrent or Masaoka stage IVA/IVB thymic carcinoma, the combination of carboplatin (AUC6) and paclitaxel (200 mg/m^2) achieved a response rate of 37.5 %, and 33 % of responses were CR (Table **18.9**). The median progression-free survival was 8.6 months [59].

Docetaxel

In a retrospective series from Japan, 13 thymic carcinoma patients received docetaxel monotherapy after becoming platinum refractory (Table **18.9**). Overall response rate was 31 % and disease control rate was 77 %. Overall survival after docetaxel monotherapy was 24 months, while progression-free survival was only 5.5 months suggesting that these patients benefited from other treatments after failing docetaxel [60].

Pemetrexed

Single-agent pemetrexed, a multi-targeted antifolate, provided a promising PFS of 45 weeks in an early report of 16 patients with previously treated thymoma (Table **18.10**). Overall response rate was 25 % and half of them were complete remissions. There were no responses among the 11 patients with thymic carcinoma and the median time to progression among those was only 5 weeks [55, 61].

S-1

In a case report, S-1 as a single agent showed dramatic activity and achieved CR in a patient with thymic carcinoma at third line of treatment. Low level of expression of TS may be associated with better efficacy of S-1 [62].

What Are the Best Chemotherapy Choices for Second-Line Treatment of Thymic Carcinoma?

Thymic carcinomas are exceedingly rare cancers. Consequently, optimal second-line treatment has not been established yet (Tables 18.9 and 18.10).

Carboplatin and paclitaxel could be a reasonable choice for those patients with thymic carcinoma previously treated with chemotherapy regimens other than carboplatin and paclitaxel. Based on studies reporting on small numbers of patients, even after failing cisplatin- and doxorubicin-based chemotherapy, patients respond to carboplatin and paclitaxel.

In addition, it should be noted that selected targeted therapies can be considered for second treatment as can be seen in the section below.

There is evidence of docetaxel, the other commonly used taxane, being effective as second- and third-line treatment of thymic carcinoma after failing cisplatin-containing chemotherapy. This raises the question of the contribution of carboplatin given together with paclitaxel or docetaxel after cisplatin failure. In a retrospective series from Japan, 13 thymic carcinoma patients received docetaxel monotherapy after becoming platinum refractory. Overall response rate was 31 % and disease control rate was 77 %. Overall survival after docetaxel monotherapy was 24 months, while progression-free survival was only 5.5 months suggesting that these patients benefited from other treatments after failing docetaxel [60].

Targeted Therapies

There are many different classes of agents tried in phase II trials for the treatment of TETs. It may be encouraging to find a certain response rate and a certain duration of response when using targeted therapies, but unless correlative studies are done simultaneously to understand why the responders are responding, we will miss the groups that will truly benefit from that agent, and perhaps worse, we will throw away a drug that will help some selected group of patients. This is particularly important for TETs, as they are such a heterogeneous group of tumors.

Currently, sunitinib is recommended among the choices for second-line treatment of thymic carcinomas and everolimus and octreotide, for both thymoma and thymic carcinomas [24, 37].

Somatostatin Receptor Analogs

Somatostatin is a naturally occurring peptide that inhibits the secretion of wide range of hormones [63]. The somatostatin analogs, octreotide, lanreotide, and their longer-acting depot forms, have played an important role in the treatment of neuroendocrine carcinomas, a tumor type that commonly overexpress somatostatin receptors [64].

A frequently overlooked fact is that somatostatin receptors are also overexpressed in non-neuroendocrine TETs, as well as in thymic neuroendocrine cancers (see the imaging section on radionuclide scintigraphy using radiolabeled octreotide). As early as in 1998, thymomas and thymic carcinomas were shown to have increased uptake by somatostatin receptor scintigraphy utilizing octreotide [27]. Somatostatin analogs, employed either alone or in combination with prednisone, were among the first targeted agents found to be active in TETs [65].

Octreotide

In 1997, successful treatment of a patient with thymoma and pure red cell aplasia with octreotide and prednisone was reported [65].

In 2002, a phase II study from Italy tested (Table **18.10**) treatment with somatostatin analogs and prednisone [66]. Octreotide (1.5 mg/day SC), and in some patients, the long-acting somatostatin analog lanreotide (30 mg every 14 days), was given with a relatively high dose of oral prednisone (0.6 mg/kg/day) for 3 months, to be followed by 0.2 mg/kg/day during follow-up. These were patients unresponsive to chemotherapy and response rate was impressive (CR 6 % and PR 31 %; only 25 % of the patients progressed during therapy). Median survival was 15 months and median time to progression was 14 months.

It was not clear whether octreotide had any contribution to these results. This was tested in a large ECOG phase II trial [67] which revealed that octreotide had some efficacy when used alone, but the results were better when combined with prednisone, though toxicity was higher as well (Table **18.10**). In this trial, all of the 32 patients with advanced thymoma and 6 patients with thymic carcinoma or carcinoid initially received octreotide alone. If, after 2 months of therapy, there was at least PR, octreotide was continued alone. If there was stable disease, then prednisone was also added. In the case of progressive disease, the patients were taken off the study. All patients in the study had increased uptake in radionuclide octreotide scan. More than 80 % of the patients previously received chemotherapy and radiotherapy. Overall response rate was 30.3 % (CR 5.3 % and PR 25 %) and 36.8 % of the patients had stable disease. The objective response rate among the patients treated with octreotide alone during the first 2 months was 10.5 %. The median PFS for octreotide alone was shorter (2 months; 95 % CI, 1.8–11.0 months) than that for patients treated with both octreotide and prednisone (9.2 months; 95 % CI, 8.1–13.9 months). The PFS was longer for patients with thymoma (8.8 months; 95 % CI, 3.7–12.3 months) than thymic carcinoma (4.5 months; 95 % CI, 1.9–9.5 months).

Longo et al. treated 11 relapsed thymoma patients and 1 patient with thymic carcinoma with long-acting octreotide (Sandostatin LAR ®) after a positive OctreoScan. Of note, 83 % received chemotherapy and 58 % received radiotherapy previously. Twenty-five percent of the patients achieved PR and 42 % had SD, which lasted a median of 41 months. The clinical benefit rate was 67 % and the median duration of clinical benefit (CR + PR + SD) was 47 months [68].

Radionuclide Treatment

Peptide receptor radioligand therapy has been used successfully against low-grade neuroendocrine tumors [69]. Encouraged by the fact that somatostatin receptors are also expressed by the majority of TETs, there are now case reports and anecdotal information that PRRT is effective in some patients with TETs, too [30, 70]. Somatostatin receptor subtype 3 was shown to be the predominant among the five somatostatin subtypes [71].

Pasireotide (SOM230) binds to SSRs 1, 2, 3, and 5. An ongoing phase II trial is currently evaluating the effect of pasireotide in a dosage of 60 mg IM every 4 weeks in adult patients with inoperable or metastatic T (Schalke NCT02021942).

mTOR: Everolimus

mTOR (mammalian target of rapamycin) is a serine/threonine kinase belonging to the PI3K/AKT signaling pathway. Activation of mTOR leads to an increase in protein synthesis, which is required for tumor growth. It is an important regulator of proliferation, response to hypoxia, and angiogenesis, and therefore it is an attractive target for cancer treatment [72].

In an exciting report from MD Anderson Cancer Center, results of ten patients with thymoma or thymic carcinoma treated in phase I trials with combinations containing mTOR inhibitors were reported. Sixty percent of these patients achieved stable disease ≥12 months or a partial response. Median time to treatment failure was 11.6 months versus 2.3 months on last conventional regimen prior to referral ($p=0.024$) [73].

In 2014, the initial results of the first 35 patients with thymoma and thymic carcinoma, all pretreated, enrolled in a phase II study, were presented (Table **18.10**). The disease control rate in patients with thymic carcinoma reached 67 %, with 8 % CR and 17 % PR. Responses were rare in thymoma (4 %), but disease stabilization was seen in 70 % of the patients. With a median follow-up of 10 months, median PFS was 12.1 months, while median OS was 24.0 months [74].

Finally, investigators at Gustave Roussy collectively reported on the outcomes of patients with TETs enrolled in various phase I trials. Results with temsirolimus, an mTOR inhibitor, appeared particularly encouraging. Among four patients, there were one CR, one PR, and two patients with SD [75]. These patients also received neratinib, an oral pan ErbB inhibitor which could be partly responsible from the response. However, at least one patient responded to temsirolimus after removal of neratinib suggesting that mTOR inhibitors alone could be effective.

Everolimus is now listed as an option for second-line treatment of TETs [24, 37].

Multi-targeted Tyrosine Kinase Inhibitors: Sunitinib

Sunitinib is an oral multi-targeted tyrosine kinase inhibitor. Its targets include VEGFR, KIT, and PDGFR among others [76]. It is the first targeted treatment that showed promise in the treatment of TETs, particularly thymic carcinoma [77], and now included among the standard second-line treatment options for thymic carcinoma [24, 37].

In 2010, responses to sunitinib in thymic squamous cell carcinomas were noted in a small number of patients [78]. In 2015, Thomas et al. reported the results of a phase II study with sunitinib on 39 patients (16 thymoma, 23 thymic carcinoma) with treatment refractory TETs (Table **18.10**). Eighty-one percent of the thymoma group and 58 % of thymic carcinoma group received at least two previous chemotherapy regimens. Partial responses were noted in 26 % and stable disease in 65 % of thymic carcinoma patients, and the median duration of response was an impressive 16.4 months. This was and still is an unprecedented result for treatment refractory thymic carcinoma. In contrast, only 6 % of thymoma patients achieved a partial response. This study established sunitinib as a standard second-line treatment for thymic carcinoma [77].

IGF-1R: Cixutumumab

Insulin-like growth factor-1 receptor (IGF-1R) is a transmembrane tyrosine kinase receptor that plays a role in the regulation of cell metabolism, growth, and survival. Thymomas and thymic carcinomas commonly stain positive for IGF-1R [79, 80]. The fully human monoclonal antibody cixutumumab binds and inactivates IGF-1R through internalization and degradation of the receptor [81]. Rajan et al. reported the results of a multicenter phase II study of cixutumumab (Table **18.10**) in previously treated advanced TETs (37 T, 12 TC) [82]. In these heavily pretreated patients, cixutumumab was well tolerated and active in the thymoma group. With a median follow-up of 24 months, the disease control rate was 89 %, and 14 % of patients experienced a partial remission with a median overall survival of 27.5 months. Tumor IFG-1R expression did not show a good correlation with response to treatment. A common side effect was autoimmune disorders. There were no responses among the thymic carcinoma group and the median time to progression was only 1.7 months.

Histone Deacetylase Inhibitor: Belinostat

In a phase I/II study, the histone deacetylase inhibitor belinostat was combined with chemotherapy containing cisplatin, doxorubicin, and cyclophosphamide, in treatment-naïve patients with TETs (thymoma, 12; thymic carcinoma, 14) (Table **18.10**). Objective response rates in thymoma and thymic carcinoma were 64 % and 21 %, respectively [83]. How do these results compare with response rates with chemotherapy alone? Clearly, it is never possible to reach a definitive conclusion by comparing the results of the past series, because of the differences in patient composition in different studies, but this is the only thing we can do at this time. The PAC chemotherapy regimen, which contains the same agents used together with belinostat but in a slightly different schedule and dose, achieved 50 % response rate in chemotherapy-naïve thymoma patients [48]. Prednisone added to this regimen achieved a response rate of 77 % as an induction chemotherapy, again in chemotherapy-naïve patients with thymoma [49]. Vincristine added to the PAC regimen, which makes it the ADOC regimen, achieved 92 % response rate in patients with thymoma [47], and 50–75 % response rate in patients with thymic carcinoma [53, 56]. These results from past series suggest that the addition of belinostat to chemotherapy backbone containing cisplatin, doxorubicin, and cyclophosphamide may not be particularly encouraging when all TETs are considered together. Whether there are groups of patients selectively benefiting from belinostat is not known yet. Of note, one of the largest phase II trials on targeted agents tested single-agent belinostat in 41 patients with advanced treatment refractory TETs ($T=25$, $TC=16$). Patients with thymoma had a not-so-exciting response rate of 8 %, but a promising TTP of 11.4 months and 2-year survival of 66 % [83, 84].

c-KIT and PDGFR: Imatinib

Imatinib did not show encouraging results in phase II studies [85–87]. In these studies, none of the patients harbored c-KIT mutations, and the presence of c-KIT overexpression did not correlate with response. No radiological response or disease stabilization was seen.

It is important to note that there are case reports of prolonged stable disease and tumor response with imatinib in patients with thymic carcinoma and c-KIT mutation [88–90]. However, c-KIT mutations are a rare finding in thymic carcinoma and even rarer in thymoma, while c-KIT expression is much more common [80].

Anti-PD1 Treatments

It was shown that programmed cell death 1 ligand (PD-L1) expression was found in 70 % of thymic carcinomas but only in 23 % of thymomas [91]. Furthermore, immunoregulatory responses in blood lymphocytes of patients with thymic carcinoma treated with sunitinib were noted to have prognostic relevance suggesting that immune response might play a role in the treatment of thymic carcinoma, perhaps even in combination with sunitinib [92].

Based on this finding, and after encouraging results achieved with anti-PD1 treatments in a wide variety of cancers including lung, colon, stomach, liver, kidney, and urothelial cancers, as well as melanoma, and Hodgkin lymphoma, at the time of this writing, a trial is currently enrolling patients with thymic carcinoma for treatment with pembrolizumab (https://clinicaltrials.gov/ct2/show/NCT02364076).

EGFR and VEGF: Gefitinib, Erlotinib, and Bevacizumab

With gefitinib [93], and erlotinib + bevacizumab [94], clinically meaningful responses were not observed, but disease stabilization was seen in some patients.

Src Inhibitor: Saracatinib

The Src family of kinases plays a role in normal thymic development as well as in the carcinogenesis of other epithelial tumors. A phase II study of saracatinib (AZD0530), an oral Src inhibitor in patients with advanced thymoma, or thymic carcinoma, did not produce any responses [95]. The median time to progression was only 5.7 and 3.6 months for thymoma and thymic carcinoma patients, respectively.

References

1. Engels EA. Epidemiology of thymoma and associated malignancies. J Thorac Oncol. 2010;5(10 Suppl 4):S260–5.
2. Rice TW, Blackstone EH. Rarest of a rare disease: challenges in advancing our knowledge of thymic carcinoma. J Thorac Cardiovasc Surg. 2015;149(1):101–2.
3. Detterbeck FC. The international thymic malignancy interest group. J Natl Compr Cancer Netw. 2013;11(5):589–93.
4. Huang J, Detterbeck FC, Wang Z, Loehrer PJ. Standard outcome measures for thymic malignancies. J Thorac Oncol. 2011;6(7 Suppl 3):S1691–7.
5. Detterbeck FC, Moran C, Huang J, Suster S, Walsh G, Kaiser L, Wick M. Which way is up? Policies and procedures for surgeons and pathologists regarding resection specimens of thymic malignancy. J Thorac Oncol. 2011;6(7 Suppl 3):S1730–8.
6. Detterbeck FC, Nicholson AG, Kondo K, Van Schil P, Moran C. The masaoka-koga stage classification for thymic malignancies: classification and definition of terms. J Thorac Oncol. 2011;6(7 Suppl 3):S1710–6.

7. Marom EM, Rosado-de-Christenson ML, Bruzzi JF, Hara M, Sonett JR, Ketai L. Standard report terms for chest computed tomography reports of anterior mediastinal masses suspicious for thymoma. J Thorac Oncol. 2011;6(7 Suppl 3):S1717–23.
8. Detterbeck F, Youssef S, Ruffini E, Okumura M. A review of prognostic factors in thymic malignancies. J Thorac Oncol. 2011;6(7 Suppl 3):S1698–704.
9. Toker A, Sonett J, Zielinski M, Rea F, Tomulescu V, Detterbeck FC. Standard terms, definitions, and policies for minimally invasive resection of thymoma. J Thorac Oncol. 2011; 6(7 Suppl 3):S1739–42.
10. Gomez D, Komaki R, Yu J, Ikushima H, Bezjak A. Radiation therapy definitions and reporting guidelines for thymic malignancies. J Thorac Oncol. 2011;6(7 Suppl 3):S1743–8.
11. Girard N, Lal R, Wakelee H, Riely GJ, Loehrer PJ. Chemotherapy definitions and policies for thymic malignancies. J Thorac Oncol. 2011;6(7 Suppl 3):S1749–55.
12. Detterbeck FC, Stratton K, Giroux D, Asamura H, Crowley J, Falkson C, et al. The IASLC/ITMIG thymic epithelial tumors staging project: proposal for an evidence-based stage classification system for the forthcoming (8th) edition of the TNM classification of malignant tumors. J Thorac Oncol. 2014;9(9 Suppl 2):S65–72.
13. Nicholson AG, Detterbeck FC, Marino M, Kim J, Stratton K, Giroux D, et al. The IASLC/ITMIG thymic epithelial tumors staging project: proposals for the T component for the forthcoming (8th) edition of the TNM classification of malignant tumors. J Thorac Oncol. 2014;9(9 Suppl 2):S73–80.
14. Kondo K, Van Schil P, Detterbeck FC, Okumura M, Stratton K, Giroux D, et al. The IASLC/ITMIG thymic epithelial tumors staging project: proposals for the N and M components for the forthcoming (8th) edition of the TNM classification of malignant tumors. J Thorac Oncol. 2014;9(9 Suppl 2):S81–7.
15. Bhora FY, Chen DJ, Detterbeck FC, Asamura H, Falkson C, Filosso PL, et al. The ITMIG/IASLC thymic epithelial tumors staging project: a proposed lymph node map for thymic epithelial tumors in the forthcoming 8th edition of the TNM classification of malignant tumors. J Thorac Oncol. 2014;9(9 Suppl 2):S88–96.
16. Benveniste MF, Korst RJ, Rajan A, Detterbeck FC, Marom EM, International Thymic Malignancy Interest Group. A practical guide from the international thymic malignancy interest group (ITMIG) regarding the radiographic assessment of treatment response of thymic epithelial tumors using modified RECIST criteria. J Thorac Oncol. 2014;9(9 Suppl 2): S119–24.
17. den Bakker MA, Roden AC, Marx A, Marino M. Histologic classification of thymoma: a practical guide for routine cases. J Thorac Oncol. 2014;9(9 Suppl 2):S125–30.
18. Rajan A, Girard N, Marx A. State of the art of genetic alterations in thymic epithelial tumors. J Thorac Oncol. 2014;9(9 Suppl 2):S131–6.
19. Weksler B, Lu B. Alterations of the immune system in thymic malignancies. J Thorac Oncol. 2014;9(9 Suppl 2):S137–42.
20. Evoli A, Lancaster E. Paraneoplastic disorders in thymoma patients. J Thorac Oncol. 2014;9(9 Suppl 2):S143–7.
21. Carter BW, Tomiyama N, Bhora FY, de Rosado CML, Nakajima J, Boiselle PM. A modern definition of mediastinal compartments. J Thorac Oncol. 2014;9(9 Suppl 2): S97–101.
22. Carter BW, Marom EM, Detterbeck FC. Approaching the patient with an anterior mediastinal mass: a guide for clinicians. J Thorac Oncol. 2014;9(9 Suppl 2):S102–9.
23. Carter BW, Okumura M, Detterbeck FC, Marom EM. Approaching the patient with an anterior mediastinal mass: a guide for radiologists. J Thorac Oncol. 2014;9(9 Suppl 2): S110–8.
24. Girard N, Ruffini E, Marx A, Faivre-Finn C, Peters S, ESMO Guidelines Committee. Thymic epithelial tumours: ESMO clinical practice guidelines for diagnosis, treatment and follow-up†. Ann Oncol. 2015;26 Suppl 5:v40–55.
25. Korst RJ, Bezjak A, Blackmon S, Choi N, Fidias P, Liu G, et al. Neoadjuvant chemoradiotherapy for locally advanced thymic tumors: a phase II, multi-institutional clinical trial. J Thorac Cardiovasc Surg. 2014;147(1):36–44, 46.e1.

26. Treglia G, Sadeghi R, Giovanella L, Cafarotti S, Filosso P, Lococo F. Is (18)F-FDG PET useful in predicting the WHO grade of malignancy in thymic epithelial tumors? A meta-analysis. Lung Cancer. 2014;86(1):5–13.
27. Lastoria S, Vergara E, Palmieri G, Acampa W, Varrella P, Caracò C, et al. In vivo detection of malignant thymic masses by indium-111-dtpa-d-phe1-octreotide scintigraphy. J Nucl Med. 1998;39(4):634–9.
28. Guidoccio F, Grosso M, Maccauro M, Orsini F, Perri M, Boni G, et al. Current role of 111in-dtpa-octreotide scintigraphy in diagnosis of thymic masses. Tumori. 2011;97(2):191–5.
29. De Luca S, Fonti R, Palmieri G, Federico P, Del Prete G, Pacelli R, et al. Combined imaging with 18F-FDG-PET/CT and 111in-labeled octreotide SPECT for evaluation of thymic epithelial tumors. Clin Nucl Med. 2013;38(5):354–8.
30. Makis W, McCann K, McEwan AJ. Thymoma treated with 177lu DOTATATE induction and maintenance PRRT. Clin Nucl Med. 2015;40(5):e278–81.
31. Hofman MS, Kong G, Neels OC, Eu P, Hong E, Hicks RJ. High management impact of ga-68 DOTATATE (gatate) PET/CT for imaging neuroendocrine and other somatostatin expressing tumours. J Med Imaging Radiat Oncol. 2012;56(1):40–7.
32. Marchevsky AM, Wick MR. Controversies in the pathology of thymoma viewed through the prism of evidence-based pathology. Oncology (Williston Park). 2012;26(10):982–4.
33. Detterbeck FC. Clinical value of the WHO classification system of thymoma. Ann Thorac Surg. 2006;81(6):2328–34.
34. Okumura M, Ohta M, Tateyama H, Nakagawa K, Matsumura A, Maeda H, et al. The world health organization histologic classification system reflects the oncologic behavior of thymoma: a clinical study of 273 patients. Cancer. 2002;94(3):624–32.
35. Falkson CB, Bezjak A, Darling G, Gregg R, Malthaner R, Maziak DE, et al. The management of thymoma: a systematic review and practice guideline. J Thorac Oncol. 2009;4(7):911–9.
36. Girard N, Mornex F, Van Houtte P, Cordier JF, van Schil P. Thymoma: a focus on current therapeutic management. J Thorac Oncol. 2009;4(1):119–26.
37. NCCN clinical practice guidelines in oncology. Accessed 31 Oct 2015.
38. Ruffini E, Detterbeck F, Van Raemdonck D, Rocco G, Thomas P, Weder W, et al. Thymic carcinoma: a cohort study of patients from the European society of thoracic surgeons database. J Thorac Oncol. 2014;9(4):541–8.
39. Weksler B, Pennathur A, Sullivan JL, Nason KS. Resection of thymoma should include nodal sampling. J Thorac Cardiovasc Surg. 2015;149(3):737–42.
40. Yamada Y, Yoshino I, Nakajima J, Miyoshi S, Ohnuki T, Suzuki M, et al. Surgical outcomes of patients with stage III thymoma in the japanese nationwide database. Ann Thorac Surg. 2015;100(3):961–7.
41. Kunitoh H, Tamura T, Shibata T, Takeda K, Katakami N, Nakagawa K, et al. A phase II trial of dose-dense chemotherapy, followed by surgical resection and/or thoracic radiotherapy, in locally advanced thymoma: report of a Japan clinical oncology group trial (JCOG 9606). Br J Cancer. 2010;103(1):6–11.
42. Hamaji M, Burt BM. Long-term outcomes of surgical and nonsurgical management of stage IV thymoma: a population-based analysis of 282 patients. Semin Thorac Cardiovasc Surg. 2015;27(1):1–3.
43. Hamaji M, Kojima F, Omasa M, Sozu T, Sato T, Chen F, et al. A meta-analysis of debulking surgery versus surgical biopsy for unresectable thymoma. Eur J Cardiothorac Surg. 2015;47(4):602–7.
44. Hishida T, Nomura S, Yano M, Asamura H, Yamashita M, Ohde Y, et al. Long-term outcome and prognostic factors of surgically treated thymic carcinoma: Results of 306 cases from a Japanese nationwide database study. Eur J Cardiothorac Surg. 2016;49(3):835–41.
45. Wright CD, Choi NC, Wain JC, Mathisen DJ, Lynch TJ, Fidias P. Induction chemoradiotherapy followed by resection for locally advanced masaoka stage III and IVA thymic tumors. Ann Thorac Surg. 2008;85(2):385–9.
46. Safieddine N, Liu G, Cuningham K, Ming T, Hwang D, Brade A, et al. Prognostic factors for cure, recurrence and long-term survival after surgical resection of thymoma. J Thorac Oncol. 2014;9(7):1018–22.

47. Fornasiero A, Daniele O, Ghiotto C, Piazza M, Fiore-Donati L, Calabró F, et al. Chemotherapy for invasive thymoma. A 13-year experience. Cancer. 1991;68(1):30–3.
48. Loehrer PJ, Kim K, Aisner SC, Livingston R, Einhorn LH, Johnson D, Blum R. Cisplatin plus doxorubicin plus cyclophosphamide in metastatic or recurrent thymoma: final results of an intergroup trial. The eastern cooperative oncology group, southwest oncology group, and southeastern cancer study group. J Clin Oncol. 1994;12(6):1164–8.
49. Kim JH, Kim BH, Kim YW, Park JC, Jung YH, Lee BO, et al. Autoimmune cholangitis in a patient with thymoma. J Gastroenterol Hepatol. 2004;19(11):1324–7.
50. Giaccone G, Ardizzoni A, Kirkpatrick A, Clerico M, Sahmoud T, van Zandwijk N. Cisplatin and etoposide combination chemotherapy for locally advanced or metastatic thymoma. A phase II study of the european organization for research and treatment of cancer lung cancer cooperative group. J Clin Oncol. 1996;14(3):814–20.
51. Loehrer PJ, Jiroutek M, Aisner S, Aisner J, Green M, Thomas CR, et al. Combined etoposide, ifosfamide, and cisplatin in the treatment of patients with advanced thymoma and thymic carcinoma: an intergroup trial. Cancer. 2001;91(11):2010–5.
52. Lemma GL, Lee JW, Aisner SC, Langer CJ, Tester WJ, Johnson DH, Loehrer PJ. Phase II study of carboplatin and paclitaxel in advanced thymoma and thymic carcinoma. J Clin Oncol. 2011;29(15):2060–5.
53. Koizumi T, Takabayashi Y, Yamagishi S, Tsushima K, Takamizawa A, Tsukadaira A, et al. Chemotherapy for advanced thymic carcinoma: clinical response to cisplatin, doxorubicin, vincristine, and cyclophosphamide (ADOC chemotherapy). Am J Clin Oncol. 2002;25(3):266–8.
54. Okuma Y, Saito M, Hosomi Y, Sakuyama T, Okamura T. Key components of chemotherapy for thymic malignancies: a systematic review and pooled analysis for anthracycline-, carboplatin- or cisplatin-based chemotherapy. J Cancer Res Clin Oncol. 2015;141(2): 323–31.
55. Liang Y, Padda SK, Riess JW, West RB, Neal JW, Wakelee HA. Pemetrexed in patients with thymic malignancies previously treated with chemotherapy. Lung Cancer. 2015; 87(1):34–8.
56. Agatsuma T, Koizumi T, Kanda S, Ito M, Urushihata K, Yamamoto H, et al. Combination chemotherapy with doxorubicin, vincristine, cyclophosphamide, and platinum compounds for advanced thymic carcinoma. J Thorac Oncol. 2011;6(12):2130–4.
57. Palmieri G, Merola G, Federico P, Petillo L, Marino M, Lalle M, et al. Preliminary results of phase II study of capecitabine and gemcitabine (CAP-GEM) in patients with metastatic pretreated thymic epithelial tumors (tets). Ann Oncol. 2010;21(6):1168–72.
58. Palmieri G, Buonerba C, Ottaviano M, Federico P, Calabrese F, Von Arx C, et al. Capecitabine plus gemcitabine in thymic epithelial tumors: final analysis of a phase II trial. Future Oncol. 2014;10(14):2141–7.
59. Furugen M, Sekine I, Tsuta K, Horinouchi H, Nokihara H, Yamamoto N, et al. Combination chemotherapy with carboplatin and paclitaxel for advanced thymic cancer. Jpn J Clin Oncol. 2011;41(8):1013–6.
60. Watanabe N, Umemura S, Niho S, Kirita K, Matsumoto S, Yoh K, et al. Docetaxel for platinum-refractory advanced thymic carcinoma. Jpn J Clin Oncol. 2015;45(7):665–9.
61. Loehrer PJ, Yiannoutsos CT, Dropcho S, Burns M, Helft P, Chiorean EG, Nelson RP. A phase II trial of pemetrexed in patients with recurrent thymoma or thymic carcinoma. ASCO Meet Abstr. 2006;24(18_Suppl):7079.
62. Kaira K, Naruse I, Imai H, Sunaga N, Hisada T, Motegi M, et al. Dramatic response of S-1 administration to chemorefractory advanced thymic cancer. Chemotherapy. 2015; 60(5–6):356–9.
63. Lamberts SW, van der Lely AJ, de Herder WW, Hofland LJ. Octreotide. N Engl J Med. 1996;334(4):246–54.
64. Kunz PL, Reidy-Lagunes D, Anthony LB, Bertino EM, Brendtro K, Chan JA, et al. Consensus guidelines for the management and treatment of neuroendocrine tumors. Pancreas. 2013;42(4):557–77.

65. Palmieri G, Lastoria S, Colao A, Vergara E, Varrella P, Biondi E, et al. Successful treatment of a patient with a thymoma and pure red-cell aplasia with octreotide and prednisone. N Engl J Med. 1997;336(4):263–5.
66. Palmieri G, Montella L, Martignetti A, Muto P, Di Vizio D, De Chiara A, Lastoria S. Somatostatin analogs and prednisone in advanced refractory thymic tumors. Cancer. 2002;94(5):1414–20.
67. Loehrer PJ, Wang W, Johnson DH, Aisner SC, Ettinger DS. Eastern Cooperative Oncology Group Phase II Trial. Octreotide alone or with prednisone in patients with advanced thymoma and thymic carcinoma: an eastern cooperative oncology group phase II trial. J Clin Oncol. 2004;22(2):293–9.
68. Longo F, De Filippis L, Zivi A, Vitolo D, Del Signore E, Gori B, et al. Efficacy and tolerability of long-acting octreotide in the treatment of thymic tumors: results of a pilot trial. Am J Clin Oncol. 2012;35(2):105–9.
69. Kwekkeboom DJ, de Herder WW, Kam BL, van Eijck CH, van Essen M, Kooij PP, et al. Treatment with the radiolabeled somatostatin analog [177 lu-dota 0, tyr3]octreotate: toxicity, efficacy, and survival. J Clin Oncol. 2008;26(13):2124–30.
70. Vasamiliette J, Hohenberger P, Schoenberg S, Diehl S, Dinter DJ, Marx A, et al. Treatment monitoring with 18F-FDG PET in metastatic thymoma after 90y-dotatoc and selective internal radiation treatment (SIRT). Hell J Nucl Med. 2009;12(3):271–3.
71. Ferone D, van Hagen MP, Kwekkeboom DJ, van Koetsveld PM, Mooy DM, Lichtenauer-Kaligis E, et al. Somatostatin receptor subtypes in human thymoma and inhibition of cell proliferation by octreotide in vitro. J Clin Endocrinol Metab. 2000;85(4):1719–26.
72. Dancey J. MTOR signaling and drug development in cancer. Nat Rev Clin Oncol. 2010;7(4):209–19.
73. Wheler J, Hong D, Swisher SG, Falchook G, Tsimberidou AM, Helgason T, et al. Thymoma patients treated in a phase I clinic at MD Anderson cancer center: responses to mtor inhibitors and molecular analyses. Oncotarget. 2013;4(6):890–8.
74. Zucali PA, De Pas TM, Palmieri G, Favaretto AG, Chella A, Tiseo M, et al. Phase II study of everolimus in patients with thymoma and thymic carcinoma previously treated with cisplatin-based chemotherapy. ASCO Meet Abstr. 2014;32(15_Suppl):7527.
75. Kossai M, Duchemann B, Boutros C, Caramella C, Hollebecque A, Angevin E, et al. Antitumor activity in advanced cancer patients with thymic malignancies enrolled in early clinical drug development programs (phase I trials) at gustave roussy. Lung Cancer. 2015;89(3):306–10.
76. O'Farrell AM, Abrams TJ, Yuen HA, Ngai TJ, Louie SG, Yee KW, et al. SU11248 is a novel FLT3 tyrosine kinase inhibitor with potent activity in vitro and in vivo. Blood. 2003;101(9):3597–605.
77. Thomas A, Rajan A, Berman A, Tomita Y, Brzezniak C, Lee MJ, et al. Sunitinib in patients with chemotherapy-refractory thymoma and thymic carcinoma: an open-label phase 2 trial. Lancet Oncol. 2015;16(2):177–86.
78. Ströbel P, Bargou R, Wolff A, Spitzer D, Manegold C, Dimitrakopoulou-Strauss A, et al. Sunitinib in metastatic thymic carcinomas: laboratory findings and initial clinical experience. Br J Cancer. 2010;103(2):196–200.
79. Girard N, Teruya-Feldstein J, Payabyab EC, Riely GJ, Rusch VW, Kris MG, Zakowski MF. Insulin-like growth factor-1 receptor expression in thymic malignancies. J Thorac Oncol. 2010;5(9):1439–46.
80. Petrini I, Zucali PA, Lee HS, Pineda MA, Meltzer PS, Walter-Rodriguez B, et al. Expression and mutational status of c-kit in thymic epithelial tumors. J Thorac Oncol. 2010;5(9):1447–53.
81. Simonelli M, Zucali PA, Suter MB, Lorenzi E, Rubino L, Fatuzzo G, et al. Targeted therapy for thymic epithelial tumors: a new horizon? Review of the literature and two cases reports. Future Oncol. 2015;11(8):1223–32.
82. Rajan A, Carter CA, Berman A, Cao L, Kelly RJ, Thomas A, et al. Cixutumumab for patients with recurrent or refractory advanced thymic epithelial tumours: a multicentre, open-label, phase 2 trial. Lancet Oncol. 2014;15(2):191–200.

83. Thomas A, Rajan A, Szabo E, Tomita Y, Carter CA, Scepura B, et al. A phase I/II trial of belinostat in combination with cisplatin, doxorubicin, and cyclophosphamide in thymic epithelial tumors: a clinical and translational study. Clin Cancer Res. 2014;20(21): 5392–402.
84. Giaccone G, Rajan A, Berman A, Kelly RJ, Szabo E, Lopez-Chavez A, et al. Phase II study of belinostat in patients with recurrent or refractory advanced thymic epithelial tumors. J Clin Oncol. 2011;29(15):2052–9.
85. Salter JT, Lewis D, Yiannoutsos C, Loehrer PJ, Risley L, Chiorean EG. Imatinib for the treatment of thymic carcinoma. ASCO Meet Abstr. 2008;26(15_Suppl):8116.
86. Giaccone G, Smit EF, van Groeningen C, Hogedoorn PC. Phase II study of imatinib in patients with WHO B3 and C thymomas. ASCO Meet Abstr. 2008;26(15_Suppl):14665.
87. Palmieri G, Buonerba C, Federico P, Formisano L, Nappi L, Di Lorenzo G, et al. Everolimus plus long-acting somatostatin analogs in thymic epithelial malignancies. World J Clin Oncol. 2012;3(7):111–5.
88. Hagemann IS, Govindan R, Javidan-Nejad C, Pfeifer JD, Cottrell CE. Stabilization of disease after targeted therapy in a thymic carcinoma with KIT mutation detected by clinical next-generation sequencing. J Thorac Oncol. 2014;9(2):e12–6.
89. Lim SH, Lee JY, Sun JM, Kim KM, Ahn JS, Ahn MJ, Park K. A new KIT gene mutation in thymic cancer and a promising response to imatinib. J Thorac Oncol. 2013; 8(10):e91–2.
90. Buti S, Donini M, Sergio P, Garagnani L, Schirosi L, Passalacqua R, Rossi G. Impressive response with imatinib in a heavily pretreated patient with metastatic c-kit mutated thymic carcinoma. J Clin Oncol. 2011;29(33):e803–5.
91. Katsuya Y, Fujita Y, Horinouchi H, Ohe Y, Watanabe S, Tsuta K. Immunohistochemical status of PD-L1 in thymoma and thymic carcinoma. Lung Cancer. 2015;88(2):154–9.
92. Marx A, Weis CA. Sunitinib in thymic carcinoma: enigmas still unresolved. Lancet Oncol. 2015;16(2):124–5.
93. Kurup A, Burns M, Dropcho S, Pao W, Loehrer PJ. Phase II study of gefitinib treatment in advanced thymic malignancies. ASCO Meet Abstr. 2005;23(16_Suppl):7068.
94. Bedano PM, Perkins S, Burns M, Kessler K, Nelson R, Schneider BP, et al. A phase II trial of erlotinib plus bevacizumab in patients with recurrent thymoma or thymic carcinoma. ASCO Meet Abstr. 2008;26(15_Suppl):19087.
95. Gubens MA, Burns M, Perkins SM, Pedro-Salcedo MS, Althouse SK, Loehrer PJ, Wakelee HA. A phase II study of saracatinib (AZD0530), a src inhibitor, administered orally daily to patients with advanced thymic malignancies. Lung Cancer. 2015;89(1):57–60.
96. Tumours of the thymus. In: Travis WD, Brambilla E, Müller-Hermelink HK, Harris CC, editors. World Health Organization Classification of Tumours: tumours of the lung, pleura, thymus and heart. Lyon: IARC Press; 2004.
97. Macchiarini P, Chella A, Ducci F, Rossi B, Testi C, Bevilacqua G, Angeletti CA. Neoadjuvant chemotherapy, surgery, and postoperative radiation therapy for invasive thymoma. Cancer. 1991;68(4):706–13.
98. Rea F, Sartori F, Loy M, Calabrò F, Fornasiero A, Daniele O, Altavilla G. Chemotherapy and operation for invasive thymoma. J Thorac Cardiovasc Surg. 1993;106(3):543–9.
99. Shin DM, Walsh GL, Komaki R, Putnam JB, Nesbitt J, Ro JY, et al. A multidisciplinary approach to therapy for unresectable malignant thymoma. Ann Intern Med. 1998;129(2): 100–4.
100. Kim ES, Putnam JB, Komaki R, Walsh GL, Ro JY, Shin HJ, et al. Phase II study of a multidisciplinary approach with induction chemotherapy, followed by surgical resection, radiation therapy, and consolidation chemotherapy for unresectable malignant thymomas: final report. Lung Cancer. 2004;44(3):369–79.
101. Park S, Ahn MJ, Ahn JS, Sun JM, Shim YM, Kim J, et al. A prospective phase II trial of induction chemotherapy with docetaxel/cisplatin for masaoka stage III/IV thymic epithelial tumors. J Thorac Oncol. 2013;8(7):959–66.

102. Kawasaki H, Taira N, Ichi T, Yohena T, Kawabata T, Ishikawa K. Weekly chemotherapy with cisplatin, vincristine, doxorubicin, and etoposide followed by surgery for thymic carcinoma. Eur J Surg Oncol. 2014;40(9):1151–5.
103. Hirai F, Yamanaka T, Taguchi K, Daga H, Ono A, Tanaka K, et al. A multicenter phase II study of carboplatin and paclitaxel for advanced thymic carcinoma: WJOG4207L. Ann Oncol. 2015;26(2):363–8.
104. Igawa S, Murakami H, Takahashi T, Nakamura Y, Tsuya A, Naito T, et al. Efficacy of chemotherapy with carboplatin and paclitaxel for unresectable thymic carcinoma. Lung Cancer. 2010;67(2):194–7.
105. Loehrer PJ, Chen M, Kim K, Aisner SC, Einhorn LH, Livingston R, Johnson D. Cisplatin, doxorubicin, and cyclophosphamide plus thoracic radiation therapy for limited-stage unresectable thymoma: an intergroup trial. J Clin Oncol. 1997;15(9):3093–9.
106. Kunitoh H, Tamura T, Shibata T, Nakagawa K, Takeda K, Nishiwaki Y, et al. A phase-ii trial of dose-dense chemotherapy in patients with disseminated thymoma: report of a Japan clinical oncology group trial (JCOG 9605). Br J Cancer. 2009;101(9):1549–54.
107. Tamiya A, Matsumura A, Tsuji T, Morimoto M, Asami K, Okishio K, et al. A pilot study of cisplatin and etoposide with and without radiotherapy for advanced malignant thymoma. Anticancer Res. 2014;34(4):2023–7.
108. Highley MS, Underhill CR, Parnis FX, Karapetis C, Rankin E, Dussek J, et al. Treatment of invasive thymoma with single-agent ifosfamide. J Clin Oncol. 1999;17(9):2737–44.
109. Yoh K, Goto K, Ishii G, Niho S, Ohmatsu H, Kubota K, et al. Weekly chemotherapy with cisplatin, vincristine, doxorubicin, and etoposide is an effective treatment for advanced thymic carcinoma. Cancer. 2003;98(5):926–31.
110. Okuma Y, Hosomi Y, Takagi Y, Iguchi M, Okamura T, Shibuya M. Cisplatin and irinotecan combination chemotherapy for advanced thymic carcinoma: evaluation of efficacy and toxicity. Lung Cancer. 2011;74(3):492–6.
111. Komatsu Y, Koizumi T, Tanabe T, Hatayama O, Yasuo M, Okada M, et al. Salvage chemotherapy with carboplatin and paclitaxel for cisplatin-resistant thymic carcinoma – three cases. Anticancer Res. 2006;26(6C):4851–5.
112. Watanabe K, Shinkai M, Goto H, Yoshikawa S, Yamaguchi N, Hara Y, et al. Chemotherapy with carboplatin and paclitaxel after failure of primary chemotherapy for advanced thymic carcinoma. A report of three cases and review of the literature. Tumori. 2013;99(4):e172–6.
113. Song Z, Zhang Y. Outcomes after surgical resection of thymic carcinoma: a study from a single tertiary referral centre. Eur J Surg Oncol. 2014;40(11):1523–7.
114. Kanda S, Koizumi T, Komatsu Y, Yoshikawa S, Okada M, Hatayama O, et al. Second-line chemotherapy of platinum compound plus CPT-11 following ADOC chemotherapy in advanced thymic carcinoma: analysis of seven cases. Anticancer Res. 2007; 27(4C):3005–8.
115. Koizumi T, Agatsuma T, Ichiyama T, Yokoyama T, Ushiki A, Komatsu Y, et al. Salvage chemotherapy with amrubicin and platinum for relapsed thymic carcinoma: experience in six cases. Med Oncol. 2010;27(2):392–6.
116. Hirai F, Seto T, Yamanaka T, Toyozawa R, Inamasu E, Kojo M, et al. Amrubicin as second-line and beyond treatment for platinum-refractory advanced thymic carcinoma. Jpn J Clin Oncol. 2013;43(10):1018–22.
117. Oshita F, Kasai T, Kurata T, Fukuda M, Yamamoto N, Ohe Y, et al. Intensive chemotherapy with cisplatin, doxorubicin, cyclophosphamide, etoposide and granulocyte colony-stimulating factor for advanced thymoma or thymic cancer: preliminary results. Jpn J Clin Oncol. 1995;25(5):208–12.
118. Grassin F, Paleiron N, André M, Caliandro R, Bretel JJ, Terrier P, et al. Combined etoposide, ifosfamide, and cisplatin in the treatment of patients with advanced thymoma and thymic carcinoma. A French experience. J Thorac Oncol. 2010;5(6):893–7.
119. Marchevsky AM, Wick MR, editors. Pathology of the Mediastinum. Cambridge University Press; 2014. p. 271).

Target Volume Delineation Guidelines in Malignant Pleural Mesothelioma

19

Gokhan Ozyigit, Pervin Hurmuz, Sezin Yuce Sari, Gozde Yazici, and Melis Gultekin

Introduction

Trimodality treatment, i.e., surgery, chemotherapy (CXT), and radiotherapy (RT), should be administered to medically fit patients with early-stage malignant pleural mesothelioma (MPM) in order to increase both local control and overall survival [1, 2]. In the conventional RT technique, the whole ipsilateral hemithorax is irradiated including all drain sites. However, this large field significantly increases the toxicity rate if curative doses are considered to be given. With innovative techniques such as intensity-modulated RT (IMRT) and arc therapies, critical structures can be protected more easily. There is no published delineation guideline for the RT treatment of MPM. However, some authors have recommended target volume delineation tips with regard to the local recurrence pattern of MPM.

Patient Simulation

The patient is immobilized with a wing board with T- or U-bar handgrip and a headrest on the computed tomography (CT) in the supine position. The scanning should be performed from the middle of the neck to the anterior superior iliac spine in order to observe both kidneys. It is clearly known that MPM has a tendency to recur at previous instrumentation sites [3]. Therefore, all drain sites should be included in the planning CT scanning. In case laparoscopy or mediastinoscopy was performed during staging and was negative, there is no need to include the port sites in the

G. Ozyigit, MD • P. Hurmuz, MD • S.Y. Sari, MD (✉) • G. Yazici, MD • M. Gultekin, MD
Department of Radiation Oncology, Faculty of Medicine, Hacettepe University, Ankara, Turkey
e-mail: gozyigit@hacettepe.edu.tr; phurmuz@yahoo.com; sezin_yuce@hotmail.com; yazicig@hacettepe.edu.tr; melisbahadir@yahoo.com

G. Ozyigit et al. (eds.), *Principles and Practice of Radiotherapy Techniques in Thoracic Malignancies*, DOI 10.1007/978-3-319-28761-4_19

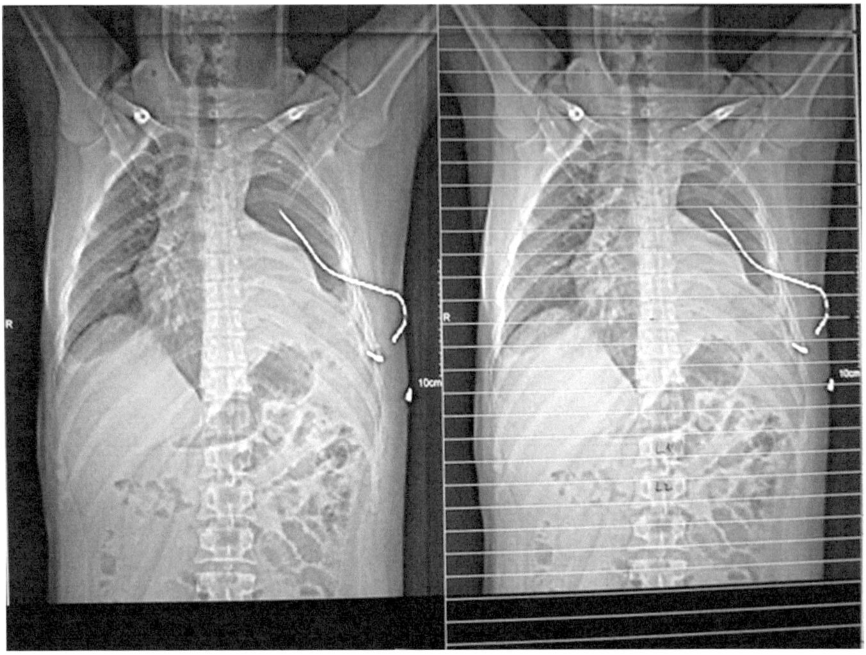

Fig. 19.1 Radiopaque wires can be used in the simulation process to identify the drain sites and surgical incisions

clinical target volume (CTV) and so in the CT scanning. Radiopaque wires can be used to identify the drain sites and surgical incisions more easily while delineating (Fig. 19.1).

Target Volume Delineation

Planning CT is used for all patients; however, fusion of the images with other diagnostic images is strongly recommended. Pehlivan et al. showed that adding positron emission tomography (PET)/CT-based delineation significantly decreased the mean gross tumor volume (GTV), CTV, and planning target volume (PTV); and this reduction was related to target volume reductions rather than nodal disease [4]. Therefore, it is recommended to take PET/CT images into account while delineating the target volumes of a patient with MPM.

The ipsilateral hemithorax and mediastinum should be included in the CTV because of the high incidence of mediastinal nodal involvement even the patient has N0 disease [5, 6]. The delineation starts from the thoracic inlet at the superior and should include the ipsilateral diaphragm at the inferior. The level of the diaphragm is variable and extra caution is needed for respiratory motion (see Chap. 3 for details on respiratory motion tracking). It is recommended that the location of the insertion of the diaphragm should be marked with radiopaque clips during surgery or suturing the "neodiaphragm" in its new position in order to guide the radiation oncologist in target delineation [7, 8]. The differentiation of the liver from pleural effusion can sometimes be troublesome; using radiopaque patches during the reconstruction of the diaphragm can facilitate making the distinction between these structures.

The medial border should include ipsilateral mediastinal lymph nodes (LNs) with the subcarinal region and trachea or should extend to the contralateral border of vertebral bodies [7, 8]. As there was no recurrence observed in the posterior mediastinal structures behind the heart, they are not necessarily contoured [6]. The anteromedial pleural space can sometimes extend to the contralateral hemithorax, and the anatomy can be destroyed during surgery. As the anteromedial pleural reflection should be included in the CTV because of marginal recurrences, this space should be defined with radiopaque clips in the intraoperative setting. On the other hand, the same space can be observed on preoperative CT scans, and its new position can be estimated on the planning CT scan. The identification of the medial border of the diaphragm crus, particularly at the inferior, can also be difficult. This region can be more easily visualized when surgical radiopaque clips are placed. In other words, the inferior border of the diaphragm, the anteromedial pleural reflection, and the diaphragm crus are the most difficult regions for accurate delineation (Fig. 19.2).

All sites of drains and ports should be included in the CTV. The delineation should be made to the skin and all regions of subcutaneous tissue disruption [9]. Generally, a tunnel under the subcutaneous fatty tissue develops following instrumentation, and this whole region should be delineated including the subscapular tissues (Fig. 19.3).

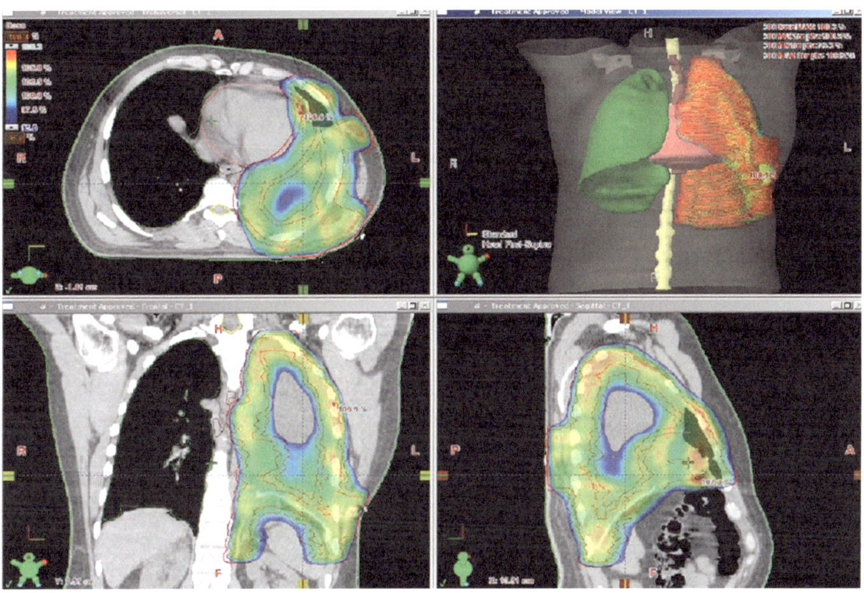

Fig. 19.2 CTV of a patient with T3N0M0 disease after EPP. The patient received 50.4 Gy to the ipsilateral pleural area. The neodiaphragm, pleural reflections, and diaphragm crus are included in the treatment field

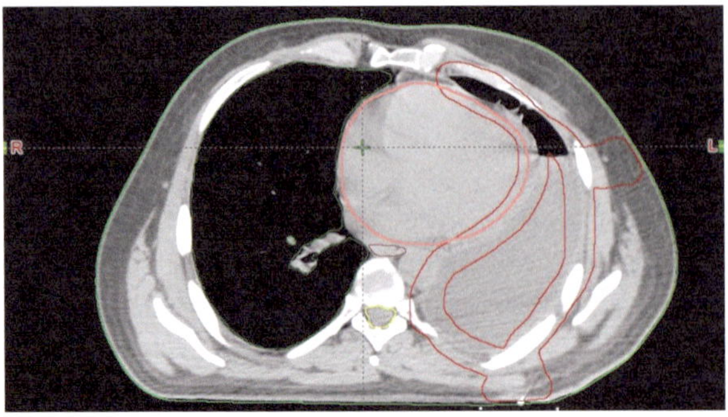

Fig. 19.3 Incisional scars should be included in the CTV

Delineation of the Organs at Risk

There are many critical organs in the thorax, and the delineation of the heart, lungs, spinal cord, and esophagus can be found in Chap. 23 in detail. Extra caution should be made on the dose constraint of the lungs as there is only one lung in patients with MPM who underwent extrapleural pneumonectomy. It has been recommended limiting the mean lung dose to <10 Gy and the volume of the lung receiving ≥20 Gy (V20) to <15 % during three-dimensional conformal RT (3D CRT) and IMRT [10].

In this chapter, the delineation of the liver and kidneys will be discussed in detail as these organs specifically receive high doses when treating patients with MPM.

Liver

Contouring

The liver should be delineated for the treatment of MPM when the whole right ipsilateral hemithorax is included in CTV. It is generally easily detectable on CT images. The medial border can sometimes be indistinguishable from the stomach or the heart unless contrast is used [11]. The whole liver should be contoured including the portal vein and excluding the gall bladder and vena cava inferior. It should be kept in mind that the liver can move with respiratory motion. It was reported that the liver can move ≥2 cm at superior-inferior direction [11].

Dose-Volume Constraints and Toxicity

Once the radiation-induced liver disease (RILD) develops, there is no effective treatment to reverse it. Therefore, prevention is the best option. The classic RILD usually presents with right upper abdominal pain. Consequently, abdominal swelling occurs due to ascites and hepatomegaly leading to weight gain. Ascites generally develops 2–4 months after RT and much earlier after concurrent chemoradiotherapy [12].

In non-classic RILD, dramatic elevation of liver enzymes and significant liver dysfunction develop.

The liver parenchyma has a parallel organization; therefore, the mean dose to a percentage of the volume is more important than the maximum dose to the whole organ. The majority of the data for dose constraints are obtained from liver irradiation. It has been clearly shown that partial irradiation causes significantly lower rates of toxicity compared to whole organ irradiation [13]. Emami et al. reported the total dose with a 5 % risk of toxicity in 5 years (TD5/5) for the whole liver 30 Gy in conventional fraction scheme [14]. In the Radiation Therapy Oncology Group (RTOG) 8405 study, no RILD was observed in 122 patients treated with 27–30 Gy to the whole liver in 1.5 Gy fractions twice daily compared to approximately 10 % in patients treated with 33 Gy with the same fractionation scheme [15].

It was reported that a mean liver dose of 25 Gy caused late liver toxicity in patients with hepatocellular carcinoma compared to none with a mean dose of 20 Gy [16]. In the same study, the total dose with a 50 % risk of toxicity in 5 years (TD50/5) for the whole, two thirds and one third of the liver were reported 43 Gy, 50 Gy, and 67 Gy; and TD5/5 were 25 Gy, 28 Gy, and 38 Gy, respectively. Kim et al. showed that V30 of the liver was the only significant factor for the development of toxicity, and the rate of hepatotoxicity significantly increased when the V30 was >60 % [17].

No RILD was observed when the mean liver dose was limited to <31 Gy in patients with unresectable liver malignancies when treated with CXT and RT [18]. The authors reported the TD5/5 and TD50/5 for the whole liver 31 Gy and 43 Gy, respectively. When RT is administered alone, the mean dose can be increased to ≤35 Gy.

The tolerance dose of the liver is higher in patients with liver metastases and cancers other than the liver because patients with primary liver cancer mostly have underlying liver disease [12]. It is recommended limiting the whole liver dose to ≤28 for metastatic and ≤30 Gy for primary disease in 2-Gy fractions and ≤21 Gy in 3-Gy fractions, respectively. The dose should be <30 Gy and <28 Gy for metastatic and primary liver cancer in partial liver irradiation [11]. In gastric cancer patients, <30 Gy has been recommended to the 70 % of the liver [19].

Kidneys

Contouring

The kidneys can be easily identified on CT images even without contrast. The whole kidney is delineated excluding the renal hilum in order to avoid the overestimation of the volume of the renal parenchyma [20]. It is important to delineate the functioning parts of the kidney, i.e., the parenchyma, rather than the collecting system [12]. It should be remembered that the kidneys can move up to 7 cm in the superior-inferior direction with respiratory motion [21].

Dose-Volume Constraints and Toxicity

Acute radiation-induced renal disease (RIRD) occurs within 6 months after RT and is usually subclinical. It can be diagnosed by urinary findings such as hematuria and proteinuria. After a latency period of 6–12 months, it can be clinical with symptoms of hypertension, lower extremity edema, and urinary abnormalities. Chronic RIRD usually develops 12–18 months after RT and presents with hypertension, anemia, increase in creatinine levels, and finally renal failure [22].

It is recommended evaluating the dose to both kidneys combined and separately [23]. The development of RIRD starts with ≥10 Gy to bilateral kidneys, and the risk rises to 50–80 % with a dose >20 Gy [24]. It was shown that the risk of renal atrophy, kidney dysfunction, and hypertension increases with >1/2 kidney receiving >20–30 Gy and 1/3 >30–40 Gy [25]. Emami et al. reported the TD5/5 and TD50/5 for the whole kidney 23 Gy and 28 Gy, respectively [14]. Cassady calculated the same parameters 18 Gy and 28 Gy, respectively, and stated that 15 Gy to the whole kidney is the threshold dose for the development of RIRD [26]. Flentje et al. reported the TD5/5 and TD50/5 17.5–21.5 Gy and 22–26 Gy, respectively [27]. Köst et al. showed that the incidence of renal dysfunction was <10 %, 40 %, and >70 % when the 10–30 %, 30–60 %, and >60 % of the kidney receives 20 Gy, and 35 %, >90 %, and >98 % when the same percentage of volumes receive 30 Gy, respectively [28]. The mean dose to at least 70 % of one normal functioning kidney was recommended to be limited <20 Gy in patients with gastric cancer [29]. Cheng et al. reported the TD5/5 of the whole kidney was 9.8 Gy with any fractionation scheme in patients treated with total body irradiation [30].

It can easily be foreseen that the use of concurrent or sequential CXT increases the risk of RIRD. Jansen et al. reported significant decrease in the function of the left kidney with a mean dose of ≥30 Gy and V20 of ≥64 % in patients with gastric cancer treated with concurrent CXT [31].

The functions of both kidneys should be evaluated prior to surgery in patients with MPM. The ipsilateral kidney is not usually considered as an organ at risk (OAR) as it is adjacent to and even sometimes inside the PTV [7]. The contralateral kidney is recommended to receive <15 Gy to 80 % of its volume [32]. It is recommended limiting the mean dose <15–18 Gy in conventional schedule. If partial kidney irradiation is the issue such as in the setting of MPM, maximal sparing of the contralateral kidney should be aimed; both kidneys should receive <18 Gy each, and if this is not possible the V6 of the contralateral kidney should be <30 % [12].

Conclusion

Trimodality scheme is the treatment of choice for MPM and RT constitutes a crucial part in it. The ipsilateral hemithorax is irradiated in patients with MPM either after surgery or in unresectable state. Although there are not many data on the delineation of the target volume in MPM, the challenging issues on contouring the whole target have clearly been identified. By following the recommendations on delineation of the target and OARs, a more satisfactory treatment can be achieved.

References

1. Rusch VW. Pleurectomy/decortication and adjuvant therapy for malignant mesothelioma. Chest. 1993;103:382S–4.
2. Gordon Jr W, Antman KH, Greenberger JS, et al. Radiation therapy in the management of patients with mesothelioma. Int J Radiat Oncol Biol Phys. 1982;8:19–25.
3. Boutin C, Rey F, Viallat JR. Prevention of malignant seeding after invasive diagnostic procedures in patients with pleural mesothelioma. A randomized trial of local radiotherapy. Chest. 1995;108:754–8.
4. Pehlivan B, Topkan E, Onal C, et al. Comparison of CT and integrated PET-CT based radiation therapy planning in patients with malignant pleural mesothelioma. Radiat Oncol. 2009;4:35.
5. Sugarbaker DJ, Garcia JP. Multimodality therapy for malignant pleural mesothelioma. Chest. 1997;112:272S–5.
6. Ahamad A, Stevens CW, Smythe WR, et al. Promising early local control of malignant pleural mesothelioma following postoperative intensity modulated radiotherapy (IMRT) to the chest. Cancer J. 2003;9:476–84.
7. Ahamad A, Stevens CW, Smythe WR, et al. Intensity-modulated radiation therapy: a novel approach to the management of malignant pleural mesothelioma. Int J Radiat Oncol Biol Phys. 2003;55:768–75.
8. Yajnik S, Rosenzweig KE, Mychalczak B, et al. Hemithoracic radiation after extrapleural pneumonectomy for malignant pleural mesothelioma. Int J Radiat Oncol Biol Phys. 2003;56:1319–26.
9. Forster KM, Smythe WR, Starkschall G, et al. Intensity-modulated radiotherapy following extrapleural pneumonectomy for the treatment of malignant mesothelioma: clinical implementation. Int J Radiat Oncol Biol Phys. 2003;55:606–16.
10. Scherpereel A, Astoul P, Baas P, et al. Guidelines of the European Respiratory Society and the European Society of Thoracic Surgeons for the management of malignant pleural mesothelioma. Eur Respir J. 2010;35:479–95.
11. Pan CC, Kavanagh BD, Dawson LA, et al. Radiation-associated liver injury. Int J Radiat Oncol Biol Phys. 2010;76:S94–100.
12. Kirkpatrick JP, Milano M, Constine LS, Vujaskovic Z, Marks LB. Late effects and QUANTEC. In: Halperin EC, Wazer D, Perez C, Brady LW, editors. Principles and practice of radiation oncology. 6th ed. Philadelphia: Lippincott Williams 2013. p. 296–328.
13. Lawrence TS, Ten Haken RK, Kessler ML, et al. The use of 3-D dose volume analysis to predict radiation hepatitis. Int J Radiat Oncol Biol Phys. 1992;23:781–8.
14. Emami B, Lyman J, Brown A, et al. Tolerance of normal tissue to therapeutic irradiation. Int J Radiat Oncol Biol Phys. 1991;21:109–22.
15. Russell AH, Clyde C, Wasserman TH, et al. Accelerated hyperfractionated hepatic irradiation in the management of patients with liver metastases: results of the RTOG dose escalating protocol. Int J Radiat Oncol Biol Phys. 1993;27:117–23.
16. Schefter TE, Kavanagh BD, Timmerman RD, et al. A phase I trial of stereotactic body radiation therapy (SBRT) for liver metastases. Int J Radiat Oncol Biol Phys. 2005;62:1371–8.
17. Kim TH, Kim DY, Park JW, et al. Dose-volumetric parameters predicting radiation-induced hepatic toxicity in unresectable hepatocellular carcinoma patients treated with three-dimensional conformal radiotherapy. Int J Radiat Oncol Biol Phys. 2007;67:225–31.
18. Dawson LA, Normolle D, Balter JM, et al. Analysis of radiation-induced liver disease using the Lyman NTCP model. Int J Radiat Oncol Biol Phys. 2002;53:810–21.
19. Czito BG, Palta M, Willett CG. Stomach cancer. In: Halperin EC, Wazer D, Perez C, Brady LW, editors. Principles and practice of radiation oncology. 6th ed. Philadelphia: Lippincott Williams 2012. p. 1165–88.
20. Goodman KA, Regine WF, Dawson LA, et al. Radiation Therapy Oncology Group consensus panel guidelines for the delineation of the clinical target volume in the postoperative treatment of pancreatic head cancer. Int J Radiat Oncol Biol Phys. 2012;83:901–8.

21. Reiff JE, Werner-Wasik M, Valicenti RK, Huq MS. Changes in the size and location of kidneys from the supine to standing positions and the implications for block placement during total body irradiation. Int J Radiat Oncol Biol Phys. 1999;45:447–9.
22. Verheij M, Dewit LG, Valdes Olmos RA, Arisz L. Evidence for a renovascular component in hypertensive patients with late radiation nephropathy. Int J Radiat Oncol Biol Phys. 1994;30:677–83.
23. Dawson LA, Kavanagh BD, Paulino AC, et al. Radiation-associated kidney injury. Int J Radiat Oncol Biol Phys. 2010;76:S108–15.
24. Schneider DP, Marti HP, Von Briel C, et al. Long-term evolution of renal function in patients with ovarian cancer after whole abdominal irradiation with or without preceding cisplatin. Ann Oncol. 1999;10:677–83.
25. Willett CG, Tepper JE, Orlow EL, Shipley WU. Renal complications secondary to radiation treatment of upper abdominal malignancies. Int J Radiat Oncol Biol Phys. 1986;12:1601–4.
26. Cassady JR. Clinical radiation nephropathy. Int J Radiat Oncol Biol Phys. 1995;31:1249–56.
27. Flentje M, Hensley F, Gademann G, et al. Renal tolerance to nonhomogenous irradiation: comparison of observed effects to predictions of normal tissue complication probability from different biophysical models. Int J Radiat Oncol Biol Phys. 1993;27:25–30.
28. Kost S, Dorr W, Keinert K, et al. Effect of dose and dose-distribution in damage to the kidney following abdominal radiotherapy. Int J Radiat Biol. 2002;78:695–702.
29. Matzinger O, Gerber E, Bernstein Z, et al. EORTC-ROG expert opinion: radiotherapy volume and treatment guidelines for neoadjuvant radiation of adenocarcinomas of the gastroesophageal junction and the stomach. Radiother Oncol. 2009;92:164–75.
30. Cheng JC, Schultheiss TE, Wong JY. Impact of drug therapy, radiation dose, and dose rate on renal toxicity following bone marrow transplantation. Int J Radiat Oncol Biol Phys. 2008;71:1436–43.
31. Jansen EP, Saunders MP, Boot H, et al. Prospective study on late renal toxicity following postoperative chemoradiotherapy in gastric cancer. Int J Radiat Oncol Biol Phys. 2007;67:781–5.
32. Senan S, van de Pol M. Considerations for post-operative radiotherapy to the hemithorax following extrapleural pneumonectomy in malignant pleural mesothelioma. Lung Cancer. 2004;45 Suppl 1:S93–6.

Modern Radiotherapy Techniques in Malignant Pleural Mesothelioma

20

Gokhan Ozyigit, Pervin Hurmuz, Sezin Yuce Sari, Gozde Yazici, and Melis Gultekin

Introduction

Malignant pleural mesothelioma (MPM) arises from the mesothelial lining of the pleural cavity, either from the visceral or parietal pleura. The pleural cavity is limited by the chest wall and ribs at the anterior, posterior, lateral, and superior, by the heart and mediastinum at the medial, and by the diaphragm at the inferior. The pleurae extend into the intrapulmonary fissures and costodiaphragmatic sulci until the level of the L4 vertebra. It can cross the midline in the costomediastinal recess.

The incidence of MPM is estimated to be 1/100,000 in the United States and 1/50,000 in Europe [1, 2]. The majority of the cases are associated with asbestos exposure [3]. The incidence of MPM increases with longer asbestos exposure; the median duration is 20 years, and the median age at diagnosis is approximately 60 years [4]. Although no direct relation was shown between MPM and smoking, people who smoke have increased risk for MPM if they are also exposed to asbestos [5]. Prior thoracic radiation exposure was also reported to increase the incidence of MPM [6]. Genetic predisposition is also an important etiological factor. In certain villages of Central Anatolia, Turkey, it was found that more than 50 % of mortalities were due to MPM. Epidemiological studies in this region revealed that houses contain a non-asbestos fiber called erionite. This fiber is present in the volcanic tuff used in the construction of houses and also found in the air of the villages [7, 8]. Intrapleural injection of erionite to animals caused MPM in in vitro studies; thus, it was concluded that erionite was the cause of MPM in these villages [9–11]. People living in these villages share the same house for a lifetime with many generations. Although all houses in this region contain a similar amount of erionite, MPM occurred only in the members of certain families living in the same house.

G. Ozyigit, MD • P. Hurmuz, MD (✉) • S.Y. Sari, MD • G. Yazici, MD • M. Gultekin, MD
Department of Radiation Oncology, Faculty of Medicine, Hacettepe University, Ankara, Turkey
e-mail: phurmuz@yahoo.com

G. Ozyigit et al. (eds.), *Principles and Practice of Radiotherapy Techniques in Thoracic Malignancies*, DOI 10.1007/978-3-319-28761-4_20

The analysis of pedigrees of these families showed that the disease is inherited in an autosomal dominant pattern [12, 13]. It is unknown whether genetics alone or together with erionite exposure is responsible for the disease, but the occurrence of MPM only in the affected families supports the importance of genetics in the etiology [14].

The most common symptoms of MPM are dyspnea, chest pain, cough, and weight loss. In more advanced disease, supraclavicular and axillary lymph nodes (LNs) can be enlarged, and even scoliosis may occur owing to the volume loss in the ipsilateral lung. As MPM has a tendency for developing along tracks of previous chest instrumentations, these sites should also be examined. Poor prognostic factors for MPM include older age, poor performance status, advanced-stage disease, the presence of chest pain, the presence of symptoms for shorter than 6 months, non-epithelioid tumor histology, the presence of LN metastasis, thrombocytosis, and less than complete resection [15].

Irregular nodularity in the pleura, pleural effusion, and loss in the lung volume can be observed on the chest X-ray. On computed tomography (CT), irregular pleural masses, invasion of adjacent structures, pleural effusion, nodularity within the fissures, mediastinal or hilar lymphadenopathy, and pericardial effusion can be seen. Magnetic resonance imaging (MRI) gives more accurate information than CT for the diagnosis and staging of MPM. Positron emission tomography (PET)/CT scanning with 18-fluoro-deoxy-glucose (FDG) has >90 % sensitivity and specificity for the diagnosis of MPM by distinguishing it from benign pleural thickening [16, 17]. The use of PET/CT is rational prior to surgery as it has been shown to upstage the disease and prevent unnecessary surgery in 40 % of patients [18]. The gold standard for pathologic diagnosis is an open pleural biopsy [19]. This can be performed by open thoracotomy or video-assisted thoracoscopic surgery (VATS).

Local recurrence (LR) is the main problem during the course of MPM [20]. The disease can spread to local and distant structures directly or by seeding throughout the pleural space and chest wall. Complete resection without an extrapleural pneumonectomy (EPP) can be difficult owing to the involvement of the visceral and parietal pleurae. The EPP is suitable for localized disease in medically fit patients. During EPP, the parietal and visceral pleurae, the involved lung, the mediastinal LNs, the diaphragm, and the pericardium in the ipsilateral hemithorax are removed en bloc. However, complete resection is not usually possible, and the superiority of EPP over limited surgery is questionable [21]. For patients with MPM, pleurectomy/decortication (P/D) is the limited surgery technique in which the parietal and visceral pleurae, the pericardium, and, when necessary, the diaphragm are removed but the lung is not. Surgery alone, even an aggressive one and even in early-stage disease, does not improve survival [22, 23]. Oncologic margins cannot be obtained by any method of surgery, particularly on the pericardium and mediastinum, so surgery alone is not curative for MPM. This leads to the fact that every surgery method is considered R1 resection [24].

Local recurrence rate was reported approximately 80 % when EPP was the only treatment; however, with additional treatment modalities, local control (LC) improves significantly. Rusch et al. reported the LR rate 13 % in patients who underwent EPP followed by 54 Gy to the hemithorax [25]. On the other hand, Baldini reported 50 % LR rate after trimodality treatment [26]. The current management of MPM is by trimodality treatment, i.e., surgery, chemotherapy (CXT), and radiotherapy (RT); this approach has been shown to improve both the overall survival (OS) and LC rates [22, 27, 28]. However, there is only one randomized prospective phase III trial on this issue. The only randomized trial has been the MARS trial which compares three cycles of induction CXT, EPP, and hemithoracic RT to best supportive care [29]. In the interim report, a trend for increased OS rate was observed in the trimodality arm. However, the final report in 2011 suggested that radical surgery in the form of EPP within trimodal therapy offers no benefit and possibly harms patients. Median survival was 14.4 months for the EPP group, whereas it was 19.5 months in patients who did not undergo EPP. Okubo et al. treated 16 patients with RT and CXT following EPP and reported the 2- and 5-year OS rates 53.3 % and 26.7 %, respectively [30]. The survival benefit was significant in stage ≤III disease. Tonoli et al. treated 56 patients with three-dimensional conformal RT (3D CRT), intensity-modulated RT (IMRT), or tomotherapy with 45–50 Gy after EPP [31]. They reported 3-year OS, disease-specific survival (DSS), disease-free survival (DFS), locoregional control (LRC), and distant metastasis-free survival (DMFS) rates 60 %, 62 %, 57 %, 90 %, and 66 %, respectively. However, as no single treatment method is curative for MPM, patients should be evaluated carefully prior to surgery by physical, radiological, and histological examination, pulmonary function test, and cardiac reserve test, not only for the suitableness for surgery but also for the administration of CXT and RT [2].

Role of Adjuvant Radiotherapy in MPM

Although EPP is performed, the nature of MPM puts the entire ipsilateral chest wall, diaphragm insertion, pericardium, mediastinum, and bronchial stump at high risk for LR owing to spillage during surgery. In the trimodality approach, the technique for conventional RT is the irradiation of the whole ipsilateral hemithorax. This RT field is very large and is adjacent to critical structures such as the contralateral lung, heart, esophagus, spinal cord, liver, and kidneys. The dose to the target is limited by these structures which decreases the outcomes for conventional RT [20, 32, 33]. To overcome this issue, newer techniques have been developed.

In Baldini et al.'s study, 49 patients underwent EPP followed by four to six cycles CXT, and 35 patients also received postoperative RT; 30.6 Gy to the hemithorax and additional 19.4 Gy boost to the gross tumor [32]. They reported that 16 patients had LR in the chest; however, 11 patients had abdominal failures which can be accepted as LR because the surgery can "abdominalize" the diaphragm. The 3-year OS rate was 34 % with no major toxicity.

A study from the Memorial Sloan Kettering Cancer Center (MSKCC) reported the median OS 18 months in 54 patients who underwent EPP and adjuvant RT [34]. The irradiation site was the ipsilateral hemithorax and all drain sites, and the dose was 54 Gy in 30 fractions with the spinal cord shielded after 41.4 Gy. Local recurrence was observed in seven patients; however, 22 patients had peritoneal or ipsilateral visceral recurrences. In the update of this study, they reported their recommendations on the field and dose in 35 patients they treated with IMRT [35]. The authors recommended starting from the superior of T1 vertebra and ending the target volume at the inferior of L2 vertebra. They limited the medial border with the contralateral border of vertebral bodies and extended it 1.5–2 cm beyond if mediastinal LNs are present. However, the medial border was moved to the ipsilateral border of vertebrae after 41.4 Gy. They blocked the liver and ipsilateral kidney in right-sided tumors and limited the heart with 19.8 Gy by blocking it after this dose in left-sided tumors. All blocked sites received boost doses with electrons. Local recurrence occurred in 13 patients; however, it is not clear whether these recurrences occurred in-field or marginally. Out of the remaining 22 patients, 17 developed regional or distant recurrence proving the need for the addition of systemic therapy.

MD Anderson Cancer Center (MDACC) reported their results of 28 patients treated with EPP followed by IMRT [36–38]. The planning target volume (PTV) included the hemithorax and ipsilateral mediastinum with all surgical clips and drain sites. The dose was 45–50 Gy to the hemithorax and 10–15 Gy boost to sites with close or positive surgical margins. No local failure was observed; however, two marginal misses were reported. The 2-year OS rate was 62 %. In the update of this study with 100 patients, locoregional failure rate was reported 13 % [39]. The 3-year OS rate was 41 % and median survival 28 months in patients with N0 disease.

Perrot et al. reported the results of 60 patients treated with induction CXT followed by EPP and adjuvant ≥50 Gy RT to the hemithorax [40]. They found the median OS 59 months and 5-year DFS rate 53 % in patients with N0 disease. Allen et al. reported that 6 of the 13 patients treated with EPP followed by adjuvant CXT and IMRT died due to treatment-related toxicity [41]. The most common cause of death was radiation pneumonitis (RP). The mean lung dose (MLD), median V5 (the volume receiving ≥5 Gy), and V20 were 15.2 Gy, 98.6 %, and 17.6 % in patients who developed RP, whereas they were 12.9 Gy, 90 %, and 10.9 % in patients who did not, respectively. In the Duke study, 13 patients with MPM were treated with IMRT, and three developed symptomatic RP with one of them being grade 5 [42]. The MLD, V5, and V20 were 11.4 Gy, 92 %, and 6.9 % in the patient who died; 7.9 Gy, 92 %, and 2.3 % for the two patients with RP; and 7.5 Gy, 66 %, and 0.2 % for others, respectively. The MDACC reported six pulmonary-related deaths out of 63 patients with MPM who were treated with IMRT, with one being due to RP [43]. In this study, V20 was found to be a significant risk factor for fatal RP, and the authors concluded that when V20 is >7 %, the risk of pulmonary death increases 42-fold. The National Comprehensive Cancer Network (NCCN) recommends limiting the MLD to 8.5 Gy and the V5 of the lung minimum.

The most recent Surveillance, Epidemiology, and End Results (SEER) database reported that pneumonectomy and RT administration are the most important predictive factors for OS rate in MPM along with epithelioid histology [44]. Patients undergoing pneumonectomy followed by RT had significantly longer median survival compared to patients treated with surgery alone (19 vs 13 months, $p=0.01$).

A study from Hacettepe University evaluated the efficacy and the toxicity of 3D CRT after EPP [45]. All 14 patients received a total median dose of 50.4 Gy to the hemithorax, whereas 11 of them received additional adjuvant chemotherapy of pemetrexed and cisplatin. Radiotherapy was generally well tolerated with few grade I–II acute toxicities. After a median 16 months of follow-up, intrathoracic control was 100 %. Six patients (43 %) developed abdominal relapse and one (7 %) developed distant metastasis (DM). The authors concluded that improved LC with 3D CRT after EPP seems to change the relapse patterns of MPM; thus, more effective systemic treatment is needed to prevent the recurrence outside the thorax.

In summary, high-dose adjuvant RT can decrease the LR rate, particularly after EPP compared to more limited surgery. Radiotherapy is well tolerated without major toxicity. However, it is important to distinguish the exact site of recurrence, i.e., true in-field or marginal. Adjuvant RT can change the pattern of relapse and CXT is required in order to decrease the rate of DM.

Role of Radiotherapy in Unresectable MPM

Radiotherapy alone is not an effective treatment method for patients with MPM. It was shown that mesothelioma cell lines have radiosensitivity similar to non-small cell lung cancer (NSCLC) cell lines and modest doses (i.e., >40 Gy) are effective for killing MPM cells [46–48]. However, this dose is still high for the critical structures adjacent to the target because the whole hemithorax and intrapulmonary fissures should be included for an accurate treatment with RT alone. The respiratory motion is the most important problem during the course of RT; the diaphragm should be included in the RT port, and it can move 2–3 cm superoinferiorly, 1–2 cm mediolaterally, and 1–1.5 cm anteroposteriorly [49]. By expanding the PTV according to these potential movements, the liver, heart, and bowel toxicity will increase significantly in right- and left-sided tumors, respectively.

Alberts et al. reported the median survival 9.6 months in 262 patients treated with different combinations of RT (45–80 Gy to the whole ipsilateral hemithorax), pleurectomy, and CXT [50]. Ball et al. administered 50 Gy to the ipsilateral hemithorax after blocking the spinal cord, and for left-sided tumors, the heart after 40 Gy, and found the median survival 9 months with grade 5 hepatitis in one and grade 5 myelopathy in one patient out of 35 [51]. In the study of Maasilta, 34 patients received high-dose definitive RT to the ipsilateral hemithorax with the spinal cord blocked after 40 Gy and the liver after 30 Gy [52]. Various RT regimens were used in this study, 55 Gy/2.2 Gy (split course) to the hemithorax and 15 Gy boost to the gross disease, 70 Gy/1.25 Gy twice daily (split course) to the hemithorax, and 35 Gy/1.25 twice daily to the hemithorax and 36 Gy/4 Gy boost to the gross disease. The authors recorded deteriorated lung functions.

The role of RT in patients with unresectable MPM is not yet clear. Radiotherapy alone is an effective choice in the palliative setting only. There is a radiation dose-response relationship; doses >40 Gy were shown to yield significant relief of symptoms [53]. Pain relief was also achieved with 20 Gy in five fractions and 30 Gy in ten fractions in another study with no difference between the RT schemes [54]. Munter et al. treated 11 patients with 40–50 Gy IMRT and reported no severe RT-related toxicity [55].

The role of IMRT and arc therapy to the pleura in patients with unresectable tumors has also been investigated. Rosenzweig et al. retrospectively analyzed 36 patients; 16 had unresectable tumors and 20 underwent P/D [56]. The median OS was 17 months and 26 months, whereas the 1- and 2-year OS rates were 75 % and 21 % and 80 % and 55 %, respectively. Grade ≥3 RP developed in 20 % of the patients. In the update of this study, the authors analyzed the patterns of failure; 1- and 2-year in-field LR rate was 56 % and 74 %, respectively [57]. The results were improved in patients who underwent P/D compared to the patients with more limited or no surgery. Marginal and distant failures were observed in 13 and 32 patients, respectively. This study revealed that although IMRT is administered, the primary site of failure remains local. Minatel et al. treated 28 patients with helical tomotherapy (HT) (50 Gy to the hemithorax and involved mediastinal LNs and 10 Gy boost to the hypermetabolic areas on PET/CT) after P/D or biopsy alone [58]. They added a 5-mm margin for PTV and restricted MLD of the contralateral lung with 7 Gy. They observed pulmonary toxicity in five patients with no grade higher than 3. They concluded that V5 of the contralateral lung significantly affected the development of RP.

Role of Radiotherapy for Drain Sites of MPM

It was shown that MPM has a tendency for recurrence along the tracks of previous chest wall instrumentation and also at the previous thoracoscopy port sites if not excised during surgery [59–61]. It is recommended limiting the number of port sites and placing them to easily excisable sites during VATS in order to reduce LR on the chest wall. This high recurrence rate on intervention sites emerged the idea whether prophylactic irradiation to these sites could reduce the recurrence rate. There are contradictory results on this issue. The first study on intervention site irradiation was held in 20 patients with 38 port sites, and the authors reported no recurrences [35–37]. Consequently, Boutin et al. compared immediate RT and observation after chest instrumentation in a total of 40 patients, and no LR was observed in patients who received 21 Gy in three fractions to drain sites, whereas 40 % of unirradiated patients developed recurrence [62]. However, other studies found no difference between two groups in regard to intervention site recurrence [63–66]. Nevertheless, in the study of Bydder et al., a single fraction of low-energy electrons was used, and all but one was in the era of historical treatment methods without using CXT [66]. De Ruysscher et al. published a survey that 84 % of RT centers preferred prophylactic intervention site irradiation in the Netherlands and Belgium, whereas Lee et al. reported that the rate was 75 % in the United Kingdom [67, 68].

There is not a randomized trial to answer the question of whether intervention site RT reduces the recurrence rate definitively. However, once recurrence occurs on the intervention site, the pain significantly deteriorates patient's quality of life and is difficult to control; so elective irradiation is generally recommended [69]. The SMART trial has been planned comparing immediate RT after chest intervention (within 42 days after intervention) to delayed RT when intervention site metastasis occurs (within 35 days after metastasis) [70]. In both arms, 21 Gy in three fractions will be administered; the CTV is intervention site + 3-cm and 2-cm margin in the immediate and delayed RT arms, respectively. The results of this randomized study can give more satisfactory results than already-published work.

Hemithoracic Radiotherapy Techniques

Treatment with Three-Dimensional Conformal Radiation Therapy

The first method of 3D CRT was from MSKCC which combined 10-MV X-rays with 13-MeV electrons and prescribed 42.5 Gy to the ipsilateral mediastinum in 18 fractions with anteroposterior (AP) and posteroanterior (PA) beams [34]. The authors used lung and liver blocks and irradiated these regions with additional 4 Gy with 13-MeV electrons. They also treated gross disease sites with a ^{125}I permanent implant. Although the dose distributions were satisfying considering the techniques available at that time, significant portions of the PTV received <50 % of the prescribed dose. With this technique, it was later reported that LR was observed in 67 % of the patients [32].

Sugarbaker et al. reported their results in 183 patients treated with adjuvant CXT and RT after EPP [27]. Seven patients died during the operation. They prescribed 30 Gy to the ipsilateral hemithorax, 40 Gy to the mediastinum, and 54 Gy to gross residual disease and positive surgical margins to the remaining 176 patients. They reported high LR rate in the ipsilateral hemithorax with 2- and 5-year OS rates 38 % and 15 %, respectively. The same authors changed their treatment policy after 2004 and started to prescribe 54 Gy to the whole hemithorax [48]. They reported that high-dose RT to the hemithorax resulted in better in-field LC; however, DM rate still remains high.

In the current 3D CRT technique, the hemithorax is irradiated by two fields, i.e., AP and PA [34, 35]. The total recommended dose is 54 Gy in 30 fractions. An abdominal block is used on both fields during the whole treatment for right-located tumors, and 1.53 Gy/day electrons are prescribed to this region. A kidney block is used during the whole treatment and the heart is blocked on the AP field after 19.8 Gy for left-located tumors. The spinal cord is shielded after 41.4 Gy on both fields. It was reported that dose homogeneity can be achieved at target volumes by 3D CRT and critical organs can be spared well.

Gupta et al. retrospectively evaluated 123 patients with MPM who were treated with 3D CRT in MSKCC between 1974 and 2003 [71]. The adjuvant external RT dose was median 42.5 Gy to the ipsilateral hemithorax, and 54 patients received intraoperative brachytherapy (BRT) with a matched peripheral dose of 160 Gy. They reported 2- and 5-year OS rates 23 % and 5 %, respectively. It was stated that

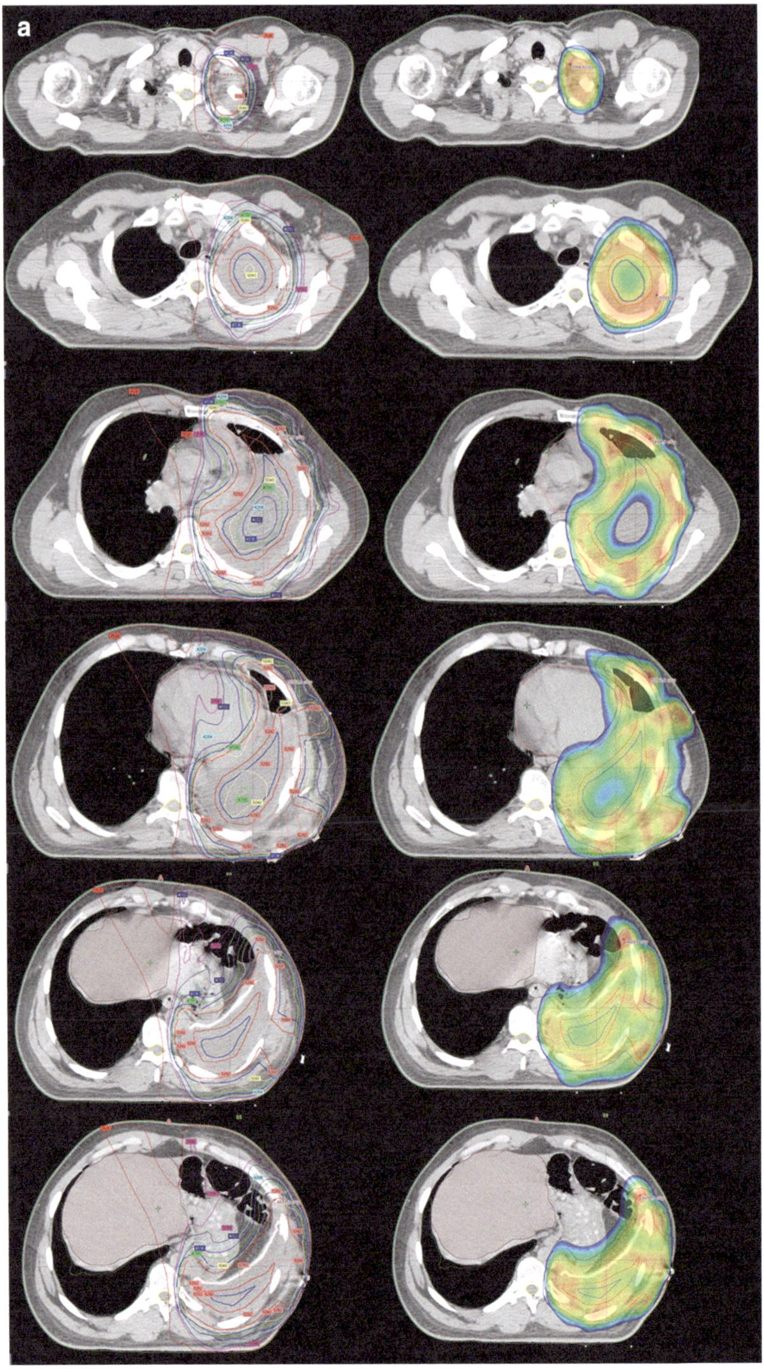

Fig. 20.1 (**a**) Intensity modulated radiotherapy (IMRT) after extrapleural pneumonectomy (EPP) in a patient with malignant pleural mesothelioma, (**b**) coronal, sagittal, and axial view of IMRT plan

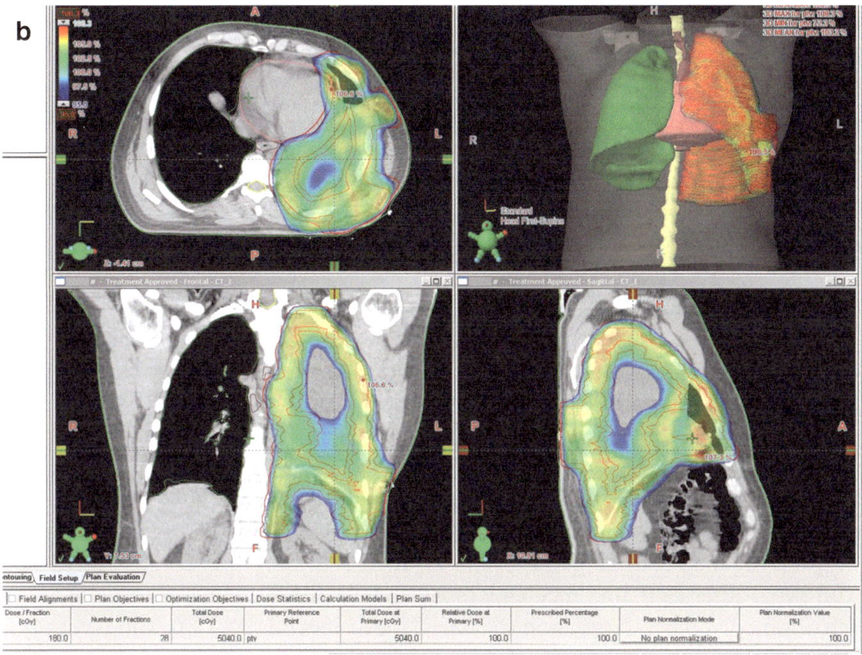

Fig. 20.1 (continued)

non-epithelioid histology; left-sided tumors; the presence of extensive residual disease after surgery, receiving BRT; and RT doses <40 Gy were poor prognostic factors for OS. Any recurrence was observed in 67 % of the patients, and 1-year LC rate was 42 %. Two patients died of RT-related toxicity during treatment, one with RP and one with cardiac toxicity. Grade 3–4 toxicity developed in 28 % of the patients.

Treatment with Intensity-Modulated Radiation Therapy

The target volume can be covered better and more homogeneously by intensity-modulated radiation therapy (IMRT) compared to 3D CRT (Fig. 20.1a, b). However, the planning step is more complicated, the treatment is longer, smaller volumes of critical structures can receive high doses, and radiation scatter to critical organs and the whole body is much higher owing to the higher number of treatment fields. Hill-Kayser et al. observed significant dose decrease in the contralateral lung, heart, and kidney when electrons and 3D CRT of 54 Gy were combined compared to 45 Gy IMRT [72]. The abdominal, heart, and spinal cord blocks were used the same as they are in 3D CRT. The authors stated that the ipsilateral kidney generally receives a high dose; so renal functions of the contralateral kidney should be adequate. Furthermore, they recommended pneumococcal prophylaxis in patients with left-located tumors as the spleen usually receives a high dose. On the other hand, in the study of Allen et al. which is the first study of IMRT for MPM, severe pulmonary toxicity with 46 % being fatal pneumonitis was reported [41]. However, the V20 of the contralateral lung was 20 % and MLD 15 Gy, and the majority of the patients also received heated intrapleural CXT which may be the reasons for the high rate of toxicity. A retrospective trial has revealed that the pulmonary toxicity due to IMRT was related to the dose to the contralateral lung [42]. It was recommended limiting the MLD and V20 of both lungs to decrease pulmonary toxicity rate [39]. Buduhan et al. treated patients with either adjuvant 3D CRT or IMRT and showed that patients who received IMRT developed significantly less LR with similar toxicity [73].

Forster et al. administered IMRT to seven patients with MPM after EPP [38]. The total dose was 50 Gy to the whole ipsilateral hemithorax and adjacent abdomen with additional 10 Gy boost dose to the regions with close or positive surgical margins. With a minimal follow-up of 13 months, two patients died due to the disease; one recurred in the ipsilateral and the other in the contralateral hemithorax, respectively. None of the recurrences was in-field. Kristensen et al. treated 26 patients with 50 Gy IMRT after neoadjuvant CXT and EPP and reported grade 5 RP in four patients whose V20 was significantly higher than the patients who did not develop RP [74]. Ahamad et al. reported 100 % in-field local control in 28 patients treated with IMRT after EPP after median 9 months, with two marginal misses, one in the anterior-medial pleural reflection and one at the ipsilateral crus [36]. The 1-year OS, DSS, and DFS were 65 %, 91 %, and 88 %, respectively. Nausea-vomiting and dyspnea were the most common toxicities. Rice et al. treated 63 patients with median 45 Gy of IMRT following EPP [39]. They reported 2- and 3-year OS 32 % and 21 %, respectively, with no major toxicity. The locoregional and in-field recurrence rates were 13 % and 5 %, respectively. van Sandick et al. reported 9 % LR in median 17 months in patients they treated with IMRT (28–34). Cho et al. treated 25 patients with T1–3N0M0 MPM with 25 Gy IMRT to the ipsilateral hemithorax in five fractions and 5 Gy concomitant boost to high-risk areas prior to EPP within 1 week [75]. They administered adjuvant CXT to patients with N2 disease. Grade ≥3 pulmonary toxicity developed in 13 and 0 patients due to surgery and IMRT, respectively. They reported 3-year OS 84 % and 13 % in patients with epithelial and biphasic tumors, respectively.

Gomez et al. retrospectively evaluated 86 patients they treated with hemithoracic IMRT after EPP [76]. They observed grade ≥3 pulmonary toxicity in 11.6 % of patients, and three of these were fatal RP. The 2-year OS and LC rates were 32 % and 55 %, respectively; LR occurred in 14 patients. Of the two patients who had LR only, the recurrence region was in the low-dose-receiving area while the other had received the full dose. Patel et al. analyzed 30 patients treated with IMRT after EPP [77]. With a median dose of 45 Gy to the ipsilateral hemithorax, they reported the 2-year rates of OS, DFS, and LC 50 %, 34 %, and 47 %, respectively. They observed RP in four patients with one being fatal. In the review by Rosenzweig, limiting the V20 of the contralateral lung to <5 % and MLD <10 Gy was recommended in the adjuvant setting of IMRT for MPM [78]. In patients with unresectable tumors, he stated that MLD can be 20 Gy. With these restrictions, grade ≥3 RP rate is 12–20 %, and grade 5 is approximately 3–8 % in the literature.

The Duke University recommends limiting the MLD of the contralateral lung dose to <9.5 Gy as the ipsilateral lung is absent after EPP [42]. However, a more conservative approach has also been recommended by the University of Pennsylvania; they limit the MLD of the contralateral lung to <9 Gy, the V5 <60 %, and the V20 <20 % [79]. Other than dose constraints, Allen et al. restricted spacing of the beams as they enter the body of the patient and decreased the dose to the contralateral lung [41, 80]. They treated the superior part of the PTV with three or four beams not passing through the contralateral lung in order to further decrease its dose. They also observed that using nine beams improves the target dose homogeneity as well as decreasing the dose to OARs.

It is crucial to measure the volumes of organs at risk (OARs) receiving low doses during IMRT. Some more recent planning systems improve the target dose homogeneity and decrease the OAR dose; however, they can underestimate the percentage of low-dose-receiving volumes due to dose scattering from the multileaf collimators (MLC) [81, 82]. Therefore, using a Monte Carlo planning algorithm-based system is recommended for IMRT because it can calculate dose distribution more accurately, particularly in the volumes receiving low dose. If Monte Carlo cannot be used, stricter V5 should be set for the contralateral lung in order to overcome the dose underestimation while using other planning systems [83].

Treatment with Arc Therapy

Recent advances in technology lead the way to more improved treatment devices. Helical tomotherapy is one of the devices administering image-guided IMRT (Fig. 20.2a, b) [84]. This technique provides a 360° gantry rotation and synchronous couch and MLC movement during radiation delivery and uses 51 separate angles for each gantry rotation in order to administer a highly conformal and homogeneous dose to the target and better spare the OARs [83].

It has been reported that HT provides a more homogeneous dose distribution and reduced OAR doses compared to linac-based IMRT in a variety of cancers [85, 86]. Sterzing et al. have shown that HT significantly increased the LC rate and decreased the fatal pulmonary toxicity rate compared to step-and-shoot IMRT while treating MPM in the adjuvant setting, without prolonging the treatment time [87]. Giraud et al. treated 24 patients with HT after EPP [88]. They used three different CTVs; CTV1 was the surgical cavity receiving 50–54 Gy, CTV2 sites with positive surgical margin receiving 4–6 Gy boost, and CTV3 the mediastinal structures adjacent to the primary tumor receiving 46 Gy. The rate of grade ≥3 RP was 16 % with a V20 <20 % and half of them were fatal. Three patients developed LR, whereas all other patients had distant failure. Sylvestre et al. treated 24 patients with median 50 Gy of HT after EPP [89]. Local recurrence was observed in two patients at a median follow-up of 24 months; and they reported grade 3 RP in two and grade 5 in two patients, respectively. Helou et al. treated 29 patients with 50 Gy HT after EPP and reported 1- and 2-year OS rates 65 % and 36 %, respectively [90]. The MLD of the contralateral lung was 11 Gy, and V20, V15, V13, V10, V5, and V2 were 5 %,

19 %, 36 %, 52 %, 98 %, and 100 %, respectively, leading to grade 3 RP in three and grade 5 two patients. The authors stated that MLD ≥10 Gy, V15 ≥15 %, and V10 ≥50 % were predictive factors for pulmonary toxicity. They also stated that three patients developed grade 3–4 esophageal toxicity; and MLD and V13, V10, and V5 significantly affected the rate of esophageal toxicity.

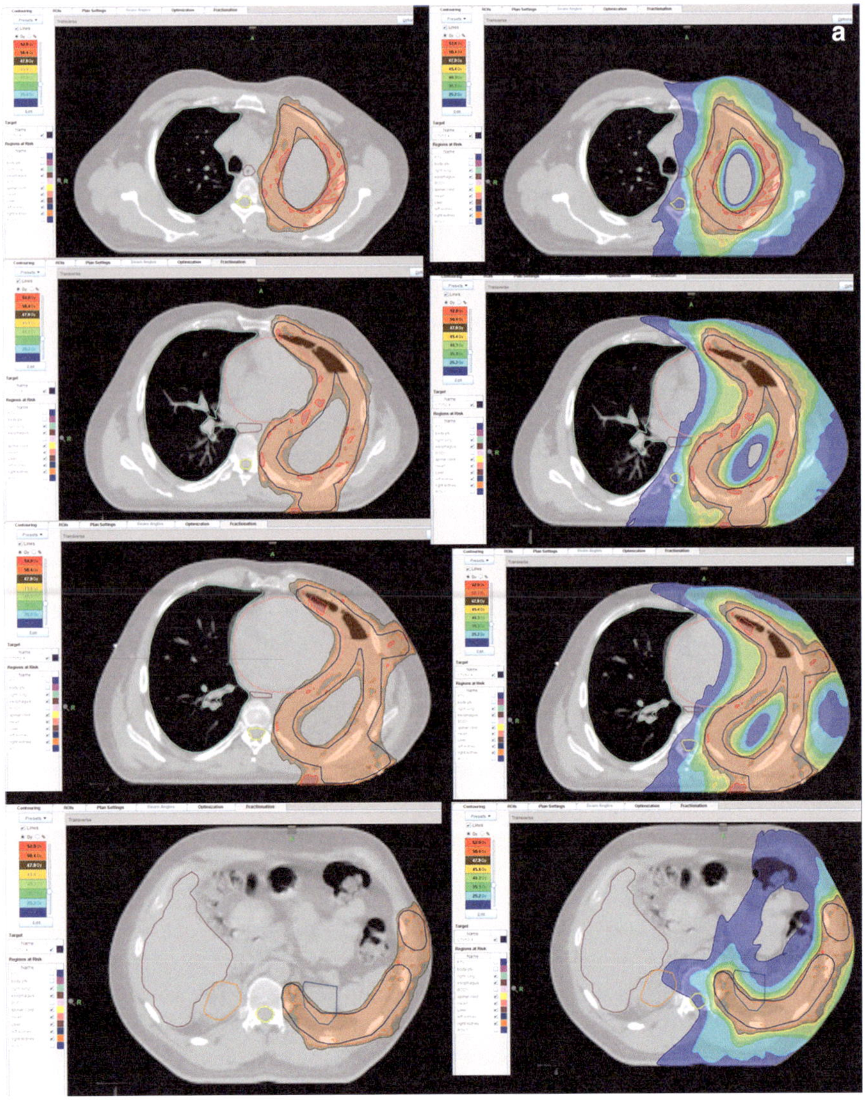

Fig. 20.2 (**a**) Tomotherapy plan after extrapleural pneumonectomy (*EPP*) in a patient with malignant pleural mesothelioma, (**b**) coronal, sagittal, and axial view of 3D CRT plan, (**c**) dose volume histogram (DVH) and dose statistics

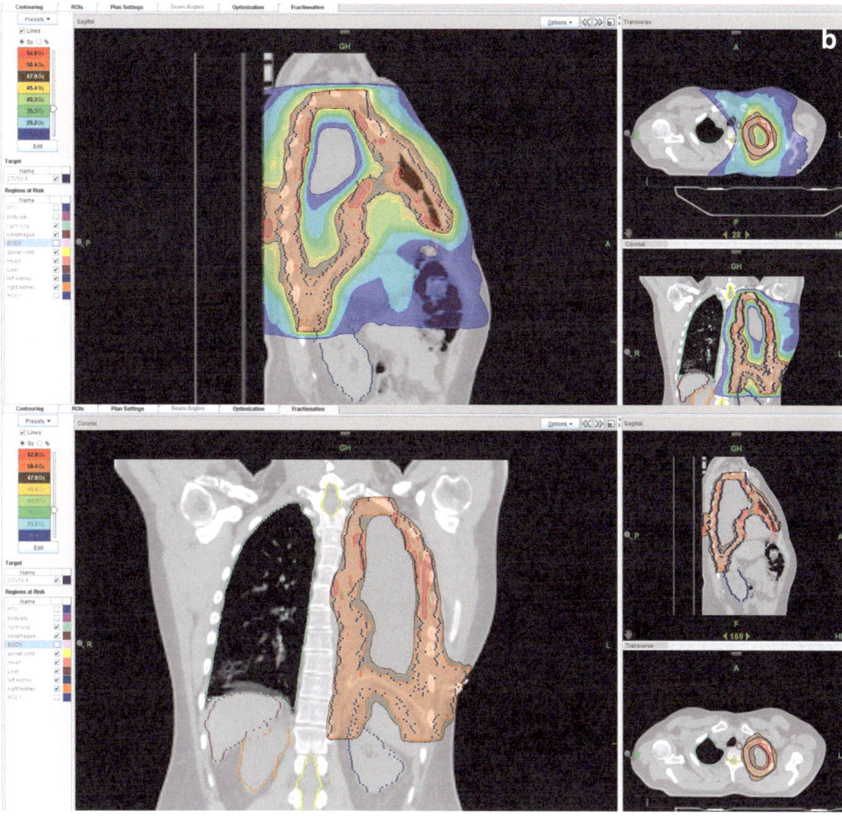

Fig. 20.2 (continued)

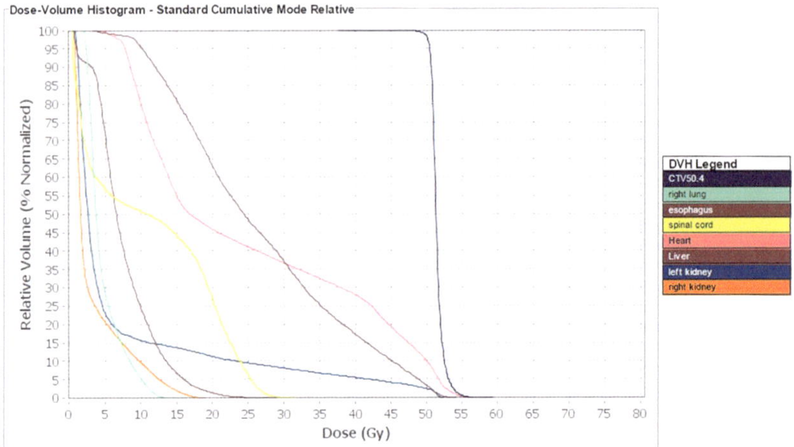

c

Target Constraints and Statistics

Name	Blocked	Use?	Importance	Overlap Priority	Max Dose Constr. [Gy]	Max Dose Pen.	DVH Vol [%]	DVH Dose [Gy]	Min Dose Constr. [Gy]	Min Dose Pen.	Max Dose [Gy]	Min Dose [Gy]	Median Dose [Gy]	Avg Dose [Gy]	StdDev Dose [Gy]	Physical Vol [cc]
CTV50.4	None	yes	1,000	1	50.40	10,000	97.00	50.40	50.40	50,000	59.34	37.65	51.31	51.46	0.90	2,207.20

Regions at Risk Constraints and Statistics

Name	Blocked	Use?	Importance	Overlap Priority	Max Dose Constr. [Gy]	Max Dose Pen.	DVH Vol [%]	DVH Dose [Gy]	DVH Pt. Pen	Max Dose [Gy]	Min Dose [Gy]	Median Dose [Gy]	Avg Dose [Gy]	StdDev Dose [Gy]	Physical Vol [cc]
PTV		no								59.34	15.77	51.12	50.54	2.61	3,448.00
body-ptv	None	yes	10,000	9	45.00	1,000	28.00	20.00	3,000	47.95	0.31	6.21	10.36	9.52	15,521.76
							55.00	5.00	3,000						
							2.50	33.00	6,000						
right lung	DIRECTIO...	yes	2,000	5	13.00	2,000	35.00	4.00	8,000	15.66	1.71	3.68	4.61	2.37	2,296.91
esophagus	None	yes	1	3	1.00	1	1.00	1.00	1	54.14	3.24	24.41	26.52	12.05	37.62
BODY	None	yes	1	10	1.00	1	1.00	1.00	1	59.34	0.20	4.33	13.88	17.02	33,036.55
spinal cord	DIRECTIO...	yes	100	6	40.00	200	1.00	1.00	1	31.79	0.46	10.94	11.41	9.45	81.55
Heart	None	yes	400	4	50.40	100	50.00	15.00	4,000	58.12	4.17	16.81	24.96	16.16	831.76
							35.00	31.00	4,000						
							15.00	46.00	4,000						
Liver	None	yes	1	7	1.00	1	1.00	1.00	1	28.93	0.60	6.53	7.55	4.32	1,521.91
left kidney	None	yes	100	2	50.40	100	8.00	25.00	100	52.38	0.92	2.56	7.27	12.02	180.44
right kidney	None	yes	1	8	1.00	1	1.00	1.00	1	18.92	0.71	1.60	3.37	3.78	147.10
ROI-1	None	yes	3,000	1	50.00	1,000	80.00	10.00	5,000	51.25	8.70	23.19	25.60	13.67	475.08
							48.00	25.00	5,000						

Fig. 20.2 (continued)

Krayenbuehl et al. treated 25 patients with MPM with 3D CRT and 14 with high conformal RT (11 IMRT and three volumetric arc therapies [VMAT]) after neoadjuvant CXT and EPP and compared the results [91]. They reported that, although not statistically significant, high conformal RT resulted in a decreased LR rate (27.3 % vs 72.7 %, $p=0.06$), and longer duration to LR (16.2 ± 3.1 months vs 10.9 ± 5.4 months, $p=0.06$), but similar OS rate. The most important difference was that high conformal RT resulted in significantly improved target coverage. Scorsetti et al. reported better target volume coverage, decreased V20 of the contralateral lung, and shorter treatment time with the RapidArc® which is another form of arc therapy, compared to linac-based IMRT [92].

Treatment with Protons and Heavy Particles

In order to decrease the doses to the OARs, proton and neutron therapies have emerged. Protons are positively charged particles with a Bragg peak showing an immediate dose decrease to zero beyond the target [93]. Although the number of patients is limited in the studies, it has been shown that protons are superior to IMRT with photons in regard to better target dose coverage and OAR sparing while treating MPM after either EPP or P/D or biopsy [94–96].

Boron neutron capture therapy (BNCT) has also been studied in patients with MPM. In BNCT, ^{10}B atoms which are not radioactive disintegrate into ^{4}He particles and ^{7}Li nuclei after they absorb low-energy (thermal) neutrons [97]. This combination of particles can deposit large amounts of energy during its very short path. The patient first receives ^{10}B-binded agents to selectively accumulate in the tumor and is irradiated with thermal neutrons. If a large gradient of ^{10}B concentration between the tumor and normal tissue cells is achieved, the thermal neutrons can selectively kill the tumor cells only. Theoretically, this makes the sparing of OARs more possible without compromising the target dose [98, 99]. Suzuki et al. reported the results of two patients with pleural tumors treated with BNCT and concluded that the tumor was stable or regressed with no grade ≥ 2 acute toxicity [100].

Patel et al. retrospectively evaluated 30 patients with MPM who received neutron RT between 1980 and 2012 [101]. They reported the median OS time 20.3 months and observed LR in 15, distant recurrence in three, and local and distant recurrence in three patients, respectively. There are no data on the toxicity of this treatment.

Conclusion

It has clearly been shown that trimodality treatment should be administered while treating MPM. The extension of the surgery does not significantly affect the LC rates, but it is obvious that all patients need adjuvant treatment even after EPP. Radiotherapy is essential in the treatment of MPM. With the improving techniques, more homogeneous dose distribution is achieved besides decreased critical organ doses. More advanced technology should be administered if possible; however, because of the low incidence of MPM, more phase III studies with higher number of patients are needed.

References

1. Connelly RR, Spirtas R, Myers MH, et al. Demographic patterns for mesothelioma in the United States. J Natl Cancer Inst. 1987;78:1053–60.
2. Scherpereel A, Astoul P, Baas P, et al. Guidelines of the European Respiratory Society and the European Society of Thoracic Surgeons for the management of malignant pleural mesothelioma. Eur Respir J. 2010;35:479–95.

3. Wagner JC, Sleggs CA, Marchand P. Diffuse pleural mesothelioma and asbestos exposure in the North Western Cape Province. Br J Ind Med. 1960;17:260–71.
4. Lanphear BP, Buncher CR. Latent period for malignant mesothelioma of occupational origin. J Occup Med. 1992;34:718–21.
5. Muscat JE, Wynder EL. Cigarette smoking, asbestos exposure, and malignant mesothelioma. Cancer Res. 1991;51:2263–7.
6. Antman KH, Corson JM, Li FP, et al. Malignant mesothelioma following radiation exposure. J Clin Oncol. 1983;1:695–700.
7. Baris I, Simonato L, Artvinli M, et al. Epidemiological and environmental evidence of the health effects of exposure to erionite fibres: a four-year study in the Cappadocian region of Turkey. Int J Cancer. 1987;39:10–7.
8. Baris YI, Sahin AA, Ozesmi M, et al. An outbreak of pleural mesothelioma and chronic fibrosing pleurisy in the village of Karain/Urgup in Anatolia. Thorax. 1978;33:181–92.
9. Wagner JC, Skidmore JW, Hill RJ, Griffiths DM. Erionite exposure and mesotheliomas in rats. Br J Cancer. 1985;51:727–30.
10. Baris B, Demir AU, Shehu V, et al. Environmental fibrous zeolite (erionite) exposure and malignant tumors other than mesothelioma. J Environ Pathol Toxicol Oncol. 1996;15:183–9.
11. Emri S, Demir A, Dogan M, et al. Lung diseases due to environmental exposures to erionite and asbestos in Turkey. Toxicol Lett. 2002;127:251–7.
12. Carbone M, Kratzke RA, Testa JR. The pathogenesis of mesothelioma. Semin Oncol. 2002;29:2–17.
13. Roushdy-Hammady I, Siegel J, Emri S, et al. Genetic-susceptibility factor and malignant mesothelioma in the Cappadocian region of Turkey. Lancet. 2001;357:444–5.
14. Pass HI, Hahn S, Vogelzang NJ, et al. Benign and malignant mesothelioma. In: DeVita V, Hellman S, editors. Cancer: principles and practice of oncology. 7th ed. Philadelphia: Lippincott Williams & Wilkins; 2001. p. 1937–64.
15. Edwards JG, Abrams KR, Leverment JN, et al. Prognostic factors for malignant mesothelioma in 142 patients: validation of CALGB and EORTC prognostic scoring systems. Thorax. 2000;55:731–5.
16. Yildirim H, Metintas M, Entok E, et al. Clinical value of fluorodeoxyglucose-positron emission tomography/computed tomography in differentiation of malignant mesothelioma from asbestos-related benign pleural disease: an observational pilot study. J Thorac Oncol. 2009;4:1480–4.
17. Benard F, Sterman D, Smith RJ, et al. Prognostic value of FDG PET imaging in malignant pleural mesothelioma. J Nucl Med. 1999;40:1241–5.
18. Wilcox BE, Subramaniam RM, Peller PJ, et al. Utility of integrated computed tomography-positron emission tomography for selection of operable malignant pleural mesothelioma. Clin Lung Cancer. 2009;10:244–8.
19. Bueno R, Reblando J, Glickman J, et al. Pleural biopsy: a reliable method for determining the diagnosis but not subtype in mesothelioma. Ann Thorac Surg. 2004;78:1774–6.
20. Rusch VW. Pleurectomy/decortication and adjuvant therapy for malignant mesothelioma. Chest. 1993;103:382S–4.
21. Treasure T, Utley M. Mesothelioma: benefit from surgical resection is questionable. J Thorac Oncol. 2007;2:885–6.
22. Calavrezos A, Koschel G, Husselmann H, et al. Malignant mesothelioma of the pleura. A prospective therapeutic study of 132 patients from 1981–1985. Klin Wochenschr. 1988;66:607–13.
23. Pass HI, Kranda K, Temeck BK, et al. Surgically debulked malignant pleural mesothelioma: results and prognostic factors. Ann Surg Oncol. 1997;4:215–22.
24. Weder W, Stahel RA, Bernhard J, et al. Multicenter trial of neo-adjuvant chemotherapy followed by extrapleural pneumonectomy in malignant pleural mesothelioma. Ann Oncol. 2007;18:1196–202.

25. Rusch VW, Rosenzweig K, Venkatraman E, et al. A phase II trial of surgical resection and adjuvant high-dose hemithoracic radiation for malignant pleural mesothelioma. J Thorac Cardiovasc Surg. 2001;122:788–95.
26. Baldini EH. External beam radiation therapy for the treatment of pleural mesothelioma. Thorac Surg Clin. 2004;14:543–8.
27. Sugarbaker DJ, Flores RM, Jaklitsch MT, et al. Resection margins, extrapleural nodal status, and cell type determine postoperative long-term survival in trimodality therapy of malignant pleural mesothelioma: results in 183 patients. J Thorac Cardiovasc Surg. 1999;117:54–63; discussion 63–55.
28. Huncharek M, Kelsey K, Mark EJ, et al. Treatment and survival in diffuse malignant pleural mesothelioma; a study of 83 cases from the Massachusetts General Hospital. Anticancer Res. 1996;16:1265–8.
29. Treasure T, Waller D, Tan C, et al. The mesothelioma and radical surgery randomized controlled trial: the mars feasibility study. J Thorac Oncol. 2009;4:1254–8.
30. Okubo K, Sonobe M, Fujinaga T, et al. Survival and relapse pattern after trimodality therapy for malignant pleural mesothelioma. Gen Thorac Cardiovasc Surg. 2009;57:585–90.
31. Tonoli S, Vitali P, Scotti V, et al. Adjuvant radiotherapy after extrapleural pneumonectomy for mesothelioma. Prospective analysis of a multi-institutional series. Radiother Oncol. 2011;101:311–5.
32. Baldini EH, Recht A, Strauss GM, et al. Patterns of failure after trimodality therapy for malignant pleural mesothelioma. Ann Thorac Surg. 1997;63:334–8.
33. Bricout PB, Engler MJ. Computerized tomography scanning and the planning of high-dose radiotherapy for pleural mesothelioma: a report of five patients. Int J Radiat Oncol Biol Phys. 1981;7:821–6.
34. Kutcher GJ, Kestler C, Greenblatt D, et al. Technique for external beam treatment for mesothelioma. Int J Radiat Oncol Biol Phys. 1987;13:1747–52.
35. Yajnik S, Rosenzweig KE, Mychalczak B, et al. Hemithoracic radiation after extrapleural pneumonectomy for malignant pleural mesothelioma. Int J Radiat Oncol Biol Phys. 2003;56:1319–26.
36. Ahamad A, Stevens CW, Smythe WR, et al. Promising early local control of malignant pleural mesothelioma following postoperative intensity modulated radiotherapy (IMRT) to the chest. Cancer J. 2003;9:476–84.
37. Ahamad A, Stevens CW, Smythe WR, et al. Intensity-modulated radiation therapy: a novel approach to the management of malignant pleural mesothelioma. Int J Radiat Oncol Biol Phys. 2003;55:768–75.
38. Forster KM, Smythe WR, Starkschall G, et al. Intensity-modulated radiotherapy following extrapleural pneumonectomy for the treatment of malignant mesothelioma: clinical implementation. Int J Radiat Oncol Biol Phys. 2003;55:606–16.
39. Rice DC, Stevens CW, Correa AM, et al. Outcomes after extrapleural pneumonectomy and intensity-modulated radiation therapy for malignant pleural mesothelioma. Ann Thorac Surg. 2007;84:1685–92; discussion 1692–1683.
40. de Perrot M, Feld R, Cho BC, et al. Trimodality therapy with induction chemotherapy followed by extrapleural pneumonectomy and adjuvant high-dose hemithoracic radiation for malignant pleural mesothelioma. J Clin Oncol. 2009;27:1413–8.
41. Allen AM, Czerminska M, Janne PA, et al. Fatal pneumonitis associated with intensity-modulated radiation therapy for mesothelioma. Int J Radiat Oncol Biol Phys. 2006;65:640–5.
42. Miles EF, Larrier NA, Kelsey CR, et al. Intensity-modulated radiotherapy for resected mesothelioma: the Duke experience. Int J Radiat Oncol Biol Phys. 2008;71:1143–50.
43. Rice DC, Smythe WR, Liao Z, et al. Dose-dependent pulmonary toxicity after postoperative intensity-modulated radiotherapy for malignant pleural mesothelioma. Int J Radiat Oncol Biol Phys. 2007;69:350–7.
44. Flores RM, Riedel E, Donington JS, et al. Frequency of use and predictors of cancer-directed surgery in the management of malignant pleural mesothelioma in a community-based

(Surveillance, Epidemiology, and End Results [SEER]) population. J Thorac Oncol. 2010;5:1649–54.
45. Hurmuz P, Akyol F, Selek U, Ozyigit G, Dogan R, Ozdemir N, Tastepe I, Kayi Cangir A, Kara M, Demirkazik F, Emri S. The efficiency and toxicity of hemithoracic radiotherapy after extra pleural pneumonectomy in malign pleural mesothelioma. Int J Hematol Oncol. 2010;1:20–6.
46. Carmichael J, Degraff WG, Gamson J, et al. Radiation sensitivity of human lung cancer cell lines. Eur J Cancer Clin Oncol. 1989;25:527–34.
47. Gordon Jr W, Antman KH, Greenberger JS, et al. Radiation therapy in the management of patients with mesothelioma. Int J Radiat Oncol Biol Phys. 1982;8:19–25.
48. Allen AM, Den R, Wong JS, et al. Influence of radiotherapy technique and dose on patterns of failure for mesothelioma patients after extrapleural pneumonectomy. Int J Radiat Oncol Biol Phys. 2007;68:1366–74.
49. Rengan R, Bonner Millar LP, Thomas Jr CR. Uncommon thoracic tumors. In: Gunderson LL, Tepper J, editors. Clinical radiation oncology. 3rd ed. Philadelphia: Elsevier Saunders; 2012. p. 859–89.
50. Alberts AS, Falkson G, Goedhals L, et al. Malignant pleural mesothelioma: a disease unaffected by current therapeutic maneuvers. J Clin Oncol. 1988;6:527–35.
51. Ball DL, Cruickshank DG. The treatment of malignant mesothelioma of the pleura: review of a 5-year experience, with special reference to radiotherapy. Am J Clin Oncol. 1990;13:4–9.
52. Maasilta P. Deterioration in lung function following hemithorax irradiation for pleural mesothelioma. Int J Radiat Oncol Biol Phys. 1991;20:433–8.
53. Rusch VW, Piantadosi S, Holmes EC. The role of extrapleural pneumonectomy in malignant pleural mesothelioma. A Lung Cancer Study Group trial. J Thorac Cardiovasc Surg. 1991;102:1–9.
54. van Ooijen B, Eggermont AM, Wiggers T. Subcutaneous tumor growth complicating the positioning of Denver shunt and intrapleural port-a-cath in mesothelioma patients. Eur J Surg Oncol. 1992;18:638–40.
55. Munter MW, Thieke C, Nikoghosyan A, et al. Inverse planned stereotactic intensity modulated radiotherapy (IMRT) in the palliative treatment of malignant mesothelioma of the pleura: the Heidelberg experience. Lung Cancer. 2005;49 Suppl 1:S83–6.
56. Rosenzweig KE, Zauderer MG, Laser B, et al. Pleural intensity-modulated radiotherapy for malignant pleural mesothelioma. Int J Radiat Oncol Biol Phys. 2012;83:1278–83.
57. Rimner A, Spratt DE, Zauderer MG, et al. Failure patterns after hemithoracic pleural intensity modulated radiation therapy for malignant pleural mesothelioma. Int J Radiat Oncol Biol Phys. 2014;90:394–401.
58. Minatel E, Trovo M, Polesel J, et al. Tomotherapy after pleurectomy/decortication or biopsy for malignant pleural mesothelioma allows the delivery of high dose of radiation in patients with intact lung. J Thorac Oncol. 2012;7:1862–6.
59. Ruffie P, Feld R, Minkin S, et al. Diffuse malignant mesothelioma of the pleura in Ontario and Quebec: a retrospective study of 332 patients. J Clin Oncol. 1989;7:1157–68.
60. Law MR, Hodson ME, Turner-Warwick M. Malignant mesothelioma of the pleura: clinical aspects and symptomatic treatment. Eur J Respir Dis. 1984;65:162–8.
61. Agarwal PP, Seely JM, Matzinger FR, et al. Pleural mesothelioma: sensitivity and incidence of needle track seeding after image-guided biopsy versus surgical biopsy. Radiology. 2006;241:589–94.
62. Boutin C, Rey F, Viallat JR. Prevention of malignant seeding after invasive diagnostic procedures in patients with pleural mesothelioma. A randomized trial of local radiotherapy. Chest. 1995;108:754–8.
63. O'Rourke N, Garcia JC, Paul J, et al. A randomised controlled trial of intervention site radiotherapy in malignant pleural mesothelioma. Radiother Oncol. 2007;84:18–22.
64. Muirhead R, O'Rourke N. Drain site radiotherapy in malignant pleural mesothelioma: a wasted resource. Eur Respir J. 2007;30:1021.

65. Chapman E, Berenstein EG, Dieguez M, Ortiz Z. Radiotherapy for malignant pleural mesothelioma. Cochrane Database of Systematic Reviews 2006, Issue 3. Art. No.: CD003880. doi:10.1002/14651858.CD003880.pub4.
66. Bydder S, Phillips M, Joseph DJ, et al. A randomised trial of single-dose radiotherapy to prevent procedure tract metastasis by malignant mesothelioma. Br J Cancer. 2004;91:9–10.
67. De Ruysscher D, Slotman B. Treatment of intervention sites of malignant pleural mesothelioma with radiotherapy: a Dutch-Belgian survey. Radiother Oncol. 2003;68:299–302.
68. Lee C, Bayman N, Swindell R, Faivre-Finn C. Prophylactic radiotherapy to intervention sites in mesothelioma: a systematic review and survey of UK practice. Lung Cancer. 2009;66:150–6.
69. Janssen-Heijnen ML, Damhuis RA, Klinkhamer PJ, et al. Increased but low incidence and poor survival of malignant mesothelioma in the southeastern part of The Netherlands since 1970: a population-based study. Eur J Cancer Prev. 1999;8:311–4.
70. Clive AO, Wilson P, Taylor H, et al. Protocol for the surgical and large bore procedures in malignant pleural mesothelioma and radiotherapy trial (SMART Trial): an RCT evaluating whether prophylactic radiotherapy reduces the incidence of procedure tract metastases. BMJ Open. 2015;5:e006673.
71. Gupta V, Mychalczak B, Krug L, et al. Hemithoracic radiation therapy after pleurectomy/decortication for malignant pleural mesothelioma. Int J Radiat Oncol Biol Phys. 2005;63:1045–52.
72. Hill-Kayser CE, Avery S, Mesina CF, et al. Hemithoracic radiotherapy after extrapleural pneumonectomy for malignant pleural mesothelioma: a dosimetric comparison of two well-described techniques. J Thorac Oncol. 2009;4:1431–7.
73. Buduhan G, Menon S, Aye R, et al. Trimodality therapy for malignant pleural mesothelioma. Ann Thorac Surg. 2009;88:870–5; discussion 876.
74. Price A. What is the role of radiotherapy in malignant pleural mesothelioma? Oncologist. 2011;16:359–65.
75. Cho BC, Feld R, Leighl N, et al. A feasibility study evaluating Surgery for Mesothelioma After Radiation Therapy: the "SMART" approach for resectable malignant pleural mesothelioma. J Thorac Oncol. 2014;9:397–402.
76. Gomez DR, Hong DS, Allen PK, et al. Patterns of failure, toxicity, and survival after extrapleural pneumonectomy and hemithoracic intensity-modulated radiation therapy for malignant pleural mesothelioma. J Thorac Oncol. 2013;8:238–45.
77. Patel PR, Yoo S, Broadwater G, et al. Effect of increasing experience on dosimetric and clinical outcomes in the management of malignant pleural mesothelioma with intensity-modulated radiation therapy. Int J Radiat Oncol Biol Phys. 2012;83:362–8.
78. Rosenzweig KE. Current readings: improvements in intensity-modulated radiation therapy for malignant pleural mesothelioma. Semin Thorac Cardiovasc Surg. 2013;25:245–50.
79. Du KL, Both S, Friedberg JS, et al. Extrapleural pneumonectomy, photodynamic therapy and intensity modulated radiation therapy for the treatment of malignant pleural mesothelioma. Cancer Biol Ther. 2010;10:425–9.
80. Allen AM, Schofield D, Hacker F, et al. Restricted field IMRT dramatically enhances IMRT planning for mesothelioma. Int J Radiat Oncol Biol Phys. 2007;69:1587–92.
81. Zhu XR, Prado K, Liu HH, et al. Intensity-modulated radiation therapy for mesothelioma: impact of multileaf collimator leaf width and pencil beam size on planning quality and delivery efficiency. Int J Radiat Oncol Biol Phys. 2005;62:1525–34.
82. Jang SY, Liu HH, Mohan R. Underestimation of low-dose radiation in treatment planning of intensity-modulated radiotherapy. Int J Radiat Oncol Biol Phys. 2008;71:1537–46.
83. Chi A, Liao Z, Nguyen NP, et al. Intensity-modulated radiotherapy after extrapleural pneumonectomy in the combined-modality treatment of malignant pleural mesothelioma. J Thorac Oncol. 2011;6:1132–41.
84. Fenwick JD, Tome WA, Soisson ET, et al. Tomotherapy and other innovative IMRT delivery systems. Semin Radiat Oncol. 2006;16:199–208.
85. Chen AM, Marsano J, Perks J, et al. Comparison of IMRT techniques in the radiotherapeutic management of head and neck cancer: is tomotherapy "better" than step-and-shoot IMRT? Technol Cancer Res Treat. 2011;10:171–7.

86. Chen YJ, Liu A, Han C, et al. Helical tomotherapy for radiotherapy in esophageal cancer: a preferred plan with better conformal target coverage and more homogeneous dose distribution. Med Dosim. 2007;32:166–71.
87. Sterzing F, Sroka-Perez G, Schubert K, et al. Evaluating target coverage and normal tissue sparing in the adjuvant radiotherapy of malignant pleural mesothelioma: helical tomotherapy compared with step-and-shoot IMRT. Radiother Oncol. 2008;86:251–7.
88. Giraud P, Sylvestre A, Zefkili S, et al. Helical tomotherapy for resected malignant pleural mesothelioma: dosimetric evaluation and toxicity. Radiother Oncol. 2011;101:303–6.
89. Sylvestre A, Mahe MA, Lisbona A, et al. Mesothelioma at era of helical tomotherapy: results of two institutions in combining chemotherapy, surgery and radiotherapy. Lung Cancer. 2011;74:486–91.
90. Helou J, Clement-Colmou K, Sylvestre A, et al. Helical tomotherapy in the treatment of malignant pleural mesothelioma: the impact of low doses on pulmonary and oesophageal toxicity. Cancer Radiother. 2013;17:755–62.
91. Krayenbuehl J, Dimmerling P, Ciernik IF, Riesterer O. Clinical outcome of postoperative highly conformal versus 3D conformal radiotherapy in patients with malignant pleural mesothelioma. Radiat Oncol. 2014;9:32.
92. Scorsetti M, Bignardi M, Clivio A, et al. Volumetric modulation arc radiotherapy compared with static gantry intensity-modulated radiotherapy for malignant pleural mesothelioma tumor: a feasibility study. Int J Radiat Oncol Biol Phys. 2010;77:942–9.
93. Suit H, Urie M. Proton beams in radiation therapy. J Natl Cancer Inst. 1992;84:155–64.
94. Krayenbuehl J, Hartmann M, Lomax AJ, et al. Proton therapy for malignant pleural mesothelioma after extrapleural pleuropneumonectomy. Int J Radiat Oncol Biol Phys. 2010;78:628–34.
95. Lorentini S, Amichetti M, Spiazzi L, et al. Adjuvant intensity-modulated proton therapy in malignant pleural mesothelioma. A comparison with intensity-modulated radiotherapy and a spot size variation assessment. Strahlenther Onkol. 2012;188:216–25.
96. Pan HY, Jiang S, Sutton J, et al. Early experience with intensity modulated proton therapy for lung-intact mesothelioma: a case series. Pract Radiat Oncol. 2015;5:e345–53.
97. Coderre JA, Morris GM. The radiation biology of boron neutron capture therapy. Radiat Res. 1999;151:1–18.
98. Suzuki M, Sakurai Y, Masunaga S, et al. Feasibility of boron neutron capture therapy (BNCT) for malignant pleural mesothelioma from a viewpoint of dose distribution analysis. Int J Radiat Oncol Biol Phys. 2006;66:1584–9.
99. Suzuki M, Sakurai Y, Masunaga S, et al. A preliminary experimental study of boron neutron capture therapy for malignant tumors spreading in thoracic cavity. Jpn J Clin Oncol. 2007;37:245–9.
100. Suzuki M, Endo K, Satoh H, et al. A novel concept of treatment of diffuse or multiple pleural tumors by boron neutron capture therapy (BNCT). Radiother Oncol. 2008;88:192–5.
101. Patel SA, Kusano AS, Truong A, et al. Fast neutron radiotherapy in the treatment of malignant pleural mesothelioma. Am J Clin Oncol. 2015;38:47–50.

Modern Surgical Techniques in Malignant Pleural Mesothelioma

21

Yusuf Kahya, Erkan Dikmen, and Ayten Kayı Cangır

Introduction

Pathologic diagnosis was based on standard histologic, histochemical, and immunohistochemical criteria in all cases.

As a positive marker of immunohistochemistry for MPM:

1. Calretinin
2. Mesothelin
3. Cytokeratin 5/6
4. D2–40

As negative:

1. Thyroid transcription factor-1
2. Carcinoembryonic antigen
3. BerEP4

Y. Kahya
Department of Thoracic Surgery, Faculty of Medicine, Ankara University, Ankara, Turkey
e-mail: dr.yusufkahya@hotmail.com

E. Dikmen, MD
Department of Thoracic Surgery, Faculty of Medicine, Hacettepe University, Ankara, Turkey
e-mail: erkandikmen@hacettepe.edu.tr

A.K. Cangır, MD (✉)
Department of Thoracic Surgery, Faculty of Medicine, Ankara University, Ankara, Turkey
e-mail: cangir@medicine.ankara.edu.tr

G. Ozyigit et al. (eds.), *Principles and Practice of Radiotherapy Techniques in Thoracic Malignancies*, DOI 10.1007/978-3-319-28761-4_21

Pretreatment evaluation for patients diagnosed with MPM is performed to stage patients and to assess whether patients are candidates for surgery. This evaluation includes the following:

1. Chest and abdominal computed tomography (CT) with contrast.
2. Cranial magnetic resonance imaging (MRI)/CT.
3. Positron emission tomography-CT (PET-CT) but only for patients being considered for surgery.
4. Video-assisted thoracic surgery (VATS) or laparoscopy can be considered if contralateral or peritoneal disease is suspected.

If surgical resection is being considered, mediastinoscopy or endobronchial ultrasonography (EBUS) fine needle aspiration (FNA) of the mediastinal lymph nodes is recommended. The following tests may be performed if suggested by imaging: (1) laparoscopy to rule out transdiaphragmatic extension (e.g., extension to the peritoneum is indicative of stage IV [unresectable] disease) and (2) chest MRI [10].

Staging is performed using the International Mesothelioma Interest Group (IMIG) TNM staging system. The staging system for malignant pleural mesothelioma is controversial. Therefore, in collaboration with IMIG, the International Association for the Study of Lung Cancer (IASLC) has decided to update the staging system for MPM by developing a large international database. The prospective MPM staging project is an international effort to study and improve the current staging system for MPM. The revised new staging system will be announced soon [9, 16].

Most patients have advanced disease at presentation. However, it is difficult to accurately stage patients before surgery. Understaging is common with PET-CT. Patients with clinical stage I to III MPM can be evaluated for surgery using the following:

1. Pulmonary function tests (PFTs) including diffusing capacity of the lung for carbon monoxide (DLCO)
2. Perfusion scanning (if forced expiratory volume in 1 s (FEV1) <80 %)
3. Cardiac stress tests, transthoracic echocardiography, and cardiac MRI
4. Routine blood examinations

Cytoreductive Surgery

It is essential that patients receive a careful assessment before surgery is performed. Surgical resection for patients with MPM can include either (1) radical pleurectomy/decortication (P/D, also known as total pleurectomy, lung-sparing surgery), which is complete removal of the involved the visceral, parietal, and pericardial of pleura and mediastinal nodes; (Fig. 21.1) or (2) extrapleural pneumonectomy (EPP) is a more aggressive procedure entailing en bloc resection of the parietal and

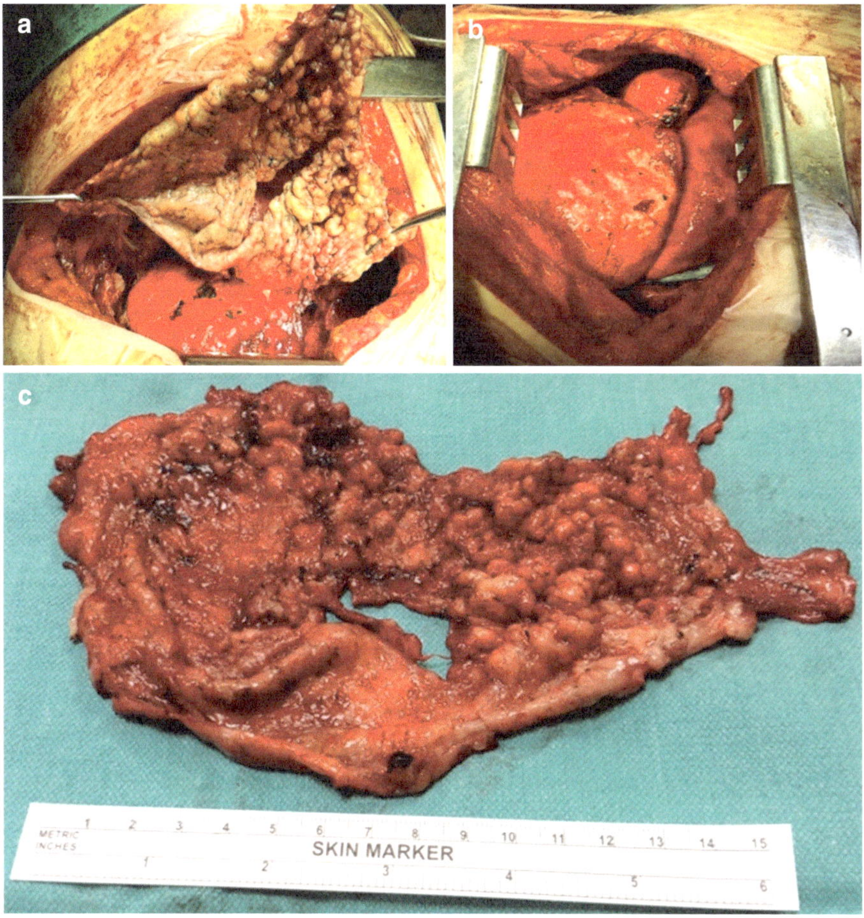

Fig. 21.1 Right P/D, operative view (**a**) lung surface after P/D (**b**) resection specimen (**c**)

visceral pleura with the enclosed lung, pericardium, ipsilateral diaphragm, and mediastinal nodes (Fig. 21.2). Extended P/D refers to the resection of the diaphragm and pericardium in addition to total pleurectomy. Mediastinal nodal dissection is recommended in patients having either P/D or EPP; at least three nodal stations should be obtained.

Surgery is recommended for select patients who require a complete cytoreduction:

1. Good performance status (PS)
2. No comorbidities
3. Patients with stage I–III disease
4. Favorable histology (i.e., epithelioid)
5. No N2 disease

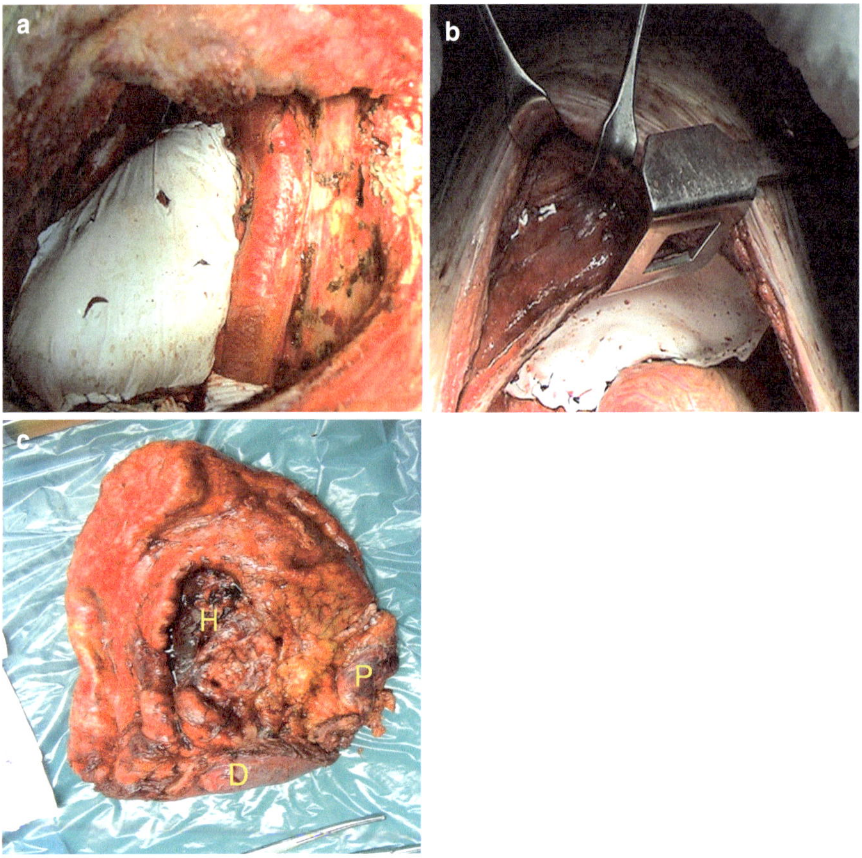

Fig. 21.2 Left EPP operative views, EPP involves the en bloc resection of the parietal and visceral pleura, lung, ipsilateral pericardium, and diaphragm with reconstruction of the latter two structures, in this case with polytetrafluoroethylene (PTFE) membrane (**a**, **b**) Resection specimen, *H* hilum, *D* diaphragm, and *P* pericardium (**c**)

But surgery is not usually recommended for patients at high risk:

1. Unfavorable histology (e.g., sarcomatoid, mixed tumors)
2. N2 disease (Data about the role of mediastinal lymph node involvement of the different case series are conflicting, but the results of the new IASLC/IMIG staging project analyzing the largest set of MPM data demonstrate that N2 disease is not a factor which influences survival significantly as compared to the N1 nodes.)
3. Patient with stage IV [4, 5, 7]

The surgical goal for MPM is cytoreductive surgery to achieve macroscopic complete resection. Neither EPP nor P/D will yield an R0 resection. The choice of surgery for MPM is controversial, because data from randomized controlled trials are not available. In patients who are medically operable, the decision about whether to do a P/D or an EPP may not be made until surgical exploration. The choice between P/D and EPP should be made based on several factors including tumor histology and distribution, pulmonary reserve, and surgical experience and expertise, as well as availability of adjuvant and intraoperative strategies. For early disease (confined to the pleural envelope and no N2 lymph node involvement) with favorable histology (epithelioid), P/D may be safer than EPP, but it is unclear which operation is oncologically better. P/D may be more appropriate for patients with advanced MPM who cannot tolerate an EPP. EPP would often be required to remove all gross tumors in patients with stages II to III MPM. However, EPP is associated

Table 21.1 Result after EPP and multimodality therapy in selected series

Author	Year	Chemotherapy	EPP (n)	TMT/ITT (%)	30 day mortality (%)	Median survival, ITT (month)
Sugarbaker	1999	Adjuvant	183	?	3.8	19
Rusch	2001	No, adj radiotherapy	62	61 %	11.3	17
Pagan	2006	Adjuvant	44	57 %	4.5	20
Weder	2007	Neoadjuvant	45	59 %	2.2	19.8
Edwars	2007	Adj/neoadjuvant	105	?	6.7	14.5
Rice	2007	Not standard	100	<63 %	8	10.2
Batirel	2008	Adjuvant	16	60 %	5	17.2
De Perrot	2009	Neoadjuvant	45	50 %	6.7	14
Krug	2009	Neoadjuvant	54	52 %	3.7	16.8
Trousse	2009	Adj/neoadjuvant	83	?	4.8	14.5
Hasani	2009	Adjuvant	18	64 %	11	20.4
Buduhan	2009	Neoadjuvant	46	69 %	4.3	24
Van Schil	2010	Neoadjuvant	42	65 %	6.5 (90d)	18.4
Rea	2013	Neoadjuvant	45	40 %	4.4	15.5

TMT/ITT percentage of patients receiving trimodality therapy by intention to treat

Table 21.2 Results after P/D in selected series

Author	Year	Chemotherapy, radiotherapy	P/D (n)	TMT/ ITT (%)	Morbidity (%)	30 day mortality (%)	Median survival, ITT (month)
Hilaris	1984	Intraoperative brachytherapy adjuvant radiotheraphy 45 Gy	41	100 %	15	0	21
Rusch	1994	Intraoperative chemotherapy adjuvant chemotherapy	28	64 %		3.5	17

(continued)

Table 21.2 (continued)

Author	Year	Chemotherapy, radiotherapy	P/D (n)	TMT/ ITT (%)	Morbidity (%)	30 day mortality (%)	Median survival, ITT (month)
Lee	2002	Adjuvant chemotherapy intraoperative and adjuvant radiotherapy 45 Gy	32	37.5 %	15	6.2	18.1
Richards	2006	Intraoperative chemotherapy	44	72 %	41	11	9
Lucchi	2007	Adjuvant chemotherapy, interleukin-2 and radiotherapy 30 Gy	49	100 %	10	0	26
Nakas	2008	Adjuvant chemotherapy prophylactic radiotherapy	51	?46 %	55	5.9	15.3
Bolukbas	2011	Adjuvant chemotherapy prophylactic radiotherapy	35	94 %	20	2.9	30
Lang-Lazdunski	2011	Adjuvant chemotherapy prophylactic radiotherapy	36	100 %	25	0	24
Friedberg	2012	Adjuvant photodynamic therapy and chemotherapy	38	100 %		2.7	31.7
Minatel	2013	Adjuvant chemotherapy and radiotherapy 50 Gy	20	95 %		0	33

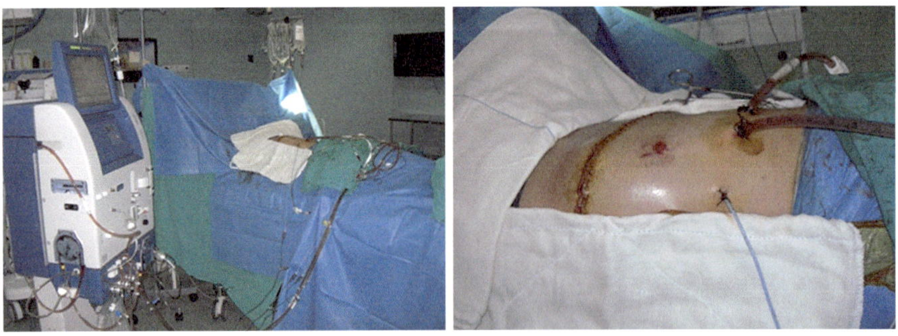

Fig. 21.3 Application of HIPEC after cytoreductive surgery

with higher morbidity and mortality. P/D is safer than EPP (Tables 21.1 and 21.2) [8, 11–15].

Intraoperative adjuvant therapy, such as heated chemotherapy (HIPEC) or photodynamic therapy, is still under investigation but may be considered as part of a reasonable multidisciplinary approach to this locally aggressive disease (Fig. 21.3) [6].

Management of MPM should take place in the setting of a multidisciplinary team with a multimodality approach. Multimodality therapy combined with surgery (EPP or P/D) has seen success with 5-year survival at select group of patients [17].

References

1. Rice D, Rusch V, Pass H, et al. Recommendations for uniform definitions of surgical techniques for malignant pleural mesothelioma: a consensus report of the International Association for the Study of Lung Cancer International Staging Committee and the International Mesothelioma Interest Group. J Thorac Oncol. 2011;6:1304–12.
2. Flores RM, Pass HI, Seshan VE, et al. Extrapleural pneumonectomy versus pleurectomy/decortication in the surgical management of malignant pleural mesothelioma: results in 663 patients. J Thorac Cardiovasc Surg. 2008;135:620–6.
3. Spaggiari L, Marulli G, Boyolato P, et al. Extrapleural pneumonectomy for malignant mesothelioma: an Italian multicenter retrospective study. Ann Thorac Surg. 2014;97:1859–65.
4. Flores RM, Riedel E, Donington JS, et al. Frequency of use and predictors of cancer-directed surgery in the management of malignant pleural mesothelioma in a community-based (Surveillance, Epidemiology, and End Results [SEER]) population. J Thorac Oncol. 2010;5:1649–54.
5. Treasure T, Lang-Lazdunski L, Waller D, et al. Extra-pleural pneumonectomy versus no extra-pleural pneumonectomy for patients with malignant pleural mesothelioma: clinical outcomes of the Mesothelioma and Radical Surgery (MARS) randomised feasibility study. Lancet Oncol. 2011;12:763–72.
6. Sugarbaker DJ, Gill RR, Yeap BY, Wolf AS, DaSilva MC, Baldini EH, et al. Hyperthermic intraoperative pleural cisplatin chemotherapy extend interval to recurrence and survival among low – risk patients with malignant pleural mesothelioma undergoing surgical macroscopic complete resection. J Thorac Cardiovasc Surg. 2013;145:955–63.
7. Sugarbaker DJ, Wolf AS, Chirieac LR, et al. Clinical and pathological features of three-year survivors of malignant pleural mesothelioma following extrapleural pneumonectomy. Eur J Cardiothorac Surg. 2011;40:298–303.
8. Lang-Lazdunski L. Surgery for malignant pleural mesothelioma: why, when and what? Lung Cancer. 2014;84:103–9.
9. Rusch VW, Giroux D. Do we need a revised staging system for malignant pleural mesothelioma? Analysis of the IASLC database. Ann Cardiothorac Surg. 2012;1:438–48.
10. Wilcox BE, Subramaniam RM, Peller PJ, et al. Utility of integrated computed tomography-positron emission tomography for selection of operable malignant pleural mesothelioma. Clin Lung Cancer. 2009;10:244–8.
11. Teh E, Fiorentino F, Tan C, Treasure T. A systematic review of lung-sparing extirpative surgery for pleural mesothelioma. J R Soc Med. 2011;104:69–80.
12. Cao C, Tian D, Park J, et al. A systematic review and meta-analysis of surgical treatments for malignant pleural mesothelioma. Lung Cancer. 2014;83:240–5.
13. Bovolato P, Casadio C, Bille A, et al. Does surgery improve survival of patients with malignant pleural mesothelioma? A multicenter retrospective analysis of 1365 consecutive patients. J Thorac Oncol. 2014;9:390–6.

14. Zauderer MG, Krug LM. The evolution of multimodality therapy for malignant pleural mesothelioma. Curr Treat Options Oncol. 2011;12:163–72.
15. Zahid I, Sharif S, Routledge T, Scarci M. Is pleurectomy and decortication superior to palliative care in the treatment of malignant pleural mesothelioma? Interact Cardiovasc Thorac Surg. 2011;12:812–7.
16. Rusch VW, Giroux D, Kennedy C, Ruffini E, Cangır AK, Rice D, Pass H, Asamura H, Waller, Edwards J, Weder W, van Meerbeeck HHJP, on behalf of the IASLC Staging Committee and participating institutions. Initial analysis of the International Association for the Study of Lung Cancer mesothelioma database. J Thorac Oncol. 2012;7:1631–9.
17. Pass HI, Giroux D, Kennedy C, Ruffini E, Cangır AK, Rice D, Asamura H, Waller D, Edwards J, Weder W, van Meerbeeck HHJP, Rusch VW, on behalf of the IASLC Staging Committee and Participating Institutions. Supplementary prognostic variables for pleural mesothelioma a report from the IASLC staging committee. J Thorac Oncol. 2014;9:856–64.

Systemic Therapies in Malignant Pleural Mesothelioma

22

Ozan Yazici and Sercan Aksoy

Introduction

In patients who were not candidate for surgery and patients with sarcomatoid MPM, systemic chemotherapy is the choice of treatment option [10]. The combination of pemetrexed with platinum (cisplatin or carboplatin) is the standard systemic chemotherapy regimen for the patients with MPM. The combination of pemetrexed and platin is shown to prolong the overall survival of patients. Therefore this regimen might be applied prior or after surgery or radiotherapy [16, 35]. The systemic therapy options for the patients with unresectable MPM will be discussed below.

First-Line Therapies

In the beginning of the twentieth century, multiple single-agent chemotherapy agents were tested in patients with MPM [24, 28]. However, the overall survival (OS) did not exceed 6–8 months. The following years, the active single agents were tested in combinations (Table 22.1).

Cisplatin Plus Pemetrexed

This combination is the most frequently preferred regimen in treatment of patients with MPM based on the results of a randomized phase III trial. In this single-blinded

O. Yazici
Department of Medical Oncology, Ankara Numune Education & Research Hospital, Sihhiye 06410, Ankara, Turkey

S. Aksoy, MD (✉)
Department of Medical Oncology, Faculty of Medicine, Hacettepe University, Ankara, Turkey
e-mail: saksoy07@yahoo.com

G. Ozyigit et al. (eds.), *Principles and Practice of Radiotherapy Techniques in Thoracic Malignancies*, DOI 10.1007/978-3-319-28761-4_22

Table 22.1 Randomized phase II and phase III trials evaluating the first- or second-line chemotherapy agents in patients with MPM

Agents	Line of therapy	Phase and randomization status	Number of patients	Progression-free survival (PFS) (Months)	*p* value	Overall survival (OS) (Months)	*p* value	Results
Pemetrexed 500 mg/m^2 plus cisplatin 75 mg/m^2 on day 1, or cisplatin 75 mg/m^2 on day 1	First	III, randomized	448	5.7 vs 3.9	0.01	12.1 vs 9.3	0.002	PFS and OS were improved in combination arm
Pemetrexed 500 mg/m^2 and carboplatin area under the plasma concentration-time curve of 5 mg/mL/min	First	II, non randomized	102	6.5	–	12.7	–	Pemetrexed plus carboplatin was active regimen
Pemetrexed 500 mg/m^2, cisplatin 75 mg/m^2 on day 1 plus bevacizumab 15 mg/kg biweekly or pemetrexed cisplatin combination without bevacizumab	First	III, randomized	445	9.6 vs 7.5	<0.01	18.8 vs 16.1	0.012	PFS and OS were improved by addition of bevacizumab to chemotherapy combination
Cisplatin 80 mg/m^2 plus raltitrexed 3 mg/m2 or cisplatin 80 mg/m^2 on day 1 alone	First	III, randomized	250	5.3 vs 4.0	0.058	11.4 vs 8.8	0.048	PFS and OS were improved in combination arm

Gemcitabine 1250 mg/m^2 on day 1 and day 8 plus cisplatin 80 mg/m^2 on day 1	First	II, non randomized	25	6	–	9.6	–	Gemcitabine plus cisplatin had moderate activity
Gemcitabine 1250 mg/m^2 on days 1 and 8, and cisplatin 75 mg/m^2 plus bevacizumab 15 mg/kg on day 1 vs gemcitabine and cisplatin plus placebo	First	II, randomized	115	6.9 vs 6	0.88	15.6 vs 14.7	0.91	PFS and OS were not improved by addition of bevacizumab to chemotherapy combination
High-dose methotrexate (3 g total dose)	First	II, non randomized	62	7.5		11		High-dose methotrexate was active regimen
Pemetrexed 500 mg/m^2 in combination with cisplatin 75 mg/m^2 or pemetrexed 500 mg/m^2 alone	Second	III, randomized	187			7.6 vs 4.1		Pemetrexed alone or in combination with cisplatin is active in second line

EMPHACIS trial, chemotherapy-naive patients, who were not suitable for surgery, were randomized to receive pemetrexed 500 mg/m^2 plus cisplatin 75 mg/m^2 on day 1, or cisplatin 75 mg/m^2 on day 1. A total of 226 patients received pemetrexed plus cisplatin, and 222 patients received cisplatin alone. The patients orally received folic acid 350–1,000 μg daily, and vitamin B12 1,000 μg was given 1–3 weeks before the first doses and was continued during study period. Vitamin supplementation was given to both study arms to maintain patient blindness. The primary end of the study was OS. In the combination arm, the response rate was 41.3 % compared to 16.7 % in cisplatin-alone arm ($p<0.0001$). In combination and control arms, median progression-free survival (PFS) was 5.7 and 3.9 months, respectively ($p=0.001$). The median OS was significantly increased by adding of pemetrexed to cisplatin chemotherapy (12.1 versus 9.3 months, $p=0.02$). In the combination arm, grade 3/4 neutropenia (27.9 %) and grade 3/4 leukopenia (17.7 %) were observed frequently compared to patients in cisplatin-alone arm. In both arms, nausea, vomiting, and fatigue were the most common toxicities. Addition of vitamin supplementation significantly reduced the toxicity without adversely affecting the survival time. In this phase III trial, OS was significantly increased in pemetrexed plus cisplatin arm compared to cisplatin-alone arm in patients with chemotherapy-naive MPM [34].

After the result of this trial was reported, the factors that predict the long OS were evaluated in multiple regression analyses. Vitamin supplementation, Karnofsky performance status, disease stage, histologic subtype, and white blood cell count are the factors effecting the OS duration [29]. Until now no standard factors are defined predicting response to pemetrexed therapy. In a retrospective study low thymidylate synthase levels were associated with longer PFS and OS. However, this result should be tested in randomized trials [23]. The combination of cisplatin plus pemetrexed is the only accepted gold-standard regimen worldwide and approved by the US Food and Drug Administration.

Carboplatin Plus Pemetrexed

In a large phase II trial, the activity of carboplatin plus pemetrexed was tested. A total of 102 patients with unresectable MPM were included in the study population. Patients received pemetrexed 500 mg/m^2 and carboplatin area under the plasma concentration-time curve of 5 mg/mL/min, repeated every 3 weeks. The objective response was achieved in 19 (18.6 %) patients. Stable disease was observed in 48 (47.0 %; 95 % CI, 37.1–57.2 %) patients. Median PFS and OS were 6.5 months and 12.7 months, respectively. The observed grade 3–4 hematological toxicities were neutropenia (9.7 %) and anemia (3.5 %). Pemetrexed and carboplatin combination was active and a well-tolerated regimen in patients with MPM. The objective response and disease control rates were similar to cisplatin and pemetrexed combination. Therefore, this regimen might be an alternative to cisplatin plus pemetrexed combination [9].

Pemetrexed-Cisplatin Plus Bevacizumab

In a phase III trial, patients with unresectable MPM were randomized to receive pemetrexed 500 mg/m^2 and cisplatin 75 mg/m^2 at day 1 plus bevacizumab 15 mg/kg biweekly (Arm B) or pemetrexed-cisplatin combination without bevacizumab (Arm A) for six cycles. In arm B patients received bevacizumab maintenance until progression or intolerable toxicity. Primary end point of the trial was OS. A total of 445 patients were randomized. In arm B (chemotherapy regimen + bevacizumab) and arm A (chemotherapy regimen), median OS was 18.8 months and 16.1 months, respectively, and difference was statistically significant (adjusted HR=0.76, [95 % CI, 0.61; 0.94], $p=0.012$). After median follow-up duration of 39 months, in patients receiving bevacizumab combination, median PFS was 9.6 months, [95 % CI, 8.5–10.6] compared to 7.5 months [95 %CI, 6.8–8.1] in patients receiving chemotherapy regimen alone (adj. HR=0.62, [95 %CI, 0.50–0.75], $p<0.0001$). Serious proteinuria (0.0 % versus 3.1 %), hypertension (0.0 % versus 23 %), and arterial thrombotic events (0.0 % vs. 2.7 %) rates were significantly higher in patients receiving bevacizumab compared to chemotherapy-alone arm [36]. The addition of bevacizumab to cisplatin and pemetrexed combination was not approved by drug regulatory authorities in Europe and the USA.

Raltitrexed Plus Cisplatin

In patients with chemotherapy-naive mesothelioma, raltitrexed plus cisplatin improved OS duration compared to cisplatin alone. This result was reported in randomized phase III trial. In this trial 250 patients were randomized to receive cisplatin 80 mg/m^2 on day 1 alone (arm A) or combined with raltitrexed 3 mg/m^2 (arm B). In raltitrexed arm objective response rate was 23.6 % compared to 13.6 % in cisplatin-alone arm ($p=0.056$). Median OS was 11.4 months (95 % CI, 10.1–15) in raltitrexed arm compared to 8.8 (95 % CI, 7.8–10.8) months in cisplatin-alone arm ($p=0.48$). In patients with measurable disease ($n=213$), objective response rate was higher in raltitrexed plus cisplatin arm compared to cisplatin-alone arm (24 % versus 14 %, $p=0.06$). Quality-of-life scales of patients were similar in both therapy arms [32]. Raltitrexed plus cisplatin prolongs the OS compared to cisplatin alone without effecting the quality of life.

Gemcitabine Plus Cisplatin

In a phase II trial, gemcitabine and cisplatin combination was evaluated in 32 patients with unresectable MPM. The results were reported for 25 patients. Gemcitabine 1,250 mg/m^2 was administered on day 1 and day 8, and cisplatin 80 mg/m^2 was administered on day 1 in a 3-week cycle with a maximum of six cycles. Four of the 25 evaluable patients had partial response (PR). Median PFS and OS were 6 months (5–7 months) and 9.6 months (95 % CI 8–12 months), respectively [31]. In another phase II trial, 35 chemo-naive patients received gemcitabine and cisplatin combination. Partial response, stable disease, and progression were detected in 9 (26 %), 14 (41 %), and 11 (32 %) patients, respectively. Median PFS and OS were 13 and 8 months, respectively. Serious emesis and vomiting was detected in 35 % of patients. Grade 3–4 anemia, thrombocytopenia, and neutropenia were observed in 24 %, 52 %, and 61 % of patients, respectively [8]. In 2008, gemcitabine plus cisplatin was evaluated in another phase II trial. Patients were randomized to receive two different chemotherapy schedules as cohort 1 (gemcitabine 1.250 mg/m^2 on days 1 and 8, with pemetrexed 500 mg/m^2 on day 8) and cohort 2 (gemcitabine 1.250 mg/m^2 on days 1 and 8, with pemetrexed 500 mg/m^2 on day 1); cycles were repeated in every 21 days. In cohort 1 and 2, 56 and 52 patients were enrolled to the study population. Response rate was 26 % and 17.1 % in cohort 1 and 2, respectively. In cohort 1 and 2, median PFS was 4.3 and 7.4 months, respectively. Median OS was 8 months for cohort 1 (1-year survival rate = 31.14 %) and 10.1 months for cohort 2 (1-year survival rate = 45.80 %) [11]. As a result gemcitabine and cisplatin combination had a moderate activity in patients with advanced MPM.

Gemcitabine-Cisplatin Plus Bevacizumab

In a phase II trial, bevacizumab was added to gemcitabine and cisplatin combination. A total of 115 patients were randomized to receive gemcitabine 1.250 mg/m^2 on days 1 and 8, cisplatin 75 mg/m^2, and bevacizumab 15 mg/kg or placebo every 21 days for six cycles and then bevacizumab or placebo maintenance until progression. In bevacizumab and placebo arm, median OS was 15.6 and 14.7 months, respectively (p=0.91). Partial response rate was similar in both therapy arms (24.5 % vs 21.8 %; p=0.74). The addition of bevacizumab to chemotherapy regimen did not improve the PFS and OS [14].

Methotrexate

In a phase II study, 63 patients with advanced MPM were treated with four to eight cycles of high-dose methotrexate (3 g total dose). A total of 60 patients had evaluable disease. Partial/complete remission and stable and progressive disease were demonstrated in 37 %, 32 %, and 32 % of patients, respectively. Median OS for all patients was 11 months. In patients with the epithelial type (n=42) and sarcomatous or mixed types, OS was 12 and 5 months, respectively. Adverse effects of methotrexate were tolerable. Five patients (8 %) terminated the therapy due to toxicity. One toxic death occurred. High-dose methotrexate was an active regimen with acceptable toxicity profile in patients with MPM [26].

Raltitrexed

Single-agent activity of raltitrexed was tested in a phase II trial. Patients received raltitrexed 3 mg/m^2 in every 3 weeks as first-line therapy. Eight cycles of raltitrexed were planned to be administered whether unacceptable toxicity or progression was observed.

A total of 24 patients were enrolled to the study. Partial response was observed in five patients (20.8 %, 95 % CI 7.1–42.2 %). Mild side effects were detected (diarrhea, nausea, vomiting, fatigue, and neutropenia). Raltitrexed has the modest activity with tolerable toxicity profile in patients with MPM as a first-line therapy [3].

Anthracycline

In a phase II study, 23 MPM patients were treated with epirubicin at the dosage of 75 mg/m^2 repeated every 3 weeks. A total of 21 patients were evaluable; responses to epirubicin were 1 partial, 11 stable diseases, and 9 progression. Median OS was 7.5 months with mild adverse events. In the current dose epirubicin had mild effects against patients with MPM [17].

Liposomal doxorubicin was evaluated in 15 patients at dose of 55 mg/m^2 every 4 weeks. Four of 15 patients had good response to therapy. The side effects were not serious [25].

Vinca Alkaloids

Twenty-nine patients were treated with weekly injections of vinorelbine 30 mg/m^2. Partial response was observed in 7 (24 %) patients, and 16 (55 %) patients had stable disease. On the other hand 6 (21 %) patients had progression. This phase II trial showed that vinorelbine had promising activity against MPM [27].

Second-Line Therapies

Single-agent chemotherapy drugs demonstrated activity in phase II trials. However, single-agent therapies did not improve the OS in patients with MPM. Therefore, these single agents were suggested to be used as a second-line chemotherapy strategy in patients with advanced MPM [33].

Cisplatin

Cisplatin was demonstrated with the most promising activity as a single agent. Therefore, it constitutes the backbone of all chemotherapy regimens until 2001 [5]. Carboplatin might be an alternative to cisplatin therapy.

Pemetrexed

Most of the trials evaluating the second-line therapies against the MPM tested either the single-agent pemetrexed or combinations of pemetrexed.

In a phase III trial, previously treated patients with MPM were randomized to receive pemetrexed 500 mg/m alone ($n=91$) or in combination with cisplatin 75 mg/m^2 ($n=96$) for a maximum of six cycles every 21 days. All patients were supported by vitamin B12, folic acid, and steroid prophylaxis. In patients receiving pemetrexed plus cisplatin, the overall response rate was 32.5 % compared to 5.5 % for patients receiving pemetrexed alone. In combination and cisplatin-alone arm, the disease control rate (response rate 4 stable disease) was 68.7 % and 46.6 %, respectively. Median OS was 7.6 months for pemetrexed plus cisplatin and 4.1 months for pemetrexed alone. This phase III trial showed that the previously treated patients with MPM might be benefited from pemetrexed alone or in combination with cisplatin [12].

In an another phase III trial, patients who relapsed after first-line therapy were assigned to receive pemetrexed 500 mg/m^2 plus best supportive care (BSC) in every 21 days or BSC alone. A total of 123 patients were randomized to pemetrexed plus BSC arm, and 120 were randomized to BSC-alone arm. Partial response rate was significantly higher in patients receiving pemetrexed compared to BSC (18.7 % vs 1.7 %, $p<0.0001$). Disease control rate was also significantly higher in pemetrexed arm (59.3 % vs 19.2 %, $p<0.0001$). In pemetrexed and BSC-alone arm, median OS was 8.4 months and 9.7 months, respectively ($p=0.74$). In multivariate regression analysis, the trend of improved OS was observed in patients responding to first-line therapy [13].

Gemcitabine and Combinations

In a post-study analysis of the first-line pemetrexed plus cisplatin versus cisplatin-alone phase III trial, the data of patients who received second-line therapy were collected. As a second-line therapy, 189 (62 %) patients were treated with single-agent therapy (48 from the pemetrexed plus cisplatin arm and 70 from cisplatin arm), while 71 patients (38 %) received combination chemotherapy (36 from the pemetrexed plus cisplatin arm and 35 from the cisplatin arm). The most commonly preferred single agent was gemcitabine. The second most commonly preferred single agent was anthracylines like doxorubicin. On the other hand gemcitabine plus cisplatin or gemcitabine plus a non-platinum agent was the most frequently administered combination regimen. In cisplatin and pemetrexed arm and cisplatin-alone arm, the patients who were treated with second-line chemotherapy had better OS duration (15.3 months vs 9.8 months for cisplatin plus pemetrexed arm, 12.2 vs 6.8 arm for cisplatin-alone arm). In regression analysis second-line chemotherapy was significantly associated with improved OS time ($p<0.001$). The adjusted hazard ratio for post-study chemotherapy over the nonpost-study chemotherapy subgroup was 0.56 (CI 0.44–0.72). In this study, it was demonstrated that gemcitabine and its combinations were reasonable second-line therapy options after pemetrexed plus cisplatin therapy in first line [18].

Gemcitabine Plus Vinorelbine

In a phase II trial, 17 patients who were treated at least one prior line of pemetrexed plus cisplatin received gemcitabine plus vinorelbine as second-line therapy. Disease control (partial response + stable disease) rate was 82 %. Median PFS and OS were 6 and 11.2 months, respectively. Grade 3–4 neutropenia (41 %) and grade 3–4 anemia (29 %) were the most common hematological adverse events [30].

Novel Therapies

Novel therapies in the management of MPM are summarized in Table 22.2.

Vorinostat

Vorinostat is a novel drug inhibiting histone deacetylase. Histone deacetylase has a role in mitosis and deoxyribonucleic acid repair. In cancer cell lines, it was demonstrated that vorinostat induces differentiation, cell cycle arrest, and apoptosis [19]. In a double-blind, randomized, placebo-controlled phase III trial, patients with MPM who progressed after one or two lines of chemotherapy were randomized 1:1 to receive vorinostat or placebo. The primary end point of the study was the OS. A total of 661 patients were enrolled to the study; 329 of them randomized to vorinostat arm whereas 332 of them on placebo arm. The vorinostat did not improve OS compared to placebo [Median OS for vorinostat and placebo: 30.7 versus 27.1 weeks, respectively (HR: 0.98 %, 95 % CI 0·83–1·17, $p=0.86$)] [15].

Table 22.2 Novel therapies in patients with MPM

Target	Agents	Number of patients	Setting	Phase	Overall Survival (OS) (Months)	*P* value
Histone deacetylase	Vorinostat vs placebo	661	Second or third	III	7.6 vs 6.8	0.86
Angiogenesis	Thalidomide	40	Second or more	II	7.6	–
Tyrosine kinase	Imatinib	25	Second or more	II	13.2	–
Programmed cell death receptor-1	Pembrolizumab[a]	25	Second or more	Ib	2–6[a]	–
Cytotoxic T-lymphocyte antigen 4	Tremelimumab	29	Second	II	10.7	–
Mammalian target of rapamycin	Everolimus	59	Second or more	II	6.3	–

[a]Sixteen patients (64 %), including all responders, remain on treatment (duration 8+ to 24+ weeks)

Thalidomide

It is an ancient teratogenic agent. However, in the last decades the anti-angiogenic effects of thalidomide were reported. In 2005, thalidomide was evaluated in a phase II trial in patients with mesothelioma. A total of 40 patients were enrolled to the study. Eleven patients (27.5 %) showed disease stabilization beyond 6 months, and the median OS was 230 days [4]. After the promising results of the phase II study, phase III maintenance therapy with thalidomide in patients with mesothelioma was conducted. In this phase III study, 222 patients with peritoneal or pleural mesothelioma were enrolled. These patients received at least four cycles of pemetrexed with or without platin as a first-line therapy and had not progressed on this treatment. Patients were assigned to receive thalidomide 200 mg/day as a maintenance ($n = 111$) or supportive care ($n = 111$) until progression. The primary end point of the study was PFS. There was no significant PFS difference in between thalidomide and active supportive care groups (median PFS in thalidomide and active supportive care group was 3.6 months versus 3.5 months) (HR: 0.95 %, 95 % CI 0.73–1.20, $p = 0.72$). Thalidomide has no beneficial effect on top of the first-line therapy in patients with pleural or peritoneal mesothelioma [6].

Imatinib

Imatinib is a tyrosine kinase inhibitor that inhibits tyrosine kinase domains of c-kit and platelet-derived growth factor. In a phase II trial, the efficacy of imatinib 400–800 mg was evaluated in 25 patients with mesothelioma. No objective responses were detected. Three patients had stable disease beyond 6 months. The median OS and PFS were 398 days (range 88–840) and 63 days (range 29–275), respectively [20]. In a pilot study 11 patients with MPM were enrolled. These patients received imatinib 200 mg b.i.d. The disease stabilization was observed in four (36.3 %) patients, whereas seven (63.6 %) patients progressed. Median PFS was 8 weeks (range 7–19) [22]. Imatinib did not improve survival in patients with MPM.

Pembrolizumab

Pembrolizumab is a highly potent inhibitor of programmed cell death receptor-1 (PD-1). By inhibiting the binding of PD-1 ligands to PD-1 receptor, T cell activation against tumor continued. PD-1 ligand was overexpressed in patients with MPM. Twenty-five patients with MPM whose tumor were stained positive for PD-1 ligands received pembrolizumab at least as second-line therapy. In 2-week cycles pembrolizumab was given at dose of 10 mg/kg until progression or unacceptable toxicity. Most of the patients (80 %) received pemetrexed and platinum combination prior to pembrolizumab therapy. In six (24 %) patients partial response was observed, whereas stable disease was detected in 13 (52 %) patients and four (16 %) patients progressed. In this study disease control rate was 76 %. Grade 3 adverse events were observed in three (12 %) patients. In patients with MPM, pembrolizumab was well tolerated and has promising results (disease control rate 76 %). In patients with MPM pembrolizumab might be evaluated in further studies [1].

Tremelimumab

Tremelimumab is an antibody against cytotoxic T-lymphocyte antigen 4 (CTLA4). It has been reported to have promising antitumor activity in different tumor types. In an open-label, single-arm phase II study, 29 patients with mesothelioma who progressed after first-line platinum doublet therapy were enrolled. Patients were given tremelimumab 15 mg/kg in every 90 days until progression or unacceptable toxicity. The primary end point of the study was objective response (complete or partial response). Three patients had partial response. Disease control rate was 31 %. The median PFS and OS were 6.2 months (95 % CI 1.3–11.1) and 10.7 months (95 % CI, 0.0–21.9), respectively. The study did not reach its primary end point. However, tremelimumab has promising clinical activity in patients with mesothelioma [7]. Tremelimumab is being evaluated in an ongoing phase III trial (NCT01843374).

m-TOR Inhibitors

In human mesothelioma cells overactivation of PIK3/m-TOR (phosphoinositide 3 kinase) pathway was reported [2]. In a phase II trial, 59 patients with MPM who received one or two lines of platinum-based therapy were given 10 mg everolimus daily. Overall response rate was 2 % [95 %CI, 0–12 %]. The median PFS and OS were 2.8 months (95 % CI: 1.8–3.4) and 6.3 months (95 % CI: 4.0–8.0), respectively. Single-agent everolimus had limited clinical activity in patients with advanced MPM [21].

References

1. Alley EW, Molife L, Santoro A et al. Clinical safety and efficacy of pembrolizumab (MK-3475) in patients with malignant pleural mesothelioma: preliminary results from KEYNOTE-028 (abstract CT103). American Association of Cancer Research 2015 meeting.
2. Altomare DA, You H, Xiao GH, Ramos-Nino ME, Skele KL, de Rienzo A, Jhanwar SC, Mossman BT, Kane AB, Testa JR. Human and mouse mesotheliomas exhibit elevated AKT/PKB activity, which can be targeted pharmacologically to inhibit tumor cell growth. Oncogene. 2005;24:6080–9.
3. Baas P, Ardizzoni A, Grossi F, Nackaerts K, Numico G, van Marck E, van de Vijver M, Monetti F, Smid-Geirnaerdt MJ, van Zandwijk N, Debruyne C, Legrand C, Giaccone G. The activity of raltitrexed (Tomudex) in malignant pleural mesothelioma: an EORTC phase II study (08992). Eur J Cancer. 2003;39:353–7.
4. Baas P, Boogerd W, Dalesio O, Haringhuizen A, Custers F, van Zandwijk N. Thalidomide in patients with malignant pleural mesothelioma. Lung Cancer. 2005;48:291–6.

5. Berghmans T, Paesmans M, Lalami Y, Louviaux I, Luce S, Mascaux C, Meert AP, Sculier JP. Activity of chemotherapy and immunotherapy on malignant mesothelioma: a systematic review of the literature with meta-analysis. Lung Cancer. 2002;38:111–21.
6. Buikhuisen WA, Burgers JA, Vincent AD, Korse CM, van Klaveren RJ, Schramel FM, Pavlakis N, Nowak AK, Custers FL, Schouwink JH, Gans SJ, Groen HJ, Strankinga WF, Baas P. Thalidomide versus active supportive care for maintenance in patients with malignant mesothelioma after first-line chemotherapy (NVALT 5): an open-label, multicentre, randomised phase 3 study. Lancet Oncol. 2013;14:543–51.
7. Calabro L, Morra A, Fonsatti E, Cutaia O, Amato G, Giannarelli D, di Giacomo AM, Danielli R, Altomonte M, Mutti L, Maio M. Tremelimumab for patients with chemotherapy-resistant advanced malignant mesothelioma: an open-label, single-arm, phase 2 trial. Lancet Oncol. 2013;14:1104–11.
8. Castagneto B, Zai S, Dongiovanni D, Muzio A, Bretti S, Numico G, Botta M, Sinaccio G. Cisplatin and gemcitabine in malignant pleural mesothelioma: a phase II study. Am J Clin Oncol. 2005;28:223–6.
9. Ceresoli GL, Zucali PA, Favaretto AG, Grossi F, Bidoli P, Del Conte G, Ceribelli A, Bearz A, Morenghi E, Cavina R, Marangolo M, Parra HJ, Santoro A. Phase II study of pemetrexed plus carboplatin in malignant pleural mesothelioma. J Clin Oncol. 2006;24:1443–8.
10. Ellis P, Davies AM, Evans WK, Haynes AE, Lloyd NS. The use of chemotherapy in patients with advanced malignant pleural mesothelioma: a systematic review and practice guideline. J Thorac Oncol. 2006;1:591–601.
11. Janne PA, Simon GR, Langer CJ, Taub RN, Dowlati A, Fidias P, Monberg M, Obasaju C, Kindler H. Phase II trial of pemetrexed and gemcitabine in chemotherapy-naive malignant pleural mesothelioma. J Clin Oncol. 2008;26:1465–71.
12. Janne PA, Wozniak AJ, Belani CP, Keohan ML, Ross HJ, Polikoff JA, Mintzer DM, Ye Z, Monberg MJ, Obasaju CK. Pemetrexed alone or in combination with cisplatin in previously treated malignant pleural mesothelioma: outcomes from a phase IIIB expanded access program. J Thorac Oncol. 2006;1:506–12.
13. Jassem J, Ramlau R, Santoro A, Schuette W, Chemaissani A, Hong S, Blatter J, Adachi S, Hanauske A, Manegold C. Phase III trial of pemetrexed plus best supportive care compared with best supportive care in previously treated patients with advanced malignant pleural mesothelioma. J Clin Oncol. 2008;26:1698–704.
14. Kindler HL, Karrison TG, Gandara DR, Lu C, Krug LM, Stevenson JP, Janne PA, Quinn DI, Koczywas MN, Brahmer JR, Albain KS, Taber DA, Armato 3rd SG, Vogelzang NJ, Chen HX, Stadler WM, Vokes EE. Multicenter, double-blind, placebo-controlled, randomized phase II trial of gemcitabine/cisplatin plus bevacizumab or placebo in patients with malignant mesothelioma. J Clin Oncol. 2012;30:2509–15.
15. Krug LM, Kindler HL, Calvert H, Manegold C, Tsao AS, Fennell D, Ohman R, Plummer R, Eberhardt WE, Fukuoka K, Gaafar RM, Lafitte JJ, Hillerdal G, Chu Q, Buikhuisen WA, Lubiniecki GM, Sun X, Smith M, Baas P. Vorinostat in patients with advanced malignant pleural mesothelioma who have progressed on previous chemotherapy (VANTAGE-014): a phase 3, double-blind, randomised, placebo-controlled trial. Lancet Oncol. 2015;16:447–56.
16. Krug LM, Pass HI, Rusch VW, Kindler HL, Sugarbaker DJ, Rosenzweig KE, Flores R, Friedberg JS, Pisters K, Monberg M, Obasaju CK, Vogelzang NJ. Multicenter phase II trial of neoadjuvant pemetrexed plus cisplatin followed by extrapleural pneumonectomy and radiation for malignant pleural mesothelioma. J Clin Oncol. 2009;27:3007–13.
17. Magri MD, Veronesi A, Foladore S, de Giovanni D, Serra C, Crismancich F, Tuveri G, Nicotra M, Tommasi M, Morassut S, et al. Epirubicin in the treatment of malignant mesothelioma: a phase II cooperative study. The North-Eastern Italian Oncology Group (GOCCNE) – Mesothelioma Committee. Tumori. 1991;77:49–51.
18. Manegold C, Symanowski J, Gatzemeier U, Reck M, von Pawel J, Kortsik C, Nackaerts K, Lianes P, Vogelzang NJ. Second-line (post-study) chemotherapy received by patients treated in the phase III trial of pemetrexed plus cisplatin versus cisplatin alone in malignant pleural mesothelioma. Ann Oncol. 2005;16:923–7.

19. Martinez-Iglesias O, Ruiz-Llorente L, Sanchez-Martinez R, Garcia L, Zambrano A, Aranda A. Histone deacetylase inhibitors: mechanism of action and therapeutic use in cancer. Clin Transl Oncol. 2008;10:395–8.
20. Mathy A, Baas P, Dalesio O, van Zandwijk N. Limited efficacy of imatinib mesylate in malignant mesothelioma: a phase II trial. Lung Cancer. 2005;50:83–6.
21. Ou SH, Moon J, Garland LL, Mack PC, Testa JR, Tsao AS, Wozniak AJ, Gandara DR. SWOG S0722: phase II study of mTOR inhibitor everolimus (RAD001) in advanced malignant pleural mesothelioma (MPM). J Thorac Oncol. 2015;10:387–91.
22. Porta C, Mutti L, Tassi G. Negative results of an Italian Group for Mesothelioma (G.I.Me.) pilot study of single-agent imatinib mesylate in malignant pleural mesothelioma. Cancer Chemother Pharmacol. 2007;59:149–50.
23. Righi L, Papotti MG, Ceppi P, Bille A, Bacillo E, Molinaro L, Ruffini E, Scagliotti GV, Selvaggi G. Thymidylate synthase but not excision repair cross-complementation group 1 tumor expression predicts outcome in patients with malignant pleural mesothelioma treated with pemetrexed-based chemotherapy. J Clin Oncol. 2010;28:1534–9.
24. Ryan CW, Herndon J, Vogelzang NJ. A review of chemotherapy trials for malignant mesothelioma. Chest. 1998;113:66S–73.
25. Skubitz KM. Phase II trial of pegylated-liposomal doxorubicin (Doxil) in mesothelioma. Cancer Invest. 2002;20:693–9.
26. Solheim OP, Saeter G, Finnanger AM, Stenwig AE. High-dose methotrexate in the treatment of malignant mesothelioma of the pleura. A phase II study. Br J Cancer. 1992;65:956–60.
27. Steele JP, Shamash J, Evans MT, Gower NH, Tischkowitz MD, Rudd RM. Phase II study of vinorelbine in patients with malignant pleural mesothelioma. J Clin Oncol. 2000;18:3912–7.
28. Sterman DH, Kaiser LR, Albelda SM. Advances in the treatment of malignant pleural mesothelioma. Chest. 1999;116:504–20.
29. Symanowski JT, Rusthoven J, Nguyen B, et al. Multiple regression analysis of prognostic variables for survival from the phase III study of pemetrexed plus cisplatin vs. cisplatin in malignant pleural mesothelioma. Proc Am Soc Clin Oncol. 2003;22:647a.
30. Toyokawa G, Takenoyama M, Hirai F, Toyozawa R, Inamasu E, Kojo M, Morodomi Y, Shiraishi Y, Takenaka T, Yamaguchi M, Shimokawa M, Seto T, Ichinose Y. Gemcitabine and vinorelbine as second-line or beyond treatment in patients with malignant pleural mesothelioma pretreated with platinum plus pemetrexed chemotherapy. Int J Clin Oncol. 2014;19:601–6.
31. van Haarst JM, Baas P, Manegold C, Schouwink JH, Burgers JA, de Bruin HG, Mooi WJ, van Klaveren RJ, de Jonge MJ, van Meerbeeck JP. Multicentre phase II study of gemcitabine and cisplatin in malignant pleural mesothelioma. Br J Cancer. 2002;86:342–5.
32. van Meerbeeck JP, Gaafar R, Manegold C, van Klaveren RJ, van Marck EA, Vincent M, Legrand C, Bottomley A, Debruyne C, Giaccone G. Randomized phase III study of cisplatin with or without raltitrexed in patients with malignant pleural mesothelioma: an intergroup study of the European Organisation for Research and Treatment of Cancer Lung Cancer Group and the National Cancer Institute of Canada. J Clin Oncol. 2005;23:6881–9.
33. Vogelzang NJ. Chemotherapy for malignant pleural mesothelioma. Lancet. 2008;371:1640–2.
34. Vogelzang NJ, Rusthoven JJ, Symanowski J, Denham C, Kaukel E, Ruffie P, Gatzemeier U, Boyer M, Emri S, Manegold C, Niyikiza C, Paoletti P. Phase III study of pemetrexed in combination with cisplatin versus cisplatin alone in patients with malignant pleural mesothelioma. J Clin Oncol. 2003;21:2636–44.
35. Weder W, Stahel RA, Bernhard J, Bodis S, Vogt P, Ballabeni P, Lardinois D, Betticher D, Schmid R, Stupp R, Ris HB, Jermann M, Mingrone W, Roth AD, Spiliopoulos A. Multicenter trial of neo-adjuvant chemotherapy followed by extrapleural pneumonectomy in malignant pleural mesothelioma. Ann Oncol. 2007;18:1196–202.
36. Zalcman G, Mazières J, Margery J et al. Bevacizumab 15mg/kg plus cisplatin-pemetrexed (CP) triplet versus CP doublet in Malignant Pleural Mesothelioma (MPM): results of the IFCT-GFPC-0701 MAPS randomized phase 3 trial. J Clin Oncol. 2015;33(suppl; abstr 7500).

Radiation-Induced Toxicities and Management Strategies in Thoracic Malignancies

23

Gokhan Ozyigit, Gozde Yazici, Sezin Yuce Sari, Melis Gultekin, and Pervin Hurmuz

Introduction

The thorax encompasses numerous OARs some of which are vital, and these organs are affected during the course of RT for intrathoracic tumors and breast malignancies. The challenging issue in the treatment of lung cancer is that the location of the primary lesion inside an OAR, lung. Therefore, the radiation dose limits for the lungs are different from other malignancies concerning the thorax.

The lungs are in close proximity to the heart and the spinal cord. For apical tumors the brachial plexus is the other critical organ, and for central tumors the esophagus, trachea, and proximal bronchial tree (PBT) are the other critical organs. The dose to the chest wall (CW) and skin should also be taken into account in patients who undergo stereotactic ablative body radiotherapy (SABR). Among these OARs the spinal cord, coronary arteries, brachial plexus, esophagus, and trachea are serial organs for which the maximum point dose affects the function of the whole organ. On the other hand, the heart is in a parallel structure, and the mean dose to a specific volume is more important than the maximum dose. In order to interpret the dose-volume histograms (DVH) precisely, the accurate delineation of OARs is crucial [1].

This chapter aims to guide the radiation oncologists in the delineation of OARs and to define the dose-volume constraints for OARs in the treatment of lung cancer. Dose-volume constraints have been derived from the studies of Emami, Radiation Therapy Oncology Group (RTOG) protocols, and the reviews of Quantitative Analyses of Normal Tissue Effects in the Clinic (QUANTEC).

G. Ozyigit, MD • G. Yazici, MD (✉) • S.Y. Sari, MD • M. Gultekin, MD • P. Hurmuz, MD
Department of Radiation Oncology, Faculty of Medicine, Hacettepe University, Ankara, Turkey
e-mail: yazicig@hacettepe.edu.tr

G. Ozyigit et al. (eds.), *Principles and Practice of Radiotherapy Techniques in Thoracic Malignancies*, DOI 10.1007/978-3-319-28761-4_23

Lung

Contouring

The RTOG proposed an atlas for the delineation of OARs in thoracic RT which is based on the 1106 trial [2]. This atlas recommends contouring both lungs using the "pulmonary window" (see Chap. 3 for details). The lungs can be delineated as separate organs as right and left; however, the evaluation of the DVH should be done after combining both lungs as a single organ. The emphysematic, collapsed, inflated, or fibrotic regions of the lungs and the small vessels beyond the hilar regions should also be contoured as normal lung tissue. The atelectatic parenchyma, the fluid, hilar regions, the trachea, main bronchus, and the PBT should be excluded from normal lung tissue delineation. The collapsed lung region can be distinguished from the gross tumor volume (GTV) easily by using intravenous contrast during computed tomography (CT) and/or positron emission tomography (PET) [2]. The target volume is subtracted from the lungs; however, different protocols subtract different target volumes to define the normal lung tissue. The RTOG 9311 trial recommends subtracting the planning target volume (PTV), while RTOG 0617 recommends the clinical target volume (CTV) to be subtracted for the delineation of lungs as OARs. The RTOG 0117, 0618, 0813, 0915, and the QUANTEC recommend the GTV to be subtracted [3–5]. Kong et al. recommended using the GTV subtracted volume as normal lung tissue based on the data from RTOG trials [2]. They also prefer dividing the lung into central and peripheral regions in SABR planning.

Dose-Volume Constraints and Toxicity

The incidence of radiation pneumonitis (RP) after conventional RT for lung cancer was reported to be 13–37 % [6]. Fortunately, RP is frequently asymptomatic and does not require intervention. It is restricted with radiologic findings in 62 % and 91 % of patients in the acute and late period, respectively [7]. In the acute period, a diffuse infiltration restricted to the RT port can be observed on the chest X-ray. The infiltration can extend outside the RT field and the trachea can deviate toward the irradiated lung in the chronic period.

Computed tomography is more sensitive in detecting lung injury after RT than chest X-rays. The patterns of RP on CT are classified as consolidative or ground-glass opacity changes with both subdivided into diffuse (>5 cm) or patchy (≤5 cm) in the acute and modified conventional, mass-like, or scar-like in the late settings, respectively [8]. Lung contraction, deviation of the mediastinal structures toward the irradiated lung, tenting of the diaphragm, and pleural thickening can be seen in the late period.

Perfusion and ventilation scintigraphy is more sensitive than chest X-rays and CT scans, particularly for the changes in lung after low doses of RT [9]. Abnormalities of perfusion and ventilation can be seen in up to 95 % and 45 % of patients, respectively [10, 11].

Acute RP develops 2–4 months after RT, and the risk is associated with total dose, fraction dose, irradiated lung volume, and other concurrent or sequential therapies as well as patient characteristics such as age, coexisting lung disease, smoking, genetic susceptibility, and poor pulmonary function test (PFT) results. In the presence of persistent nonproductive cough, dyspnea, or low-grade fever, high-dose oral corticosteroids are used for 4–8 weeks to alleviate the symptoms. Rapid response is common in approximately 80 % of the patients [12]. In more severe cases, intravenous corticosteroids with oxygen support and even hospitalization may be required.

Emami et al. reported estimations for tolerance doses based on studies with two-dimensional RT (2-D RT) [13]. They defined TD5/5 as the tolerance dose with a risk of 5 % complication rate at 5 years and recommended a maximum of 45 Gy for the 1/3, 30 Gy for the 2/3, and 17.5 Gy for the 3/3 of the lung, respectively.

In the era of three-dimensional (3-D RT) and intensity modulated RT (IMRT), the dose to the percentage volume can be evaluated precisely. The mean lung dose (MLD) and the percentage of the total lung volume irradiated with a specific minimum dose such as V5 (i.e., the lung volume that receives ≥5 Gy), V13, V20, V30, and V40 have been used to define the tolerance limits in different trials. Although it was shown that MLD predicts the toxicity more accurately then Vx, it was also reported that V13 is more predictive when the MLD is >20 Gy or V13 is >50 % [14]. A study from the Memorial Sloan-Kettering Cancer Center (MSKCC) showed that the risk of RP is 50 % and 5 % when the MLD is ≥26 Gy and ≤12 Gy and V13 of the ipsilateral lung >80 % and >40 %, respectively [15]. The same center also showed that the risk of grade ≥3 lung toxicity increases from 4 % to 38 % when the V25 increases from <30 % to >30 %, respectively [16]. They specified the most important predictors for RP as MLD, V5 to V40 of the total, ipsilateral, and lower lung, with V5 to V20 of the ipsilateral lung being the most predictive [15, 17].

Marks et al. reported that when the V20 is ≤30 %, the RP risk is <20 %, and the risk of symptomatic RP increases to 40 % from 5 % when the MLD increases to 27 Gy from 7 Gy [5]. Graham et al. reported that symptomatic RP is 0 % when the V20 is <22 %; however, it increases to 36 % when the V20 is >40 % [18]. Princess Margaret Hospital has recommended keeping the V20 ≤30–35 % and the MLD ≤20–23 Gy in order to minimize the risk of RP [19].

Washington University reported the 2-year risk of RP 36 %, 13 %, 7 %, and 0 % when the V20 is >40 %, 32–40 %, 22–31 %, and <22 %, respectively [18]. A study from the same center also showed that the risk is significantly correlated with D30 to D40 (the dose delivered to the 30 % and 40 % volume of the lung, respectively) and V5 to V15 and V70 to V75 [20]. The M.D. Anderson Cancer Center (MDACC) reported that the MLD and V5 to V65 were the most significant predictors for the risk of RP; the risk of grade ≥3 RP was increased to 38 % from 3 % when the V5 is increased to >42 % from ≤42 % [21]. The Mayo Clinic found that the risk of RP was 10–20 % when the V10 is 32–43 %, V13 29–39 %, V15 27–34 %, and V20 21–31 %, respectively, which revealed that V10 to V13 are the most significant predictors [22]. The QUANTEC recommends the MLD <20 % and V20 <30–35 % in patients with non-small cell lung cancer (NSCLC) [5].

Patients receiving concurrent chemoradiotherapy (CRT) have an increased risk of RP. The Duke University reported the risk of grade ≥1 RP 24 % and 6 % when the V30 is >18 % and <18 %, respectively, in a group of patients in which 18 % received CRT [23]. A Japanese study also reported increased risk with increased MLD; 44 %, 27 %, 16 %, and 10 % when the MLD is >30 Gy, 21–30 Gy, 10–20 Gy, and <10 Gy, respectively, in patients who underwent CRT [24].

Tumor location is also a factor for the development of RP. The MSKCC reported that the risk of RP was increased in tumors located in lower lobes compared to upper lobe lesions [15]. The Washington University also found that the location of the tumor was the most significant predictor of RP [20].

It was shown that the risk of RP is lower with IMRT treatment [25–27]. However, the dose to small volumes of the lungs should be evaluated more carefully in this setting. A study from the MDACC reported the risk of grade ≥3 RP 21 % and 2 % when the V5 is >70 % and ≤70 Gy, respectively [25]. The studies in patients with mesothelioma also revealed better toxicity results with IMRT. No RP was reported in patients whose MLD, V5, and V20 were 12.9 Gy, 90 %, and 10.9 %, respectively [28]. The same values for patients who did not develop RP were 7.5 Gy, 66 %, and 0.2 %, respectively, in another study [29]. The MDACC study revealed that the risk of pulmonary death is increased to 42-fold when the V20 is >7 % [30]. Willner et al. reported that the risk of RP increases when the volume of ipsilateral lung receiving >40 Gy increases and <10 Gy decreases [17]. Murshed et al. reported 7 % and 10 % reduction with IMRT in the V10 and V20, respectively, compared to 3-D RT [31]. This also led to a decrease more than 2 Gy in the MLD and 10 % reduction in the risk of RP. However, the V5 increased, possibly due to the increase in monitor units (MUs) and the leakage from the multileaf collimators (MLCs). When using IMRT, the step-and-shoot technique can reduce MUs significantly compared to the sliding window technique.

In the treatment with SABR, smaller volumes of lung are irradiated and the incidence of RP is lower [32]. In a meta-analysis of studies on SABR, the rate of grade ≥3 RP was reported 2 % [33]. However, large volumes of lung are irradiated to low doses because of beam numbers [34]. In the RTOG 0236 study, 8 % of the patients with stage I NSCLC who received SABR developed RP, and the authors recommended limiting the <10 % of the lung volume to 20 Gy [35]. Nyman et al. compared the incidence of RP in patients with T1-2 N0 NSCLC who received SABR (3 × 22 Gy) and conventional RT (35 × 2 Gy) and reported decreased toxicity rates for SABR (16 % vs 34 %) [36]. Barriger et al. reported the risk of grade ≥2 RP 17 % and 4 % when the MLD was >4 Gy and ≤4 Gy, and 16 % and 4 % when the V20 was >4 % and ≤4 Gy, respectively [37]. The American Association of Physicists in Medicine (AAPM) Task Group 101 report recommends that the 10 and 15 cc of bilateral lungs should receive 7.4 and 7 Gy in one fraction, 12.4 and 11.6 Gy in three fractions, and 13.5 and 12.5 Gy in five fractions at maximum, respectively [38].

Patients with large tumors or interstitial lung disease (ILD) are at higher risk for the development of RP. It was shown that RP risk was 26 % in patients with large tumors (PTV >80 cc) who underwent SABR, and the risk was increased with the increased volume of contralateral lung receiving low dose (≥5 Gy) [39]. Similarly, the risk of grade ≥4 RP after SABR was significantly higher in patients with ILD (26 %) compared to patients without ILD (3 %) [40].

Pulmonary functions are not largely affected by the administration of SABR [41, 42]. In the RTOG 0236 study, no statistically significant difference between the pre- and posttreatment PFTs was reported [43].

It is generally accepted to limit the V20 <40 % of total lung volume in patients receiving RT alone, <35 % in patients receiving CRT alone, and <20 % in patients receiving CRT after surgery. It is also recommended keeping V10 <40 % in the latter group of patients [44].

Heart

Contouring

According to Feng et al. who developed a heart atlas for the prediction of radiation exposure in breast cancer patients, the whole heart, its chambers, great vessels, cardiac valves, conduction system, and coronary arteries should be delineated (Fig. 23.1) [45]. However, as the life expectancy of patients with lung cancer is much shorter than patients with breast cancer, there is no recommendation on detailed contouring in these patients as there is not enough time to encounter most complications.

The optimal windowing in CT slices for the delineation of the heart is the level of 50 and window of 500 Hounsfield Unit (HU), whereas it is 50 and 150 HU, respectively, for the great vessels [45]. The RTOG recommends that the heart should be contoured along with the pericardial sac. The base (superior part) of the heart starts at the level of the inferior border of the left pulmonary artery and continues until the diaphragm appears. The pericardium comprises pericardial fatty tissue, great vessels, heart chambers, normal recesses, and pericardial effusion if applicable. The delineation of the pericardium begins at 5–6 mm above the top of the aortic arch and ends at the last slice of the apex of the heart.

The delineation of great vessels is recommended but not mandated by RTOG. They are recommended to be contoured separately from the heart, using "mediastinal windowing" (see Chap. 3 for details) by which the walls and muscular layers of the vessels can be seen more accurately. The delineation starts from at least 3 cm above the superior border of the PTV (or from the level of the aortic arch, depending on which is superior) and ends at least 3 cm below the inferior border of the PTV. The superior vena cava and aorta are delineated for the treatment of right and left lung tumors, respectively. For either side tumors, the ipsilateral pulmonary artery is also contoured.

The RTOG guideline for the delineation of OARs in intrathoracic malignancies does not include recommendations for the coronary arteries, heart chambers, and valves. They are included in the delineation of the pericardium in this atlas. If required these structures can be delineated by following the recommendations in the heart atlas developed by Feng et al. [45].

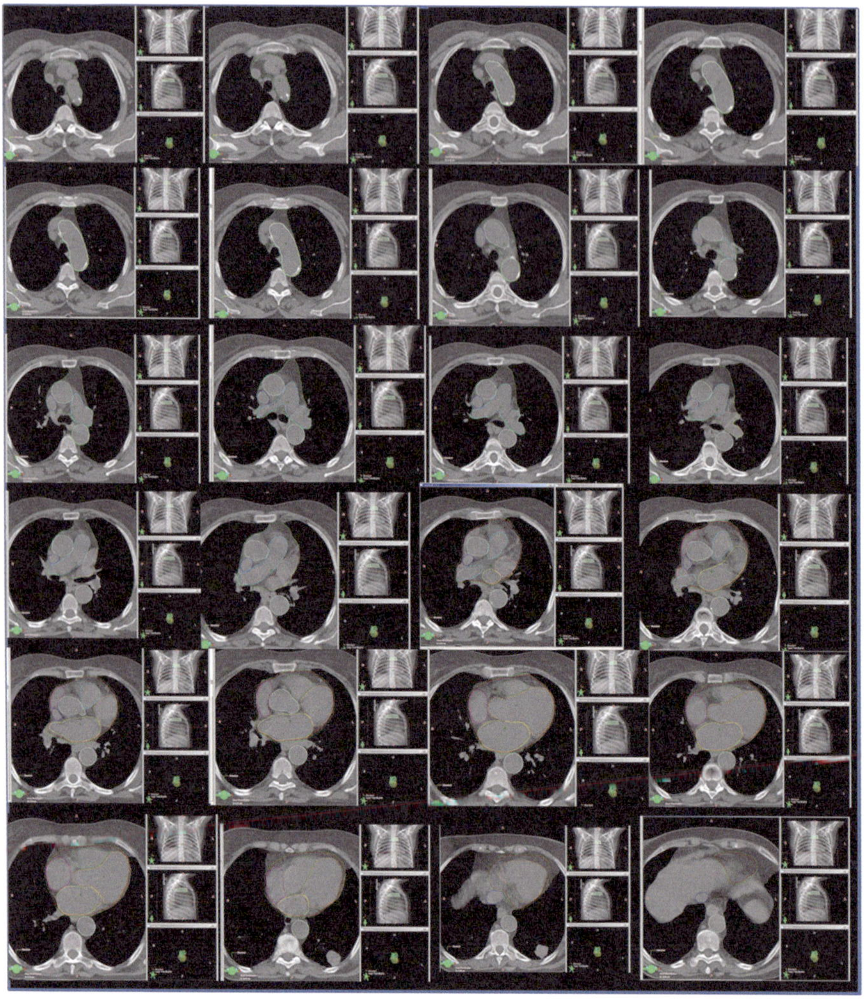

Fig. 23.1 Delineation of heart

Dose-Volume Constraints and Toxicity

As the survival is longer, most data on dose-volume constraints for the heart have been obtained from patients with breast cancer and lymphoma. Cardiac morbidity and mortality rates after RT for intrathoracic malignancies are associated with total dose, fraction dose, irradiated volume of the heart, and patient characteristics [46]. The most common acute radiation-induced toxicity is pericarditis which is usually transient. However, it can progress to be chronic and lead to fibrosis, pericardial effusion, and constrictive pericarditis. The incidence of radiation-induced pericarditis is strongly associated with the irradiated volume of the heart [47].

Emami et al. estimated the TD5/5 40 Gy for 3/3, 45 Gy for 2/3, and 60 Gy for 1/3 of the heart, respectively, when conventional RT is administered [13]. It was reported that the risk of pericarditis increases when >50 % of the heart is irradiated and the volume of the heart treated with ≥30 Gy increases [48, 49]. The QUANTEC reported that the risk of pericarditis is <15 % when the mean heart dose is <26 Gy and V30 is <46 % [46]. It was also stated that the risk of cardiac mortality at 5 years is <1 % when the V25 is >10 %. It has been recommended limiting the V50 of the heart <50 % [50]. V40 and V50 of the heart were reduced in patients who were treated with IMRT [31]. The RTOG 0236 trial has recommended limiting the maximum point dose to the heart to 30 Gy in patients treated with SABR [35].

Coronary artery disease, myocardial infarction, and congestive heart failure may develop in the chronic period. The University of Michigan has recommended the mean and maximum dose for the left anterior descending artery (LAD) <5 Gy and <15 Gy, respectively [51].

Postoperative RT for lung cancer was shown to increase mortality rate due to unknown causes by 6 % [52]. On the other hand, adjuvant RT increased cardiac mortality rate threefold in a study where 5 % of the patients who underwent postoperative RT were succumbed to cardiac disease [53].

Shafman et al. recommend using non-axial beams rather than axial to decrease the dose that the heart receives incidentally, particularly in patients with lower lobe tumors and positive lymph nodes [54]. They suggest that using non-axial beams can decrease the irradiated volume of the heart.

Esophagus

Contouring

According to the RTOG atlas, delineation of the esophagus starts from the inferior border of the cricoid cartilage and ends at the gastroesophageal junction (Fig. 23.2). The mediastinal window on CT allows us to see the mucosa, submucosa, and muscular layers of the esophagus. Oral contrast use is not recommended unless the esophagus wall is surrounded by the tumor. If oral contrast is going to be used, the esophagus is defined as a soft tissue to minimize the contrast effect [2].

Dose-Volume Constraints and Toxicity

Acute esophageal toxicity is observed as dysphagia, odynophagia, or dysmotility, whereas necrosis, fistula, or stricture can be seen in the late period. The incidence of grade ≥3 acute esophagitis is 1.3 % in patients treated with conventional fractionation [55]. It was shown that induction and concurrent chemotherapy increases the risk of severe acute esophagitis [56, 57]. Acute grade ≥3 esophagitis is observed in 15–25 % of the patients, particularly in those receiving CRT. Dysphagia usually

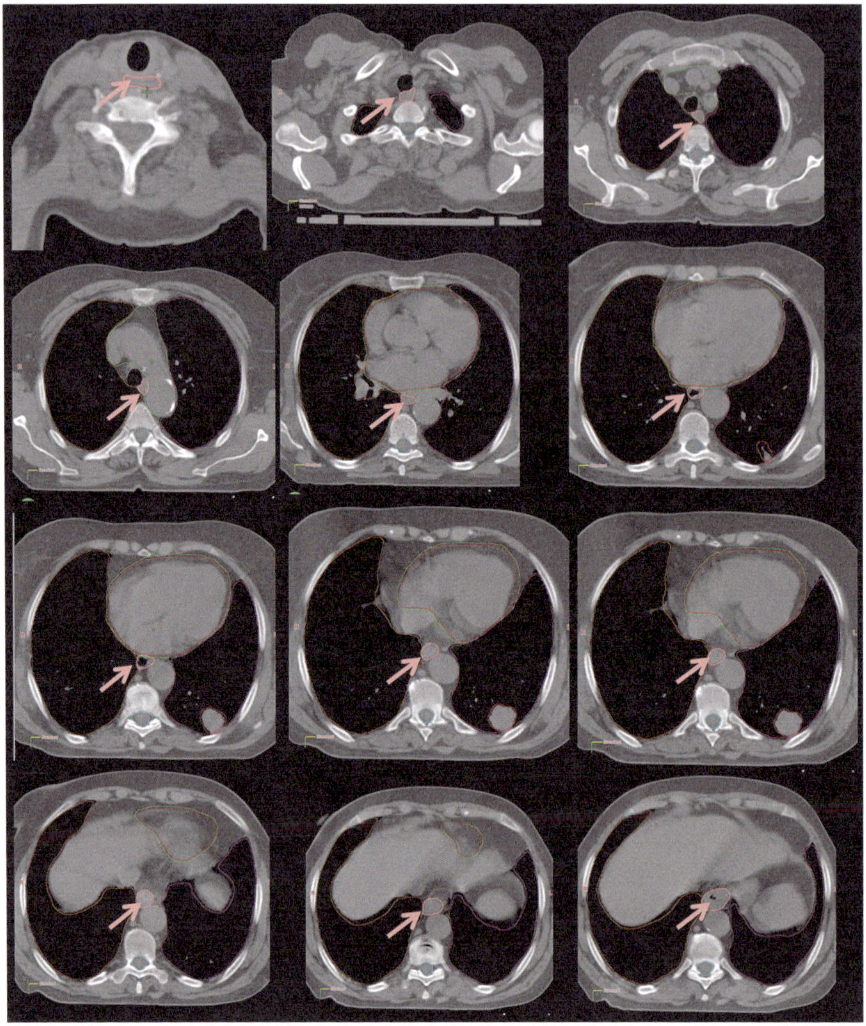

Fig. 23.2 Delineation of esophagus (*arrow* shows esophagus)

starts within the second or third week of RT where the total dose reaches 18–21 Gy [55]. It may progress to odynophagia and then to constant pain which may require gastric tube and even parenteral nutrition. Acute esophagitis generally recovers 1–3 weeks after the completion of RT. In the late-setting fibrosis, ulceration, stricture, fistula, and perforation may occur 3–8 weeks after RT. Grade ≥3 late toxicity can develop in <5 % of the patients [58, 59].

Chemotherapeutic agents such as adriamycin and gemcitabine can cause severe esophagitis when used concurrently or sequentially with RT [60–62]. Furthermore, hyperfractionated and accelerated regimens of RT also leads to increased rate and duration of severe acute esophagitis [57, 63–66].

Emami et al. estimated the maximum doses for the 1/3, 2/3, and 3/3 of the esophagus 60 Gy, 58 Gy, and 55 Gy, respectively [13]. The QUANTEC paper reported that the risk of grade ≥3 esophagitis is <20 % when the mean esophagus dose was <34 Gy [67]. It was also stated that when the V35 is <50 %, V50 is <40 %, and V70 is <20 %, the risk of esophagitis decreases. The RTOG 0617 also recommends the mean dose to the esophagus <34 Gy [68]. It is recommended to limit the length of esophagus receiving 60 Gy <16 cm [50].

The Washington University reported that the rate of grade ≥3 acute and late esophagitis increases when the maximum dose (Dmax) is >58 Gy, mean dose >34 Gy, and when concurrent CRT is administered [58]. The Duke University specified the significant predictors of late esophagitis as V50, the length of esophagus that receives >50–60 Gy, the surface dose that receives (S50) ≥50 Gy, and the circumferential Dmax >80 Gy [69]. The rate of late esophagitis was found approximately 30 % when the V50 or S50 was >32 % or when >3.2 cm of the esophagus received >50 Gy; however, the rate of acute esophagitis was not affected. Another study from the same center showed that the circumference of the esophagus receiving ≥50 Gy and ≥55 Gy, maximal percentage of circumference receiving ≥60–80 Gy, and 75 % of the circumference receiving ≥70 Gy were correlated with late esophageal toxicity and also stated that the most significant predictor of late toxicity was the presence of acute toxicity [70].

The RTOG 9311 trial compared three doses in patients who received RT alone (arm 1: 90.3 Gy total and V20 of the lungs <25 %; arm 2: 83.8 Gy total and V20 25–37 %; and arm 3: 77.4 Gy total and V20 >37 %) [3]. The maximum dose to the 1/3 of the esophagus was 65 Gy, to 2/3 58 Gy, and to 3/3 55 Gy in this study, respectively. No severe acute esophagitis was observed in any treatment arm. However, late esophageal toxicity was increased with higher total doses. The RTOG 0117 trial compared patients who received IMRT and 3-D RT both with concurrent paclitaxel and carboplatin chemotherapy [71, 72]. With a mean dose to the esophagus <32 Gy and V55 of the esophagus <28 %, it was possible to significantly decrease the dose to the esophagus with IMRT up to 80 Gy total dose. The V40 and V50 of the esophagus were decreased in patients who underwent IMRT [31]. The RTOG trial has recommended limiting the maximum point dose to the esophagus to 27 Gy in patients treated with SABR [35].

Spinal Cord

Contouring

The RTOG atlas recommends contouring the spinal cord limited by the bony structures of the spinal canal [2]. The delineation starts at the inferior border of the cricoid cartilage or inferior to the skull base in apical tumors, until the inferior border of the body of the lumbar (L)2 vertebra. The entire spinal canal should be delineated; however, the neural foramens are not included. Some RTOG trials recommend starting to delineate the spinal cord from 10 cm superior to the PTV and continue until 10 cm inferior to it. However, the expansion can go beyond the end of the spinal canal and even the range of the CT scan if this method is used. Kong et al. recommend using magnetic resonance imaging (MRI) for tumors in the vicinity of the spinal cord when treated with SABR [2].

Dose-Volume Constraints and Toxicity

Myelopathy is defined as grade ≥2 myelitis. Acute radiation-induced spinal cord toxicity is generally encountered as the transient Lhermitte syndrome which typically starts 2–4 months after RT and cannot be classified as "myelopathy" as the symptoms are mild. Radiation myelopathy generally develops more than 6 months after RT [73]. It starts within the white matter due to either direct or secondary to microvascular damage [74]. The symptoms are usually presented as numbness, tingling, and reduced sensitivity to temperature in the lower extremities. It may progress to weakness resulting in foot drop. Chronic progressive myelopathy can be observed 9–15 months after RT but fortunately is rare. It is observed as paresis, bladder, and rectal incontinence, and even complete paralysis. Sensory losses may recover over a period of time; however, motor losses are usually irreversible [75].

It is known that increased length of irradiated spinal cord is associated with an increased risk of myelopathy. Emami et al. recommended the maximum doses as 50 Gy to 5 cm, 50 Gy to 10 cm, and 47 Gy to 20 cm of the spinal cord, respectively [13]. The tolerance of the spinal cord is also affected by patient characteristics such as age, congenital abnormalities, and comorbidities as well as neurotoxic chemotherapeutic agents and oxygen level [76].

Schultheiss et al. reported that the risk of radiation myelopathy is 5 % between conventional fraction doses of 57 and 61 Gy [77]. Wong et al. observed no myelopathy after 50 Gy in 25 fractions [78]. The RTOG limits the maximum dose with 45–50 Gy. It was calculated that the risk of myelopathy is 0.03 % when the maximum dose is <45 Gy [79]. The QUANTEC paper, on the other hand, reported that increased maximum dose from 50 to 60 Gy and 69 Gy increases the risk of myelopathy from 0.2 % to 6 % and 50 %, respectively [80]. It was also shown that the thoracic (T) cord is more radioresistant than the cervical (C) cord [81]. However, no difference in the duration of latency was shown between T and C cords.

It is well known that the repair of subacute injury of the spinal cord is slower than many other tissues [82]. No unexpected myelopathy was reported after two fractions in a day with at least 6–8 h between them. Jeremic reported no myelopathies after 50.6 Gy in 1.1 Gy fractions in the C cord and 50.4 Gy in 1.2 Gy fractions in the T cord [83, 84]. However, studies with three to four fractions a day reported unexpected myelopathies [85, 86].

By using more developed technologies such as IMRT or proton therapy, small volumes of the spinal cord can receive higher doses than would be intolerable for the whole cord [87]. Depending on this, it has been stated that small portions of the spinal cord may tolerate higher doses up to 60 Gy [74].

In studies of SABR, it was reported that a maximum dose of 13 Gy in a single fraction or 20 Gy in three fractions is safe with <1 % risk of myelopathy [35]. The RTOG 0631 study which administers SABR to spine metastases limits the D10 and D0.35 ml with 10 Gy and Dmax with 14 Gy [88].

Brachial Plexus

Contouring

The delineation of the brachial plexus is only required for upper lobe tumors and contouring only the ipsilateral brachial plexus is sufficient (Fig. 23.3). The

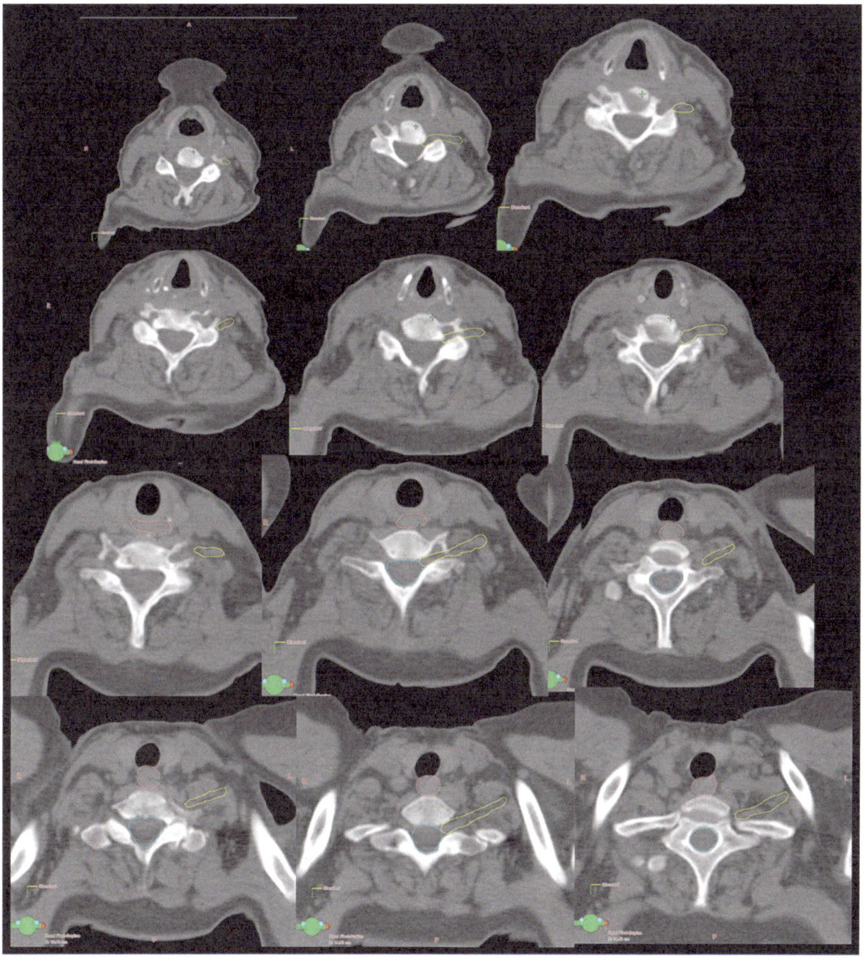

Fig. 23.3 Delineation of brachial plexus

delineation starts from the superior of the C5 vertebra to the superior of the T2 vertebra, including the spinal nerves exiting the neural foramens. Timmerman has shown an easy way to identify the brachial plexus in the ongoing RTOG 1106 trial. According to "Timmerman's trick"; the vein, artery, and nerves lie over the first rib and under the clavicle, and by finding this plane, you can delineate the neurovascular tissues on all CT slices. The contouring should extend at least 3 cm above the PTV. Although RTOG 0618 trial has recommended including the subclavian and axillary vessels, the ongoing 1106 study has contoured the nerves according to the CT anatomy on every other CT slice. Contrast use will facilitate the contouring by making the arteries more visible. If the brachial plexus is involved by the tumor and cannot be identified, contralateral brachial plexus can be used to find the involved one more easily.

Hall et al. proposed an atlas for the delineation of brachial plexus in patients with head and neck cancer treated with IMRT [89]. This atlas can be adapted for patients with lung cancer. The authors have recommended following these steps; first, one should find and delineate the C5, T1, and T2 vertebrae, the subclavian and axillary neurovascular bundles, and anterior and middle scalene muscles from the C5 vertebra to their insertions onto the first rib. The next step is to delineate the brachial plexus by using a 5 mm diameter paint tool, starting from the neural foramina from C5 to T1 vertebra, extending from the lateral aspect of the spinal canal to the space between the anterior and middle scalene muscles. In CT slices where the neural foramen does not exist, only the space mentioned above is delineated. Delineation continues until the middle scalene muscle ends at the subclavian neurovascular bundle. The brachial plexus is delineated inferior and lateral to the posterior aspect of the neurovascular bundle and until the inferior to the clavicular head. The medial border is the first and second ribs.

Dose-Volume Constraints and Toxicity

Based on its poorly described diagnosis, radiation-induced brachial plexopathy (BP) has somewhat low incidence. The reason for the development of BP is demyelination resulting in the loss of axons [90]. The early transient BP may develop during RT or weeks or months after the completion of RT [91]. It usually resolves spontaneously and can occur at low doses. Late BP develops years after RT; has more significant symptoms such as hyperesthesia, paresthesia, and weakness of the affected arm and shoulder; and can even progress to total paralysis.

Emami et al. reported the TD5/5 for the 1/3 of the brachial plexus 62 Gy, for 2/3 61 Gy, and for 3/3 60 Gy, respectively [13]. Late toxicity develops if the maximum dose of the brachial plexus exceeds 60–66 Gy [89]. The RTOG 0617 study recommends keeping the maximum dose <66 Gy, whereas the RTOG 0972/Cancer and Leukemia Group B (CALGB) 36050 study advises the V20 is kept ≤35 % [68, 92]. Eblan et al. reported five cases of radiation-induced BP in

80 patients with apical NSCLC who received ≥50 Gy to the primary tumor, and the median onset of toxicity was 11 months [93]. They stated that the rate of BP was 9 % in patients who were estimated to have received >60 Gy to the ipsilateral brachial plexus. They estimated the rates of radiation-induced BP at 1 and 3 years 8 % and 17 %, respectively. In this study, no patients who received ≤78 Gy to the ipsilateral brachial plexus developed toxicity. The mean V66, V76, and V80 were 51 %, 39 %, and 22 %, respectively, in patients who developed radiation-induced BP. They also reported the V76 of >1 cc of the ipsilateral brachial plexus as the strongest predictor for the development of BP. Amini et al. reported the results in 90 patients with unresectable NSCLC in upper lobes who received CRT [94]. The rate of grade 1 BP was 16 %, and grade ≥2 7 % in these patients with median 70 Gy to the brachial plexus. The most important predictive factors for the development of BP were the presence of prior BP, a median dose of >69 Gy to the brachial plexus, and a maximum dose of >75 Gy to 2 cm^3 of the brachial plexus.

Brachial plexopathy can also be observed in patients who receive SABR for apical lung tumors. The RTOG trial limits the maximum point dose to the ipsilateral brachial plexus to 24 Gy [35]. The Indiana University reported 7 BPs in 37 apical tumors median 7 months after RT with median 30 Gy to the brachial plexus [95]. The risk of grade 2–4 BP was increased to 46 % from 8 % when the maximum dose increased to >26 Gy from ≤26 Gy. The AAPM Task Group 101 recommends the maximum point dose and maximum dose to 3 cc of the brachial plexus 17.5 Gy and 14 Gy in a single fraction, 24 Gy and 20.4 Gy in three fractions, and 30.5 Gy and 27 Gy in five fractions of SABR, respectively [38].

Chest Wall and Ribs

Contouring

Chest wall can easily be delineated by expanding 2 cm lateral, anterior, and posterior to the ipsilateral lung and excluding the lung itself [2, 96]. The medial border of the CW ends at the lateral border of the sternum on the anterior and at the lateral border of vertebral bodies including the spinal nerve roots on the posterior (Fig. 23.4). The contour includes intercostal muscles and nerves but excludes the vertebral bodies, sternum, skin, and other muscles. Auto-delineation can be made by the auto-expansion of the ipsilateral lung. The delineation of the CW should start 3 cm superior to the PTV and end 3 cm inferior to it.

Shaikh et al. reviewed the delineation of the CW and ribs in various SABR studies [97]. The most common method for contouring the CW is 3 cm expansion from the ipsilateral lung including the roots of thoracic nerves and intercostal muscles while excluding the mediastinal structures, lung, and vertebral bodies. The ongoing RTOG 1021 and 0915 trials have recommended delineating the ribs within 5 cm of the PTV by outlining the bone and marrow and contouring adjacent ribs as one structure excluding the intercostal spaces.

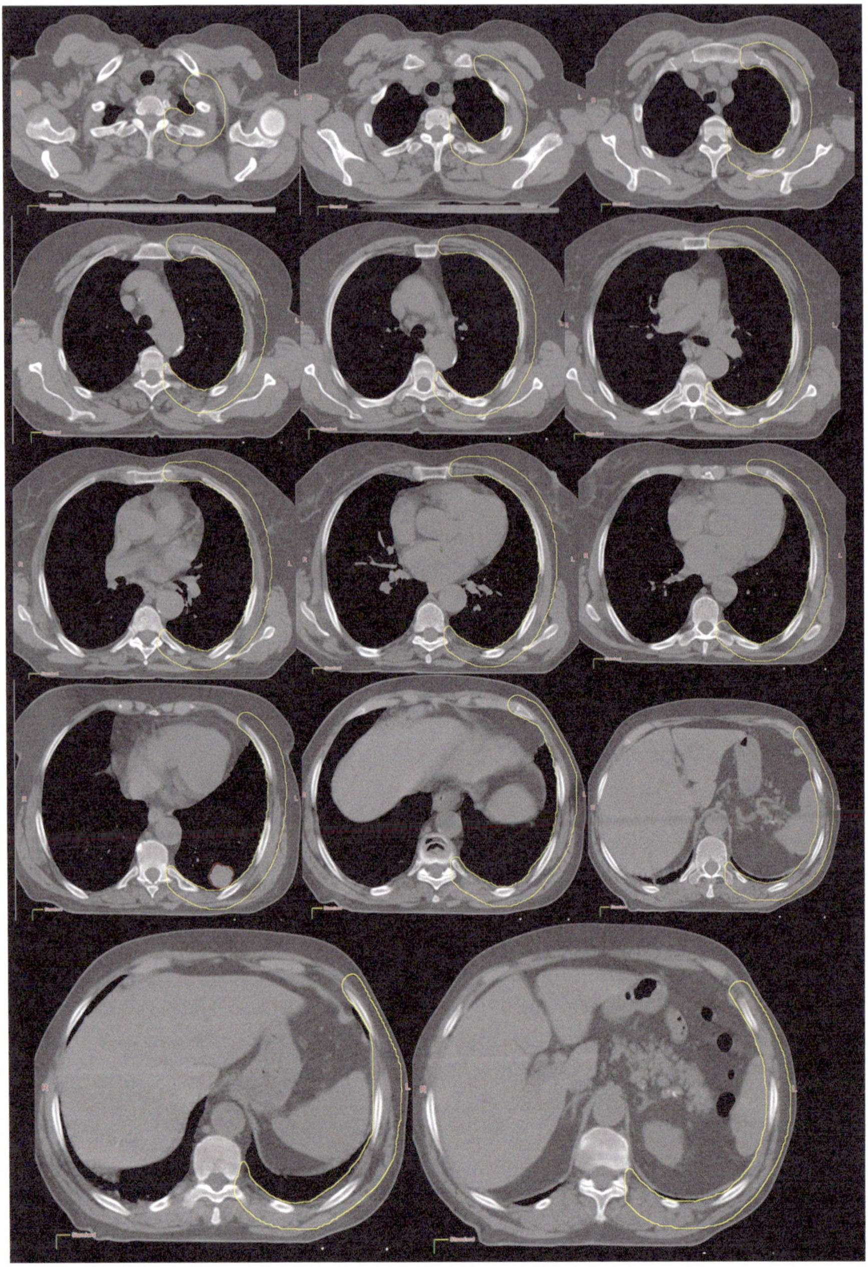

Fig. 23.4 Delineation of chest wall

Dose-Volume Constraints and Toxicity

Chest wall toxicity should particularly be considered in patients treated with SABR which is preferred in medically inoperable in patients with early stage lung cancer. The symptoms generally develop several months after the completion of RT and can be observed as CW pain which is due to the injury of the intercostal nerves, or rib fracture which is usually asymptomatic. Recent studies held in breast cancer patients treated with conventionally fractionated RT have reported the rates of rib fracture 0.3–3.6 % [98, 99]. It was shown that rib fractures can occur with point doses as low as 33 Gy [100].

Voroney et al. reported 11 CW toxicities and 7 rib fractures in 42 medically inoperable patients with NSCLC treated with SABR doses of 54–60 Gy in three fractions [100]. On the other hand, rates of CW toxicity and rib fracture were reported 11.4 % and 1.6 %, respectively, when 55 Gy was delivered in five fractions [101]. Coroller et al. reported the rate of CW toxicity 8.3 % and rib fracture 6.9 % in 69 patients receiving 54 Gy in three fractions or 50–60 Gy in five fractions [102]. In the review of Shaikh et al. which evaluated CW toxicity in 12 SABR studies, the rates of CW pain and rib fracture were 0–46 % and 0–39 %, respectively, with doses of 18–72 Gy in 3–24 fractions [97]. Andolino et al. reported that the rates of CW pain and rib fracture were increased in patients who received a maximum dose of 50 Gy to the CW and ribs [103]. Stephans et al. found that no patients developed CW toxicity when the point dose to the CW was <67.5 Gy, and the risk was higher when 60 Gy in three fractions was administered compared to 50 Gy in five fractions [104].

It was reported that the volume of the CW receiving >30 Gy during SABR is a predictor for the development of severe pain and rib fracture [105]. The authors stated that the risk of CW toxicity was 30 % when 35 cm^3 of the CW received 30 Gy and recommended that the V30 of the CW should be <30 cm^3 in three to five fractions. Creach et al. found that when the V30 is >0.7 % and V40 is >0.19 %, the risk of CW toxicity is 15 % [106]. Hoppe et al. reported 14 % grade >2 acute skin toxicity in 50 patients with early stage NSCLC who were treated with SABR, and the maximum back skin dose, distance between the tumor and the skin, and the number of beams were predictive factors for the development of toxicity [107].

The volume receiving high-dose RT is also crucial for the development of CW toxicity. Taremi et al. reported that the risk of rib fracture is 50 % when the D0.5 cc of the rib is ≥60 Gy, and they proposed a calculation algorithm for the risk of development of CW toxicity according to patient age and gender and D0.5 cc of the CW [108]. Pettersson et al., on the other hand, found that the D2 of the rib ≥27.3 Gy was associated with the same risk [109]. Andolino et al. reported that D5 >40 Gy and D15 >40 Gy result in 10 % and 30 % rate of rib fracture, respectively [103]. Kim et al. found that D8 >58 Gy was associated with a 50 % risk of rib fracture [110]. The RTOG recommends the maximum point dose of the ribs 30 Gy in one or 40 Gy four fractions, respectively.

Trachea and Proximal Bronchial Tree

Contouring

The delineation of the trachea and PBT is recommended in patients with lung cancer but not mandated (Fig. 23.5). The PBT starts at 2 cm above the carina and includes the distal 2 cm of the trachea, the carina, bilateral main bronchi, bilateral upper lobe bronchi, the intermedius bronchus and middle lobe bronchus of the right

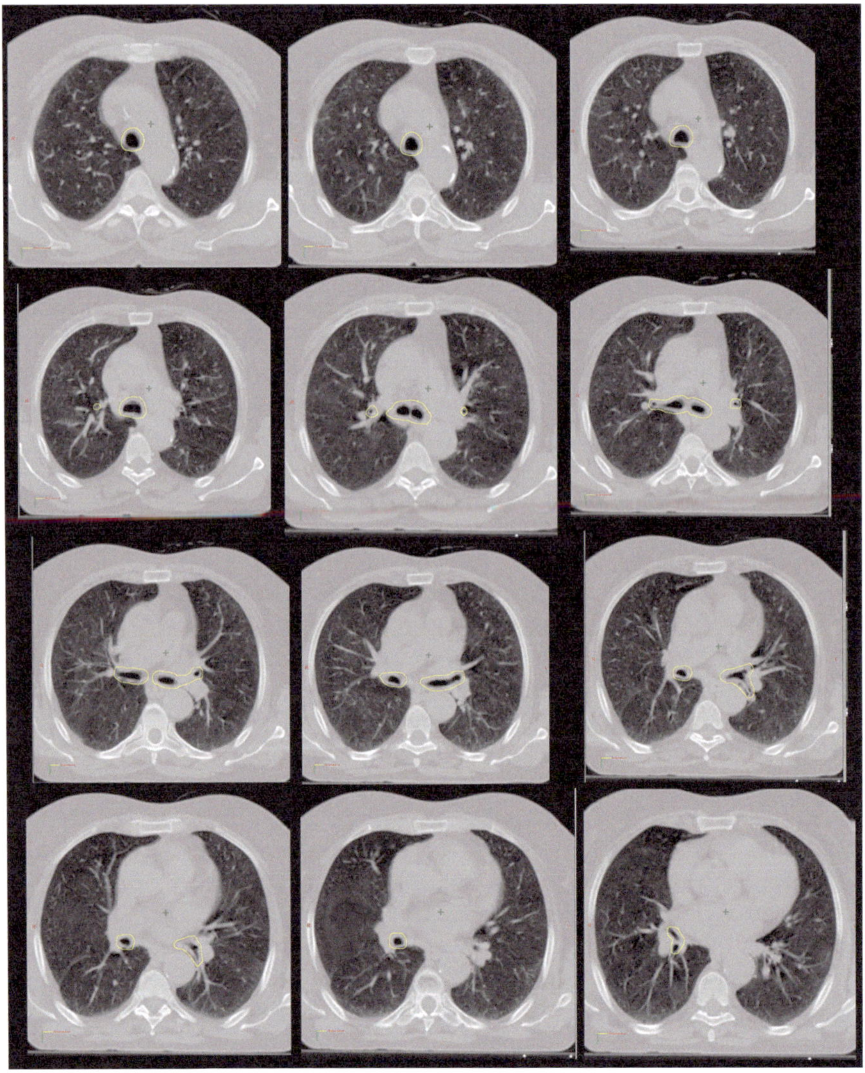

Fig. 23.5 Delineation of trachea and proximal bronchial tree

lung, the lingular bronchus of the left lung, and bilateral lower lobe bronchi. The mediastinal windowing should be used on the CT scan to clearly see the mucosa, submucosa, and cartilage rings and airway channels of these structures [2]. The whole bronchial tree can be contoured as one structure. The delineation can be done by expanding the lobar bronchus by 2 mm, the main bronchus by 3 mm, and the trachea by 4 mm. The RTOG 0618 trial recommends ending the delineation of the lobar bronchi at the level of a segmental bifurcation [34].

Dose-Volume Constraints and Toxicity

The risk for the development of PBT toxicity is associated with the distance of the tumor to bronchi and total and fraction dose of RT. It has been clearly shown that central lesions are at higher risk for PBT toxicity [32]. Fakiris et al. treated 70 patients with medically inoperable early stage lung cancer with 54 Gy SABR in three fractions, and severe central airway toxicity was observed in 10.4 % and 27.3 % of patients with peripheral and central tumors, respectively [111]. The rate of grade 3–4 PBT toxicity was reported <9 % in a review of 315 patients with central lung tumors treated by SABR, and it was concluded that the treatment-related mortality significantly decreased when the lower biologically effective dose (BED) was ≤210 Gy [112]. The QUANTEC paper has recommended limiting the dose to the central airways to ≤80 Gy in order to reduce the risk of PBT toxicity [113].

The AAPM Task Group 101 recommends the maximum point dose and maximum dose to 4 cc of PBT 20.2 Gy and 10.5 Gy in a single fraction, 30 Gy and 15 Gy in three fractions, and 40 Gy and 16.5 Gy in five fractions, respectively, in patients treated with SABR [38]. The RTOG 0236 trial limits the maximum point dose to the trachea and ipsilateral bronchus to 30 Gy [35].

Conclusion

Most data on toxicity of RT in lung cancer patients are based on conventional fractionation. Data on more developed techniques have been accumulated. It is important to apply the recommended dose-volume constraints for lung cancer patients in order to minimize toxicity.

References

1. Li XA, Tai A, Arthur DW, et al. Variability of target and normal structure delineation for breast cancer radiotherapy: an RTOG Multi-Institutional and Multiobserver Study. Int J Radiat Oncol Biol Phys. 2009;73:944–51.
2. Kong FM, Ritter T, Quint DJ, et al. Consideration of dose limits for organs at risk of thoracic radiotherapy: atlas for lung, proximal bronchial tree, esophagus, spinal cord, ribs, and brachial plexus. Int J Radiat Oncol Biol Phys. 2011;81:1442–57.
3. Bradley JGM, Winter K, Purdy JA, Komaki R, Roa WH, Ryu JK, Bosch W, Emami B. Toxicity and outcome results of RTOG 9311: a phase I-II dose-escalation study using

three-dimensional conformal radiotherapy in patients with inoperable non-small-cell lung carcinoma. Int J Radiat Oncol Biol Phys. 2005;61:318–28.
4. Bradley JD, Bae K, Graham MV, et al. Primary analysis of the phase II component of a phase I/II dose intensification study using three-dimensional conformal radiation therapy and concurrent chemotherapy for patients with inoperable non-small-cell lung cancer: RTOG 0117. J Clin Oncol. 2010;28:2475–80.
5. Marks LB, Bentzen SM, Deasy JO, et al. Radiation dose-volume effects in the lung. Int J Radiat Oncol Biol Phys. 2010;76:S70–6.
6. Rodrigues G, Lock M, D'Souza D, et al. Prediction of radiation pneumonitis by dose – volume histogram parameters in lung cancer – a systematic review. Radiother Oncol. 2004;71:127–38.
7. Huang K, Dahele M, Senan S, et al. Radiographic changes after lung stereotactic ablative radiotherapy (SABR) – can we distinguish recurrence from fibrosis? A systematic review of the literature. Radiother Oncol. 2012;102:335–42.
8. Palma DA, Senan S, Haasbeek CJ, et al. Radiological and clinical pneumonitis after stereotactic lung radiotherapy: a matched analysis of three-dimensional conformal and volumetric-modulated arc therapy techniques. Int J Radiat Oncol Biol Phys. 2011;80:506–13.
9. Shapiro SJ, Shapiro SD, Mill WB, Campbell EJ. Prospective study of long-term pulmonary manifestations of mantle irradiation. Int J Radiat Oncol Biol Phys. 1990;19:707–14.
10. Bell J, McGivern D, Bullimore J, et al. Diagnostic imaging of post-irradiation changes in the chest. Clin Radiol. 1988;39:109–19.
11. Marks LB, Spencer DP, Bentel GC, et al. The utility of SPECT lung perfusion scans in minimizing and assessing the physiologic consequences of thoracic irradiation. Int J Radiat Oncol Biol Phys. 1993;26:659–68.
12. Movsas B, Raffin TA, Epstein AH, Link Jr CJ. Pulmonary radiation injury. Chest. 1997;111:1061–76.
13. Emami B, Lyman J, Brown A, et al. Tolerance of normal tissue to therapeutic irradiation. Int J Radiat Oncol Biol Phys. 1991;21:109–22.
14. Seppenwoolde Y, Lebesque JV, de Jaeger K, et al. Comparing different NTCP models that predict the incidence of radiation pneumonitis. Normal tissue complication probability. Int J Radiat Oncol Biol Phys. 2003;55:724–35.
15. Yorke ED, Jackson A, Rosenzweig KE, et al. Dose-volume factors contributing to the incidence of radiation pneumonitis in non-small-cell lung cancer patients treated with three-dimensional conformal radiation therapy. Int J Radiat Oncol Biol Phys. 2002;54:329–39.
16. Armstrong J, Raben A, Zelefsky M, et al. Promising survival with three-dimensional conformal radiation therapy for non-small cell lung cancer. Radiother Oncol. 1997;44:17–22.
17. Willner J, Jost A, Baier K, Flentje M. A little to a lot or a lot to a little? An analysis of pneumonitis risk from dose-volume histogram parameters of the lung in patients with lung cancer treated with 3-D conformal radiotherapy. Strahlenther Onkol. 2003;179:548–56.
18. Graham MV, Purdy JA, Emami B, et al. Clinical dose-volume histogram analysis for pneumonitis after 3D treatment for non-small cell lung cancer (NSCLC). Int J Radiat Oncol Biol Phys. 1999;45:323–9.
19. Koh ES, Sun A, Tran TH, et al. Clinical dose-volume histogram analysis in predicting radiation pneumonitis in Hodgkin's lymphoma. Int J Radiat Oncol Biol Phys. 2006;66:223–8.
20. Hope AJ, Lindsay PE, El Naqa I, et al. Modeling radiation pneumonitis risk with clinical, dosimetric, and spatial parameters. Int J Radiat Oncol Biol Phys. 2006;65:112–24.
21. Wang S, Liao Z, Wei X, et al. Analysis of clinical and dosimetric factors associated with treatment-related pneumonitis (TRP) in patients with non-small-cell lung cancer (NSCLC) treated with concurrent chemotherapy and three-dimensional conformal radiotherapy (3D-CRT). Int J Radiat Oncol Biol Phys. 2006;66:1399–407.
22. Schallenkamp JM, Miller RC, Brinkmann DH, et al. Incidence of radiation pneumonitis after thoracic irradiation: dose-volume correlates. Int J Radiat Oncol Biol Phys. 2007;67:410–6.

23. Hernando ML, Marks LB, Bentel GC, et al. Radiation-induced pulmonary toxicity: a dose-volume histogram analysis in 201 patients with lung cancer. Int J Radiat Oncol Biol Phys. 2001;51:650–9.
24. Tsujino K, Hirota S, Endo M, et al. Predictive value of dose-volume histogram parameters for predicting radiation pneumonitis after concurrent chemoradiation for lung cancer. Int J Radiat Oncol Biol Phys. 2003;55:110–5.
25. Liao ZX, Komaki RR, Thames Jr HD, et al. Influence of technologic advances on outcomes in patients with unresectable, locally advanced non-small-cell lung cancer receiving concomitant chemoradiotherapy. Int J Radiat Oncol Biol Phys. 2010;76:775–81.
26. Sura S, Gupta V, Yorke E, et al. Intensity-modulated radiation therapy (IMRT) for inoperable non-small cell lung cancer: the Memorial Sloan-Kettering Cancer Center (MSKCC) experience. Radiother Oncol. 2008;87:17–23.
27. Yom SS, Liao Z, Liu HH, et al. Initial evaluation of treatment-related pneumonitis in advanced-stage non-small-cell lung cancer patients treated with concurrent chemotherapy and intensity-modulated radiotherapy. Int J Radiat Oncol Biol Phys. 2007;68:94–102.
28. Allen AM, Czerminska M, Janne PA, et al. Fatal pneumonitis associated with intensity-modulated radiation therapy for mesothelioma. Int J Radiat Oncol Biol Phys. 2006;65:640–5.
29. Miles EF, Larrier NA, Kelsey CR, et al. Intensity-modulated radiotherapy for resected mesothelioma: the Duke experience. Int J Radiat Oncol Biol Phys. 2008;71:1143–50.
30. Rice DC, Smythe WR, Liao Z, et al. Dose-dependent pulmonary toxicity after postoperative intensity-modulated radiotherapy for malignant pleural mesothelioma. Int J Radiat Oncol Biol Phys. 2007;69:350–7.
31. Murshed H, Liu HH, Liao Z, et al. Dose and volume reduction for normal lung using intensity-modulated radiotherapy for advanced-stage non-small-cell lung cancer. Int J Radiat Oncol Biol Phys. 2004;58:1258–67.
32. Timmerman R, McGarry R, Yiannoutsos C, et al. Excessive toxicity when treating central tumors in a phase II study of stereotactic body radiation therapy for medically inoperable early-stage lung cancer. J Clin Oncol. 2006;24:4833–9.
33. Grutters JP, Kessels AG, Pijls-Johannesma M, et al. Comparison of the effectiveness of radiotherapy with photons, protons and carbon-ions for non-small cell lung cancer: a meta-analysis. Radiother Oncol. 2010;95:32–40.
34. Timmerman RD, Park C, Kavanagh BD. The North American experience with stereotactic body radiation therapy in non-small cell lung cancer. J Thorac Oncol. 2007;2:S101–12.
35. Timmerman R, Paulus R, Galvin J, et al. Stereotactic body radiation therapy for inoperable early stage lung cancer. JAMA. 2010;303:1070–6.
36. Nyman J, HA, Lund JA, et al. SPACE – a randomized study of SBRT vs conventional fractionated radiotherapy in medically inoperable stage I NSCLC [abstract]. In: European Society for Radiotherapy and Oncology Annual Meeting, Vienna, Austria. 2014.
37. Barriger RB, Forquer JA, Brabham JG, et al. A dose-volume analysis of radiation pneumonitis in non-small cell lung cancer patients treated with stereotactic body radiation therapy. Int J Radiat Oncol Biol Phys. 2012;82:457–62.
38. Benedict SH, Yenice KM, Followill D, et al. Stereotactic body radiation therapy: the report of AAPM Task Group 101. Med Phys. 2010;37:4078–101.
39. Ong CL, Palma D, Verbakel WF, et al. Treatment of large stage I-II lung tumors using stereotactic body radiotherapy (SBRT): planning considerations and early toxicity. Radiother Oncol. 2010;97:431–6.
40. Takeda A, Sanuki N, Enomoto T, Kunieda E. Subclinical interstitial lung disease: is it a risk factor for fatal radiation pneumonitis following stereotactic body radiotherapy? Lung Cancer. 2014;83:112.
41. Takeda A, Enomoto T, Sanuki N, et al. Reassessment of declines in pulmonary function >/=1 year after stereotactic body radiotherapy. Chest. 2013;143:130–7.
42. Stephans KL, Djemil T, Reddy CA, et al. Comprehensive analysis of pulmonary function Test (PFT) changes after stereotactic body radiotherapy (SBRT) for stage I lung cancer in medically inoperable patients. J Thorac Oncol. 2009;4:838–44.

43. Stanic S, Paulus R, Timmerman RD, et al. No clinically significant changes in pulmonary function following stereotactic body radiation therapy for early- stage peripheral non-small cell lung cancer: an analysis of RTOG 0236. Int J Radiat Oncol Biol Phys. 2014;88:1092–9.
44. Lee HK, Vaporciyan AA, Cox JD, et al. Postoperative pulmonary complications after preoperative chemoradiation for esophageal carcinoma: correlation with pulmonary dose-volume histogram parameters. Int J Radiat Oncol Biol Phys. 2003;57:1317–22.
45. Feng M, Moran JM, Koelling T, et al. Development and validation of a heart atlas to study cardiac exposure to radiation following treatment for breast cancer. Int J Radiat Oncol Biol Phys. 2011;79:10–8.
46. Gagliardi G, Constine LS, Moiseenko V, et al. Radiation dose-volume effects in the heart. Int J Radiat Oncol Biol Phys. 2010;76:S77–85.
47. Carmel RJ, Kaplan HS. Mantle irradiation in Hodgkin's disease. An analysis of technique, tumor eradication, and complications. Cancer. 1976;37:2813–25.
48. Stewart JR, Fajardo LF. Dose response in human and experimental radiation-induced heart disease. Application of the nominal standard dose (NSD) concept. Radiology. 1971;99:403–8.
49. Martel MK, Sahijdak WM, Ten Haken RK, et al. Fraction size and dose parameters related to the incidence of pericardial effusions. Int J Radiat Oncol Biol Phys. 1998;40:155–61.
50. Komaki R, LH, Murshed H. Lung cancer. In: Chao CKS editor. Practical essentials of intensity modulated radiation therapy. Lippincott Williams & Wilkins, Philadelphia, 2nd ed. 2005. pp. 255–275.
51. Jagsi R, Moran J, Marsh R, et al. Evaluation of four techniques using intensity-modulated radiation therapy for comprehensive locoregional irradiation of breast cancer. Int J Radiat Oncol Biol Phys. 2010;78:1594–603.
52. Group PM-aT. Postoperative radiotherapy in non-small cell lung cancer: systematic review and meta-analysis of individual patient data from nine randomised controlled trials. Lancet. 1998;352:257–63.
53. Dautzenberg B, Arriagada R, Chammard AB, et al. A controlled study of postoperative radiotherapy for patients with completely resected nonsmall cell lung carcinoma. Groupe d'Etude et de Traitement des Cancers Bronchiques. Cancer. 1999;86:265–73.
54. Shafman TD, Yu X, Vujaskovic Z, et al. Radiation-induced lung and heart toxicity. In: Jeremić B, editor. Advances in radiation oncology in lung cancer. New York/Berlin: Springer; 2005. p. 351–66.
55. Werner-Wasik M. Radiation therapy-related toxicity: esophagus. In: Jeremic B, editor. Advances in radiation oncology in lung cancer. New York/Berlin: Springer; 2006. p. 373–82.
56. Werner-Wasik M, Pequignot E, Leeper D, et al. Predictors of severe esophagitis include use of concurrent chemotherapy, but not the length of irradiated esophagus: a multivariate analysis of patients with lung cancer treated with nonoperative therapy. Int J Radiat Oncol Biol Phys. 2000;48:689–96.
57. Byhardt RW, Scott C, Sause WT, et al. Response, toxicity, failure patterns, and survival in five Radiation Therapy Oncology Group (RTOG) trials of sequential and/or concurrent chemotherapy and radiotherapy for locally advanced non-small-cell carcinoma of the lung. Int J Radiat Oncol Biol Phys. 1998;42:469–78.
58. Singh AK, Lockett MA, Bradley JD. Predictors of radiation-induced esophageal toxicity in patients with non-small-cell lung cancer treated with three-dimensional conformal radiotherapy. Int J Radiat Oncol Biol Phys. 2003;55:337–41.
59. Qiao WB, Zhao YH, Zhao YB, Wang RZ. Clinical and dosimetric factors of radiation-induced esophageal injury: radiation-induced esophageal toxicity. World J Gastroenterol. 2005;11:2626–9.
60. Boal DK, Newburger PE, Teele RL. Esophagitis induced by combined radiation and adriamycin. AJR Am J Roentgenol. 1979;132:567–70.

61. Umsawasdi T, Valdivieso M, Barkley Jr HT, et al. Esophageal complications from combined chemoradiotherapy (cyclophosphamide + Adriamycin + cisplatin + XRT) in the treatment of non-small cell lung cancer. Int J Radiat Oncol Biol Phys. 1985;11:511–9.
62. Vokes EE, Herndon 2nd JE, Crawford J, et al. Randomized phase II study of cisplatin with gemcitabine or paclitaxel or vinorelbine as induction chemotherapy followed by concomitant chemoradiotherapy for stage IIIB non-small-cell lung cancer: cancer and leukemia group B study 9431. J Clin Oncol. 2002;20:4191–8.
63. Ball D, Bishop J, Smith J, et al. A phase III study of accelerated radiotherapy with and without carboplatin in nonsmall cell lung cancer: an interim toxicity analysis of the first 100 patients. Int J Radiat Oncol Biol Phys. 1995;31:267–72.
64. Werner-Wasik M, Paulus R, Curran Jr WJ, Byhardt R. Acute esophagitis and late lung toxicity in concurrent chemoradiotherapy trials in patients with locally advanced non-small-cell lung cancer: analysis of the radiation therapy oncology group (RTOG) database. Clin Lung Cancer. 2011;12:245–51.
65. Saunders MI, Dische S, Barrett A, et al. Randomised multicentre trials of CHART vs conventional radiotherapy in head and neck and non-small-cell lung cancer: an interim report. CHART Steering Committee. Br J Cancer. 1996;73:1455–62.
66. Dubray B, Livartowski A, Beuzeboc P, et al. Combined chemoradiation for locally advanced nonsmall cell lung cancer. J Infus Chemother. 1995;5:195–6.
67. Werner-Wasik M, Yorke E, Deasy J, et al. Radiation dose-volume effects in the esophagus. Int J Radiat Oncol Biol Phys. 2010;76:S86–93.
68. Bradley JD, Paulus R, Komaki R, et al. Standard-dose versus high-dose conformal radiotherapy with concurrent and consolidation carboplatin plus paclitaxel with or without cetuximab for patients with stage IIIA or IIIB non-small-cell lung cancer (RTOG 0617): a randomised, two-by-two factorial phase 3 study. Lancet Oncol. 2015;16: 187–99.
69. Maguire PD, Sibley GS, Zhou SM, et al. Clinical and dosimetric predictors of radiation-induced esophageal toxicity. Int J Radiat Oncol Biol Phys. 1999;45:97–103.
70. Ahn SJ, Kahn D, Zhou S, et al. Dosimetric and clinical predictors for radiation-induced esophageal injury. Int J Radiat Oncol Biol Phys. 2005;61:335–47.
71. De Gersem WR, Derycke S, De Wagter C, De Neve WC. Optimization of beam weights in conformal radiotherapy planning of stage III non-small cell lung cancer: effects on therapeutic ratio. Int J Radiat Oncol Biol Phys. 2000;47:255–60.
72. Derycke S, De Gersem WR, Van Duyse BB, De Neve WC. Conformal radiotherapy of Stage III non-small cell lung cancer: a class solution involving non-coplanar intensity-modulated beams. Int J Radiat Oncol Biol Phys. 1998;41:771–7.
73. Abbatucci JS, Delozier T, Quint R, et al. Radiation myelopathy of the cervical spinal cord: time, dose and volume factors. Int J Radiat Oncol Biol Phys. 1978;4:239–48.
74. Schultheiss TE. Spinal cord. In: Jeremic B, editor. Advances in radiation oncology in lung cancer. New York/Berlin: Springer; 2006. p. 367–72.
75. Ang KK, Stephens LC. Prevention and management of radiation myelopathy. Oncology (Williston Park). 1994;8:71–6; discussion 78, 81–72.
76. Coy P, Dolman CL. Radiation myelopathy in relation to oxygen level. Br J Radiol. 1971;44:705–7.
77. Schultheiss TE. Spinal cord radiation tolerance. Int J Radiat Oncol Biol Phys. 1994;30:735–6.
78. Wong CS, Van Dyk J, Milosevic M, Laperriere NJ. Radiation myelopathy following single courses of radiotherapy and retreatment. Int J Radiat Oncol Biol Phys. 1994;30:575–81.
79. Schultheiss TE. The radiation dose-response of the human spinal cord. Int J Radiat Oncol Biol Phys. 2008;71:1455–9.
80. Kirkpatrick JP, van der Kogel AJ, Schultheiss TE. Radiation dose-volume effects in the spinal cord. Int J Radiat Oncol Biol Phys. 2010;76:S42–9.

81. Kirkpatrick JP, Milano M, Constine LS, et al. Late effects and QUANTEC. In: Halperin EC, editor. Perez and Brady's principle and practice of radiation oncology. 6th ed. Philadelphia: Lippincott Williams & Wilkins; 2013. p. 296–328.
82. Ang KK, Jiang GL, Guttenberger R, et al. Impact of spinal cord repair kinetics on the practice of altered fractionation schedules. Radiother Oncol. 1992;25:287–94.
83. Jeremic B, Shibamoto Y, Milicic B, et al. Absence of thoracic radiation myelitis after hyperfractionated radiation therapy with and without concurrent chemotherapy for stage III nonsmall-cell lung cancer. Int J Radiat Oncol Biol Phys. 1998;40:343–6.
84. Jeremic B, Shibamoto Y, Igrutinovic I. Absence of cervical radiation myelitis after hyperfractionated radiation therapy with and without concurrent chemotherapy for locally advanced, unresectable, nonmetastatic squamous cell carcinoma of the head and neck. J Cancer Res Clin Oncol. 2001;127:687–91.
85. Dische S, Saunders MI. Continuous, hyperfractionated, accelerated radiotherapy (CHART): an interim report upon late morbidity. Radiother Oncol. 1989;16:65–72.
86. Wong CS, Van Dyk J, Simpson WJ. Myelopathy following hyperfractionated accelerated radiotherapy for anaplastic thyroid carcinoma. Radiother Oncol. 1991;20:3–9.
87. Debus J, Hug EB, Liebsch NJ, et al. Brainstem tolerance to conformal radiotherapy of skull base tumors. Int J Radiat Oncol Biol Phys. 1997;39:967–75.
88. Ryu S, Pugh SL, Gerszten PC, et al. RTOG 0631 phase 2/3 study of image guided stereotactic radiosurgery for localized (1–3) spine metastases: phase 2 results. Pract Radiat Oncol. 2014;4:76–81.
89. Hall WH, Guiou M, Lee NY, et al. Development and validation of a standardized method for contouring the brachial plexus: preliminary dosimetric analysis among patients treated with IMRT for head-and-neck cancer. Int J Radiat Oncol Biol Phys. 2008;72:1362–7.
90. Ferrante MA. Brachial plexopathies: classification, causes, and consequences. Muscle Nerve. 2004;30:547–68.
91. Churn M, Clough V, Slater A. Early onset of bilateral brachial plexopathy during mantle radiotherapy for Hodgkin's disease. Clin Oncol (R Coll Radiol). 2000;12:289–91.
92. Lilenbaum R, Samuels M, Wang X, et al. A phase II study of induction chemotherapy followed by thoracic radiotherapy and erlotinib in poor-risk stage III non-small-cell lung cancer: results of CALGB 30605 (Alliance)/RTOG 0972 (NRG). J Thorac Oncol. 2015;10:143–7.
93. Eblan MJ, Corradetti MN, Lukens JN, et al. Brachial plexopathy in apical non-small cell lung cancer treated with definitive radiation: dosimetric analysis and clinical implications. Int J Radiat Oncol Biol Phys. 2013;85:175–81.
94. Amini A, Yang J, Williamson R, et al. Dose constraints to prevent radiation-induced brachial plexopathy in patients treated for lung cancer. Int J Radiat Oncol Biol Phys. 2012;82:e391–8.
95. Forquer JA, Fakiris AJ, Timmerman RD, et al. Brachial plexopathy from stereotactic body radiotherapy in early-stage NSCLC: dose-limiting toxicity in apical tumor sites. Radiother Oncol. 2009;93:408–13.
96. Mutter RW, Liu F, Abreu A, et al. Dose-volume parameters predict for the development of chest wall pain after stereotactic body radiation for lung cancer. Int J Radiat Oncol Biol Phys. 2012;82:1783–90.
97. Shaikh T, Turaka A. Predictors and management of chest wall toxicity after lung stereotactic body radiotherapy. Cancer Treat Rev. 2014;40:1215–20.
98. Smith GL, Xu Y, Buchholz TA, et al. Association between treatment with brachytherapy vs whole-breast irradiation and subsequent mastectomy, complications, and survival among older women with invasive breast cancer. JAMA. 2012;307:1827–37.
99. Meric F, Buchholz TA, Mirza NQ, et al. Long-term complications associated with breast-conservation surgery and radiotherapy. Ann Surg Oncol. 2002;9:543–9.
100. Voroney JP, Hope A, Dahele MR, et al. Chest wall pain and rib fracture after stereotactic radiotherapy for peripheral non-small cell lung cancer. J Thorac Oncol. 2009;4:1035–7.

101. Bongers EM, Haasbeek CJ, Lagerwaard FJ, et al. Incidence and risk factors for chest wall toxicity after risk-adapted stereotactic radiotherapy for early-stage lung cancer. J Thorac Oncol. 2011;6:2052–7.
102. Coroller TP, Mak RH, Lewis JH, et al. Low incidence of chest wall pain with a risk-adapted lung stereotactic body radiation therapy approach using three or five fractions based on chest wall dosimetry. PLoS ONE. 2014;9:e94859.
103. Andolino DL, Forquer JA, Henderson MA, et al. Chest wall toxicity after stereotactic body radiotherapy for malignant lesions of the lung and liver. Int J Radiat Oncol Biol Phys. 2011;80:692–7.
104. Stephans KL, Djemil T, Tendulkar RD, et al. Prediction of chest wall toxicity from lung stereotactic body radiotherapy (SBRT). Int J Radiat Oncol Biol Phys. 2012;82:974–80.
105. Dunlap NE, Cai J, Biedermann GB, et al. Chest wall volume receiving >30 Gy predicts risk of severe pain and/or rib fracture after lung stereotactic body radiotherapy. Int J Radiat Oncol Biol Phys. 2010;76:796–801.
106. Creach KM, El Naqa I, Bradley JD, et al. Dosimetric predictors of chest wall pain after lung stereotactic body radiotherapy. Radiother Oncol. 2012;104:23–7.
107. Hoppe BS, Laser B, Kowalski AV, et al. Acute skin toxicity following stereotactic body radiation therapy for stage I non-small-cell lung cancer: who's at risk? Int J Radiat Oncol Biol Phys. 2008;72:1283–6.
108. Taremi M, Hope A, Lindsay P, et al. Predictors of radiotherapy induced bone injury (RIBI) after stereotactic lung radiotherapy. Radiat Oncol. 2012;7:159.
109. Pettersson N, Nyman J, Johansson KA. Radiation-induced rib fractures after hypofractionated stereotactic body radiation therapy of non-small cell lung cancer: a dose- and volume-response analysis. Radiother Oncol. 2009;91:360–8.
110. Kim SS, Song SY, Kwak J, et al. Clinical prognostic factors and grading system for rib fracture following stereotactic body radiation therapy (SBRT) in patients with peripheral lung tumors. Lung Cancer. 2013;79:161–6.
111. Fakiris AJ, McGarry RC, Yiannoutsos CT, et al. Stereotactic body radiation therapy for early-stage non-small-cell lung carcinoma: four-year results of a prospective phase II study. Int J Radiat Oncol Biol Phys. 2009;75:677–82.
112. Senthi S, Haasbeek CJ, Slotman BJ, Senan S. Outcomes of stereotactic ablative radiotherapy for central lung tumours: a systematic review. Radiother Oncol. 2013;106:276–82.
113. Hara R, Itami J, Komiyama T, et al. Serum levels of KL-6 for predicting the occurrence of radiation pneumonitis after stereotactic radiotherapy for lung tumors. Chest. 2004;125:340–4.

Quality Assurance of Modern Radiotherapy Techniques in Thoracic Malignancies

24

Christopher Nelson, Steven Kirsner, Yucel Saglam, and Vildan Alpan

Introduction

Radiation treatment of tumors in the thoracic region has evolved substantially over the years. Past methods of treatment were very simple and included several fixed aperture beams to deliver the prescribed dose to the tumor. With the advent of intensity-modulated radiation therapy (IMRT) and volumetric-modulated arc therapy (VMAT), the complexity of such treatments has evolved. These types of treatments use the multi-leaf collimator to create a sequence of small apertures to deliver a high dose to the tumor. The treatment plans are created so that a high dose is given to the target while keeping the dose to organs at low risk. This requires a treatment planning system (TPS) that has the capabilities of inverse planning to generate such treatment fields. The inverse planning engine uses as input contours of the targets and OARs to generate an optimal plan. With new technologies comes a new set of quality assurance (QA) tasks that need to be performed to ensure that what is being planned in the TPS is actually what is delivered to the patient.

Complicating this task of treating tumors located in the thoracic region is that this anatomical region is constantly moving with respiration. Tumors that are subject to respiratory motion have to be treated and this motion should be accounted for when simulating and treating the patient. In this chapter, we will cover the simulation, planning, and treatment of tumors located in the thoracic region along with strategies

C. Nelson, PhD (✉) • S. Kirsner, MS
Department of Radiation Physics, The University of Texas MD Anderson Cancer Center, 7007 Bertner Avenue, 1MC10.2345, Unit 1639, Houston, TX 77054, USA
e-mail: chnelson@mdanderson.org; skirsner@mdanderson.org

Y. Saglam • V. Alpan
Department of Radiation Oncology, American Hospital, Güzelbahçe Sokak, No:20, Tesvikiye, Istanbul 34365, Turkey
e-mail: yucels@amerikanhastanesi.org

G. Ozyigit et al. (eds.), *Principles and Practice of Radiotherapy Techniques in Thoracic Malignancies*, DOI 10.1007/978-3-319-28761-4_24

to mitigate tumor motion. In addition we will discuss the QA methods of each component of the radiation therapy process when treating tumors in the thoracic region.

Patient Simulation

Setup and Immobilization

Prior to beginning radiation treatment, all patients undergo a 3D CT simulation. CT simulation allows us to visualize the tumor and other anatomy in 3D. CT numbers are proportional to electron density, which is necessary in heterogeneous dose calculation algorithms. Patients are brought to the simulator and positioned on the CT couch. At this point, immobilization devices are created to make sure that the patient can be set up in a reproducible position for treatment. Patient immobilization is a key component to the radiation treatment process. Complex treatments are good only if they are treating the area that is intended. That includes setting the patient up in an accurate, reproducible, and comfortable manner for the patient so that they can be positioned in the exact same way each day they come for treatment. Typical immobilization devices for thoracic malignancies include a t-bar and vac-loc bag for upper body immobilization [1–3]. The choice of vac-loc bag varies; for stereotactic simulation, the vac-loc bag will typically wrap around the patient higher than those chosen for conventional fractionation. Another device that may be used for patients whose tumor moves during respiration is the use of a compression device. These devices as the name implies compress the patient's abdomen, so that the diaphragm motion is limited which can be a beneficial strategy to reduce tumor motion [2]. These immobilization devices must comfortably allow the patient to be positioned reproducibly each day during the course of radiation therapy.

Image Acquisition

Once the immobilization device has been made, acquisition of the CT data set begins. The patient's anatomy in the thoracic region including the tumor and the organs at risk move during respiration, this motion should be accounted for during the simulation. This can be accomplished in one of four ways: (1) acquire a slow scan CT while the patient breathes freely, (2) acquire CT data while the patient executes a breath hold maneuver, (3) acquire a respiratory-correlated CT data set, commonly referred to as a 4DCT, and (4) acquire a respiratory gated CT data set.

The first method of acquisition as the name implies is a traditional CT scan through the thorax while the patient breathes normally. For this method, the acquisition is relatively slow compared to that of a diagnostic scan. The slow scan allows areas moving with respiration to be imaged and captures the motion in the images. Structures that move fast with respect to the scan speed will have blurred edges.

This technique however, does not directly account for respiratory motion during imaging process, which must be accounted for during treatment planning. While all imaging procedures are prone to motion artifacts, these artifacts are more likely to present themselves in this technique because respiratory motion is not accounted for during acquisition.

The second approach to 3D-imaging in the thoracic region is acquiring the CT data set while the patient executes a breath hold maneuver [4, 5]. During this acquisition, the patient is instructed to hold their breath, and while the patient executes this breath hold maneuver the CT acquisition occurs. Breath hold scans are typically fast and can capture anatomy in its current state at the time of the acquisition. A well-executed breath hold acquisition should result in less motion-related artifacts than the free-breathing acquisition. However, if the patient is going to be treated using the breath hold technique, reproducibility of anatomy during breath hold needs to be examined. This can be accomplished by acquiring multiple breath hold scans and comparing the anatomy. Not all patients are candidates for breath hold imaging/treatment technique. Some patients cannot physically tolerate the breath hold procedure and some cannot comprehend/understand the instructions. One must keep in mind that if the patient has trouble tolerating the breath hold procedure at simulation, this same breath hold procedure will have to be repeated each day during the course of radiation treatment.

The third method of respiratory-correlated 3D imaging is the acquisition of a 4DCT[6, 7]. In this imaging technique, the patient's respiration is monitored during image acquisition while the patient breathes normally. The imaging technique is setup so that each axial section of anatomy is oversampled relative to the patient's breathing cycle. The section of anatomy that was imaged can then be correlated to the phase of the respiratory cycle and can be used to generate a series of 3D CT image sets which we refer to as a 4DCT. There are two different approaches to 4DCT generation each of which are vendor specific. The first approach is implemented on the GE CT scanners (GE Healthcare, Waukesha, WI), in which the 4DCT is acquired in axial mode. During this imaging application each couch position is oversampled with respect to the respiratory cycle. The images are reconstructed and sorted based upon the respiratory phase. The second approach implemented by Philips CT scanners (Philips Healthcare, Cleveland, OH) is when the patient is scanned using a helical acquisition. For this acquisition, the raw projection data are binned based upon the respiratory phase, and the binned projections are then reconstructed into different CT data sets. The end result of either approach to 4DCT acquisition is a series of images that are correlated to the respiratory phase.

The fourth and final technique to account for tumor motion is a respiratory gated CT scan [8, 9]. For this image acquisition the patient's respiration is monitored and the phase of the breathing cycle is chosen in which one wants the data collected. When the respiratory signal enters within a particular phase window, the CT scan is acquired and when the respiratory signal leaves this phase window, the CT acquisition is paused. The result of this imaging technique is a 3D CT data set which is acquired only within a particular range of respiratory phases.

Respiratory Monitoring Devices

It is important to note that both the free-breathing and breath hold acquisition can be performed without any additional hardware to monitor patient's respiration. However, to achieve a reproducible level of breath hold, the breath hold CT is acquired while the patient's respiration is monitored by an external device (of which some can be used during 4DCT acquisition). There are three common methods of monitoring patient's respiration during the CT simulation. These three approaches are vendor specific. The first technique involves using the vertical displacement of the thorax as a surrogate for the patient's breathing cycle. This motion is monitored using an infrared camera and external fiducials. This device allows monitoring of the thorax expansion/contraction and therefore the volume of air in and out of the patient's lungs as the patient breathes. This use of external fiducials to monitor respiration is implemented when using the Varian RPM system (Varian Medical Systems, Milpitas, CA). Respiration monitoring using the bellows system (records thorax expansion/contraction) is implemented on the Philips platform (Philips Medical Systems, Cleveland, OH). The bellows system consists of a strap wrapped around the patient connected to an air bladder. The change in pressure of the air bladder is measured and is used as the respiratory signal. The third method of respiration monitoring is done by the active breathing control system implemented by Elekta (Elekta Ltd, Crawley, UK) which utilizes and measures the volume of air as the patient breathes as the respiratory signal. Each respiratory monitoring system functions to generate a signal to either enable image acquisition or to enable beam delivery and there are pros and cons to each system but one must consider which system is used during image acquisition and which system is used during delivery. The RPM system can be used for both image acquisitions during 4DCT and breath hold for both Philips and GE scanners. If delivering a breath hold or a gated treatment, the RPM system can be used on Varian linear accelerators. The Bellows system is implemented only on the Philips Scanners, while it can be used to monitor patient respiration during breath hold and 4DCT acquisition, it does not interface with any of the linear accelerators. The ABC system is on a rolling cart, and while the signal cannot be used to reconstruct 4DCT images from either Philips or GE, it can be used to monitor a patient's respiration during a breath hold acquisition. This integrated setup can be used on Elekta linear accelerators during treatment delivery.

Quality Assurance of CT Simulators

CT simulators differ from diagnostic CT scanners in two main ways: (1) a flat couch insert to mimic the couch top of the linear accelerator and (2) an external laser system used to mark points and isocenters on the patient and aid in patient setup. A routine quality assurance program should be implemented to ensure the imaging device is operating safely and producing high quality and accurate images. In addition, the CT simulator components (lasers and associated software) should be tested to make sure they are functioning properly. The key components of a CT simulator QA program include dose measurements of the different scan protocols, spatial accuracy of CT images, image quality (contrast, noise, etc.), and accuracy of both internal lasers of the CT scanner and the external lasers and associated software. In addition, the accuracy of the CT numbers produced by the different CT scan protocols is very important. CT numbers are used to convert the CT data set into electron density which is used in heterogeneous dose calculations. The ability of the CT scanner to generate accurate CT numbers is essential to accurately computing dose to the patient during treatment planning. Quality assurance of the external lasers used to align and mark patients should be performed to evaluate the accuracy of the position, skewedness, and the ability to accurately mark a point and have the lasers move to that point. This is extremely important for an inaccurate external laser system could lead to setup errors on the treatment machine. Frequency and further details of a CT simulator QA program can be found in AAPM Task Group 66 [10].

A comprehensive QA program is necessary for the simulation of all treatment sites, not just sites located in the thorax. The use of respiratory-correlated imaging requires a separate QA program. This program should be designed to ensure that imaging using any type of respiratory correlation techniques yields accurate information. Such tests include but are not limited to validating the accuracy of the respiratory trace and validating the geometry of moving objects during simulation [11, 12].

The final component of the CT simulator QA program is to verify the accuracy of the data transfer of the simulation data to the treatment planning computer. If the information collected at simulation doesn't transfer to the treatment planning computer accurately, then the accuracy of the plan will be compromised and could result in delivery errors. Since there are many manufacturers of simulation equipment and treatment planning computers, a mixed environment is common. Therefore, testing the ability of the different devices to communicate with each other is essential [13].

Patient Planning

Historically, lung tumors were treated with either an AP/PA beam arrangement and/or a series of oblique beams. Treatment plans were run utilizing manually collected single contours and calculations were performed with the use of heterogeneity corrections. As technology has evolved, so have the treatment planning strategies. Complex treatment plans using IMRT and VMAT with full heterogeneity corrections has now become the standard [14–16]. The advances in imaging techniques and delivery techniques have aided in supporting the evolvement of treatment of tumors in the thoracic region. 4DCT for example allows for the acquisition of full volumetric data sets that show the movement of tumors in the thorax with respiration. With this imaging technology we are able to obtain a better overall picture of what is happening to the anatomy of the patient during respiration. This understanding allows one to be able to create target volumes that encapsulate the tumor during motion, what is referred to as an internal target volume (ITV)[17]. The advances in the technology of imaging have been complemented by the improvements and advanced technology in treatment delivery. The primary focus on this improved technology has been the advent and development of the multi-leaf collimator (MLC). IMRT and VMAT utilize the MLC on the linear accelerator to create small and complex beam apertures to deliver a high dose to the target while minimizing dose to surrounding tissues. These delivery methods are now the standard of care for patients with lung cancer and other thoracic malignancies. All of these advanced delivery techniques require a treatment planning system that can perform accurate dose calculations utilizing full heterogeneity corrections.

Consideration of Tumor Margins During the Planning Process

The type of imaging modality used at simulation, the treatment method to be used, the amount of tumor motion, and setup uncertainties should dictate the size of the margins placed on the tumor volume when generating the treatment plan. These margins are necessary to account for the fact that the tumor is not in the *exact* position it was at simulation for the reasons described above. Accounting for these uncertainties and/or tumor motion will ensure that the tumor will receive the full prescribed dose. ICRU 62[17] describes a series of target volumes that are generated during the planning process. The first of which is the gross tumor volume (GTV), which is the gross disease visible on the CT data set. The clinical target volume (CTV) is generated by adding a margin around the GTV to account for microscopic disease that is not visible on the CT scan. An internal margin (IM) is added to the CTV to account for tumor and physiological motion to generate the internal target volume (ITV). Finally, expanding the ITV by a margin to account for geometric uncertainties in treatment generates the planning target volume (PTV).

When considering an IM for the ITV generation, you must carefully consider the limitations of your imaging procedure. Patients imaged utilizing a free-breathing, slow speed CT scan will have the tumor motion accounted for in the CT set. In this acquisition, the tumor edges will not be well defined but blurred. Contouring this blurred representation of the tumor in essence encapsulates any tumor motion that occurred during the simulation. If a 4DCT data set is used for planning, it is possible to generate an average CT data set and a maximum intensity projection (MIP) data set to aid in the planning process. The average and MIP CT data sets are the average and maximum voxel values, respectively, of each phase of the 4DCT data set that was generated. Similar to the slow speed CT acquisition, the average data set will have motion artifacts on areas located near a density interface. The MIP data set does not have these artifacts, instead when the MIP is created, the voxel across each phase with the highest CT number is used for this data set. The tumor on the MIP data set in areas of high density surrounded by areas of low density will be representative of the envelope of tumor motion, which can be used to aid the physician in the contouring process.

Similar to the imaging process, the type of treatment and the immobilization devices used will also play a role in how treatment margins will be used to generate the PTV [18–20]. If margins are going to be reduced during the planning process, an increase in the imaging is used to verify this reduced margin. The use of daily setup verification images will become necessary.

Practice of Plan Quality Evaluation

It is the physician's responsibility to make clinical decisions regarding plan generation and plan evaluation. Upon completion of the treatment planning process, it is the physicist's responsibility to ensure the overall quality of the treatment plan [21]. This involves several tasks, (1) overall physics evaluation of the treatment plan, (2) evaluation of planning criteria and dose volume constraints, and (3) independent verification of the dose calculation.

To evaluate the plan from a physics perspective, one must understand the limitations of the dose calculation algorithm. While this is not a comprehensive list of questions to ask for each treatment plan, the following provide examples of what should be evaluated as part of a physics plan check. Is the proper dose prescribed by the physician displayed on the CT slices in the treatment plan? Is the proper dose per fraction and number of fractions correct along with the correct energy? Is the dose normalization point located within the beam apertures and positioned where there is electronic equilibrium? Are the beams entering the patient on an overly sloped surface? Are the beam apertures sufficiently sized or over modulated to ensure an accurate dose calculation? Was the correct CT data set used for dose computation? Was tumor motion properly accounted for in the planning process either by contours or motion management strategies? Were heterogeneous dose calculations used? These by no means are a complete list of items to look for, but it is the physicist's responsibility to ensure that what is generated by the TPS accurately depicts the intentions of the directives given by the physician. Published DVH criteria are available for reference [22]; however, an institution may wish to develop and implement their own set of DVH criteria. In this case these criteria must be spelled out in the treatment planning directives. While there are circumstances where the DVH criteria may not be met, good clinical practice should include a review of the DVH constraints of each plan that is generated. If a DVH criterion is outside of those used in clinical practice, this should be discussed with the physician before the initiation of treatment.

TPS Dose Calculation Verification

Generating a treatment plan that is an accurate representation of what the linear accelerator can actually deliver first requires accurate imaging information and secondly requires accurate beam modeling. Validating the treatment planning system's beam model is a critical component to the radiotherapy process [23, 24]. This task is completed prior to the release of the treatment planning for use in the clinical environment. A major component of the beam model verification and commissioning involves the verification of the dose computation algorithm [25, 26]. For static beams, common practice is to perform a hand calculation of the monitor unit settings based on basic machine parameters, percent depth doses (PDDs), or tissue-maximum ratios (TMRs), output factors, inverse square correction, etc. This can be done either manually or with the use of automated software to perform such tasks. For more complex delivery techniques such as IMRT or VMAT deliveries where many irregularly shaped beam apertures are used in the patient's treatment, measurements should be performed by delivering actual treatments planned with the linear accelerator. Several software vendors make products that can compute dose for IMRT and VMAT fields as a second check on the MU settings and the dose delivered. Once the commissioning of the beam modeling process is complete, a routine QA program should be implemented. This comprehensive QA program should verify that the treatment planning system continues to perform as it did at the time of acceptance and commissioning of the system. The initial commissioning of the system as well as the QA program should include the following: (1) verification that the CT to density table is generated properly, (2) the TPS is able to accurately compute dose to simple and complex geometry fields as compared with measured data, (3) output factors generated by the TPS are accurate, (4) the contouring tools still perform accurately, (5) DVH generation remains accurate, and (6) data transfer to the record and verify system maintains the integrity of the intended treatment fields. These tests should be performed on a routine basis and are particularly important after an upgrade to the TPS software is made. Finally, in all cases, for every patient and independent check of the treatment plan should be performed. This can be done with simple manual calculations of MU settings for simple cases. These manual calculations are prone to errors in that a typical photon beam in the thoracic cavity traverses different areas of density often traveling between areas having different densities. In addition, irregularly shaped, small fields will lead to inaccurate hand calculation of MU settings. Recently, secondary check software programs have been developed that are capable of a full 3D heterogeneous dose calculation. Such systems similar to the TPS will perform a full 3D dose calculation and independently compute the MU settings. These systems can provide information on both MU and dose calculations as well as DVH information. Such comprehensive systems are a valuable tool in verifying the TPS dose calculation [27, 28]

Pretreatment Patient-Specific QA

The final component of QA of treatment delivery as it pertains to tumors being treated in the thoracic region is patient-specific pretreatment QA, commonly referred to as IMRT or VMAT QA. Once the treatment plan has been generated, the actual planned treatment should be delivered and the dose measured prior to the patient beginning their course of radiotherapy. This measured dose should be compared to the dose computed in the TPS to verify that what was planned is actually being delivered. This can be accomplished using different methodologies, but the purpose is to measure the dose delivered from treatment machine and compare it to the treatment planning system to verify the accuracy of complex treatments [29–34]. Ion chamber and film and arrays of diodes/ion chambers are common techniques of measuring dose from IMRT fields to verify that the delivered dose agrees with the planned dose prior to the patient starting treatment. Another method used of verifying patient dose prior to delivery is to use the EPID to measure the dose, known as portal dosimetry. This system as the name implies uses the MV portal imager to acquire fluence patterns of the patient's treatment fields. This information can be used to compute the dose and compare it to the TPS. A final method of verifying treatment fields prior to delivery is the use of a log file-based system. These systems capture the log files generated from the treatment machine and compute dose to the patient CT data set, which can be compared to the dose computed in the TPS.

There are advantages and disadvantages to each of these systems which are briefly discussed below. Ion chambers are considered the standard in dose measurement for accuracy; the drawback of such a system is the lack of spatial resolution. If a single ion chamber is used for measurement, then only a single point is being verified. If a single ion chamber is used to verify dose, it is commonly done in conjunction with a film measurement. Arrays of ion chambers and diodes can be used but these systems still suffer from the lack of spatial resolution. Diodes also exhibit nonlinear energy dependence and suffer radiation damage. These may need to be recalibrated periodically to accurately measure the dose. Unlike point measurement dosimeters, film is a good method of measuring dose with high spatial resolution. Film is readily available; however it requires a film processor to develop. Film results are dependent upon processing conditions and may vary from one batch of film to another. Portal dosimetry like film provides good spatial resolution but relies on the MV detector to be properly calibrated in order to compute an accurate dose. Ion chamber, film, and diode measurements discussed are direct measurement, i.e., a device is placed in the treatment beam and dose is measured. Log file-based IMRT and VMAT QA is different in that no direct measurement is occurring [35–37]. These systems take the log files of the treatment machine and compute dose using an independent computation algorithm. If commissioned properly IMRT and VMAT QA using log files and an independent dose calculation algorithm provide an independent check on the TPS, which is the purpose of pretreatment QA. This technique gives you 3D dose comparisons as computed on a heterogeneous data set.

Regardless of which method is used, it is important that the dose is verified before the patients begin treatment. IMRT and VMAT QA not only verify that the TPS dose calculation is accurate but also can catch data transfer errors or data entry errors from the TPS to the treatment machine. They can also be used to check if the treatment that is planned is actually deliverable on the linear accelerator. For example if a multi-segment treatment field did not transfer to the machine properly or a field parameter was incorrectly edited, this would result in a delivery error. A comprehensive pretreatment QA program should be in place to catch such errors.

Patient Setup and Delivery

Setup and Pretreatment Imaging

Prior to patient treatment delivery, the patient must be setup accurately to make sure the intended planned dose is delivered to the patient. The patient's position on the treatment couch must be the same as that in the simulation and planning process to guarantee that the dose is delivered accurately. The patient is initially set up by aligning the setup marks placed at the time of simulation with the machine isocenter utilizing the laser system in the treatment room. Following this initial rough alignment, image guidance is used to fine-tune the position of the tumor relative to the machine's isocenter. Image guidance is accomplished using MV portal imaging, kV planar imaging, or CBCT acquisition. For MV portal imaging, the low energy photon beam is used to image the patient in the treatment position. The MV panel is extended and used to acquire the image from the transmission photons through the patient. Open field images, treatment portals, and a combination of open and treatment portals can be used to verify the patient positioning prior to treatment. For kV imaging, a kV tube is either mounted to the linear accelerator or within the treatment room. kV planar images can be acquired and can be used to set up the patient prior to treatment delivery. Both planar MV and kV images are useful for imaging and aligning the patient to a bony anatomy. In addition to kV images, the gantry-mounted kV imaging systems can be used to acquire a cone beam CT, or CBCT. Whereas traditional CT scanners image the patient using a very small aperture, the CBCT is acquired on the imaging panel using broad-beam geometry. This CBCT acquisition takes on the order of 1–2 min, and the reconstructed images can be used to see both bony landmarks and soft tissue for daily alignment.

QA of Imaging Systems

The use of these imaging systems requires a stringent QA program to ensure that the system is (1) still functioning properly, (2) performing safely, and (3) that image quality remains at a high, acceptable level [12]. The QA program should include daily and monthly tests. They should include testing of the collisional interlocks of both the EPID and the kV imaging system as well as the accuracy of the mechanical positioning and center of each imaging device. The accuracy of the shifts indicated by the imaging systems should be tested on both a daily and monthly basis for the kV system, both planar and CBCT mode. Tests should also be developed to make sure that the digital accuracy of the kV system remains acceptable. This includes the geometric magnification and the scaling accuracy. Image quality of the imagers is of great importance for the system is being used to determine the accuracy of a patient setup. The image quality tests involve both the kV and MV systems. To evaluate the image quality of systems, an image should be of a phantom that contains the following test modules: (1) spatial resolution, (2) contrast resolution, and (3) image uniformity and noise. For routine CBCT QA, a phantom that has tests for (1) spatial resolution, (2) contrast, (3) uniformity and noise, (4) geometric distortion, and (5) Hounsfield units (HU) constancy should be used. These tests should be performed on a monthly basis and the results should be compared as a constancy check to the results obtained when the system was commissioned.

QA of Delivery Systems

While advanced simulation and planning techniques are crucial to developing a treatment plan for the patient, it is crucial to verify that the delivery system (linear accelerator) is capable of accurately delivering the treatment. Therefore, it is imperative that a quality assurance program is in place to make sure that your linear accelerator is performing safely and accurately. A QA program is an essential part of any basic linear accelerator function and will not be discussed here. However, with advancing technologies, additional care must be taken to validate that the MLC and delivery system can accurately deliver what was planned when IMRT and VMAT treatments are being delivered. Therefore, it is important to implement and maintain a rigorous MLC QA program on top of traditional accelerator QA. Several components of the MLC need to be tested; these should be done on a weekly and monthly basis per the recommendations of the AAPM Task Group 142 [12]. These include but are not limited to: accuracy of the leaf position both mechanically and per the radiation fields, MLC leaf speed, MLC leaf gap, dose rate versus both leaf speed and gantry speed [12, 38–40]. These tests are designed to evaluate the output of the machine while different delivery parameters are varied. For example, different combinations of dose rate and gantry speed are used to deliver a series of uniform strips to the imaging plane. In addition to standard MLC tests, with the advent of VMAT, one must ensure that for both low dose segments and low dose rates, the linear accelerator is capable of accurately delivering dose. This should include both MU linearity and dose rate linearity at both low MU settings and low dose rates. This should be tested on an annual basis to ensure that the delivery system is still accurately delivering treatments. With increased imaging during the course of treatment, the evaluation of imaging dose for commonly used techniques should be evaluated. In addition to routine MLC QA, a patient-specific pretreatment QA program should be in place to verify that what was planned is both deliverable and the dosimetry of this plan is accurate.

If respiratory-correlated treatment is to be used in the clinical setting, routine QA of such devices needs to be performed [12]. This includes data transfer from one system to the other, safety test, and quality assurance to ensure overall proper function of the respiratory monitoring interface. Such QA can be performed to verify the accuracy of output and energy of the treatment machine during both a gated and non-gated treatment delivery.

End-to-End Testing of the Treatment Process

A good practice before beginning complex treatment of the thoracic region is an end-to-end test of the system. This should be done first as a dry run to ensure that each component of the treatment process works properly and that different data management systems communicate properly. This should be done with each imaging and treatment method to verify basic workflows and functionality. For example, a CT scan of a phantom should be acquired, sent to the TPS, and a plan generated. The plan and associated images should be sent to the record and verify system, and the phantom should be placed on the treatment couch, imaged for setup, and treatment should be delivered. If special treatment techniques are to be used such as a respiratory monitoring system, these should be tested at this time as well. After verifying that each system in place is working, a second end-to-end test should be performed to independently evaluate the accuracy in delivery of your radiation therapy treatment process [41]. Third parties conduct such tests and a phantom is sent to the site. The physicist will simulate, plan, and deliver a treatment to this phantom. Inside the phantom are dosimeters that measure the dose delivered. When the phantom is sent back, the dose is determined from the dosimeters and is compared to what your planning system predicted. This is a good end-to-end test to make sure that you have both an accurate beam model and that your linear accelerator is accurately delivering the prescribed treatments. This information should be used as an independent verification of the entire radiotherapy process before beginning to treat patients with new technologies.

Conclusion

In this chapter, we have discussed from the physics perspective key components necessary to treat tumors in the thoracic region. A lot of the discussion is not limited to only this treatment site but to other treatment sites as well. Over the years, technology has advanced in every component of radiotherapy delivery. Immobilization and simulation, imaging, treatment planning, and delivery all have evolved to allow the delivery of very complex treatment to the patient. With the advent of such technologies, it is the physicists' responsibility to ensure that it is implemented and used within context of its capabilities and to fully understand each component of the radiation therapy delivery process. A rigorous QA program is essential to verify that each component of the radiation therapy process is operating safely and as intended. This chapter provided an overview of some main areas of QA needed when treating patients in the thoracic region, and each institution's QA program should be custom tailored depending on which type of treatment and imaging is being used.

References

1. Halperin R, et al. Setup reproducibility in radiation therapy for lung cancer: a comparison between T-bar and expanded foam immobilization devices. Int J Radiat Oncol Biol Phys. 1999;43(1):211–6.

2. Negoro Y, et al. The effectiveness of an immobilization device in conformal radiotherapy for lung tumor: reduction of respiratory tumor movement and evaluation of the daily setup accuracy. Int J Radiat Oncol Biol Phys. 2001;50(4):889–98.
3. Fuss M, et al. Repositioning accuracy of a commercially available double-vacuum whole body immobilization system for stereotactic body radiation therapy. Technol Cancer Res Treat. 2004;3(1):59–67.
4. Mah D, et al. Technical aspects of the deep inspiration breath-hold technique in the treatment of thoracic cancer. Int J Radiat Oncol Biol Phys. 2000;48(4):1175–85.
5. Rosenzweig KE, et al. The deep inspiration breath-hold technique in the treatment of inoperable non-small-cell lung cancer. Int J Radiat Oncol Biol Phys. 2000;48(1):81–7.
6. Keall PJ, et al. Acquiring 4D thoracic CT scans using a multislice helical method. Phys Med Biol. 2004;49(10):2053–67.
7. Vedam SS, et al. Acquiring a four-dimensional computed tomography dataset using an external respiratory signal. Phys Med Biol. 2003;48(1):45–62.
8. Giraud P, et al. Reduction of organ motion in lung tumors with respiratory gating. Lung Cancer. 2006;51(1):41–51.
9. Wagman R, et al. Respiratory gating for liver tumors: use in dose escalation. Int J Radiat Oncol Biol Phys. 2003;55(3):659–68.
10. Mutic S, et al. Quality assurance for computed-tomography simulators and the computed-tomography-simulation process: report of the AAPM Radiation Therapy Committee Task Group No. 66. Med Phys. 2003;30(10):2762–92.
11. Jiang SB, Wolfgang J, Mageras GS. Quality assurance challenges for motion-adaptive radiation therapy: gating, breath holding, and four-dimensional computed tomography. Int J Radiat Oncol Biol Phys. 2008;71(1 Suppl):S103–7.
12. Klein EE, et al. Task Group 142 report: quality assurance of medical accelerators. Med Phys. 2009;36(9):4197–212.
13. Siochi RA, et al. Information technology resource management in radiation oncology. J Appl Clin Med Phys. 2009;10(4):3116.
14. Yu CX. Intensity-modulated arc therapy with dynamic multileaf collimation: an alternative to tomotherapy. Phys Med Biol. 1995;40(9):1435–49.
15. Cao D, et al. Comparison of plan quality provided by intensity-modulated arc therapy and helical tomotherapy. Int J Radiat Oncol Biol Phys. 2007;69(1):240–50.
16. Fukumoto S, et al. Small-volume image-guided radiotherapy using hypofractionated, coplanar, and noncoplanar multiple fields for patients with inoperable stage I nonsmall cell lung carcinomas. Cancer. 2002;95(7):1546–53.
17. ICRU, ICRU Report 62, prescribing, recording and reporting photon beam therapy (Supplement to ICRU Report 50), in International Commission on Radiation Units and Measurements 1999, ICRU: Bethesda.
18. Oh YK, et al. Assessment of setup uncertainties for various tumor sites when using daily CBCT for more than 2200 VMAT treatments. J Appl Clin Med Phys. 2014;15(2):4418.
19. Schmidhalter D, et al. Assessment of patient setup errors in IGRT in combination with a six degrees of freedom couch. Z Med Phys. 2014;24(2):112–22.
20. Huang CY, et al. Six degrees-of-freedom prostate and lung tumor motion measurements using kilovoltage intrafraction monitoring. Int J Radiat Oncol Biol Phys. 2015;91(2):368–75.
21. Fraass B, et al. American Association of Physicists in Medicine Radiation Therapy Committee Task Group 53: quality assurance for clinical radiotherapy treatment planning. Med Phys. 1998;25(10):1773–829.
22. Lee TF, Fang FM. Quantitative analysis of normal tissue effects in the clinic (QUANTEC) guideline validation using quality of life questionnaire datasets for parotid gland constraints to avoid causing xerostomia during head-and-neck radiotherapy. Radiother Oncol. 2013;106(3):352–8.
23. Van Dyk J, et al. Commissioning and quality assurance of treatment planning computers. Int J Radiat Oncol Biol Phys. 1993;26(2):261–73.
24. Ten Haken RK, Fraass BA. Quality assurance in 3-D treatment planning. Front Radiat Ther Oncol. 1996;29:104–14.

25. Stern RL, et al. Verification of monitor unit calculations for non-IMRT clinical radiotherapy: report of AAPM Task Group 114. Med Phys. 2011;38(1):504–30.
26. Gibbons JP, et al. Monitor unit calculations for external photon and electron beams: report of the AAPM Therapy Physics Committee Task Group No. 71. Med Phys. 2014;41(3):031501.
27. Butts JR, Foster AE. Comparison of commercially available three-dimensional treatment planning algorithms for monitor unit calculations in the presence of heterogeneities. J Appl Clin Med Phys. 2001;2(1):32–41.
28. Chan J, et al. Comparison of monitor unit calculations performed with a 3D computerized planning system and independent "hand" calculations: results of three years clinical experience. J Appl Clin Med Phys. 2002;3(4):293–301.
29. Low DA, et al. Dosimetry tools and techniques for IMRT. Med Phys. 2011;38(3):1313–38.
30. Ravichandran R, et al. Need of patient-specific quality assurance and pretreatment verification program for special plans in radiotherapy. J Med Phys. 2011;36(3):181–3.
31. O'Daniel J, et al. Volumetric-modulated arc therapy: effective and efficient end-to-end patient-specific quality assurance. Int J Radiat Oncol Biol Phys. 2012;82(5):1567–74.
32. Krishnamurthy K, et al. Formulation and initial experience on patient specific quality assurance for clinical implementation of dynamic IMRT. Gulf J Oncolog. 2009;5:44–8.
33. Schreibmann E, et al. Patient-specific quality assurance method for VMAT treatment delivery. Med Phys. 2009;36(10):4530–5.
34. Anjum MN, et al. IMRT quality assurance using a second treatment planning system. Med Dosim. 2010;35(4):274–9.
35. Calvo-Ortega JF, et al. A varian DynaLog file-based procedure for patient dose-volume histogram-based IMRT QA. J Appl Clin Med Phys. 2014;15(2):4665.
36. Rangaraj D, et al. Catching errors with patient-specific pretreatment machine log file analysis. Pract Radiat Oncol. 2013;3(2):80–90.
37. Litzenberg DW, Moran JM, Fraass BA. Verification of dynamic and segmental IMRT delivery by dynamic log file analysis. J Appl Clin Med Phys. 2002;3(2):63–72.
38. Chui CS, Spirou S, LoSasso T. Testing of dynamic multileaf collimation. Med Phys. 1996;23(5):635–41.
39. Mamalui-Hunter M, Li H, Low DA. MLC quality assurance using EPID: a fitting technique with subpixel precision. Med Phys. 2008;35(6):2347–55.
40. Bayouth JE, Wendt D, Morrill SM. MLC quality assurance techniques for IMRT applications. Med Phys. 2003;30(5):743–50.
41. Molineu A, et al. Design and implementation of an anthropomorphic quality assurance phantom for intensity-modulated radiation therapy for the Radiation Therapy Oncology Group. Int J Radiat Oncol Biol Phys. 2005;63(2):577–83.

Index

G. Ozyigit et al. (eds.), *Principles and Practice of Radiotherapy Techniques in Thoracic Malignancies*, DOI 10.1007/978-3-319-28761-4

MIX
Papier aus verantwortungsvollen Quellen
Paper from responsible sources
FSC® C105338

If you have any concerns about our products,
you can contact us on
ProductSafety@springernature.com

In case Publisher is established outside the EU,
the EU authorized representative is:
Springer Nature Customer Service Center GmbH
Europaplatz 3, 69115 Heidelberg, Germany

Printed by Libri Plureos GmbH
in Hamburg, Germany